1998
YEAR BOOK OF
SURGERY®

Statement of Purpose

The YEAR BOOK Service

The YEAR BOOK series was devised in 1901 by practicing health professionals who observed that the literature of medicine and related disciplines had become so voluminous that no one individual could read and place in perspective every potential advance in a major specialty. In the final decade of the 20th century, this recognition is more acutely true than it was in 1901.

More than merely a series of books, YEAR BOOK volumes are the tangible results of a unique service designed to accomplish the following:

- to *survey* a wide range of journals of proven value
- to *select* from those journals papers representing significant advances and statements of important clinical principles
- to provide *abstracts* of those articles that are readable, convenient summaries of their key points
- to provide *commentary* about those articles to place them in perspective

These publications grow out of a unique process that calls on the talents of outstanding authorities in clinical and fundamental disciplines, trained literature specialists, and professional writers, all supported by the resources of Mosby, the world's preeminent publisher for the health professions.

The Literature Base

Mosby and its editors survey approximately 500 journals published worldwide, covering the full range of the health professions. On an annual basis, the publisher examines usage patterns and polls its expert authorities to add new journals to the literature base and to delete journals that are no longer useful as potential YEAR BOOK sources.

The Literature Survey

The publisher's team of literature specialists, all of whom are trained and experienced health professionals, examines every original, peer-reviewed article in each journal issue. More than 250,000 articles per year are scanned systematically, including title, text, illustrations, tables, and references. Each scan is compared, article by article, to the search strategies that the publisher has developed in consultation with the 270 outside experts who form the pool of YEAR BOOK editors. A given article may be reviewed by any number of editors, from one to a dozen or more, regardless of the discipline for which the paper was originally published. In turn, each editor who receives the article reviews it to determine whether the article should be included in the YEAR BOOK. This decision is based on the article's inherent quality, its probable usefulness to readers of that YEAR BOOK, and the editor's goal to represent a balanced picture of a given field in each volume of the YEAR BOOK. In addition, the editor indicates when to include figures and tables from the article to help the YEAR BOOK reader better understand the information.

Of the quarter million articles scanned each year, only 5% are selected for detailed analysis within the YEAR BOOK series, thereby assuring readers of the high value of every selection.

The Abstract

The publisher's abstracting staff is headed by a seasoned medical professional and includes individuals with training in the life sciences, medicine, and other areas, plus extensive experience in writing for the health professions and related industries. Each selected article is assigned to a specific writer on this abstracting staff. The abstracter, guided in many cases by notations supplied by the expert editor, writes a structured, condensed summary designed so that the reader can rapidly acquire the essential information contained in the article.

The Commentary

The YEAR BOOK editorial boards, sometimes assisted by guest commentators, write comments that place each article in perspective for the reader. This provides the reader with the equivalent of a personal consultation with a leading international authority—an opportunity to better understand the value of the article and to benefit from the authority's thought processes in assessing the article.

Additional Editorial Features

The editorial boards of each YEAR BOOK organize the abstracts and comments to provide a logical and satisfying sequence of information. To enhance the organization, editors also provide introductions to sections or individual chapters, comments linking a number of abstracts, citations to additional literature, and other features.

The published YEAR BOOK contains enhanced bibliographic citations for each selected article, including extended listings of multiple authors and identification of author affiliations. Each YEAR BOOK contains a Table of Contents specific to that year's volume. From year to year, the Table of Contents for a given YEAR BOOK will vary depending on developments within the field.

Every YEAR BOOK contains a list of the journals from which papers have been selected. This list represents a subset of approximately 500 journals surveyed by the publisher and occasionally reflects a particularly pertinent article from a journal that is not surveyed on a routine basis.

Finally, each volume contains a comprehensive subject index and an index to authors of each selected paper.

The 1998 Year Book Series

Year Book of Allergy, Asthma, and Clinical Immunology: Drs. Rosenwasser, Borish, Boguniewicz, Nelson, Routes, and Spahn

Year Book of Anesthesiology and Pain Management®: Drs. Tinker, Abram, Chestnut, Roizen, Rothenberg, and Wood

Year Book of Cardiology®: Drs. Schlant, Collins, Gersh, Graham, Kaplan, and Waldo

Year Book of Chiropractic®: Dr. Lawrence

Year Book of Critical Care Medicine®: Drs. Parrillo, Balk, Calvin, Franklin, and Shapiro

Year Book of Dentistry®: Drs. Meskin, Berry, Jeffcoat, Leinfelder, Roser, Summitt, and Zakariasen

Year Book of Dermatologic Surgery®: Drs. Greenway, Barrett, Papadopoulos, and Whitaker

Year Book of Dermatology®: Dr. Thiers

Year Book of Diagnostic Radiology®: Drs. Osborn, Groskin, Dalinka, Maynard, Pentecost, Rebner, Ros, Smirniotopoulos, and Young

Year Book of Drug Therapy®: Drs. Lasagna and Weintraub

Year Book of Emergency Medicine®: Drs. Wagner, Dronen, Davidson, King, Niemann, and Roberts

Year Book of Endocrinology®: Drs. Bagdade, Braverman, Horton, Kannan, Landsberg, Molitch, Morley, Nathan, Odell, Poehlman, Rogol, and Ryan

Year Book of Family Practice®: Drs. Berg, Bowman, Davidson, Dexter, and Scherger

Year Book of Gastroenterology®: Drs. Aliperti and Fleshman

Year Book of Geriatrics and Gerontology®: Drs. Burton, Beck, Ostwald, Rabins, Reuben, Roth, Shapiro, and Whitehouse

Year Book of Hand Surgery®: Drs. Amadio and Hentz

Year Book of Hematology®: Drs. Spivak, Bell, Ness, Quesenberry, Wiernik, and Horowitz

Year Book of Infectious Diseases: Drs. Keusch, Barza, Bennish, Poutsiaka, Skolnik, and Snydman

Year Book of Medicine®: Drs. Cline, Frishman, Jett, Klahr, Malawista, Mandell, McCallum, and Utiger

Year Book of Neonatal and Perinatal Medicine®: Drs. Fanaroff, Maisels, and Stevenson

Year Book of Nephrology, Hypertension, and Mineral Metabolism: Drs. Schwab, Bennett, Emmett, Hostetter, Kumar, and Toto

Year Book of Neurology and Neurosurgery®: Drs. Bradley and Gibbs

Year Book of Nuclear Medicine®: Drs. Gottschalk, Blaufox, Neumann, Strauss, and Zubal

Year Book of Obstetrics, Gynecology, and Women's Health: Drs. Mishell, Herbst, and Kirschbaum

Year Book of Occupational and Environmental Medicine®: Drs. Emmett, Frank, Gochfeld, and Hessl

Year Book of Oncology®: Drs. Ozols, Eisenberg, Glatstein, Loehrer, and Tallman

Year Book of Ophthalmology®: Drs. Wilson, Augsburger, Cohen, Eagle, Grossman, Laibson, Maguire, Nelson, Penne, Rapuano, Sergott, Spaeth, Tipperman, Ms. Gosfield, and Ms. Salmon

Year Book of Orthopedics®: Drs. Morrey, Beauchamp, Currier, Tolo, Trigg, and Swiontkowski

Year Book of Otolaryngology–Head and Neck Surgery®: Drs. Paparella and Holt

Year Book of Pathology and Laboratory Medicine®: Drs. Raab, Cohen, Olson, Sirgi, and Stanley

Year Book of Pediatrics®: Dr. Stockman

Year Book of Plastic, Reconstructive, and Aesthetic Surgery®: Drs. Miller, Bartlett, Garner, McKinney, Ruberg, Salisbury, and Smith

Year Book of Psychiatry and Applied Mental Health®: Drs. Talbott, Ballenger, Frances, Lydiard, Meltzer, Schowalter, and Tasman

Year Book of Pulmonary Disease®: Drs. Jett, Maurer, Ryu, Strollo, and Wenzel

Year Book of Rheumatology®: Drs. Panush, Hadler, LeRoy, Liang, Reichlin, Simon, and Weinblatt

Year Book of Sports Medicine®: Drs. Shephard, Drinkwater, Eichner, Torg, Alexander, and Mr. George

Year Book of Surgery®: Drs. Copeland, Bland, Deitch, Eberlein, Howard, Luce, Seeger, Souba, and Sugarbaker

Year Book of Thoracic and Cardiovascular Surgery®: Drs. Ginsberg, Wechsler, and Williams

Year Book of Urology®: Drs. Andriole and Coplen

Year Book of Vascular Surgery®: Dr. Porter

1998

The Year Book of SURGERY®

Editor-in-Chief

Edward M. Copeland III, M.D.

The Edward R. Woodward Professor and Chairman, Department of Surgery, University of Florida College of Medicine, Gainesville, Florida

Mosby

St. Louis Baltimore Boston Carlsbad Naples New York Philadelphia Portland London
Madrid Mexico City Singapore Sydney Tokyo Toronto Wiesbaden

Mosby
Dedicated to Publishing Excellence

A Times Mirror Company

Associate Publisher: Cynthia Baudendistel
Developmental Editor: Gary O'Brien
Manager, Periodical Editing: Kirk Swearingen
Production Editor: Pat Costigan
Project Supervisor, Production: Joy Moore
Production Assistant: Karie House
Manager, Literature Services: Idelle L. Winer
Illustrations and Permissions Specialist: Steve Ramay

1998 EDITION

Printed in the United States of America
Composition by Reed Technology and Information Services, Inc.
Printing/binding by Maple-Vail

Mosby, Inc.
11830 Westline Industrial Drive
St. Louis, MO 63146

International Standard Serial Number: 0090-3671
International Standard Book Number: 0–8151-9743-8

Editors

Editorial Board

Kirby I. Bland, M.D.

J. Murray Beardsley Professor and Chairman, Department of Surgery, Professor of Medical Sciences, Brown University School of Medicine; Surgeon-in-Chief, Rhode Island Hospital, Providence, Rhode Island

Edwin A. Deitch, M.D.

Professor and Chairman, Department of Surgery, UMD-New Jersey Medical School, Newark, New Jersey

Timothy J. Eberlein, M.D.

Bixby Professor and Chairman, Department of Surgery, Professor of Pathology and Immunology, Washington University School of Medicine; Surgeon-in-Chief, Barnes-Jewish Hospital, St. Louis Children's Hospital, Veterans Administration Hospital, St. Louis, Missouri

Richard J. Howard, M.D., Ph.D.

Robert H. and Kathleen M. Axline Professor of Surgery, University of Florida College of Medicine, Shands Hospital at the University of Florida, Gainesville, Florida

Edward A. Luce, M.D.

Kiehn-Desprez Professor and Chief of Plastic Surgery, Case-Western Reserve and University Hospital, Cleveland, Ohio

James M. Seeger, M.D.

Professor and Chief, Section of Vascular Surgery, Department of Surgery, University of Florida College of Medicine, Gainesville, Florida

Wiley W. Souba, M.D., Sc.D.

Chief, Division of Surgical Oncology, Deputy Director, Massachusetts General Hospital Cancer Center, Director, Surgical Oncology Research Laboratories; Director, Nutrition Support Service, Massachusetts General Hospital; Professor of Surgery, Harvard Medical School; Professor of Nutrition, Harvard School of Public Health, Boston, Massachusetts

David J. Sugarbaker, M.D.

Associate Professor of Surgery, Harvard Medical School; Chief, Division of Thoracic Surgery, Brigham and Women's Hospital, Chief of Surgical Services, Dana Farber Cancer Institute, Boston, Massachusetts

Contributing Editors

Joseph F. Amaral, M.D.

Associate Professor of Surgery, Brown University School of Medicine; Director of Laparoscopic Surgery, Rhode Island Hospital, Providence, Rhode Island

William G. Cioffi, M.D.

Associate Professor of Surgery, Brown University School of Medicine; Chief of Trauma and Burns, Rhode Island Hospital, Providence, Rhode Island

Francois I. Luks, M.D.
Associate Professor of Surgery and Pediatrics, Brown University School of Medicine; Attending Pediatric Surgeon, Hasbro Children's Hospital and Rhode Island Hospital, Providence, Rhode Island

Victor E. Pricolo, M.D.
Associate Professor of Surgery, Brown University School of Medicine; Director of Gastrointestinal and Colorectal Surgery, Rhode Island Hospital, Providence, Rhode Island

H. Hank Simms, M.D.
Associate Professor of Surgery, Brown University School of Medicine; Chief, Division of Surgical Critical Care, Department of Surgery, Rhode Island Hospital, Providence, Rhode Island

Table of Contents

Journals Represented

Mosby and its editors survey approximately 500 U.S. and foreign medical and allied health journals. From these journals, the editors select the articles to be abstracted. Journals represented in this YEAR BOOK are listed below.

Academic Medicine
American Heart Journal
American Journal of Gastroenterology
American Journal of Infection Control
American Journal of Kidney Diseases
American Journal of Pathology
American Journal of Physiology
American Journal of Respiratory and Critical Care Medicine
American Journal of Roentgenology
American Journal of Surgery
American Surgeon
Annals of Burns and Fire Disasters
Annals of Otology, Rhinology, and Laryngology
Annals of Plastic Surgery
Annals of Surgery
Annals of Surgical Oncology
Annals of Thoracic Surgery
Annals of Vascular Surgery
Annals of the Royal College of Surgeons of England
Archives of Otolaryngology—Head and Neck Surgery
Archives of Surgery
Breast Journal
British Journal of Cancer
British Journal of Plastic Surgery
British Journal of Surgery
Burns
Canadian Journal of Anaesthesia
Cancer
Chest
Circulation
Clinical Infectious Diseases
Clinical Pediatrics
Critical Science
Clinical Transplantation
Critical Care Medicine
Diabetes
Diabetes Care
Diseases of the Colon and Rectum
European Journal of Surgery
European Respiratory Journal
Gastroenterology
Gut
Head and Neck
Hepatology
Infection Control and Hospital Epidemiology
Israel Journal of Medical Sciences
Journal of Bone and Joint Surgery (American Volume)

Journal of Burn Care and Rehabilitation
Journal of Clinical Investigation
Journal of Clinical Oncology
Journal of Computer Assisted Tomography
Journal of Experimental Medicine
Journal of Immunology
Journal of Neurosurgery
Journal of Pathology
Journal of Pediatric Surgery
Journal of Pediatrics
Journal of Reconstructive Microsurgery
Journal of Surgical Oncology
Journal of Surgical Research
Journal of Thoracic and Cardiovascular Surgery
Journal of Trauma
Journal of Trauma: Injury, Infection, and Critical Care
Journal of Urology
Journal of Vascular Surgery
Journal of the American Academy of Dermatology
Journal of the American College of Surgeons
Journal of the American Medical Association
Kidney International
Laboratory Investigation
Mayo Clinic Proceedings
Metabolism: Clinical and Experimental
New England Journal of Medicine
Nutrition
Otolaryngology–Head and Neck Surgery
Plastic and Reconstructive Surgery
Radiology
SHOCK
Scandinavian Journal of Plastic and Reconstructive Hand Surgery
Scandinavian Journal of Thoracic and Cardiovascular Surgery
Surgery
The Laryngoscope Journal
Transplantation
Western Journal of Medicine
World Journal of Surgery
Wound Repair and Regeneration

Standard Abbreviations

The following terms are abbreviated in this edition: acquired immunodeficiency syndrome (AIDS), cardiopulmonary resuscitation (CPR), central nervous system (CNS), cerebrospinal fluid (CSF), computed tomography (CT), deoxyribonucleic acid (DNA), electrocardiography (ECG), health maintenance organization (HMO), human immunodeficiency virus (HIV), intensive care unit (ICU), intramuscular (IM), intravenous (IV), magnetic resonance (MR) imaging (MRI), and ribonucleic acid (RNA).

NOTE

The YEAR BOOK OF SURGERY is a literature survey service providing abstracts of articles published in the professional literature. Every effort is made to assure the accuracy of the information presented in these pages. Neither the editor nor the publisher of the YEAR BOOK OF SURGERY can be responsible for errors in the original materials. The editors' comments are their own opinions. Mention of specific products within this publication does not constitute endorsement.

To facilitate the use of the YEAR BOOK OF SURGERY as a reference tool, all illustrations and tables included in this publication are now identified as they appear in the original article. This change is meant to help the reader recognize that any illustration or table appearing in the YEAR BOOK OF SURGERY may be only one of many in the original article. For this reason, figure and table numbers appear to be out of sequence within the YEAR BOOK OF SURGERY.

1 General Considerations

Introduction

From 1986 to 1995, clinical departments of academic institutions in geographic areas of high managed care penetration had a proportionately lower growth in National Institutes of Health awards than did clinical departments in areas of minimal managed care penetration. Surgeons are being called on to provide even more of the financial resources for their academic institutions because of reduced reimbursement from providers. Consequently, a surgeon's chance for extramural funding for research may be more severely hampered than for members of other medical disciplines. In addition, reimbursement from HMOs in some geographic areas may be spuriously low because the capitation rates are based on healthy patients who preselect an HMO provider. At the same time that these market forces are having a negative impact on the time and money of the surgeon, hospital administrators are rapidly proliferating.

The emphasis placed on training generalist physicians has eroded surgical clerkships during medical school. Surgical knowledge has been shown to equate to the volume of clinical training. A fail-safe method of preselecting medical students to be excellent surgical residents has yet to be developed, further emphasizing the need for a surgical core of knowledge to be imparted to students during their medical school education.

Clinical pathways have become a popular and effective method of reducing costs for some surgical procedures. A thorough history and physical examination may eliminate the need for all preoperative tests for elective surgical procedures if the patient is deemed healthy. Washing hands with soap may reduce bacteria on the hands more than scrubbing with a brush, the latter being a higher-cost item for the operating suite. Another challenge to an axiom was the need for perioperative steroids in patients taking long-term doses of prednisone. Regulatory action by the Food and Drug Administration will govern the use of mammography and, thereby, limit the use of stereotactic breast biopsy to those physicians who meet appropriate criteria.

Personal and professional profiles are being developed as predictors of malpractice risks. Multivariate analysis has shown that permanent disability is the only factor associated with payment of a malpractice suit.

Payment was unrelated to an adverse event, even one caused by negligence. Personality profiles of patients who do and do not get breast augmentation are quite different. Could one group be innately more daily litigious than the other? If the items in this paragraph seem stressful, you should know that the daily level of mental stress has been shown to trigger myocardial ischemia.

Edward M. Copeland III, M.D.

Relationship Between National Institutes of Health Research Awards to US Medical Schools and Managed Care Market Penetration

Moy E, Mazzaschi AJ, Levin RJ, et al (Assoc of American Med Colleges, Washington, DC)

JAMA 278:217–221, 1997 1–1

Introduction.—To help support core academic programs, undergraduate and graduate medical education, and biomedical research, medical schools in the United States have traditionally relied on clinical revenues generated by their faculty. In 1993, this clinical support was estimated to be $2.4 billion. The capability of medical schools to maintain their research base may be jeopardized as managed care entities negotiate discounted fees with the faculty practice plans and teaching hospitals that support medical schools. Greater difficulty may be experienced in competing for peer-reviewed, externally funded research grants in schools with high managed care penetration if faculty have less time to conduct research, have less seed money with which to initiate new research projects, or leave these institutions altogether. To test the hypothesis that the rate of growth in awards to medical schools was lower for medical schools located in markets with high managed care penetration than for schools located in markets with lower penetration, data on research awards to medical schools from the National Institutes of Health (NIH) were used.

Methods.—Each medical school was matched to a market for which information about health maintenance organization penetration in 1995 was available. Each medical school was examined for the annual extramural research grant that was awarded by the NIH. In schools located in markets with low, medium, and high managed care penetration, a comparison was conducted of the growth in total awards by the NIH, traditional research project awards, traditional research project awards to clinical and basic science departments, and changes in institutional ranking by the NIH awards.

Results.—From 1986 to 1990, medical schools in all markets had comparable rates of growth in awards from the NIH. Slower growth in dollar amounts of numbers of awards from the NIH was seen in medical schools in markets with high managed care penetration after 1990 when compared with medical schools that were in markets with low or medium managed care penetration. A loss of the share of NIH awards, equal to $98 million in 1995, and lower institutional ranking by NIH awards were associated with a slower growth for schools in high managed care markets. In high managed care markets, the slower growth of traditional research project awards to clinical departments in medical schools can explain much of this revenue loss.

Conclusion.—An inverse relationship was found between managed care penetration among U.S. medical schools and a growth in awards by the NIH. It remains to be determined whether this association is causal.

► The balance between research and patient care in surgical departments has been tipped toward clinical practice for many years because of the difficulty academic surgeons have in obtaining "protected time." Nevertheless, quality research funded by the NIH has emanated from surgical departments. Surgical researchers have learned how to manage their schedules so that they can run a successful research laboratory and continue to practice clinical medicine without taking blocks of time (e.g., every other month) away from patient care. Members of other clinical disciplines, especially medicine, can learn from these surgeons' experiences. The luxury of providing clinical service for only 3 months of the year and doing full time research for the other 9 months may soon be a thing of the past, unless a research grant fully funds the investigator's salary. Cross-subsidization of the research salaries and laboratory expenses from clinical income of other faculty members is no longer possible.

We may soon see a different trend. NIH grants from clinical departments in areas heavily penetrated by managed care may actually increase disproportionately because investigators who have excellent scientific projects will be stimulated to have their science funded through NIH rather than through excess clinical income.

E.M. Copeland III, M.D.

Differential Clinical Workloads Among Faculty at a Major Academic Health Center

Zelenock GB, Stanley JC, More RA, et al (Univ of Michigan, Ann Arbor)

Ann Surg 226:336–347, 1997 — 1–2

Background.—Because of managed health care, academic medical centers are moving away from providing complex care and toward providing more primary health care activities. This change will undoubtedly affect a health center's revenues and practice incentives for individual physicians. How physician workloads at one institution have changed with the growth of managed care was evaluated.

Methods.—The University of Michigan Medical Center encompasses 4 hospitals (including medical-surgical, women's, pediatric and neonatal, and eye hospitals), a psychiatric unit, inpatient rehabilitation, and a large outpatient multispeciality group and 12 community clinics. For each of these operating units, medical center records from 1981 to 1995 were examined to determine the number of admissions, discharges, clinic visits, and operations for each department; the roster for each department; the

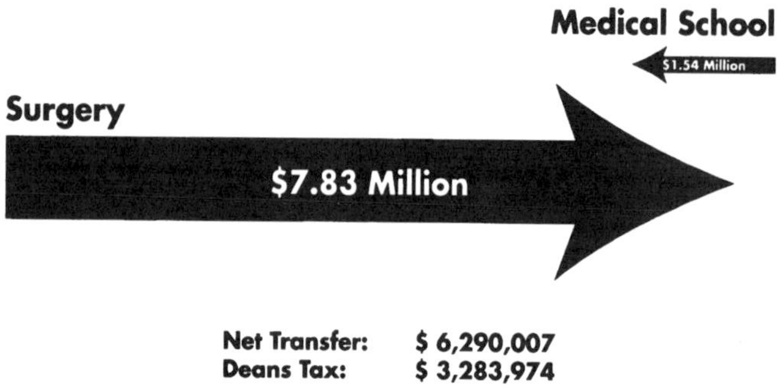

FIGURE 10.—The University of Michigan Medical School provided $1.54 million in support of Department of Surgery educational programs. The Department of Surgery provided $7.83 million to the medical school. (Courtesy of Zelenock GB, Stanley JC, More RA, et al: Differential clinical workloads among faculty at a major academic health center. *Ann Surg* 26:336–347, 1997.)

number of operations and operative hours of both departments and individual surgeons; financial data; and research space and funding data.

Findings.—The Department of Internal Medicine accounted for 30% of all full-time hospital physicians, and the Department of Surgery accounted for 11% of staff. From 1981 to 1995, Internal Medicine, Psychiatry, and Surgery saw great increases (greater than 50%) in admissions, whereas admissions were decreased for Ophthalmology (50% fewer) and Otolaryngology (8% fewer). The Department of Surgery accounted for the most hospital admissions and discharges (33%) and the second-most number of outpatient visits (16%, second only to Internal Medicine). In 1995 compared to 1981, the Department of Surgery had a 249% increase in the number of operations performed; in fact, the Department of Surgery performed more operations than the Deparments of Ophthalmology, Otolaryngology, and Obstetrics-Gynecology combined. This represented a 30% increase in operations per individual Department of Surgery surgeon per year. In 1995, the Department of Surgery contributed substantially more monies to the medical school (Fig 10) and the hospital (Fig 11) than they received in funding from these 2 entities.

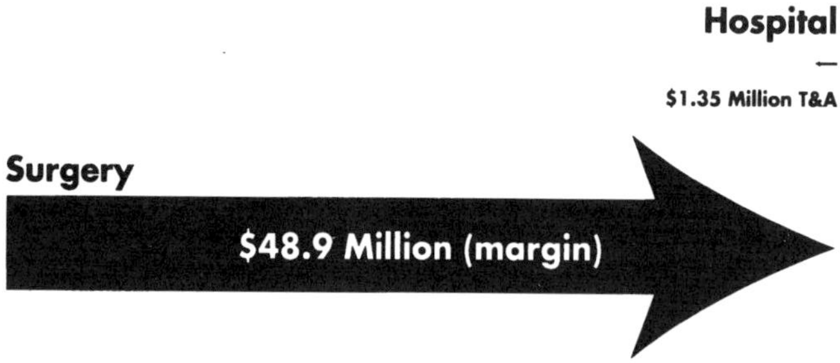

FIGURE 11.—The University of Michigan Hospital provided $1.35 million of teaching and administration funds to the Department of Surgery in support of graduate medical education. Surgical activity generates $240 million in hospital revenue, accounting for $48.9 million margin to the hospital from inpatient activity. (Courtesy of Zelenock GB, Stanley JC, More RA, et al: Differential clinical workloads among faculty at a major academic health center. *Ann Surg* 26:336–347, 1997.)

Conclusions.—The Department of Surgery experienced an increase in workload and an increase in departmental financial support of medical school and hospital activities, while receiving substantially less revenue support from these sources in return. Over the course of the study, managed care did have an effect in decreasing specialty visits and increasing primary care activities. As this trend continues, and as workloads of surgeons continue to increase, academic health centers must ensure that the contribution of the department of surgery is not lessened or impinged upon by restructuring.

▶ The financial support provided to the academic complex at the University of Michigan mimics by percentage the support provided by the Department of Surgery at the University of Florida College of Medicine. I would guess these figures would be similar for most state programs that include a university hospital admitting private patients. The enthusiasm these institutions have for spending money to expand primary care practice may be somewhat misguided. My practice has not yet been enhanced by these expansions. If surgery is the financial "backbone" of state academic health centers, wouldn't money be wisely spent ensuring that surgery practices are maintained? To do so will require knowledge of the referral patterns to departments of surgery that developed before establishment of institutionally owned referral networks of generalists. These already established surgery referral networks may not all be abolished by managed care, especially when patient choice remains an option.

E.M. Copeland III, M.D.

The Medicare-HMO Revolving Door: The Healthy Go In and the Sick Go Out

Morgan RO, Virnig BA, DeVito CA, et al (Univ of Miami, Fla; George Washington Univ, Washington, DC)

N Engl J Med 337:169–175, 1997 1–3

Introduction.—A reduction in the length of stay and the number of bed-days associated with the traditional fee-for-service system has been credited to HMOs serving Medicare beneficiaries. The growth in the costs of health care for the elderly is assumed to increase more slowly with HMOs; however, recently, this assumption has been questioned. There is a theory that selective enrollment of healthier Medicare recipients benefits HMOs and that sicker patients are more likely to withdraw from Medicare HMOs, which would raise the average fee-for-service costs.

Methods.—To examine differences in the use of in-patient medical services by 375,406 beneficiaries in the Medicare fee-for-service system, 48,380 HMO enrollees before enrollment, and 23,870 HMO enrollees after withdrawal, investigators studied Medicare enrollment and inpatient billing records from a 3-year period. It was also determined whether the pattern of use after withdrawal persisted over time and whether these differences were related to demographic characteristics.

Results.—During the year before enrollment, the rate of use of inpatient services in the HMO-enrollment group was 66% of the rate of the fee-for-service group. After withdrawal, the rate in the HMO-withdrawal group was 180% of that in the fee-for-service group. Those who withdrew from HMOs had a higher rate of admissions than the fee-for-service beneficiaries. At least 1 inpatient stay was found in twice as many beneficiaries in the HMO-withdrawal group, and they had twice as many inpatient days and twice the inpatient hospital payments when compared with those who remained in the fee-for-service system.

Conclusion.—With respect to HMO enrollment and withdrawal, there is marked selection biases. The effectiveness of the Medicare managed care system is undermined by these biases. The need for longitudinal and population-based studies is highlighted. There is a strong suggestion that those who withdraw from HMOs move into the fee-for-service system to obtain needed services, then return to Medicare HMOs after they are healthier. There is also a greater proportion of younger individuals who are low-use beneficiaries using Medicare HMOs.

► This study was done on Medicare recipients in South Florida and clearly shows that patients who select an HMO need fewer medical services. During the time period of this study, HMO patients were capitated by a percent of a cost of Medicare patients in a fee-for-service plan. Because medical care costs were high in the non-HMO patients, the capitated rate for HMO patients was probably spuriously high, thereby making a capitated Medicare HMO contract attractive.

I suspect, however, that Medicare fee-for-service reimbursement will soon reflect the rate of medical service utilization by the healthier HMO patients. Then both fee-for-service and capitated reimbursement for Medicare patients will be spuriously low. Medicare capitation rates should be based on the health needs of the entire Medicare population in a given geographical area, not on a subset of patients who preselect a plan based on the status of their health care needs.

E.M. Copeland III, M.D.

Costs of Care and Administration at For-Profit and Other Hospitals in the United States

Woolhandler S, Himmelstein DU (Cambridge Hosp, Mass; Harvard Med School, Boston)

N Engl J Med 336:769–774, 1997 1–4

Background.—Studies performed in 1990 showed that administrative costs accounted for one fourth of total U.S. hospital costs, a proportion nearly double that found in Canada. Past studies have documented high costs—particularly administrative costs—at for-profit hospitals. This study used Medicare data to compare administrative costs of for-profit and other types of hospitals.

Methods.—The analysis included fiscal-year 1994 data on administrative costs at 6,227 nonfederal hospitals and on total inpatient care costs at 5,201 acute care hospitals. Data from 1990 were considered as well. Administrative costs were compared for private not-for-profit, for-profit, and public hospitals. The findings were adjusted for type and size of hospital, geographic area, and proportion of revenues for outpatient care. The data on inpatient care costs were adjusted for local wages, reporting periods, and case mix.

Results.—Administrative costs as a percentage of total hospital costs rose from 24.8% in 1990 to 26.0% in 1994. For-profit hospitals saw a greater increase, 2.2%, to a total of 34.0%. The increase was 1.2%, to a total of 24.5%, for private not-for-profit hospitals, and 0.6%, to a total of 22.9%, for public hospitals. At psychiatric hospitals, administrative costs were 37.5% overall and 44.4% at for-profit hospitals. At rehabilitation hospitals, the figures were 33.0% and 37.7%, respectively. On multivariate analysis, for-profit status raised administrative costs as a proportion of total spending by 7.9% compared with public hospitals and by 5.7% compared with private not-for-profit hospitals. Adjusted cost per discharge at acute care hospitals was $8,115 at for-profit hospitals vs. $7,490 at private not-for-profit and $6,507 at public hospitals. The administrative component of these costs per discharge was $2,289, $1,809, and $1,432, respectively.

The findings were little affected when alternative methods of allocating capital and maintenance costs were considered, nor were they related to a small number of high-cost hospitals. For-profit hospitals had higher costs across geographic ranges and hospital sizes. For 75 hospitals that switched to for-profit ownership between 1990 and 1994, administrative costs increased by an average of 2.5%, compared with a 0.4% increase at 105 hospitals that switched to not-for-profit or public status during that period. Wage and salary costs were lower at for-profit, short-term general hospitals. Almost all of this difference was related to lower compensation costs for clinical personnel.

Conclusions.—For-profit hospitals have higher administrative costs and higher costs per inpatient day and per discharge than do private not-for-profit hospitals. The cost data considered may underestimate total overhead. It is uncertain why administrative costs are rising so quickly at for-profit hospitals—the shortened lengths of stay at these institutions have not led to lower costs per admission. Market forces appear to be "upsizing," rather than downsizing, administration. The findings question whether our recent reliance on market forces to lower health care costs is having the desired effect.

▶ Woodhandler and Himmelstein have confirmed what those of us who walk the halls of our hospitals have known for sometime: the "suits" are increasing. Ironically, the people who are charged with lowering health care costs have actually raised them while, at the same time, lowering the number of personnel who tend to the personal needs of patients. The patient is the ultimate loser, being pushed away from the hospital, having limited time with a designated physician, and paying a larger insurance premium to support individuals who do not participate in the resolution of their illnesses. How can so many tolerate the actions of so few?

E.M. Copeland III, M.D.

The Relationship of Clinical Knowledge to Months of Clinical Training Among Medical Students

Vosti KL, Bloch DA, Jacobs CD (Stanford Univ, Calif)
Acad Med 72:305–307, 1997 1–5

Background.—In traditional medical school programs, students spend almost equal amounts of time in preclinical and clinical training. The effects of changes in the time spent in clinical training have not been examined. The medical school at Stanford University has a flexible curriculum, and there is a wide range in the time that students are in clinical training. This provides an opportunity to test 2 hypotheses: (1) that there is a correlation between the number of months in clinical training and percentile scores on the United States Medical Licensing Examination Step 2, and (2) that percentile scores on this part of the examination are significantly correlated with time spent in clinical training.

Methods.—For 217 graduates of Stanford University School of Medicine, the number of months in clinical training and percentile scores on the United States Medical Licensing Examination Step 2 was determined. Percentile scores on subsections of the Medical College Admission Test and on the National Board of Medical Examiners Part 1 or United States Medical Licensing Examination Step 1 also were calculated.

Results.—The number of months students were in clinical training was between 12 and 23, with a median of 18. There was a very significant association between more months in clinical training and higher scores on Step 2. There was a significant but weaker correlation between scores on Step 1. When scores for Step 1 and for each subsection of the Medical College Admission Test were used in the regression model, the correlation with Step 2 scores did not measurably decrease.

Discussion.—A very significant association was found between the amount of clinical training of medical students and clinical knowledge. Although there is currently concern about the high cost of medical education, decreasing the amount of clinical training may not be a sound solution.

▶ Although this study equates overall clinical knowledge with volume of clinical training, the same results would be found if only surgical knowledge were equated to the volume of surgical training. The current emphasis on the production of generalist physicians has eroded the time spent in surgical clerkships in many institutions. Early diagnosis of surgical illness with appropriate intervention is critical to the reduction in postoperative morbidity and mortality.

Medical school is the only place a physician ever has the opportunity to study a discipline in a protected environment. The results of this study indicate that a better quality of clinical knowledge comes from appropriate clinical exposure. The argument can be made that generalist physicians should have intense exposure to surgical diseases in medical school because they will spend the remainder of their professional lives practicing general medicine. The reverse is true for those students selecting surgery as a discipline. They should take as much specialty and general medicine as possible because never again will the opportunity be available to learn in a structured environment.

E.M. Copeland III, M.D.

The Relationship Between Criteria Used to Select Residents and Performance During Residency

Papp KK, Polk HC, Richardson JD (Univ of Louisville, Ky)

Am J Surg 173:326–329, 1997 1–6

Introduction.—Reports vary regarding the relationship between performance during medical school and performance during residency. Admission variables were analyzed to determine whether they could be used to predict general success during residency.

Methods.—Faculty members were asked to make separate evaluations of residents' knowledge, technical skills, maturity, judgment, and overall ability. Evaluations were made twice with 16 months between evaluations. These evaluations were compared with results of the American Board of Surgery In-Training Examination (ABSITE), medical school class rank, honors received, and various professional and personal activities. General surgical residents were compared with those who chose surgical specialties.

Results.—Reliability of grades assigned with 16 months intervening was high. There was no significant relationship between the rank order assigned before residency and the rank order based on performance after residency. Residents in the top and bottom 10 of their class did not differ significantly. Eight residents in the top 10 and 3 in the bottom 10 chose to remain in general surgery. The ABSITE score for the first year of residency could not be predicted from medical school class rank.

Conclusion.—There was no single predictor of success of surgical residency based on admission data. Residents' interpersonal and technical skills and qualities of character were not well reflected in candidates' credentials at admission, but they had a significant role in faculty perception of success during surgical residency.

► The attempt to perfect a system to reliably produce the best residents from the initial pool of applicants has been unsuccessful. Usually, however, the studies have been conducted in highly competitive residency programs that attract the best resident applicants (almost all from the upper one third of the class). I wonder what the results would be if a study were done of a program with students from a lower part of the class and multiple foreign medical graduates. The simple screening of applicants for class rank and the practice of only interviewing those applicants in the top portion of the class may result in a homogenous group of trainees who are difficult to distinguish from one another, regardless of the criteria used.

E.M. Copeland III, M.D.

Impact of a Clinical Guidelines Program for Breast and Colon Cancer in a French Cancer Center

Ray-Coquard I, Philip T, Lehmann M, et al (Centre Leon Berard, Lyon, France; Fédération Nationale des Centres de Lutte Contre le Cancer, Paris)
JAMA 278:1591–1595, 1997 1–7

Introduction.—Clinical practice guidelines are being promoted to reduce unnecessary costs in health care services and to assist clinical decision making. A comprehensive cancer center in France implemented clinical practice guidelines in 1993 and 1994. The guidelines were based on analysis of the literature and the consensus of intrainstitutional experts. The guidelines were created to help community based oncologists in their decision making, to optimize health benefit, to ensure rational chemotherapy drug prescriptions, to minimize inappropriate variation in practice, and to provide leadership for cancer treatment. Institutional computerized records of patients with breast or colon cancer were reviewed for a before-and-after study.

Methods.—One hundred women with localized breast cancer and 158 with colon cancer were reviewed from records of 1993 and 1995. To assess compliance with clinical practice guidelines, medical decisions on these records were analyzed. To determine the scientific evidence for noncompliant decisions, a systematic search of the literature was performed.

Results.—There were 350 of 375 available medical decisions that could be assessed. In 1995, the compliance rate with clinical practice guidelines for breast cancer was significantly higher than in 1993 (54% vs. 19%). In 1995, the compliance rate for colon cancer was significantly higher than in 1993 (70% vs. 50%). In 1995, 68% of medical decisions for breast cancer conformed with the clinical practice guidelines or were judged to be based on scientific evidence, whereas 42% of medical decisions for breast cancer were based on clinical practice guidelines. In 1995, 81% of medical decisions for colon cancer were judged to be based on scientific evidence or conformed to the clinical practice guidelines; in 1993, 71% of medical decisions for colon cancer were based on clinical practice guidelines.

Conclusion.—For both cancers, compliance rates were significantly higher in 1995. Significant changes in medical practice seem to result from the development and implementation of clinical practice guidelines; however, this study did not demonstrate a causal relationship between the guidelines and the changes.

▶ Clinical guidelines or "pathways" have become popular and have been proven effective for certain surgical diseases such as those requiring hip replacement or vascular surgery. Usually, these patients are treated with only 1 therapeutic modality. The French cancer center study is important because it required compliance from several different medical disciplines (surgery, medical oncology, and radiation therapy). Impact on treatment was greater for breast cancer than for colon cancer, probably because only surgery and medical oncology were involved in the treatment of colon cancer. Thus, there were fewer physicians to order tests. Reduction in unnecessary preoperative and postoperative tests alone—such as carcinoembryonic antigen, CA 15-3, and bone scans for stage I breast cancer—make the clinical guidelines cost effective. The other disease for which too many staging tests are frequently ordered is melanoma. The Society for Surgical Oncology has developed clinical guidelines for the treatment of solid tumors and has published them in recent issues of the *Journal of Surgical Oncology*.

E.M. Copeland III, M.D.

Outcomes of Patients With No Laboratory Assessment Before Anesthesia and a Surgical Procedure

Narr BJ, Warner ME, Schroeder DR, et al (Mayo Clin, Rochester, Minn)

Mayo Clin Proc 72:505–509, 1997 1–8

Purpose.—Previous studies have found that preoperative tests have little or no effect on the outcomes of anesthesia and surgery. The authors' center has therefore stopped performing routine preoperative screening tests in healthy surgical patients younger than 40 years. The effect of this policy change on perioperative morbidity was assessed.

Methods.—The retrospective study included review of the medical records of 56,119 patients who underwent surgical or diagnostic procedures with anesthesia during 1 calendar year. Of these, 5,120 patients underwent no laboratory tests within 90 days before their elective surgical procedure. A random sample of 1,044 such patients was analyzed to demonstrate the absence of preoperative tests, presence of preexisting disease, type of anesthetic used, and intraoperative and postoperative test outcomes. The patients' median age was 21 years (range, 0–95 years). The study was designed to demonstrate, with a 95% confidence level, that true morbidity was less than 0.4%.

Results.—None of the patients died or experienced major morbidity. Although blood typing and screening were performed in 10 patients, none required blood transfusion. During surgery, 17 laboratory tests were performed and 1 electrocardiogram (ECG) was obtained; the results were abnormal in 3 of these. Of 44 blood tests performed postoperatively, 5 patients showed abnormal results, most often low hemoglobin levels. One of the 2 ECGs performed postoperatively showed premature ventricular contractions; otherwise, both were normal. None of the intraoperative or postoperative tests altered the patients' medical or surgical management. One patient undergoing outpatient surgery had unexpected blood loss and was hospitalized for observation.

Conclusions.—This study demonstrates the absence of perioperative morbidity in patients undergoing no laboratory tests before anesthesia and surgery. As long as the history and physical examination show no preoperative indications for laboratory tests, anesthesia and surgery can be safely performed without routine testing. Intraoperative and postoperative tests can be ordered as indicated.

▶ This study differs from others of this type in that many of these patients had no prior testing at all. The patients were deemed healthy by preoperative history and physical examination. Anyone who has had a patient evaluated by the staff at the Mayo Clinic realizes the extensive nature of the history and physical examination done at that institution. A parallel piece of information not included is how many patients who appeared healthy, other than for their surgical problem, had an indication for testing identified by the preoperative evaluation? And did the results of these tests affect the patient's course at the Clinic?

Unless a physician's preoperative history and physical examination are as thorough as is done at the Mayo Clinic, the results obtained in this study may not be duplicated.

E.M. Copeland III, M.D.

A Randomized Trial of Surgical Scrubbing With a Brush Compared to Antiseptic Soap Alone

Loeb MB, Wilcox L, Smaill F, et al (McMaster Univ, Hamilton, Ont, Canada)
Am J Infect Control 25:11–15, 1997 1–9

Objective.—Although use of a scrub brush is standard practice in preoperative cleansing, the brush may actually increase transfer of bacteria by exposing bacterial flora of deeper layers. A randomized, crossover study was undertaken to compare the effectiveness of surgical scrub vs. soap alone in reducing hand bacterial counts.

Methods.—Bacterial specimen counts were obtained by the standard glove fluid sampling procedure before, immediately after, and 45 minutes after 15 healthy adult volunteers performed a 5-minute surgical wash using 15 mL of 4% chlorhexidine soap and isopropyl alcohol with or without a brush. After a 1-week washout period, the volunteers were crossed over, and the experiment was repeated. Culture results were compared statistically.

Results.—At 45 minutes, bacteria were detected on the hands of 7 volunteers after scrubbing but not after washing with soap alone. Bacteria were detected on the hands of 3 volunteers after washing but not after scrubbing. Absolute reduction of baseline bacterial counts was greater in 5 volunteers 45 minutes after scrubbing than after washing; was greater in 5 volunteers 45 minutes after washing than after scrubbing; and was similar in 5 volunteers 45 minutes later, regardless of whether they washed or scrubbed.

Conclusion.—Although the study was small, it demonstrated that reduction in hand bacterial levels was similar for washing and scrubbing. This study measured absolute reduction of hand bacterial levels. Whether these reductions were clinically significant is unknown. Prospective studies of surgical infection rates after using soap alone are necessary.

► In front of most scrub sinks there are a selection of scrub vehicles, usually at least 2 types of soap and brushes. Most surgeons are not going to alter their scrub technique if infection in their patients is not a problem. Nevertheless, the cost savings incurred by scrubbing with soap alone should be considered.

E.M. Copeland, III, M.D.

A Double-blind Study of Perioperative Steroid Requirements in Secondary Adrenal Insufficiency

Glowniak JV, Loriaux DL (Oregon Health Sciences Univ, Portland)

Surgery 121:123–129, 1997 1–10

Objective.—To prevent perioperative hypotension, recommendations call for giving large doses of adrenocorticotropic hormone (ACTH) or cortisone before surgery to patients who have been taking supraphysiologic doses of cortisone. How much glucocorticoid is necessary has never been determined. Results were presented regarding a double-blind study of patients undergoing elective operations who had been treated with glucocorticoids. One group was treated with the recommended increased dose of cortisol, and the other group was treated with saline.

Methods.—Patients taking prednisone for at least 2 months were screened for adrenal insufficiency before elective surgery. Patients with 60-minute cortisol levels below 20 μ/dL were defined as having adrenal insufficiency. Of the 17 patients enrolled in the study, 6 received an IV injection of 100 mg cortisol in normal saline 1 hour before surgery and IV injections of 25 mg cortisol every 6 hours after surgery for 2 days and then every 12 hours for 1 day. Twelve patients (1 patient was studied twice) received injections of saline. Age, cortisol levels, and perioperative blood pressures and pulse rates were statistically compared between groups.

Results.—One patient in each group experienced hypotension. Blood pressures and pulse rates did not differ significantly between groups during the postoperative period.

Conclusion.—The size of the study was small because most patients were taking doses of prednisone too small to compromise adrenal function. No patients taking prednisone doses of 5 to 7.5 mg daily had compromised adrenal function. Some patients taking 10 mg prednisone per day had normal adrenal responses. Patients taking large enough doses of glucocorticoids to cause adrenal insufficiency did not require supplemental glucocorticoids to prevent perioperative hypotension.

▶ Studies that challenge contemporary methods of management are not frequent, even though the data upon which the management strategies are based may be meager. I have always been nervous when operating upon a patient who uses steroids chronically, and I have been dogmatic about the use of "replacement" steroids. Because of the results of this study, I will be less rigid in my insistence on additional steroid medication, but I doubt that I will abandon additional steroids entirely. It is important to point out that each patient in this study continued to get the usual daily dose of steroids and that none of the patients had complications postoperatively, which would have imposed an additional stress (and possibly, the need for additional steroids).

E.M. Copeland III, M.D.

The Mammography Quality Standards Act and Interventional Mammography Procedures

Houn F, Finder C (Johns Hopkins Med School, Baltimore, Md; Food and Drug Administration, Rockville, Md)

J Am Coll Surg 82:14–18, 1997 1–11

Background.—In 1992, Congress passed the Mammography Quality Standards Act (MQSA), administered by the Food and Drug Administration (FDA), and requiring all mammography facilities to meet certain quality standards and obtain FDA accreditation. The MQSA defines its jurisdiction in terms of facilities and diagnostic activities including stereotactic needle biopsy, galactography, X-ray–guided needle localizations of the breast, and other procedures using X-rays.

Screening and Diagnostic Mammography.—Personnel must be licensed, board certified, or have 2 months of radiation instruction and training in interpretation of radiographs, have 40 hours of continuing education, have read at least 240 mammograms within 6 months, read an average of 40 mammograms per month during 24 months, and have at least 15 hours of continuing medical education (CME) credits during a period of 3 years. A facility must be FDA certified and accredited by an approved state or not-for-profit organization that reviews images, quality control programs, and personnel records.

Interventional Mammography.—The goal of regulation is to balance public health needs with access to and availability of services and costs to patients and practitioners. The FDA will publish proposed regulations to improve national performance of this diagnostic technique.

Conclusions.—The purpose of FDA regulation of mammography procedures is to maximize the public health benefit in a cost-effective way and minimize the adverse impact of regulations.

▶ The current enthusiasm of surgeons for stereotactic breast biopsy could be tempered by the FDA regulations that govern the use of mammography. No doubt, these regulations will mimic, to some degree, regulations currently in place for screening and diagnostic mammography (in my opinion, a wise decision). Anyone who uses mammography for diagnostic biopsy purposes should have proven competency in interpreting mammogram radiographs. Breast ultrasonography is, no doubt, a somewhat easier technique to master, but it, like any operator-dependent technique, should require skilled training before clinical application.

E.M. Copeland III, M.D.

Characteristics of Surgeons With High and Low Malpractice Claims Rates

Adamson TE, Baldwin DC Jr, Sheehan TJ, et al (Univ of California, San Francisco; American Med Assoc, Chicago; Univ of Connecticut, Farmington; et al)

West J Med 166:37–44, 1997 1–12

Objective.—At least two thirds of malpractice claims are settled without payment. To determine the relationship between the number of malpractice claims and personal, educational, and practice characteristics, the malpractice experiences of 148 orthopedic surgeons, 115 obstetric-gynecologic surgeons, and 164 other surgeons were examined.

Methods.—The surgeons were all members of the Cooperative of American Physicians, an interindemnity liability-protection trust. They were divided into 4 categories: no claims, those with 0.13 or less mean claims per year, active members with 0.54 to 0.61 mean claims per year, and those terminated because of high claim experience of 0.90 to 1.4 mean claims per year. The no- or low-claims group encompassed 62% of the orthopedists and obstetricians-gynecologists, 82% of the otolaryngologists, 25% of the neurosurgeons, and 19% of the cardiothoracic surgeons. Information on physician characteristics was obtained from biographical profiles, medical schools, boards, the trust's records, and questionnaires filled out and returned by 293 of the nonterminated physicians. A subset of surgeons filled out Rest's Defining Issues Test (DIT) to assess the relationship between clinical performance and moral reasoning.

Results.—The average age of the all-male cohort was 53 years. Terminated orthopedic surgeons were significantly younger (49 years) than other surgeons. Obstetrician-gynecologists were significantly less likely to have been born in the United States, and orthopedic surgeons were significantly more likely to be in the no-claims or low-claims group. Surgeons who were terminated were significantly more likely to have attended medical school outside of the United States or Canada, somewhat less likely to have completed a fellowship, significantly less likely to be board certified, significantly less likely to have a clinical faculty appointment, significantly more likely to be a member of several professional societies, significantly less likely to be members of the American College of Surgeons, and significantly more likely to be in solo practice. Orthopedists with no or low claims were more likely to employ registered nurses than nonprofessional personnel. Orthopedists with fewer or no claims were more likely to have higher DIT scores, and more had religious affiliations.

Conclusion.—Increased collegial interaction, a United States or Canadian medical school education, and being born in the United States (for orthopedic surgeons) appear to decrease significantly the malpractice experience of surgeons. A better understanding of the reasons behind malpractice claims needs to be built into education programs at the medical school level and should be re-emphasized through continuing education programs.

► The identification of extent of training, professional collegiality, and moral fiber as risk indicators for malpractice claims could be used by insurance companies to limit access to liability insurance, by HMOs to select physicians for contract, and by hospital committees as credentialing criteria. This study collected a portion of the data by questionnaire and, consequently, falls prey to all the criticisms and inaccuracies of such a data-gathering mechanism. Nevertheless, it does give a possible glimpse into the future on the methods by which personality and practice profiles may be used to dictate outcomes prospectively.

E.M. Copeland III, M.D.

Relation Between Negligent Adverse Events and the Outcomes of Medical-Malpractice Litigation

Brennan TA, Sox CM, Burstin HR (Harvard School of Public Health, Boston)
N Engl J Med 335:1963–1967, 1996 1–13

Introduction.—Malpractice research indicates that many medical injuries caused by physician negligence do not lead to claims, although many of the claims that are filed do not involve any medical injury or demonstrable physician negligence. However, the litigation system can still be accurate if compensation is awarded only for the cases in which it is merited. Factors predicting payment to plaintiffs were studied to assess the relation between negligent adverse events and the outcomes of malpractice litigation.

Methods.—The investigators followed 51 litigated medical malpractice claims for 10 years to see if the malpractice insurer had closed the case. The outcome of each case was predicted on the basis of detailed case summaries obtained from the insurers. The litigation files were reviewed if the actual outcome differed from the predicted outcome.

TABLE 3.—Logistic-Regression Analysis of Predictors That a Claim Would Be Settled in Favor of the Plaintiff

Predictor*	Odds Ratio (95% confidence interval)	P Value
Permanent disability	29.7 (1.41–621.4)	0.03
Negligent adverse event	0.2 (0.01–4.1)	0.32
Adverse event	0.7 (0.1–7.1)	0.79
Low income	0.1 (0.0–1.5)	0.10
Black race	1.0 (0.1–15.0)	0.97
Age		
<21 yr	0.6 (0.0–10.6)	0.73
>59 yr	1.8 (0.2–17.5)	0.61

*The comparison groups were no permanent disability, no adverse event, high income, non-black race, and age of 21–59 years. We also controlled for the diagnosis-related groups (DRG) category as a measure of the severity of disease, and for the specialty of the physician. These variables are further defined in the Methods section.

(Reprinted by permission of *The New England Journal of Medicine* from Brennan TA, Sox CM, Burstin HR: Relation between negligent adverse events and the outcomes of medical-malpractice litigation. *N Engl J Med* 335:1963–1967, 1996.)

Results.—Forty-six of the 51 cases were closed at the time of the review. Twenty-four cases were classified as involving no adverse event; of these, 10 were settled for the plaintiff, with a mean payment of nearly $29,000. Also settled for the plaintiff were 6 of 13 cases involving adverse events but no negligence, with a mean payment of about $98,000, and 5 of 9 cases involving adverse events caused by negligence, with a mean payment of $67,000. These included 7 of 8 claims involving permanent disability, with a mean payment of $201,250. Permanent disability was the only factor significantly associated with payment on multivariate analysis (Table 3). Payment was unrelated to adverse events of any type, including those caused by negligence.

Conclusions.—In malpractice cases, the size of the payment is related to the severity of the patient's disability, not to the occurrence of an adverse event or an adverse event caused by negligence. The results question the reliance on determinations of negligence when considering compensation for medical injury. No-fault compensation and other malpractice litigation reforms may be more effective in compensating injured patients and avoiding preventable medical injuries.

► The long-term follow-up (10 years) of these alleged malpractice cases gives the best determinant of reasons for monetary settlement. Over a lengthy period of time, a disability that resulted from a physician-patient encounter dictated the settlement amount whether resulting from a negligent act or not. A consensus opinion seems to exist that the physician-patient relationship also dictates the willingness to sue. It would be interesting to know how many settlements resulting in a disability *not* from negligence occur in cases with good physician-patient rapport. If disability remained a significant variable in this setting, then the evidence that our tort system is no longer measuring true malpractice would be even stronger.

E.M. Copeland III, M.D.

Characteristics of Women With and Without Breast Augmentation

Cook LS, Daling JR, Voigt LF, et al (Fred Hutchinson Cancer Research Ctr, Seattle; Univ of Washington, Seattle; Univ of Utah, Salt Lake City; et al)

JAMA 277:1612–1617, 1997 1–14

Objective.—Although silicone breast implants have been associated with myriad illnesses, most epidemiologic studies have failed to establish a connection. Because the characteristics of women with and without implants may be different and therefore may confound epidemiologic studies, interviews were conducted to identify any differences between the 2 groups.

Methods.—The case-control cross-sectional analysis involved personal structured interviews with 80 women who received breast augmentation between the ages of 17 and 49 years and 3,490 women who did not. Records of major life events and photographs of oral contraceptive and hormone preparations were used to enhance recall of past exposures.

Results.—Women with implants were better educated and less likely to be overweight. They were more likely to drink and smoke, to be younger at first pregnancy, and to be younger at first birth. They were more likely to have had a history of pregnancy terminations, to have had a first-degree relative with breast cancer, to have used oral contraceptives and to have used them longer, to have had more lifetime sexual partners, and to have used hair dyes.

Conclusions.—Limitations of this study include the small number of women with implants and the level of response among women, which varied between 70.7% and 76.7%. These findings show that the characteristics of women with breast implants are possibly very different from those of women without breast implants and illustrate the potential confounding factors in any analysis of the risk of breast augmentation.

► This study was conducted by personal interview with most of the participants rather than the usual reliance on a questionnaire (which makes the data more reliable). The only conclusion reached is that the population of women who have had augmentation mammaplasty differ in many respects from a selected cohort of women who have not had the procedure. Such information should be built into decisions such as the relationship of silicone to various disease processes before setting in motion our product liability system.

E.M. Copeland III, M.D.

Effects of Mental Stress on Myocardial Ischemia During Daily Life

Gullette ECD, Blumenthal JA, Babyak M, et al (Duke Univ, Durham, NC; Ohio State Univ, Columbus; Uniformed Services Univ, Bethesda, Md)

JAMA 277:1521–1526, 1997 1–15

Objective.—Myocardial ischemia, an important indicator of future cardiac events in patients with coronary artery disease (CAD), can be triggered by stress. The effect of generalized vs. specific emotional stress on initiation of ischemia was determined prospectively by the case-crossover method.

Methods.—Ambulatory ECG monitoring was performed during a 48-hour period on 132 patients with CAD and recent evidence of exercise-induced ischemia. Patients received no anti-ischemic medication and kept a diary of major activities during the monitoring period. Information about emotional arousal, time of day, and physical activity level were correlated with ST-segment episodes.

Results.—Two of the 58 patients who had myocardial ischemia during the monitoring period were excluded from the study. No physical activity was recorded for 2,311 of the 2,760 hours during the monitoring period. Although most patients did not report high levels of negative emotions, the percentage of ischemic hours was highest during high levels of negative emotions that included 101 hours of tension levels greater than 2, 98 hours of high frustration, and 28 hours of sadness. The percentage of ischemic hours was lower during high levels of positive emotions. Unadjusted relative risk for high levels of negative emotions was 3.0 for tension, 2.9 for sadness, and 2.6 for frustration. When adjusted for time and day and level of activity, the relative risk diminished to 2.2 for all 3 emotions.

Conclusions.—These findings indicate that everyday mental stress can trigger myocardial ischemia. Stress management techniques are recommended and should be evaluated for use in CAD patients.

► The patients in this study had CAD, and mental stress correlated with coronary ischemia. The results of this and other confirmatory studies should be transferred to the workplace. Training supervisors to limit stress for their employees may be more important than stress management training for the employees. The more difficult question is what role does stress play in the initial development of CAD. With the current public health interest in disease prevention, stress management should be practiced more often.

E.M. Copeland III, M.D.

2 Critical Care

Introduction

Clinical pathways, patient care algorithms, and *best practices* are terms that have emerged over the last decade as medicine responds to internal and external economic and societal demands. Thus, it is only fitting that this year's selections begin with an article showing how the literature can be used to modify or direct clinical practice. The practice of basing patient-care decisions on solid research findings, known as *evidence-based medicine,* is a potentially powerful method of improving patient care. In the selected abstract, the strengths and the weaknesses of evidence-based medicine are illustrated in a clinical scenario that deals with using diagnostic tests to assess weaning in ICU patients. Because of the importance of this subject, I encourage everyone to read this article in its entirety. The next abstract is a long-term outcome study of patients who survived an episode of severe sepsis. This paper was chosen because it clearly documents that sepsis not only increases acute mortality but also increases the risk of death for up to 5 years after the septic episode. This unexpected finding that an episode of severe sepsis may have adverse effects on long-term survival is disturbing, and, if verified by other studies, will require intensive investigation.

In the ICU, many aspects of care are directed at specific organs. Thus, in the remainder of this section, the chosen abstracts have been organized by organ systems, beginning with the lung. The first two lung articles deal with the use of the prone position in treating patients with refractory acute respiratory distress syndrome. Taken together, these two studies provide experimental and clinical evidence that prone positioning may improve patient outcome. However, prone positioning has some disadvantages, including the risks of aspiration and inadvertent extubation. An alternative strategy, based on similar physiologic principles, is the use of continuous bed rotation to prevent ventilator-induced pulmonary complications, such as atelectasis and pneumonitis. This approach is discussed in the last of the pulmonary articles. The next group of articles, dealing with cardiovascular and oxygen transport variables, begins with a study evaluating intensive care physicians' knowledge of right-heart pulmonary artery (PA) catheterization. The results of this study indicate that a relatively high number of ICU physicians have major deficiencies in their knowledge of PA catheters and the data generated with their use. These results are sobering and have important implications. First, one should not take one's knowledge of PA catheters for granted, and second, a widely published article reviewed last year showing worse outcomes for patients receiving PA catheters[1] may relate to the knowledge base of the catheter users rather than to the catheters themselves. The next two articles deal with a new technical spin, that is, using spectral analysis of systemic arterial pressure and heart rate as prognostic tools.

Despite the increasing amount of data to the contrary, some clinicians persist in using inotropic agents to drive cardiac output to supranormal levels with the hope of improving outcome. The well-controlled clinical trial by Hayes et al. indicates that this policy of using inotropes, especially at high doses, to drive cardiac output is associated with an *increase*, rather than a decrease, in mortality. It is now past time to accept the fact that inotropes should not be used to drive cardiac output to exceptionally high levels in the volume-resuscitated patient. On the other hand, as shown in the clinical study by Axler et al., the bolus volume of crystalloid required to obtain a hemodynamic response is much greater than the 250–500 mL of salt solution frequently given. In the light of the study by Fitzgerald et al., another controversy that may require reexamination is the transfusion of red blood cells to improve oxygen consumption in septic patients. Their findings indicate that one reason red blood cell transfusions fail to increase oxygen consumption is that old blood is transfused. Since old red cells have lost the ability to deform, they are more likely to become trapped in the microcirculation than fresh red cells, thereby impairing their ability to deliver oxygen to the tissues. Because of the importance of ensuring that organ blood flow is adequate in the critically ill, methods for assessing organ-specific blood flow are being developed and tested. As described by Maynard et al., the use of lidocaine as a marker of adequacy of liver blood flow is one such test. The last of the organ-related articles indicates that recovery from experimental renal failure is better when a subject is fed enterally than parenterally. This is one more piece of evidence supporting the use of enteral over parenteral alimentation in the critically ill.

Studies on the biology of sepsis and organ failure continue to provide interesting insights. Consequently, two studies that describe novel experimental therapeutic approaches to sepsis and multiple organ failure are included. Also included is a study implicating nitric oxide as a key mediator in gut injury during endotoxemia. Lastly, a study is included indicating that failure of pulmonary neutrophils from endotoxin-challenged animals may contribute to lung injury. This concept, that inflammatory stimuli result not only in activation of neutrophils but also increase their life span, may help explain why, in certain circumstances, inflammation becomes excessive and why the normal signals to shut down the inflammatory response fail.

Edwin A. Deitch, M.D.

Reference

1. Conners AF Jr, Speroff T, Dawson NV, et al: The effectiveness of right heart catheterization in the initial care of critically ill patients. *JAMA* 276:889–897, 1996.

How to Use Diagnostic Test Articles in the Intensive Care Unit: Diagnosing Weanability Using f/Vt

Jaeschke RZ, Meade MO, Guyatt GH, et al (McMaster Univ, Hamilton, Ont, Canada; Univ of Toronto; Univ of Western Ontario, London, Canada)

Crit Care Med 25:1514–1521, 1997 2–1

Objective.—In the diagnostic process, the physician generates a set of hypotheses, then gathers additional information to modify these hypotheses. Information is obtained from a variety of sources that function as diagnostic tests, including the history, the physical examination, and laboratory studies. Diagnostic tests can be profitably translated from research studies if the study population is similar to the patients being treated, if the results are compared in independent and blinded fashion to a standard test, and if the standard test was studied in all patients. The application of diagnostic test research to the ICU setting was discussed, using the example of diagnosing weanability using respiratory frequency divided by tidal volume (f/Vt).

Discussion.—The article considered the example of a 45-year-old man with gallstone pancreatitis complicated by septic shock, acute renal failure, acute respiratory distress syndrome, and pancreatic phlegmon. When switched from pressure-control to assist-control ventilation 3 days earlier, the patient's inspired oxygen requirement fell from 90% to 35%. He was off inotropic support and did not require dialysis for 1 week. Two residents disagreed as to whether the patient was ready to be weaned from

TABLE 1.—Critical Appraisal of Studies of Diagnostic Tests

I. Are the results of the study valid?
   1. Was there an independent, blind comparison with a reference standard?
   2. Did the patient sample include an appropriate spectrum of patients to whom the diagnostic test will be applied in clinical practice?
   3. Did the results of the test being evaluated influence the decision to perform the reference standard?

II. What are the results?
   1. Are likelihood ratios, sensitivity, and specificity for the test results presented, or data necessary for their calculation provided?

III. Will the results help me in caring for my patients?
   1. Were the methods for performing the test described in sufficient detail to permit replication?
   2. Will the reproducibility of the test result and its interpretation be satisfactory in my setting?
   3. Are the results applicable to my patient?
   4. Will the results change my management?
   5. Will patients be better off as a result of the test?

(Courtesy of Jaeschke FZ, Meade MO, Guyatt GH, et al: How to use diagnostic test articles in the intensive care unit: Diagnosing weanability using f/Vt. *Crit Care Med* 25 [9]:1514–1521, 1997.)

TABLE 5.—Comparison of the Results of a Diagnostic Test (f/VT) With the Results of a Reference Standard (Successful Weaning), Using Different Cutoffs for f/VT

f/VT Category	Weaning Trial: Successful Weaning	Weaning Trial: Unsuccessful Weaning	Likelihood Ratio
<80	29	3	7.53
80–100	6	6	0.77
>100	1	19	0.04
Total	36	28	

Abbreviations: f, respiratory frequency; *VT,* tidal volume.
(Courtesy of Jaeschke FZ, Meade MO, Guyatt GH, et al: How to use diagnostic test articles in the intensive care unit: Diagnosing weanability using f/VT. *Crit Care Med* 25 [9]:1514–1521, 1997.)

mechanical ventilation and extubated, and asked for help in settling the issue. In considering the question, a study was recalled using f/Vt to diagnose weanability.

Critical appraisal of this study must consider the criteria mentioned above. The validity of the study depends on the study population, the text exposure, and the measured outcomes (Table 1). If the study meets these quality criteria, the findings can be used in the form of sensitivity, specificity, and likelihood ratios to assess changes in the probability of the target condition, depending on the test results (Table 5). The level of clinical relevance will be higher if the study is performed and interpreted under circumstances comparable to the clinical setting.

Conclusions.—The approach of using diagnostic test research articles in guiding ICU care was discussed, with the example of using f/Vt to assess the likelihood of weaning from mechanical ventilation. The representativeness of the study population, the presence of an independent reference standard, and the universal application of the standard were key criteria for evaluating study validity.

▶ Evidence-based medicine is an emerging discipline that enables clinicians to appropriately analyze the published literature and use this analysis in deciding how to modify their practices. This "how to" article was chosen because it illustrates in a step-by-step manner the key points (Table 1) one should follow when trying to decide whether a diagnostic test should be incorporated in one's clinical practice. The example chosen was the use of the respiratory frequency/tidal volume (f/Vt) ratio to predict weanability. In this diagnostic test, the patient is allowed to breathe for 1 minute on a t-tube, and the patient's respiratory rate is divided by the patient's tidal volume. The subsequent f/Vt ratio is computed and used to predict weanability. As shown in Table 5, this ratio can be used to provide a reasonably good prediction of whether a patient will be successfully weaned.

My goal in choosing this article was not to critique the f/Vt ratio, but to bring the process of evidence-based medicine to your attention. I highly recommend that you read the original article and experiment with using this process in your evaluation of the literature. If you do, I believe you will be pleased with the result.

E.A. Deitch, M.D.

Magnitude and Duration of the Effect of Sepsis on Survival

Quartin AA, for the Dept of Veterans Affairs Systemic Sepsis Cooperative Studies Group (Univ of Miami, Fla)

JAMA 277:1058–1063, 1997 2–2

Introduction.—Sepsis is an acute and deadly disease, with most studies addressing outcomes of 30 days or fewer. Since the long-term risk of death after a septic insult is unknown, the current study evaluated the magnitude and duration of the effect of a septic episode on long-term patient survival after discharge from the hospital.

Methods.—The study included 1,505 patients who had probable sepsis and were screened for inclusion in the Department of Veterans Affairs Cooperative Study of Corticosteroids in Systemic Sepsis during the 1980s. The controls were 91,830 nonpsychiatric patients free of infection who had been discharged from the same medical centers during the same approximate time span as the sepsis group. During the 8 years following the index hospitalization, the 2 groups were compared for mortality based on a proportional hazards model constructed from the characteristics of the control group. The relative contributions of sepsis and underlying disease to mortality were assessed.

Results.—Throughout the 8-year follow-up period, risk of death was higher for the patients with sepsis than it was for the control group. One-year mortality from nonseptic causes among patients with sepsis, as predicted from the model, was 26%. This figure was similar for patients with uncomplicated or severe sepsis or septic shock. For the first 5 years after screening, the daily risk of death for patients with sepsis was greater than predicted by the model. Thereafter, risk was similar to that observed in patients with similar underlying disease but without sepsis. For the first year, the hazard rate associated with sepsis rose along with the severity of the septic episode. For patients in the septic group who survived for 30 days, mean life span was reduced from a predicted 8.03 years to 4.08 years. Within the first year, there were 192 more deaths than predicted among 30-day survivors. At 5 years, there were 51 more deaths than predicted among 1-year survivors.

Conclusions.—Sepsis increases mortality risk not only within the first 30 days but also for up to 5 years after the septic episode. This is so, even with adjustment for comorbid conditions. The severity of sepsis influences the risk of death for the first year after the episode. Studies of treatment for sepsis should consider the possible long-term benefits because some treatments may improve long-term survival without demonstrating any apparent immediate benefits.

► One limitation of ICU care is the potential failure of ICU physicians and consultants to institute long-term follow up of the patients they treat. Therefore, most outcome studies of ICU patients with sepsis have focused on short-term or 30-day survival rates. Although it is well recognized that sepsis in the ICU is associated with a 30% to 50% 30-day mortality rate, there is limited information on the natural history of the disease in patients who survive to be discharged. Thus, the value of this long-term outcomes study is the fact that it clearly shows that the risk of patients who survive sepsis dying after hospital discharge is greatly increased during an 8-year follow-up period when compared with patients without sepsis with similar comorbidities.

E.A. Deitch, M.D.

Influence of Prone Position on the Extent and Distribution of Lung Injury in a High Tidal Volume Oleic Acid Model of Acute Respiratory Distress Syndrome

Broccard AF, Shapiro RS, Schmitz LL, et al (Univ of Minnesota, St Paul; Hennepin County Med Ctr, Minneapolis, Minn)
Crit Care Med 25:16–27, 1997 2–3

Introduction.—Ventilator-induced lung injury may be more intense or extensive in the lower lung zones. An experiment was devised to determine the influence of position on the extent and distribution of lung injury in an oleic acid canine model of acute respiratory distress syndrome, using mechanical ventilation with high tidal volumes and positive end-expiratory pressure (PEEP).

Methods.—Twelve adult dogs were anesthetized, then injected with oleic acid. Ninety minutes after lung injury was induced with oleic acid, the animals were randomized to be ventilated for 4 hours in either the prone or supine position while using the identical ventilatory pattern (FIO_2 0.6, PEEP 10 cm or more of water and a tidal volume that generated a peak transpulmonary pressure of 35 cm of water when implemented in the supine position). The tidal volumes, FIO_2, and PEEP were kept constant and the pulmonary artery occlusion pressure was held between 4 and 6 mm Hg, regardless of the dogs' position. At protocol completion, the animals were killed and the lungs excised for gravimetric determination (wet/dry weight ratio) and histologic score. Changes over time in the static pressure-volume curve of the lungs (taken in the supine position) were assessed.

Results.—Both groups were similar in hemodynamic and respiratory variables and lung static-volume curves at baseline. At completion of the experiment, the lung gravimetric data in the 2 groups were similar, indicating a similar extent of edema. Histologic abnormalities were signifi-

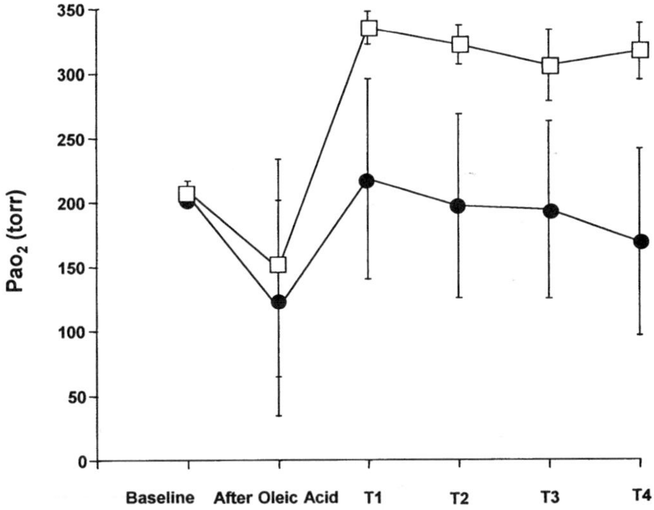

FIGURE 5.—Changes in Pao_2 over time in prone (*squares*) and supine (*circles*) dogs. Mean Pao_2 values are reported with their corresponding 95% confidence intervals. Partial pressure of arterial oxygen improved in both groups after ventilation with high transpulmonary pressure, and positive end-expiratory pressure was implemented (*T1–T4*: 1–4 hours after the beginning of ventilation). However, the improvement was significantly and consistently higher in the prone group. To convert torr to kPa, multiply the value by 0.1333. (Courtesy of Broccard AF, Shapiro RS, Schmitz LL, et al: Influence of prone position on the extent and distribution of lung injury in a high tidal volume oleic acid model of acute respiratory distress syndrome. *Crit Care Med* 25:16–27, 1997.)

cantly less in the prone than in the supine group (Fig 5). There were marked differences in the extent and severity in the dependent regions of the lungs. There was significant improvement in static lung compliance in the prone, but not the supine group.

Conclusion.—In an animal model of oleic acid-induced lung injury, dogs ventilated with high tidal volume and PEEP had less extensive histologic injury in the prone position than in the supine position. The distribution of histologic abnormalities is altered in the prone position.

Dramatic Effect on Oxygenation in Patients With Severe Acute Lung Insufficiency Treated in the Prone Position

Mure M, Martling C-R, Lindahl SGE (Karolinska Hosp and Inst, Stockholm)
Crit Care Med 25:1539–1544, 1997 2–4

Introduction.—A clinical follow-up study was conducted to confirm the positive effect on gas exchange achieved by treating patients with impaired respiratory function in the prone position. Although this finding was first presented in 1974, few reports since then have evaluated patients treated in the prone position.

Methods.—At the study institution, the prone position has for several years been the routine treatment position for patients with severe lung insufficiency. Thirteen patients treated in the ICU were the subjects of this

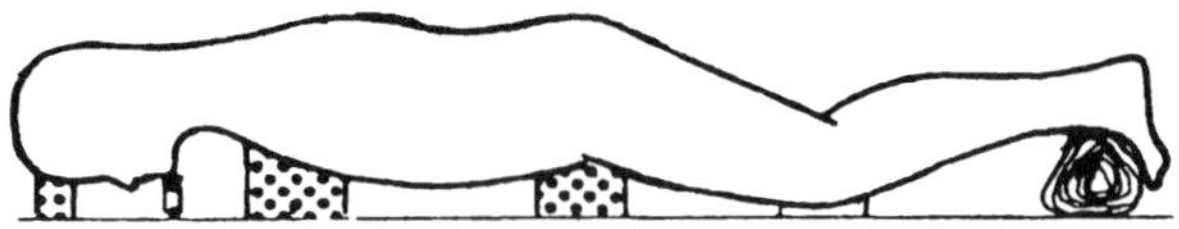

FIGURE 1.—When prone, patients should be supported by foam rubber pads under the upper thorax and pelvis. The head should be supported under the chin, cheeks, and forehead. It is essential that pressure on the eye bulbs be avoided at all times. (Courtesy of Mure M, Martling C-R, Lindahl SGE: Dramatic effect on oxygenation in patients with severe acute lung insufficiency treated in the prone position. *Crit Care Med* 25[9]:1539–1544, 1997.)

study. Two had severe burns, 3 had experienced multiple trauma, 5 had septicemia, 2 were diagnosed with intoxication, and 1 had aspiration pneumonia. Severe hypoxia was present in 11 patients. Treatment in the prone position was performed without changing any ventilatory settings other than fraction of inspired oxygen. Care must be taken to anchor the endotracheal tube securely while the patient is prone, provide supports, and protect the eyes (Fig 1).

Results.—Overall, 12 of 13 patients responded to treatment in the prone position. Oxygenation indices increased each time that the 12 responding patients were treated in this manner, except for 1 patient whose oxygenation index did not improve the third time he was turned. In 5 patients, the oxygenation indices decreased upon return to the supine position. The 2 patients who did not meet criteria for severe hypoxia responded moderately to the prone position. The single patient who failed to respond to that position, an alcoholic with severe liver disease, died of gram-negative septicemia. The alveolar-arterial oxygen gradient decreased significantly when patients were in the prone position. Nine patients survived; none of the deaths were attributed to impaired gas exchange.

Conclusion.—Twelve of 13 patients, including 11 with severe hypoxia, had significant improvement in impaired gas exchange when treated in the prone position. Because extracorporeal membrane oxygenation was not required in any case, the prone position should be tried before other more complex modalities are ordered.

▶ The concept that patients with acute respiratory distress syndrome (ARDS) might benefit from being placed in the prone position is receiving increasing attention on the basis of both clinical and experimental studies. For example, it is known from CT-based patient studies that the dependent portion of the lung is disproportionately affected in early ARDS. This clinical information combined with the observation that placing animals in the prone position limits ventilator-induced pulmonary damage has led to a further series of clinical and experimental studies investigating the potential benefits of prone positioning in limiting pulmonary dysfunction in injured lungs. Two such studies were chosen to illustrate this potentially important clinical strategy.

In the experimental study by Broccard et al. (Abstract 2–3), the authors convincingly showed that prone positioning reduced lung damage and improved pulmonary compliance and oxygenation in a dog model of lung injury. There are 2 major potential explanations for why the prone position protects against ventilator-induced injury and limits pulmonary damage in injured lungs. The first reason is based on the fact that blood flow and hydrostatic pressure is greatest in the dependent regions of the lung, and this increased pressure potentiates edema, atelectasis, and tissue injury. In the prone position, there is a reduction of pleural pressure in the dorsal lung regions that limits edema formation and consequently injury. The second reason the supine position has been thought to potentiate lung injury is that, in the supine position, atelectasis results in repeated tidal opening and recollapse in dependent lung segments resulting in surfactant depletion and thereby increasing alveolar sheer forces and lung damage. When shifting from the supine to the prone position is done, alveolar ventilation becomes more uniform and thus limits atelectasis and alveolar over and under distention, thereby preserving lung function.

The case series by Mure et al. (Abstract 2–4) is the most detailed clinical study on the physiologic effect of prone positioning on pulmonary function in mechanically ventilated patients with ARDS published to date. This study clearly documents that placing patients with profound respiratrory failure in the prone position improves oxygenation when other more traditional ventilatory maneuvers have failed.

These 2 studies highlight the potential benefits of the prone position in situations of severe lung injury. They strongly suggest that rolling patients with respiratory failure onto their stomachs may be an important way of improving lung function and limiting lung injury. Although this strategy has some potential dangers (aspiration or inadvertent extubation) and may seem counterintuitive, it appears to work.

E.A. Deitch, M.D.

Effects of Continuous Bed Rotation and Prolonged Mechanical Ventilation on Healthy, Adult Baboons

Anzueto A, Peters JI, Seidner SR, et al (Univ of Texas, San Antonio; Southwest Found for Biomedical Research, San Antonio, Tex; Kinetic Concepts Inc, San Antonio, Tex)

Crit Care Med 25:1560–1564, 1997 2–5

Introduction.—Complications related to mechanical ventilation are an important cause of morbidity and mortality. There is evidence that conventional volume-controlled mechanical ventilation induces lung injury. Ventilator-induced lung damage is dependent on peak inspiratory pressures, high tidal volumes, and the distribution of tidal volumes within the lungs. A prospective study in adult baboons examined the hypothesis that continuous bed rotation would reduce the frequency of pulmonary complications during prolonged mechanical ventilation.

Methods.—Twelve healthy adult male baboons were mechanically ventilated for 11 days by means of a volume-cycled ventilator. Five underwent continuous bed rotation therapy to 45 degrees and 7 had no bed rotation. The animals had been anesthetized, sedated, and paralyzed and were monitored during the ventilation study with pulmonary and peripheral arterial catheters. Hemodynamics, pulmonary function, lung volume, and arterial blood gases were measured daily. Chest radiographs were obtained each day, and bronchoalveolar lavage was performed at days 0, 7, and 11.

Results.—Neither group exhibited any significant changes in hemodynamics, gas exchange, or pulmonary function during the study period. In 6 of the 7 control animals, radiologic patchy atelectasis developed, and 2 had persistent radiographic changes by day 11, despite increased peak inspiratory pressures, changes in positive end-expiratory pressure, and aggressive pulmonary toilet. Controls also had a significant increase in bronchoalveolar lavage neutrophils at days 7 and 11; all had areas of bronchiolitis, with surrounding bronchopneumonia in 5 of 7 animals. Baboons allotted to continuous bed rotation had no radiologic or morphologic abnormalities.

Conclusion.—Animals assigned to bed rotation during mechanical ventilation had significantly lowered ventilator peak pressures and bronchoalveolar lavage neutrophils compared with control animals. Baboons in the bed rotation protocol had normal lung morphology during 11 days of mechanical ventilation, whereas controls exhibited atelectasis, increased concentrations of bronchoalveolar lavage neutrophils, and mild pneumonitis.

▶ This study evaluating the effect of continuous rotation on baboons ventilated for 11 days was designed to address the clinical controversy over whether continuous bed rotation will reduce the frequency of mechanical ventilation–induced pulmonary complications, including atelectasis and pneumonitis. This controversy is based on the fact that whereas several clinical trials found continuous rotation to be beneficial, others did not.

Because of the heterogeneity of the patients enrolled in these trials and their frequent co-morbidities, review of the clinical data is problematic. Consequently, there is value in testing the effect of continuous rotation in a clinically realistic animal model. The authors have done just that in this study, and their results indicate that this therapeutic approach does prevent ventilator-associated pulmonary injury and atelectasis. A second strong point of this study is that the described model will be useful in dissecting out the mechanisms by which automated turning prevents pulmonary complications.

Determining whether automated, continuous bed rotation will be as effective as placing patients with adult respiratory distress syndrome in the prone position is the next question that must be addressed, because placing patients in the prone position is technically more demanding, is less comfortable for the patient, and is associated with more potential complications. Until then, it is important to remember that immobility and stasis are bad for the lungs as well as the rest of the body, and any movement is better than no movement at all.

E.A. Deitch, M.D.

Intensive Care Physicans' Insufficient Knowledge of Right-Heart Catheterization at the Bedside: Time to Act?

Gnaegi A, Feihl F, Perret C (Lausanne Univ, Switzerland)

Crit Care Med 25:213–220, 1997 2–6

Background.—Although pulmonary artery (PA) catheters are widely used in intensive care medicine, there is no scientific proof of their clinical benefit. Like any medical technique, PA catheterization must be performed correctly if it is to favorably influence patient outcome. A recent North American study demonstrated variable knowledge about pulmonary artery catheter use among intensive care physicians. European intensive care physicians were tested on their knowledge of PA catheters.

Methods.—The study included 535 critical care physicians working in 86 French, Swiss, or Belgian ICUs. Forty-three percent of respondents were still in training, while 57% had completed their postgraduate training. The physicians were given a 31-item questionnaire regarding all aspects of bedside PA catheterization, including technical aspects of measurements, calculation of derived values, hemodynamic interpretation, catheter insertion, complications, and influence on therapy. The questionnaires were administered anonymously, to all physicians simultaneously, and without forewarning. The questionnaire was well validated, having been used in the North American study cited above.

Results.—Sixty-eight percent of respondents in training and 36% of those who had completed their training believed that they had inadequate knowledge about the PA catheter. The mean percentage of correct responses was 72% overall—67% for physicians in training and 76% for those who had completed their training. For physicians in training, the lower quartile value was 57%, the median value 70%, and the upper quartile value 77%. For physicians who had completed training, these values were 70%, 80%, and 87%, respectively. On multivariate analysis, independent predictors of a high score on the questionnaire were working in a university hospital ICU, believing that one's knowledge about PA catheters was adequate, and being responsible for supervising catheter insertions. However, there was no subgroup of physicians with consistently good knowledge. Many respondents gave incorrect answers to questions reflecting basic knowledge. For example, about half could not correctly identify PA occlusion pressure from a clear chart recording.

Conclusion.—European and North American studies have shown that ICU physicians may have inadequate knowledge about PA catheters. This deficiency should be addressed by revised accreditation policies and teaching practices. The authors call for more research to assess ICU physicians' knowledge of other complicated, expensive techniques with the potential for patient harm, such as mechanical ventilation and continuous venovenous hemodiafiltration.

▶ This article was chosen because the results indicate that a relatively high number of ICU physicians have major deficiencies in knowledge regarding pulmonary artery catheters. This finding is important because suboptimal knowledge about these catheters or the data they generate will lead to errors in patient care. Lest one say that this is a European study and U.S. physicians know more, it is important to know that a similar study was performed in the United States and Canada several years ago and the results were strikingly similar.[1] In fact, the Europeans did better (72% vs. 67% correct).

So what is the message? The message is that one should not take for granted ones knowledge regarding these catheters. In fact (who knows?), the poor results observed in a recent clinical trial when pulmonary artery catheters were used[2] may have been related, to some degree, to a lack of knowledge by the catheter "insertees" rather than to the catheters themselves.

E.A. Deitch, M.D.

References

1. Iberti JT, Fischer EP, Leibowitz AB, et al: A multicenter study of physicians' knowledge of the pulmonary artery catheter. *JAMA* 264:2928–2932, 1990.
2. Connors AF, Speraff T, Dawson NV, et al: The effectiveness of right heart catheterization in the initial care of critically ill patients. *JAMA* 276:889–897, 1996.

Spectral Analysis of Systemic Arterial Pressure and Heart Rate Signals as a Prognostic Tool for the Prediction of Patient Outcome in the Intensive Care Unit

Yien H-W, Hseu S-S, Lee L-C, et al (Veterans General Hosp-Taipei, Taiwan; Natl Yang-Ming Univ, Taipei, Taiwan)

Crit Care Med 25:258–266, 1997 2–7

Background.—Several techniques have been evaluated for use in aiding decisions about withdrawing or continuing care for patients in the ICU. Although systemic arterial pressure and heart rate are routinely monitored clinical indices, they are usually kept within a physiologic range and are, thus, not useful for predicting patient outcome. This study sought to determine whether changes in the spectra of systemic arterial pressure and in heart rate (HR) signals are useful in predicting the outcomes of adult patients in the ICU.

Methods.—The prospective study included 52 patients in an adult ICU. Each patient's demographic, diagnostic, and survival data were recorded. Acute Physiology and Chronic Health Evaluation II scores were calculated each day. Also, the patients underwent continuous, on-line, and real time spectral analysis of systemic arterial pressure and HR signals. These analyses were performed every day over at least 30 minutes between 10 PM and midnight. The data were used to calculate the average power density values of the high-frequency, low-frequency, and very–low-frequency components of the systemic arterial pressure and HR signals.

Results.—Twenty-five patients survived and 27 died. Patients who survived tended to have progressively increasing power density values in both the low-frequency and very–low-frequency components of the systemic arterial pressure and HR signals. Patients who had decreasing power density values in these spectral components were likely to experience clinical deterioration and death. The survivors and nonsurvivors were similar in terms of mean systemic arterial pressure, heart rate, systemic vascular resistance, and cardiac index.

Conclusion.—In the ICU, power spectral analysis of systemic arterial pressure and HR signals appears to be a useful technique of patient monitoring. It may become a new prognostic tool for predicting patient outcome and, thus, in making decisions about continuing or withdrawing care for critically ill patients.

Experimental Human Endotoxemia Increases Cardiac Regularity: Results From a Prospective, Randomized, Crossover Trial

Godin PJ, Fleisher LA, Eidsath A, et al (Natl Insts of Health, Bethesda, Md; Johns Hopkins Med Insts, Baltimore, Md; Washington Univ, St Louis, Mo)

Crit Care Med 24:1117–1124, 1996 2–8

Introduction.—Based on previous research, the authors hypothesize that the disruption of communication between organs observed in multiple organ system dysfunction syndrome (MODS) is caused by mediator excess. If so, the predecessors of MODS will disrupt normal interorgan communication. An experimental study was performed in humans to see if endotoxemia is linked to loss of physiologic beat-to-beat variability in heart rate.

Methods.—The prospective, randomized, crossover study included 12 healthy volunteers. They were assigned to receive IV *Escherichia coli* endotoxin or placebo, with or without pretreatment with oral ibuprofen. During each trial, ECGs were continuously recorded and digitized using series of 1,000-beat epochs of R-R intervals over 8 hours. Three different measures of heart rate variability were used: standard deviation, power spectra, and approximate entropy, representing variability in the time domain, frequency domain, and regularity, respectively.

Results.—All 3 measures showed reduced variability in response to endotoxin. Pretreatment with ibuprofen blocked the fever and symptoms caused by endotoxin administration. However, the reduction in heart rate variability was still significant (Fig 1).

Conclusion.—By all measures, experimental endotoxemia in humans causes reduced heart rate variability. The findings support the authors' hypothesis concerning MODS, which involves physiologic uncoupling of vital organ systems. There may be a threshold of oscillator uncoupling beyond which recoupling is not possible, and this may be the point of pathophysiologic irreversibility in MODS and other disease states.

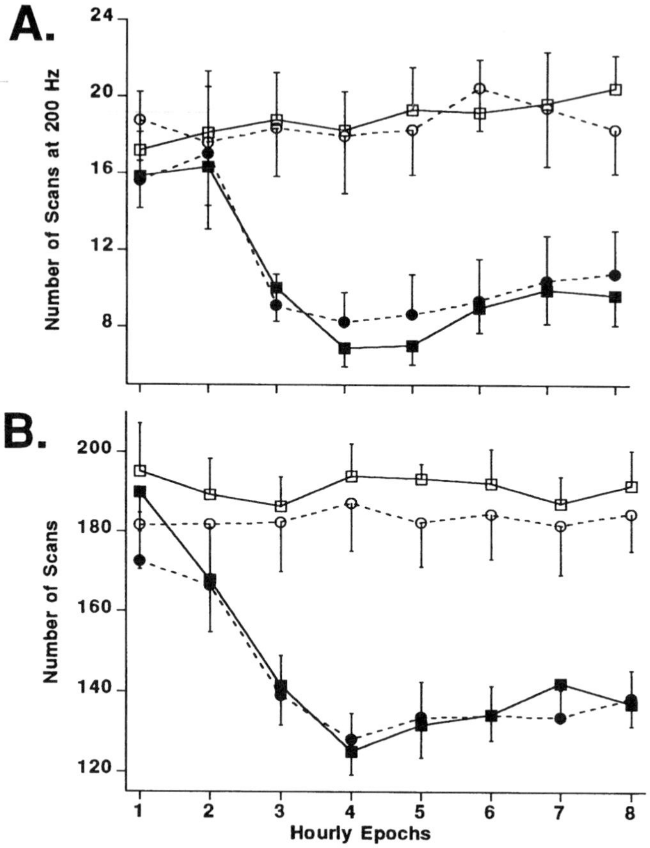

FIGURE 1.—Heart rate increases (B[p = 0.0001]) and heart rate standard deviation decreases (A[p = 0.0001]) after endotoxin administration. Increases in heart rate are shown in terms of decreases in R-R interval length, which is given as number of scans at 200 Hz (interval duration = number of scans × 0.005 sec/scan). These responses occurred after endotoxin/ibuprofen in the absence of fever and symptoms. Experimental groups are symbolized: *solid squares*, endotoxin placebo; *open squares*, saline/placebo; *solid circles*, endotoxin/ibuprofen; *open circles*, saline/ibuprofen. Data are presented as mean ± standard error of the mean. (Courtesy of Godin PJ, Fleisher LA, Eidsath A, et al: Experimental human endotoxemia increases cardiac regularity: Results from a prospective, randomized, crossover trial. *Crit Care Med* 24:1117–1124, 1996.)

▶ In the first study (Abstract 2–7), by means of sophisticated computer analysis the authors were able to use quantitative changes in the beat-to-beat "spectral power" of patients HR and systemic arterial pressure to discriminate between survivors and nonsurvivors. Interestingly, the nonsurvivors lost the normal beat-to-beat variations in the low-frequency and very-low-frequency spectral components of their HR and blood pressure. That is, the spectral power curve became flat and lost the normal hills and peaks observed in the survivors. Thus, loss of normal variability between beats was a bad prognostic sign. Most importantly, the predictive spectral changes in HR and systemic arterial pressure were observed at a time when other physiologic variables were similar between the groups.

In the second study (Abstract 2–8), in which normal volunteers were challenged with endotoxin, the authors found that endotoxemia is associated with a loss of physiologic beat-to-beat variability in several parameters of the HR. The rationale for this study was the hypothesis that during sepsis interorgan interactions are disrupted or uncoupled. As explained by the authors, the heart is a biological oscillator, as aspects of its activity vary periodically with time. Although clinically, HR is recorded as an average number, this average number hides a normal variation in beat-to-beat intervals. Because the heart is mechanically and biologically coupled with other biological oscillator systems—such as the lungs and brain, which contribute to cardiac variability—loss of cardiac beat-to-beat variability after endotoxin challenge does support the authors basic tenet that during sepsis interorgan communication is reduced.

These 2 studies are interesting perhaps and complex certainly, but why are they important? First of all, if the approach used in the study by Yien et al. pans out, it could revolutionize prognostication. Secondly, as illustrated by the second study, this methodology may provide a new way of studying the biology of sepsis.

E.A. Deitch, M.D.

Oxygen Transport Patterns in Patients With Sepsis Syndrome or Septic Shock: Influence of Treatment and Relationship to Outcome

Hayes MA, Timmins AC, Yau EHS, et al (St Bartholomew's and Homerton Hosps, London; Charing Cross Hosp, London)

Crit Care Med 25:926–936, 1997 2–9

Introduction.—Numerous studies of critically ill patients report improved survival rates for those with early increases in cardiac index and higher levels of oxygen delivery and oxygen consumption. Despite this relationship, there is controversy over the value of treatment aimed at improving oxygen transport patterns. Patients with sepsis syndrome or septic shock, managed according to 2 different treatment regimens, were studied retrospectively to characterize the hemodynamic and oxygen transport patterns of survivors and nonsurvivors.

Methods.—Seventy-eight patients with sepsis syndrome or septic shock were drawn retrospectively from a randomized trial of patients at risk of multiple organ failure. All patients received controlled oxygen therapy on admission to the ICU. If volume expansion to an optimal pulmonary artery occlusion pressure did not achieve therapeutic goals (cardiac index greater than 4.5 L/min/m^2, oxygen delivery of more than 600 mL/min/m^2, and oxygen consumption of more than 170 mL/min/m^2), patients were randomly assigned to treatment or control groups. The treatment group received dobutamine (5–200 µg/kg/min) to increase cardiac index and oxygen delivery; controls were given dobutamine only if the cardiac index was less than 2.8 L/min/m^2. All patients received norepinephrine (0.05–10 µg/kg/min) if required to maintain mean arterial pressure at 80 mm Hg.

Measurements of hemodynamic, oxygen transport, and lactate values were obtained at frequent intervals.

Results.—In both treatment and control groups, survivors significantly increased cardiac index and oxygen delivery in response to maximal resuscitation. They also showed a significant increase in oxygen consumption, despite an associated decrease in oxygen extraction. Nonsurvivors from both groups exhibited significant increases in cardiac index and oxygen delivery, but oxygen extraction decreased and oxygen consumption was unchanged. Compared to survivors, nonsurvivors had significantly lower maximum increases in oxygen delivery and oxygen consumption and exhibited persistently high lactate concentrations.

Conclusion.—Survivors and nonsurvivors of septic syndrome and septic shock had qualitatively similar hemodynamic and oxygen transport responses, whether allocated to dobutamine or control groups. But in both groups, survivors responded with greater increases in cardiac index, left ventricular stroke work index, and oxygen delivery, and their lactate concentrations were lower.

▶ This article asked the question: Is increasing oxygen delivery to supranormal levels helpful in patients with sepsis and septic shock? On the basis of the authors' results, the answer is a resounding NO. The strength of this study is that the authors evaluated only patients who *did not* have supranormal levels of oxygen delivery spontaneously after full volume resuscitation. Although it was not mentioned in the abstract, the mortality rate of the patients treated with dobutamine was higher (58% vs. 33%) than that of the patients not receiving inotropic support aimed at increasing oxygen delivery. This increased mortality in the dobutamine-treated patients occurred even though the 2 groups were similar clinically and the predicted mortality rate was lower in the dobutamine than in the control group (predicted mortality 36% in the dobutamine group vs. 44% in the control group).

This study clearly indicates that the use of inotropic agents (especially at high doses) in fully volume-resuscitated patients does not increase survival. Thus, although there is a relationship between the attainment of supranormal levels of oxygen delivery and consumption with survival, the converse does not appear to be true, that is, driving up oxygen delivery with inotropes to supranormal levels in the volume-resuscitated patient is not effective in improving survival. In conclusion, based on this and similar studies in the literature, the use of inotropes to increase oxygen delivery to supranormal levels does not appear to be very wise.

E.A. Deitch, M.D.

Small Hemodynamic Effect of Typical Rapid Volume Infusions in Critically Ill Patients

Axler O, Tousignant C, Thompson CR, et al (Univ of British Columbia, Vancouver, Canada; Université Paris V)

Crit Care Med 25:965–970, 1997 2–10

Introduction.—Rapid volume infusions are frequently administered to critically ill patients, yet the effectiveness of this clinical intervention is uncertain. Data are also lacking on the extent to which rapid volume infusions are ordered in the ICU and what volumes of solutions are typically employed. In the first part of this study, the volume and composition of all rapid volume infusions ordered over a 1-month period in 2 separate ICUs were recorded. The effects of rapid volume infusion in 13 critically ill patients were then studied prospectively.

Methods.—Data on the volume and composition of infusions were collected retrospectively from bedside charts in the 2 ICUs. The 13 patients studied prospectively were mechanically ventilated and had both a pulmonary artery flotation catheter and a radial or femoral artery catheter placed as part of their clinical management. Patients were studied when a volume infusion was planned to detect potential hypovolemia or to assist in weaning inotropic/vasoactive drug infusions. The effect of rapid volume infusion was determined by measuring hemodynamics and left ventricular end-diastolic area.

Results.—During the 1-month survey period, 159 rapid volume infusions were given during 470 patient days. The average rapid volume infusion administered was 390 mL; normal saline was the most frequently infused fluid. In the 13 study patients, a rapid volume infusion of 500 mL had little effect. Mean arterial pressure, cardiac output, and right atrial pressure showed no statistically significant increases. Also unchanged were mean pulmonary arterial pressure, heart rate, mixed venous oxygen satu-

TABLE 3.—Modeling the Effect of a Normal Saline Infusion (100 mL/min) Using Simbiosis

		Simulated Computerized Progressive Fluid Loading and Its Effects on Hemodynamics			
	Baseline	500 mL	1000 mL	1500 mL	2000 mL
Blood volume (L)	5.75	6.25	6.75	7.24	7.70
MAP (mm Hg)	93	93	92	92	92
Cardiac output (L/min)	5.2	5.8	6.5	7.0	7.3
Heart rate (beats/min)	70	71	72	72	73
PAOP (mm Hg)	6.7	8.3	10.4	12.2	13.9
RAP (mm Hg)	5	6	8	9	11

Note: Simbiosis is a computerized system including a hemodynamics software and consisting of a simulated fluid loading to observe the progressive modifications on hemodynamics. The parallel increase in blood volume, filling pressures, and cardiac output can be observed, starting from a normal hemodynamic status.

Abbreviations: MAP, mean arterial pressure; *PAOP*, pulmonary artery occlusion pressure; *RAP*, right atrial pressure.

(Courtesy of Axler O, Tousignant C, Thompson CR, et al: Small hemodynamic effect of typical rapid volume infusions in critically ill patients. *Crit Care Med* 25[6]:965–970, 1997.)

ration, and whole body oxygen delivery and consumption. There was a slight but significant increase in mean pulmonary artery occlusion pressure, from 12.9 to 14.7 mm Hg.

Conclusion.—Patients admitted to the ICU for more than 12 hours often receive rapid volume infusions, but the volumes typically used are small and have little effect on hemodynamics or left ventricular areas. For these infusions to be effective, many patients may require larger volumes (Table 3) to be infused rapidly.

▶ The idea behind this study is that if one is going to give a volume challenge, the fluid volume administered should be great enough that a response will occur. The authors point out that traditional volume challenges (250–500 mL) given in clinical practice are not sufficient to induce a physiologic response. When one considers the fact that only about 25% of a crystalloid volume bolus remains in the intravascular space, it is not surprising that small volume boluses are frequently not sufficient to produce an increase in blood pressure or wedge pressure even in hypovolemic patients.

One interesting component of this manuscript is a table (see abstract), illustrating the relationship between the volume of fluid administered and the anticipated hemodynamic response. From this table, it can be seen that a bolus of up to 1 or 2 L of fluid may need to be given to observe a significant physiologic response. What this means is that it may take more fluid than is commonly appreciated to raise the blood pressure or wedge pressure of a patient with a decreased intravascular volume.

E.A. Deitch, M.D.

Transfusing Red Blood Cells Stored in Citrate Phosphate Dextrose Adenine-1 for 28 Days Fails to Improve Tissue Oxygenation in Rats

Fitzgerald RD, Martin CM, Dietz GE, et al (Univ of Western Ontario, Canada; London Health Sciences Centre)

Crit Care Med 25:726–732, 1997 2–11

Introduction.—The goal of transfusing red blood cells in patients with sepsis syndrome is to increase systemic oxygen uptake by maintaining hemoglobin concentrations greater than 100 g/L. Some studies, however, suggest that this practice may be ineffective. The hypothesis that the failure to improve tissue oxygenation results from an interaction between duration of red blood cell storage and an injured microcirculation in sepsis was tested.

Methods.—The prospective study employed an animal model in which 37 male Sprague-Dawley rats were randomly allocated to sham laparotomy or cecal ligation and perforation. Twenty-four hours later, the animals had supply-dependency of systemic oxygen uptake induced by isovolemic hemodilution. After recovery, they were again randomized to receive either "fresh" rat red blood cells, stored for 1–3 days, or "old" rat red blood cells, stored for 28 days. The effects of treatment with red blood cells were evaluated by measuring changes in systemic oxygen uptake.

Results.—All cecal ligation and perforation animals exhibited signs of generalized peritonitis 24 hours after laparotomy; the sham animals had no detectable signs of disease. There was no demonstrable group effect of cecal ligation and perforation on systemic oxygen uptake, systemic oxygen delivery, systemic oxygen extraction, or lactate concentration after red blood cell transfusion. But when combined groups of animals receiving either fresh or old red blood cells were compared, only rats transfused with fresh red blood cells showed a significant increase in systemic oxygen uptake (from a mean of 1.62 mL/100 g/min after hemodilution to a mean of 2.10 mL/100 g/min after transfusion). The increase in systemic oxygen delivery was marginally better in the fresh red blood cell transfusion group than in the old red blood cell transfusion group.

Conclusion.—Rat red blood cells that were stored for 28 days in citrate phosphate dextrose adenine-1 impaired the ability of transfusion therapy to improve tissue oxygenation in rats randomized to sham laparotomy or to cecal ligation and perforation. The failure of "old" transfused red blood cells may be related to the effect of storage on red blood cell deformability.

► The concept behind this study was the authors' belief that the failure of red blood cell transfusions to increase oxygen consumption in septic patients might be related to the fact that "old" blood is transfused. The physiologic principles and clinical rationale behind this hypothesis are as follows: first, red blood cells stored for 15 or more days lose the ability to deform and thus have a greater likelihood of becoming trapped in the microcirculation. This possibility is increased in septic patients, because the sepsis syndrome is characterized by a systemic microcirculatory injury, which further decreases capillary cross-sectional area. Second, in a previous clinical study, the authors found that transfusing septic patients with blood stored for more than 12–15 days was associated with an unexpected decrease in gastrointestinal intramucosal pH,[1] indicating that transfusion decreased intestinal oxygenation rather than improving it.

As demonstrated in the data, the authors were correct in that oxygen consumption was not increased in the rats receiving "old" blood. If further studies verify these provocative findings, then the traditional blood bank policy of transfusing the oldest units first would need to be re-evaluated until a more effective method of red blood cell storage is developed.

E.A. Deitch, M.D.

Reference

1. Marik PE, Sibbald WJ: Effect of stored-blood transfusion on oxygen delivery in patients with sepsis. *JAMA* 269:3024–3029, 1993.

Liver Function and Splanchnic Ischemia in Critically Ill Patients

Maynard ND, Bihari DJ, Dalton RN, et al (Guy's Hosp, London)
Chest 111:180–187, 1997 2–12

Background.—Recent studies have examined the potential roles of the GI tract and liver in the pathogenesis of multiple organ failure. Hepatic dysfunction is common in critically ill patients, and it could be an important contributor to systemic injury. Early detection of significant hepatic dysfunction might enable treatment, thus reducing morbidity and mortality. However, this purpose is not served by conventional liver tests. This study used 2 dynamic, flow-dependent tests of liver function—systemic clearance of indocyanine green (ICG) and metabolism of lidocaine to monoethylglycinexylidide (MEGX)—to study the link between splanchnic ischemia and hepatic dysfunction.

Methods.—The prospective study included 27 consecutive ICU patients with signs of inadequate tissue perfusion. All had a pulmonary artery catheter and mechanical ventilation in place. During the first 3 days after ICU admission, hepatic MEGX formation and systemic clearance of ICG were measured to assess liver function. Standard liver function tests were performed for comparison. The findings were correlated with tonometric measurements of gastric intramucosal pH (pHim) and with patient outcome.

Results.—Patients who lived and died were not significantly different in levels of bilirubin, aspartate aminotransferase, alkaline phosphatase, or prothrombin, or in ICG clearance. On the third ICU day, median MEGX level was 16 ng/mL in the patients who survived vs. 2.4 ng/mL in those who died. For nonsurvivors, the median MEGX level decreased from 21 ng/mL on the first ICU day to 2.4 ng/mL on the third day. The measured MEGX level was significantly correlated to pHim, and the changes in the 2 measurements over time were significantly correlated with each other. The best predictors of death vs. survival were MEGX formation and gastric pHim.

Conclusions.—In critically ill patients, the development of hepatic dysfunction appears to be related to poor outcome, probably because of a mismatch between hepatic metabolic demand and blood flow. For these patients, the MEGX formation test may represent a highly effective test of liver function and blood flow. Combined with gastric pHim measurement, it provides crucial data on the adequacy of oxygenation to the liver, which is apparently critical for survival. Treatment for inadequate splanchnic oxygenation could significantly reduce morbidity and improve survival.

▶ The limitations of measurements of whole body oxygen delivery and the recognition that inadequate organ perfusion can cause or contribute to the development of organ dysfunction and multiple organ failure has led a number of investigators to attempt to find ways to measure organ specific blood flow in the critically ill. One well-described technique is the use of gastric tonometry to measure intestinal blood flow. Because of the key role of the liver, these authors have tested whether blood-flow dependent assays of liver function could be used in the ICU to assess the adequacy of liver perfusion. Their results indicate that measuring the rate of conversion of lidocaine to MEGX may be such a test. Currently, the MEGX test is used to assess liver graft function after transplantation. Based on these preliminary results, it is possible that this test may find a role in the ICU population as well.

E.A. Deitch, M.D.

Recovery From Ischemic Acute Renal Failure Is Improved With Enteral Compared With Parenteral Nutrition

Mouser JF, Hak EB, Kuhl DA, et al (Univ of Connecticut, Storrs; Univ of Tennessee, Memphis)

Crit Care Med 25:1748–1754, 1997 2–13

Purpose.—There are continued questions about the effects of amino acids on the recovery of renal function in acutely injured patients, and about the use of parenteral nutrition in this situation. If amino acid administration is increased, tubular cell energy demands for solute transport will increase as well; if the demand exceeds the supply, the result may be worsening of ischemic injury. The amount, form, and route of protein administration may therefore play an important role in recovery from ischemic acute renal failure. The effects of enteral vs. parenteral nutrition on renal function after acute ischemic renal failure were studied in rats.

Methods.—In a randomized experimental study, male Sprague-Dawley rats received 7 days of isocaloric nutrition, supplying 160 nonprotein kcal/kg/day, or isonitrogenous nutrition, supplying 1.4 g of nitrogen/kg/day. Ten animals received enteral nutrition via a gastrostomy tube, while 11 received parenteral nutrition via a jugular vein catheter. At the end of 7 days, the rats underwent right nephrectomy and pedicle occlusion of the left kidney for 45 minutes. Feedings were started again after 1 hour, and continued for 3 days. Various measurements of renal function were compared at that time.

Results.—The percentage increase in creatinine clearance from day 9 to 11 was 490% in the enteral nutrition group vs. 208% in the parenteral nutrition group. The enteral group had greater urinary protein excretion. On histologic study, the number of dystrophic tubular calcifications was greater in the parenteral group than in the enteral group: 50 vs. 3 per 10 high-power fields.

Conclusions.—In rats subjected to ischemic acute renal failure, renal function is better for those receiving continuous enteral nutrition than for those receiving parenteral nutrition. The differences observed in this study may result from quantitative and qualitative differences in amino acid delivery to the kidney before and after ischemia. Whatever the explanation, patients at high risk of acute renal failure should receive enteral nutrition to maximize their recovery of renal function.

▶ This study indicates that animals fed enterally recover from acute ischemic renal failure better than animals fed a similar diet parenterally. Simply stated, this is one more bit of evidence favoring the enteral over the parenteral route of alimentation. As such, the article is worthy of note.

The results aside, one might wonder why the authors even thought to do this study. The answer lies in the physiology of amino acid clearance. When amino acids are given parenterally, a significant portion of the elevated plasma levels of amino acids reach the kidney and must be actively reabsorbed by the renal tubular cells. This renal reabsorption is energy dependent, and the resulting increase in renal tubular work and energy demand can worsen a renal injury. In contrast, amino acids taken enterally are cleared by the liver and do not reach the kidney, thereby limiting renal work. This study is a nice example of physiology at work and illustrates how knowing basic physiologic principles can pay potential clinical dividends.

E.A. Deitch, M.D.

Tyrphostin AG 556 Improves Survival and Reduces Multiorgan Failure in Canine *Escherichia coli* Peritonitis

Sevransky JE, Shaked G, Novogrodsky A, et al (NIH, Bethesda, Md; Tel Aviv Univ, Israel; Hebrew Univ of Jerusalem, Israel)

J Clin Invest 99:1966–1973, 1997 2–14

Introduction.—The incidence of septic syndrome has increased in the last decade, and mortality rates remain high. Some new therapies under investigation are directed against proinflammatory cytokines such as tumor necrosis factor-alpha and interleukin 1. Because many of the known cellular effects of cytokines can be blocked by tyrosine kinase inhibitors, an experimental study was designed to investigate the therapeutic value of tyrphostins, a family of tyrosine kinase inhibitors, in a canine model of gram-negative septic shock.

Methods.—Four animals were entered into the study each week for 2.5 weeks. After the animals were infected intraperitoneally with *Escherichia coli* 0111:B4, they were randomly assigned in a blinded fashion to tyrphostin treatment (AG 556 or AG 126) or to a control condition. All received supplemental oxygen, fluids, and antibiotics. The animals were observed for 28 days or until death; any animal killed before completion of the 28-day study was considered a nonsurvivor and included in the analysis.

Results.—All animals exhibited typical signs of sepsis during the 4 days after surgery. Seven animals had to be killed at periods ranging from 20 to 48 hours because of intractable seizures or respiratory failure; 1 was killed on day 17. Survival times were significantly better in the AG 556-treated group than in the control group. And compared to controls, animals that received AG 556 exhibited improved mean arterial pressure, left ventricular ejection fraction, cardiac output, oxygen delivery, and alveolar-arterial oxygen gradient during the first 48 hours after *E. coli* infection. Although treatment with AG 556 had no significant effect on the clearance of endotoxin or bacteria from the blood, this tyrosine kinase inhibitor did significantly lower serum tumor necrosis factor levels.

Conclusion.—Tyrphostin AG 556, administered in addition to standard sepsis therapies, significantly improved survival in a canine model of gram-negative bacterial peritonitis. By inhibiting cell signaling pathways and subsequent cytokine production, AG 556 reduced the pulmonary, cardiac, and vascular abnormalities characteristic of sepsis and prevented the development of multiple organ dysfunction.

► In light of the failure of numerous anticytokine/antiendotoxin agents to improve survival in human clinical trials, one might ask why was this preclinical animal trial testing of yet another agent chosen. The answer is not just that a novel agent was used and that it was effective in improving survival. That by itself is not enough. The reason is that this agent (a tyrosine kinase inhibitor) was effective in an animal model that was clinically relevant, and the animals received supportive therapy that is similar to what patients would receive, i.e. antibiotics, fluids, and supplemental oxygen. The use of a clinically relevant animal model to verify the efficacy of a potential therapeutic agent before initiating clinical trials may seem obvious. However, the failure to employ realistic preclinical (animal) models of sepsis was an almost uniform failing of essentially all of the agents that failed when tested in clinical trials. Thus, not only do tyrosine kinase inhibitors appear to improve survival, they are one of only a few agents that have been shown to do so when tested in as rigorous a model as was used in this study.

The rationale for using tyrosine kinase inhibitors is that the signal for cells, such as macrophages, to produce inflammatory agents (cytokine and eicosanoids) occurs via tyrosine kinase signaling pathways. Thus, by blocking tyrosine kinase activity, these agents block the production of various proinflammatory agents and thus limit the septic response. Although it is too early to tell if this class of agents will be beneficial in patients, there is hope, because they are effective in well-designed experimental models.

E.A. Deitch, M.D.

Elimination of Various Subpopulations of Macrophages and the Development of Multiple-Organ Dysfunction Syndrome in Mice

Nieuwenhuijzen GAP, Knapen MFCM, Hendriks T, et al (Academic Hosp Nijmegen, The Netherlands)

Arch Surg 132:533–539, 1997 2–15

Introduction.—Although macrophages perform a number of activities in normal host-defense mechanisms, the excessive activation of macrophages appears to induce a generalized dysregulated excessive inflammatory response. Several reports have ascribed a special pathophysiologic role to specific macrophage subpopulations in certain disease processes, including multiple-organ dysfunction syndrome (MODS). The role of specific macrophage subpopulations in the development of zymosan-induced MODS was evaluated in an experimental study.

Methods.—The randomized trial used male C57Bl/6 mice that had a zymosan suspension administered intraperitoneally (IP) in a dose of 1 mg/g of body weight. Before or after the zymosan challenge, multilamellar liposomes containing dichloromethylene bisphosphonate (Cl_2MBP) were administered to the animals in order to eliminate macrophage subpopulations. A group of control mice received only zymosan. Intratracheal, IV, and IP administration induced elimination of alveolar, liver and splenic, and peritoneal and omental macrophages, respectively. All surviving mice were killed at day 12, and relative organ weights (ROW) were calculated from the lungs, liver, spleen, and kidneys.

Results.—The IV administration of liposomes that contained Cl_2MBP had no significant effect on body weight, temperature, or mortality rate, but the ROW of the liver was significantly decreased. The elimination of liver and splenic macrophages after zymosan challenge led to an increased ROW of the lung and a decreased ROW of the liver. Death was completely prevented when the liposomes that contained Cl_2MBP were administered intratracheally before zymosan challenge; mortality was increased from 50% to 90% when these liposomes were administered IP before zymosan challenge. When administered IP, liposomes that contained Cl_2MBP did not change body weight, temperature, or ROW.

Conclusion.—In this experimental model, the elimination of certain macrophage subpopulations and their elimination on specific time points had differential effects. Selective elimination of any subpopulation, either before or after zymosan challenge, could not prevent organ damage and death. This suggests that specific macrophage subpopulations may have different roles, either protective or detrimental, in the development of MODS.

► This article was chosen to illustrate the complexity of modulating the host's inflammatory response as well as to illustrate that modulation of macrophage populations located in different organs and anatomical locations may have different effects on survival after an inflammatory insult. Basically, what the authors have shown is that elimination of alveolar macrophages decreases mortality, whereas elimination of peritoneal macrophages increases mortality after an IP challenge with the inflammatory agent zymosan.

Thus, although it is clear that an uncontrolled inflammatory response is deleterious and contributes to the development of acute respiratory distress syndrome and MODS, studies such as this one indicate that not all macrophage populations exert similar effects. Instead, certain macrophage populations may exert a protective effect, whereas others potentiate organ dysfunction and death. Thus, in considering the potential clinical use of agents directed at reducing macrophage activity, the route of drug delivery as well as the macrophage populations affected will have to be considered. It seems the more we learn about the host's inflammatory response, the more complicated it gets.

E.A. Deitch, M.D.

Bacterial Translocation Is Inhibited in Inducible Nitric Oxide Synthase Knockout Mice After Endotoxin Challenge but Not in a Model of Bacterial Overgrowth

Mishima S, Xu D, Lu Q, et al (UMDNJ, Newark)

Arch Surg 132:1190–1195, 1997 2–16

Introduction.—There is evidence that organ damage resulting from lipopolysaccharide (LPS) challenge can be influenced or prevented by nitric oxide (NO) and NO synthase (NOS) inhibitors. Previous experiments have suggested that activation of inducible NOS (iNOS) mediates endotoxin-induced gut injury and bacterial translocation (BT). This hypothesis was tested in a study of mice lacking the iNOS gene.

Methods.—An *Escherichia coli* LPS or saline challenge was administered intraperitoneally to 45 wild-type (iNOS +/+) or homozygous mutant "iNOS knockout" (iNOS −/−) mice. Further experiments were conduced using an *E. coli* overgrowth model of BT.

Results.—Lipopolysaccharide challenge led to BT to the mesenteric lymph nodes in 87.5% of wild-type mice vs. none of the iNOS knockout mice. The wild-type mice showed high levels of nitrite and nitrate in the liver, ileum, and blood. The bacterial overgrowth experiments showed BT to the mesenteric lymph nodes in all mice in both groups.

Conclusions.—Lipopolysaccharide challenge does not lead to BT in iNOS knockout mice. Thus LPS-induced BT appears to require an LPS-induced increase in iNOS activity. In contrast, in a bacterial overgrowth model, iNOS activation does not appear necessary for BT to occur.

► Bacterial translocation and gut origin sepsis has been implicated in the clinical development of sepsis and multiple organ failure. Although a number of mediators have been identified as being associated with gut barrier failure in septic states, it is unclear which of these putative mediators are causally involved in the disease process. Knowing which of these numerous mediators are critically involved in inducing gut barrier failure and knowing which should be specifically targeted is an important first step in developing an effective therapeutic agent. By using genetically altered mice that do not contain the iNOS gene, this study unambiguously shows that excessive NO production is a key factor in sepsis-induced loss of gut barrier function. Studies such as this one, using genetically altered animal models, are likely to provide unique and important preclinical information that can ultimately be used to improve clinical care. For this reason, it is essential that all of us become familar with the emerging molecular biological tools.

E.A. Deitch, M.D.

MCP-1 Protects Mice in Lethal Endotoxemia

Zisman DA, Kunkel SL, Strieter RM, et al (Univ of Michigan, Ann Arbor)
J Clin Invest 99:2832–2836, 1997 2–17

Introduction.—Many of the pathophysiologic events in sepsis are mediated by lipopolysaccharide (LPS), a major cell wall component of gram-negative bacterial organisms. The release of host-derived proinflammatory cytokines, tumor necrosis factor-α (TNF-α), interleukin (IL)-1β, and interferon (IFN)-γ, is stimulated by LPS, and these cytokines either directly or indirectly mediate many of the hemodynamic and inflammatory changes of sepsis. Endotoxin-challenged mice were studied to assess the role of monocyte chemoattractant protein-1 (MCP-1) as a mediator of sepsis. Recent studies suggest that MCP-1 possesses important anti-inflammatory properties, both in vivo and in vitro.

Methods.—Female CD-1 mice were administered either 750 μg or 1 mg LPS (intraperitoneally in 1 mL of saline). Control animals were given equal amounts of saline. In passive immunization experiments, 0.5 mL rabbit antimurine MCP-1 was administered 2 hours before endotoxin treatment. The mice were killed at designated time points and their blood and organs prepared for assessment of cytokine protein expression.

Results.—The administration of LPS caused a rapid and substantial increase in MCP-1 levels. In comparison with control animals, the maximal increases of MCP-1 levels in liver and lung represented a 10- and 42-fold increase. Passive immunization of mice with rabbit antimurine MCP-1 antiserum before endotoxin administration led to a striking increase in LPS-induced mortality (65% in anti–MCP-1-treated animals vs. 10% in controls). Endotoxin-challenged mice that received anti-MCP-1 antibodies exhibited increases in peak TNF-α and IL-12 levels and a trend toward lower serum levels of IL-10. In contrast, the intraperitoneal administration of recombinant murine MCP-1 significantly protected mice from the lethal effects of endotoxin and led to increases in IL-10 levels, decreases in IL-12 levels, and a trend toward decreased levels of TNF.

Discussion.—This is the first study to demonstrate that MCP-1, a member of the chemokine family, has marked anti-inflammatory properties in vivo. Endotoxin-induced mortality was significantly increased in animals pretreated with anti-MCP-1 serum, whereas the administration of murine MCP-1 provided substantial protection against the lethal effects of LPS. The protective mechanism of MCP-1 appears to involve a shifting of balance between pro- and anti-inflammatory cytokines.

► Monocyte chemoattractant protein-1 is 1 of a family of chemoattractant proteins that share common properties, such as the ability to attract and activate macrophages and other inflammatory cells. Through these actions, chemokines are believed to be important proinflammatory factors, which contribute to the induction of the inflammatory response. Because MCP-1 is increased in patients with sepsis, can be induced by the injection of endotoxin in human volunteers, and reaches high levels in animal models of infection and sepsis, it was commonly believed that MCP-1 was one of the host-derived factors that contributes to systemic inflammatory response syndrome and consequently acute respiratory distress syndrome and organ failure. Yet, on the basis of some recent studies, it appears that MCP-1, in contrast to other chemokines, may posses anti-inflammatory properties. Consequently, the authors tested the effects of giving and blocking MCP-1 in an endotoxin sepsis model. Their observation, that MCP-1 protected the animals and appeared to have anti-inflammatory properties, indicates that an increased level of MCP-1 is beneficial rather than harmful.

Although these results are interesting in themselves, they also send us the important message that one must exert caution in interpreting the results of associations between circulating factors and clinical end points. Specifically, because MCP-1 was increased in patients with sepsis and there was human data documenting that the increase in plasma MCP-1 levels was proportional to the severity of shock, it was logical to conclude that high levels of MCP-1 were bad. On the basis of this logic, neutralization of MCP-1 should improve outcome. However, when this concept was tested, the results indicated that increased levels of MCP-1 were beneficial rather than harmful. Thus, it now appears possible that the increase in MCP-1 observed in patients with severe sepsis represents the patients' attempts to protect themselves from an over-exuberant inflammatory response. So what is the take-home message? It is that we must be careful in interpreting associations because they may be misleading. It is wise to remember that Mother Nature can be tricky and that simplistic assumptions may be wrong.

E.A. Deitch, M.D.

Impaired Apoptotic Death Signaling in Inflammatory Lung Neutrophils Is Associated With Decreased Expression of Interleukin-1beta Converting Enzyme Family Proteases (Caspases)

Watson RWG, Rotstein OD, Parodo J, et al (Univ of Toronto)

Surgery 122:163–172, 1997 2–18

Introduction.—The membrane proteins Fas and tumor necrosis factor receptor 1 (TNFR1), through downstream activation of interleukin-1β converting enzyme (ICE) proteins, are responsible for signaling for cell apoptosis. For neutrophils that transmigrate to an inflammatory focus, spontaneous cell death by apoptosis is significantly delayed. This is despite the abundant stimulus for apoptosis observed in the inflammatory response. The susceptibility of transmigrating neutrophils to apoptosis induced by Fas and TNFR1 was studied.

Methods.—The study used Sprague-Dawley rats killed 4 hours after intratracheal challenge with lipopolysaccharide, 500 μg. Neutrophils were isolated from both the systemic circulation and from bronchoalveolar lavage fluid. These cells were then incubated for 24 hours with or without agonistic antibodies to Fas or TNF. Flow cytometry was used to evaluate apoptosis and Fas expression, while Western blotting was done to measure expression of antiapoptotic (Bcl-2) and proaptotic (ICE and CPP32) proteins.

Results.—Apoptosis was significantly delayed in neutrophils isolated from the bronchoalveolar lavage fluid, which had transmigrated to the lung after LPS challenge. The lung neutrophils also showed no apoptotic response to anti-Fas antibody or TNF-α. There was no change in expression of Fas, although expression of TNFR1 was reduced. Neutrophils from either location did not express Bcl-2. Lung neutrophils showed significantly reduced expression of ICE, in both its pro- and active forms, and of CPP32 in its active form. Fas- and TNFR1-induced apoptosis was incompletely blocked by a specific ICE inhibitor.

Conclusions.—Inflammatory neutrophils are resistant to Fas- and TNFR1-induced apoptosis, the findings suggest. This resistance is accompanied by increased expression of proaptotic proteins. During episodes of acute inflammation, functional survival of neutrophils may be extended via reduced responsiveness to apoptotic stimuli. This phenomenon could be involved in the tissue injury observed in patients with acute respiratory distress syndrome.

▶ The idea behind this technical paper is that all cells contain genetic programs that turn on "suicide-inducing" genes resulting in the cell undergoing spontaneous cell death (known as apoptosis) in the presence of specific signals. Thus, one take-home message of this set of experiments is that once neutrophils have been recruited to a tissue or organ, in this case the lung, the response to suicide-inducing signals is altered and the cells are now less likely to undergo spontaneous cell death. Based on this work and other recently published articles, the net result of this failure of activated neutrophils to die could be an increase in pulmonary injury because these activated neutrophils continue to produce and secrete tissue-injurious substances.

In essence, studies investigating the biology of apoptosis are providing important insights into the biology of inflammation and inflammatory-mediated organ injury. As more information is gained, it is likely that therapeutic strategies may emerge that could aid in controlling an excessive inflammation response and thereby limit tissue injury and organ failure.

E.A. Deitch, M.D.

3 Burns

Introduction

As in years past, the clinical issues in burn care remain focused on wound healing, infection, nutrition, smoke inhalation, and rehabilitation. Since, in many ways, the first line of battle in burn care is fought at the level of the burn wound, the first group of articles in this year's selections deals with the burn wound. The ideal replacement for deeply burned skin is the patient's own skin or autografts. However, in patients with large burns, there are frequently insufficient donor sites to allow for rapid wound closure, and this lack of donor sites contributes to patient morbidity and mortality. A number of products are being manufactured and strategies tested to overcome this hurdle. One example of this strategy is the article by Hunt et al. describing the results of a clinical trial comparing cadaver skin vs. a new product called Dermagraft-TC, which consists of neonatal fibroblasts grown on a synthetic wound dressing, as temporary coverage of excised burn wounds. As illustrated in the article *by Reagan et al.*, a second wound-care strategy currently being tested is the use of dermal grafts to improve the functional and cosmetic results of cultured epithelial autografts or as a substrate on which widely meshed thin autografts can be placed. Although more work needs to be done, as illustrated by these and similar articles, progress is being made. Another major unsolved wound-related factor that limits full recovery from a thermal injury is the development of hypertrophic scarring or contracture formation. A primary reason for the failure to develop effective means of preventing excessive post-burn scarring is our limited understanding of the basic biology of hypertrophic scar formation. Thus, included in this year's selections is a potentially exciting human study indicating that an imbalance between stimulatory and inhibitory cytokine production may play a major causal role in hypertrophic scar formation. Two articles dealing with practical issues in wound care are also presented. The first documents that the incidence of wound infections is not increased by decreasing burn wound cleansings and dressing changes from twice daily to once daily. By following the recommendations of this clinical study, one can reduce patient discomfort and save money at the same time. The second article describes the use of oral ketamine to reduce pain and anxiety during dressing changes in pediatric burn patients.

It has been recognized for several decades that a burn injury induces a greater hypermetabolic response than any other stress and is associated with profound losses of lean body mass. Because of the association between weight loss and infection, as well as impaired wound healing, an important component of burn care is nutritional support. As illustrated in the article by Raff et al., it is now recognized that immediate enteral feeding of burn patients is both safe and effective. In fact, as described in the clinical study by Wolf et al., the development of enteral feeding intolerance is more a sign of infection than a consequence of the burn injury and should be viewed as such. In fact, in a study not included in this year's selections, early enteral feeding appears to be effective in preventing burn-induced stress ulcer bleeding.[1] Nonetheless, despite aggressive attempts at feeding patients with major thermal injuries, weight loss and muscle weakness are still common occurrences. Thus, the recent report by Demling et al. stating that the administration of the anabolic hormone oxandrolone increases weight, improves muscle strength, and increases endurance is both important and impressive.

The remaining articles include a potpourri of topics. The first—documenting that colonization of burn patients with methacillin-resistant *Staphylococcus aureus* (MRSA) or *Staphylococcus epidermidis* (MRSE), in contrast to gram-negative enterics, does not increase morbidity or mortality—illustrates an important point. That is, since all burn patients will be colonized with bacteria, it is better to be colonized with low-virulence organisms, such as MRSA or MRSE, than more virulent gram-negative bacteria, even if these low-virulence organisms are methacillin resistant. Because I have always wondered why so many severely burned patients manifest acute changes in their sensorium, I have included an intriguing clinical study that may answer this question. Specifically, the authors found that, after a major thermal injury, intracranial pressure is increased and cerebral blood flow is decreased. The remaining 2 articles chosen cover topics in immunology and burn-induced pulmonary dysfunction.

Edwin A. Deitch, M.D.

Reference

1. Raff T, Germann G, Hartmann B: The value of early enteral nutrition in the prophylaxis of stress ulceration in the severely burned patient. *Burns* 23:313–318, 1997.

A Multicenter Clinical Trial of a Biosynthetic Skin Replacement, Dermagraft-TC, Compared With Cryopreserved Human Cadaver Skin for Temporary Coverage of Excised Burn Wounds

Purdue GF, Hunt JL, Still JM Jr, et al (Univ of Texas, Dallas; Augusta Regional Med Ctr, Ga; Shriners Burn Inst, Galveston, Tex, et al)
J Burn Care Rehabil 18:52–57, 1997 3–1

Introduction.—For burn patients who require temporary wound coverage—whether because of limited autologous donor sites or medical reasons—fresh or cryopreserved human cadaver allograft material is the "gold standard." However, there are numerous problems associated with the use of allografts. Dermagraft-TC (DG-TC; Advanced Tissue Sciences, Inc.) is a new product consisting of human neonatal fibroblasts grown on the synthetic wound dressing Biobrane. Placed as a temporary skin replacement, DG-TC functions like epidermis to protect the wound beneath. This article reported on a multicenter clinical trial comparing DG-TC with cryopreserved human allograft for temporary closure of excised burn wounds.

Methods.—The study included 66 patients undergoing surgical excision of burn wounds. The patients had a mean 44% of total body surface area burned, including full-thickness burns over 28% of total body surface area. On each patient, 2 comparable sites were selected and randomized to be covered with DG-TC or cryopreserved human allograft. After coverage, the 2 sites were treated in the same way. When indicated, at least 5 days after placement, the skin covering was removed. At that time, the wound beds were evaluated and prepared for grafting. The main endpoint was the percentage of autograft take at 14 days.

Results.—Fourteen-day postautograft take was 95% in wounds treated with DG-TC and 93% in those treated with allograft. After adjustment for age, autograft thickness, mesh ratio, sex, and race, the results were as good or better with DG-TC. There was no significant difference in adherence or fluid accumulation during temporary coverage. On the day the temporary coverage was removed, the investigators expressed a significantly higher level of satisfaction with DG-TC. Allograft was significantly more likely to require excision, and wounds covered with allograft were significantly more likely to bleed. There were no problems with sloughing of DG-TC and no apparent adverse effects of its use.

Conclusions.—In patients with excised burn wounds, DG-TC is as good or better than cryopreserved human allograft for temporary coverage. The new biosynthetic skin replacement provides good results in terms of autograft take and is easier to remove and causes less bleeding than allograft. Dermagraft-TC has an excellent safety profile with a high benefit-to-risk ratio for the indication reported here.

► The ideal replacement for deeply burned skin is the patient's own skin. However, in patients with large burns, there may not be enough donor sites to allow expeditious burn wound closure. In fact, not uncommonly, it is the lack of available donor sites that limits the ability to close the burn wound, rather than the size of the burn. For this reason, a major area of burn research has been devoted to the development of temporary and permanent skin substitutes.

This multicenter clinical trial describes the results with DG-TC, 1 such temporary skin substitute. Dermagraft-TC is 1 of a number of products under construction that are designed to be used to temporarily close the excised burn wound until sufficient autograft is available for definitive wound closure. This particular product is composed of Biobrane onto which neonatal fibroblasts have been seeded and allowed to form a dermal matrix. The

Biobrane acts as an artificial epidermis; it protects the underlying wound while the dermal matrix facilitates adherence to the excised wound bed.

Although the study was limited to patients with moderate-sized burns, it does appear that the DG-TC was superior to cryopreserved human cadaver skin in a number of regards. Hopefully, further clinical trials will verify the clinical utility of this product.

E.A. Deitch, M.D.

Analysis of Cellular and Decellular Allogeneic Dermal Grafts for the Treatment of Full-thickness Wounds in a Porcine Model

Reagan BJ, Madden MR, Huo J, et al (New York Hosp–Cornell Burn Ctr)

J Trauma: Injury Infect Crit Care 43:458–466, 1997 3–2

Introduction.—In the absence of available donor skin in patients with burn injuries, wounds must close by contraction and epithelialization. This can lead to scarring and can predispose the wound to overwhelming bacterial invasion. There is a great need for a reliable skin substitute. Cryopreserved cellular and decellularized porcine allogeneic dermal grafts (CADGs or DADGs) were used in conjunction with an overlying thin split-thickness autograft (STSG) in a 1-step technique.

Methods.—The effect of CADG and DADG allogeneic dermis on graft take, wound contraction, inflammation, and cosmetic outcome was assessed in a porcine model. Control mirror-image wounds were created and treated with thin STSG alone. Biopsy specimens were obtained at 2, 5, and 8 weeks, and scar assessment was conducted at 10 weeks by physical therapists unaware of which treatment had been used.

Results.—The percent of take of autografts overlying CADGs or DADGs was similar to that of control sites. Wound contraction and cosmetic outcome were not altered by CADGs, but DADG treatment inhibited wound contraction and significantly enhanced cosmetic outcome in 10 of 12 paired wounds.

Conclusion.—The use of CADGs and DADGs allowed simultaneous engraftment of an overlying thin STSG. Wound contraction and cosmetic outcome were unchanged by CADGs, but DADGs significantly diminished wound contraction and improved cosmetic outcome of full-thickness wounds in a porcine mode. Burn care may reach another level of improvement with DADGs.

► Coverage of burned skin by conventional split-thickness skin grafts is limited by donor-site availability. Hence, when patients require massive areas of their bodies to be grafted (i.e., more than 60% to 70% of the body surface area), one must use either widely expanded skin grafts or, in some cases, cultured epithelial autografts (CEA). The use of widely expanded skin grafts (i.e., 3:1 or greater) is associated with significant scarring, contractures, and a poor cosmetic result. The use of CEAs has its own set of problems, including expense, a 21–28-day lag time from initial harvesting of skin biopsy specimens to usable grafts, variable capability of the grafts to take, and, in many cases, poor long-term results. Consequently, much attention has been focused on the development of dermal grafts that can be used to improve the functional and cosmetic results of CEAs or that can be used as a substrate on which widely meshed thin autografts can be placed. Several such products are in various stages of development. This experimental study illustrates the potential capability of porcine allogeneic dermal grafts to limit contracture formation and to improve the cosmetic results of meshed, thin skin grafts in a porcine model. Of clinical importance is the fact that porcine dermal grafts are effective when used in other species besides the pig, as similar results have been observed using porcine dermis to enhance widely expanded skin grafts in a rat model.[1]

Based on the high level of activity in this field, it is likely that it is only a matter of time before established materials and techniques are available that will allow the successful transplantation of allogeneic dermis or dermal substitutes to our patients. When this time arrives, it will be possible to significantly improve the cosmetic and functional results when resurfacing the burn wound in patients with large thermal injuries.

E.A. Deitch, M.D.

Reference

1. Wang HJ, Chen TM, Cheng TY: Use of a porcine dermis template to enhance widely expanded mesh autologous split-thickness skin graft growth: Preliminary report. *J Trauma* 42:177–182, 1997.

Cytokine Production in Patients With Hypertrophic Burn Scars

Polo M, Ko F, Busillo F, et al (Univ of South Florida, Tampa; Bay Pines VA Med Ctr, Fla)
J Burn Care Rehabil 18:477–482, 1997 3–3

Introduction.—An imbalance between stimulatory and inhibitory cytokines could cause the failure of wounds to heal or the production of excessive fibrosis. Keloid formation is associated with altered levels of certain immunomodulatory cytokines. It may be that a similar imbalance in the production of cytokines by immune cells may be the mechanism responsible for the formation of proliferative scars in patients with thermal injuries. Cytokine production was assessed in 10 patients with burn injuries and severe hypertrophic scarring and in 10 patients with burn injuries and minimal or normal scarring to determine the significance of the immune system in the formation of proliferative burn scars.

Methods.—Patients in both groups had received their injuries at least 6 months before entry into the study. Peripheral blood mononuclear cells (PBMCs) were isolated in all patients and incubated with and without antigenic or mitogenic stimulation. The supernatants from this process were assayed by enzyme-linked immunosorbent assay techniques for production of various cytokines.

TABLE 1.—Enzyme-linked Immunosorbent Assay Results of Cytokine Production by Unstimulated PBMC

	IL-1 (pg/ml)	IL-2 (pg/ml)	IL-6 (pg/ml)	TNF-α (pg/ml)	TGF-β (pg/ml)	IFN-α (pg/ml)	IFN-γ (pg/ml)
Hypertrophic Scar	*197.27 ± 57.82	27.30 ± 9.63	*937.5 ± 137.2	*582.3 ± 223.0	*20.92 ± 1.39	10.60 ± 2.07	—
Normal Scar	50.69 ± 18.01	44.82 ± 23.16	463.6 ± 93.2	69.3 ± 35.0	15.68 ± 1.96	6.47± 1.27	—

Note: All values are mean plus or minus standard error of the mean and are expressed in picograms of protein per milliliter of supernatant.
$P < 0.05$.
Abbreviations: PBMC, peripheral blood mononuclear cells; *IL*, interleukin; *TNF*, tumor necrosis factor; *TGF*, transforming growth factor; *IFN*, interferon.
(Courtesy of Polo M, Ko F, Busillo F, et al: Cytokine production in patients with hypertrophic burn scars. *J Burn Care Rehabil* 18:477–482, 1997.)

Results.—The production of interleukin-1 (IL-1), IL-6, tumor necrosis factor α and transforming growth factor (TGF)-β_2 by unstimulated PBMCs was significantly increased in patients with proliferative scar formation compared with controls (Table 1). The production of TGF-β_2 by stimulated PBMCs was also significantly increased in patients with proliferative scar formation compared with controls.

Conclusion.—These findings indicate that the immune system has a significant role in hypertrophic burn scar formation. Increased production of proinflammatory cytokines by resting mononuclear cells and TGF-β_2 may be responsible for accumulation of excess scar tissue.

▶ Unfortunately, one of the most common factors limiting full recovery from a thermal injury is the development of hypertrophic scars and contractures. Although great strides have been made in many areas of burn care, the ability to prevent or treat hypertrophic burn scar formation has not advanced much since the institution of pressure garments in the 1970s. One reason for this failure is the lack of understanding of the basic biological principles of scar formation. Secondly, our ability to experimentally investigate this disease process is limited by the fact that hypertrophic scar formation observed in patients does not occur in experimental animals. Nonetheless, this state of affairs is changing. One example of progress being made is the recognition that the immune response and continued inflammation appear to play a critical role in the pathogenesis of human scarring.

The current study focuses on this potential relationship between the immune response and scar formation and examines the hypothesis that an imbalance between stimulatory and inhibitory cyokine production may result in excessive fibrosis. This concept was supported by the authors' results, which showed that immune cells from patients with burn injuries and hypertrophic burn scars produced greater amounts of cytokines and TGF-β (stimulant for collagen production) than did the cells of patients without hypertrophic burn scars. Based on this observation and other results in the literature, their proposal—that patients with burn injuries who have hypertrophic burn scars may be in a prolonged hyperimmune state and that this hyperimmune state contributes to increased scar formation—appears quite plausible. If this notion proves to be true, future therapy for hypertrophic burn scars may include agents to down-regulate an excessive immune response.

E.A. Deitch, M.D.

Once-Daily Wound Cleansing and Dressing Change: Efficacy and Cost
Sheridan RL, Petras L, Lydon M, et al (Harvard Med School, Boston; Massachusetts Gen Hosp, Boston)
J Burn Care Rehabil 18:139–140, 1997 3–4

Introduction.—Dressing changes for burn patients are associated with considerable pain and expense. Children with burns are usually managed with a twice-daily schedule of wound cleansing and dressing change. A prospective study was conducted to determine whether a once-daily schedule would be as effective for children with burns of 30% or less of the body surface.

Methods.—One hundred children were enrolled in the study: 50 allocated to standard twice-daily dressing changes and 50 to a once-daily dressing change. The study and control groups were similar in mean age (4.4 and 3.7 years, respectively), burn size (11.2% and 11.1%), and length of stay (16.2 and 17.2 days). All patients had their wounds dressed in 8-ply gauze that was wet every 2 hours with 0.5% aqueous silver nitrate. Full-thickness wounds were excised and generally sheet-autografted within 5 days of the burn injury.

Results.—The incidence of infections of all types was low, and once-daily and twice-daily dressing groups were similar in number of wound infections, pneumonias, urinary tract infections, and bacteremias. Surgery to graft a portion of the wound was required in 34% of the study group and 46% of controls, not a significant difference. All children survived and were discharged home. The total cost of supplies for a single dressing change was $7.21. In addition to this savings, the once-daily regimen reduced nursing staff time and expense and the potential for complications related to pain medication. And importantly, the children had only 1 painful dressing change per day.

Conclusion.—For children treated as inpatients for burns of 30% or less body surface, once-a-day wound cleansing and dressing change yielded the same benefits as a twice-daily schedule and saved costs and staff time. The patients, their parents, and the nursing staff were enthusiastic about the once-daily regimen, now the standard method of managing burns of this size at the study institution.

► Tradition, plus the adage, "If a little is good, more is better," is being reevaluated in all areas of patient care as strategies to safely reduce costs are being examined. This simple and practical, but important, study illustrates the fact that 1 more tradition in burn care may have lost its mystique in the face of data.

E.A. Deitch, M.D.

Superiority of Oral Ketamine as an Analgesic and Sedative for Wound Care Procedures in the Pediatric Patient With Burns

Humphries Y, Melson M, Gore D (Med College of Virginia, Richmond)

J Burn Care Rehabil 18:34–36, 1997 3–5

Introduction.—Managing pain and anxiety in pediatric patients with burns involves a delicate balance between excessive and inadequate medication. Intravenous ketamine offers effective sedative, analgesic, and amnestic properties for primary closure of lacerations in children. The effectiveness of oral ketamine during wound care procedures for burns was evaluated in 19 pediatric patients.

Methods.—Patients were randomized to receive either an oral suspension of ketamine or acetaminophen with codeine phosphate and diphenhydramine (controls) 20 minutes before wound care procedures. Nurses rated sedation and pain intensity and recorded complications and length of time for returning to baseline mental status.

Results.—Patients who received ketamine had more than a 400% reduction in pain and a 360% improvement in sedation, compared with controls. Recovery time to baseline was significantly longer in the ketamine group (Table 2). One patient in the ketamine group experienced nystagmus and 1 patient each in the control group had urinary retention and vomiting, respectively (10% vs. 22%).

Conclusion.—Compared with oral acetaminophen with codeine phosphate and diphenhydramine, analgesia and sedation were significantly improved by using oral ketamine in pediatric patients undergoing wound care procedures.

► In this study, the authors have shown that the use of oral ketamine for wound care is superior to a narcotic regimen. The study is important because satisfactory control of the pain and anxiety associated with burn wound care—especially in children—remains a major unsolved problem, in spite of the large number of therapeutic approaches that have been tried over the last 20 years. The fact that ketamine has analgesic, sedative, hypnotic, and amnestic properties and does not lead to respiratory depres-

TABLE 2.—Results

	Ketamine	Codeine/ diphenhydramine
Ramsey scale (0 no sedation vs 6 heavily sedated)	3.3 ± 0.5	0.9 ± 0.1*
Visual algometer (0 no pain vs 10 very painful)	1.7 ± 0.8	7.1 ± 0.9*
Recovery time (min)	80 ± 13	22 ± 9*
Complications	1/10 (10%)	2/9 (22%)

Note: Values are mean ± standard error of the mean.

*$P < 0.05$ Comparison by Student's independent t test.

(Courtesy of Humphries Y, Melson M, Gore D: Superiority of oral ketamine as an analgesic and sedative for wound care procedures in the pediatric patient with burns. *Burn Care Rehab* 18:34–36, 1997.)

sion makes this agent especially attractive for children, as the side effect of severe hallucinations occasionally observed in adults is not commonly observed in children. The availability of ketamine as an oral elixir that can be administered 20 minutes before burn wound care has the potential to improve the experience, not just for the patient but for the family and the nurses and physicians as well.

E.A. Deitch, M.D.

Early Intragastric Feeding of Seriously Burned and Long-Term Ventilated Patients: A Review of 55 Patients

Raff T, Hartmann B, Germann G (BG-Unfallklinik Ludwigshafen, Germany)
Burns 23:19–25, 1997 3–6

Background.—Previous studies have shown that early intragastric postburn feeding is more beneficial for burn patients than late feeding. However, because of concern over possible complications of immediate feeding, this concept has been questioned. The feasibility of early gastric feeding for burn patients on long-term ventilation was assessed, including whether the patients' caloric needs can be met through the intragastric route within the first 72 hours after injury. The influence of delayed feeding, including its effect on morbidity and mortality, was evaluated as well.

Methods.—The retrospective study included 55 consecutive burn patients who were receiving mechanical ventilation for more than 5 days. All had an abbreviated burn severity index of 7 or greater; mean total body surface area burned was 44%. The feeding protocol called for all patients to have a 12F to 14F nasogastric tube placed at admission. After tube position was confirmed, tube feeding with a commercial enteric formula was started as soon as possible. If the residual gastric volume was less than the feeding rate (20 to 40 mL/hr), feeding was considered successful.

Results.—Gastric tube feeding was successful in 82% of patients, permitting the calculated caloric requirements to be delivered within 72 hours. The mean interval between injury and the start of tube feeding in this group was 11.5 hours, compared with 32.4 hours in the 10 patients in whom early intragastric feeding failed. When enteral feeding was started within 18 hours after the burn, it met the patients' caloric needs 92% of the time (44 of 48 patients). Mortality was significantly reduced for patients with successful early intragastric feeding. The patients with successful vs. failed early intragastric feeding were comparable in their incidence of severe sepsis or septic shock.

Conclusions.—Early intragastric feeding can be successfully initiated in patients with severe burns. If feeding is not started within 18 hours after the burn, it is less likely to be successful later on. With early intragastric feeding, the patients' calculated caloric needs can usually be delivered within 72 hours. Nursing skill and experience has a major influence on the success and safety of the gastric feeding protocol described in this study.

▶ That enteral feeding is clinically more beneficial that parenteral feeding has been generally accepted, since multiple prospective randomized clinical trials in diverse patient populations indicated that enterally fed patients have fewer infections and, in general, a significantly shortened hospital course. The value of this study of severely burned, ventilated patients is twofold. First, it verifies the safety and efficacy of early enteral feeding begun within 18 hours of injury and, secondly, it shows that intragastric feeding works.

These results fit with my own experience that the early institution of gastric feeding is both safe and effective[1] and helps to dispel the myth that one cannot feed the stomach in the severely injured. To my way of thinking, there are 2 major reasons to feed the patient gastrically whenever possible. First, gastric feeding is more physiologic than jejunal feeding and, secondly, it is easier. My advice is to review the feeding protocol used by the authors and try it. Your patients might like it.

E.A. Deitch, M.D.

Reference

1. McDonald WS, Sharp CW, Deitch EA: Immediate enteral feeding in burn patients is safe and effective. *Ann Surg* 213:177–183, 1991.

Enteral Feeding Intolerance: An Indicator of Sepsis-associated Mortality in Burned Children

Wolf SE, Jeschke MG, Rose JK, et al (Univ of Texas, Galveston)

Arch Surg 132:1310–1314, 1997 3–7

Background.—Infections are common after massive burns and can lead to complications or death. Thrombocytopenia and hyperglycemia are useful indicators of sepsis, but the results of confirmatory cultures are usually not available for at least 48 hours. Other clinical indicators of sepsis are needed to guide treatment decisions in this situation. Enteral feeding intolerance (EFI) was evaluated as an indicator of sepsis and increased mortality in severely burned children.

Methods.—The survey study included 91 children in a pediatric burn unit with burns covering more than 80% of total body surface area. Factors reflecting EFI were sought, including gastric residuals of greater than 150 mL/hr and uncontrollable diarrhea of greater 2,500 mL/day. The presence of thrombocytopenia, hyperglycemia, and positive blood culture results were noted as well.

Results.—Thirteen patients had EFI plus sepsis, 5 had sepsis without EFI, and 2 had EFI without sepsis. Contingency table analysis suggested an association between EFI and sepsis. Mortality was 77% for patients with EFI plus sepsis, 60% for those with sepsis alone, and 50% for those with EFI alone, compared with 8% for those with neither EFI nor sepsis. Before the development of sepsis, EFI was noted in 70% of patients, thrombocytopenia in 64%, and hyperglycemia in 66%.

Conclusions.—In massively burned children, EFI is associated with the development of sepsis and with increased mortality. In most cases, EFI is noted before infecting organisms are noted in the blood. The frequency of pre-sepsis EFI is similar to that of thrombocytopenia and hyperglycemia. When EFI occurs in a child with greater than 80% total body surface area burns, it should prompt a search for a focus of infection.

► One can look at a glass as half full or half empty, depending on one's biases. Based on my bias, I choose to look at the glass as half full in this study. Why half full? The answer is that over 80% of these 91 massively-burned children tolerated enteral feedings. This message that even massively injured patients will tolerate enteral feedings if the feedings are begun early is very important. Another important point of this article is the fact that enteral feeding intolerance occurred prior to the onset of sepsis in the majority of the septic patients. This observation further points to gut failure as an important prognostic factor in assessing outcome. Remember, feed early and if enteral feeding intolerance occurs, look for an infectious etiology.

E.A. Deitch, M.D.

Oxandrolone, an Anabolic Steroid, Significantly Increases the Rate of Weight Gain in the Recovery Phase After Major Burns

Demling RH, DeSanti L (Brigham and Women's Hosp, Boston; Braintree Rehabilitation Hosp, Boston)

J Trauma: Injury Infect Crit Care 43:47–51, 1997 3–8

Introduction.—Patients with major burn injury are at risk for severe catabolism and loss of lean body mass. A 10% decrease in lean body mass is associated with impaired immune function, and a decrease of 20% lowers the rate of wound healing. Because muscle loss occurs despite optimum nutrition, oxandrolone, an anabolic steroid shown to restore muscle mass in other catabolic disorders, was added to a standard high-protein diet administered to burn-injured patients.

Methods.—The study group included patients with a deep burn injury affecting 30% to 50% of total body surface. All were treated with a standard protocol during the acute care phase and were anticipated to require at least 3 weeks of inpatient rehabilitation care during the recovery phase. After transfer to the rehabilitation center, patients were divided into 3 groups. Six patients received a high-protein, high-calorie ad libitum oral diet and a protein supplement designed to achieve the needed 2 g/kg/day of protein. Seven patients followed the same diet as the first group, but with the addition of oxandrolone (10 mg orally twice a day). A retrospective group of 10 patients was also studied; these patients had been given a high-calorie, high-protein diet with a protein content of 1.3–1.4 g/kg/day. Physical therapists caring for the patients recorded body weight and assessed muscle strength and endurance at least twice each week.

Results.—The 3 patient groups were similar in age and burn size. Despite optimum nutrition and early wound closure, the mean weight loss for all patients during the catabolic phase was 11%. The oxandrolone-protein group had an average weight gain of 14.5 lb and a physical therapy index of 8.8 of recovery during the first 3 weeks. Both values were significantly greater than corresponding values in the high-protein alone group (mean 7.5 lb and a function index of 7.0) and the retrospective group (mean 4.4 lb and a function index of 4.1). Daily caloric intake did not differ between the groups.

Conclusion.—Current treatment of the profound catabolism occurring after major burns reduces the loss of lean body mass, but patients with large burns still have a significant deficit in muscle mass when they enter the recovery phase. The addition of oxandrolone to a high-protein diet significantly increased weight and improved muscle strength and endurance during the early recovery phase.

► The observation that the provision of an anabolic steroid in combination with a high-protein, low-fat diet significantly speeds up weight gain and exercise-induced improvement in muscle function after a *major* thermal injury is both important and impressive. Clearly, one of the major consequences of the catabolism of a major thermal injury is prolonged weakness and easy fatigability that may limit a patient's ability to return to work and/or resume normal social activities for a period of 6–12 months. Nutritional strategies that improve the rate of return of muscle strength and foster lean muscle weight gain can have a significant clinical impact, thus, the importance of this controlled pilot-type study indicating that oxandrolone (10 mg twice daily) is an effective anabolic agent.

Oxandralone is a testosterone analogue without significant androgenic activity and has been used successfully in patients with hepatitis and AIDS. Perhaps future studies will document that this agent is effective in postoperative and trauma patients as well. I hope so, because prolonged disability is a major problem in these subpopulations of patients as well as in patients with major thermal injuries.

E.A. Deitch, M.D.

Much Ado About Nothing: Methicillin-resistant *Staphylococcus aureus*

Shannon T, Edgar P, Villarreal C, et al (Univ of Texas, Galveston; Shriners Burns Inst, Galveston, Tex)

J Burn Care Rehabil 18:326–331, 1997 3–9

Background.—Many studies have addressed the methicillin-resistant staphylococci—both *Staphylococcus aureus* (MRSA) and *Staphylococcus epidermidis* (MRSE)—and their putative role in nosocomial infections. Although the true incidence of methicillin-resistant strains has changed little, their incidence relative to all other strains has increased. Morbidity and death will continue to be a major focus because of cost-containment issues and to guide microbiologic studies. The incidence, morbidity, mortality, and cost factors of MRSA and MRSE in the ICU setting were analyzed.

Methods and Findings.—The 4-year study included 214 documented infections for patients with burn wounds. Of nearly 17,000 bacterial isolates studied, 82% were staphylococci. About one fourth of *S. aureus* isolates were MRSA, whereas more than three fourths of *S. epidermidis* isolates were MRSE. Only 34% of the total organisms isolated were gram negative. Of the gram-negative isolates, 34% were *Pseudomonas aeruginosa* and 20% were *Escherichia coli.* In a further analysis, the morbidity, mortality, and cost factors related to MRSA-MRSE vs. gram-negative infections were compared.

The results showed only minor morbidity and mortality for MRSA infections. The staphylococci were usually treated with a single antimicrobial drug—51% of MRSA-MRSE infections were adequately covered with vancomycin. In contrast, the gram-negative infections were more serious, usually requiring 2 drugs with daily monitoring to ensure proper antibiotic therapy. The 47 gram-negative infections in this series required an additional 10 to 15 days in the hospital, with antibiotic costs of nearly $300/day. The use of aztreonam with ticarcillin-clavulanate helped to minimize toxicity and other adverse effects.

Conclusions.—The emphasis on methicillin-resistant staphylococcal infections in the ICU may obscure the presence of more serious gram-negative infections. The current preoccupation with MRSA or MRSE infection does not appear to be justified. Although it is clearly important to deal with infections in burn patients, the main motivating factor should be the final outcome or quality of care along with the choice of the most appropriate antibiotic therapy.

▶ I like the title of this article. It brings some common sense and clinical reality into an all too often "buzz-word" scenario, that is, the patient infected or colonized with MRSA or MRSE. While it is true that antibiotic-resistant organisms reflect a potential threat and demand strict adherence to isolation guidelines to prevent the spread of these bacteria to other patients, it is also true that not all antibiotic-resistant bacteria are virulent. Such is the case with MRSA and MRSE. In fact, as shown by the authors, it is better to be colonized with MRSA or MRSE than gram-negative organisms. So the next time you find that one of your patients is colonized with an antibiotic-resistant organism, be happy if it is MRSA or MRSE.

E.A. Deitch, M.D.

Cerebral Oedema After Extensive Thermal Injury: Prognostic Significance of Early Intracranial and Cerebral Perfusion Pressures

Gueugniaud PY, Jauffray M, Bertin-Maghit M, et al (Univ of Lyons, France)
Ann Burns Fire Disasters 10:72–77, 1997 3–10

Introduction.—Patients who have sustained severe burns require massive fluid resuscitation, which leads to extensive edema in both burned skin and vital organs. The concept of burn encephalopathy was created to describe the occurrence of neurologic abnormalities after burn injury, but this complication is largely unexplained. A prospective study was conducted to monitor intracranial pressure (ICP) and cerebral perfusion pressure (CPP) in patients with extensive thermal injury.

Methods.—Study participants were adult patients with a percentage of total burn surface area of greater than 60% and a unit burn score index greater than 220. The ICP monitoring was set up as soon as possible, using an epidural screw in a nonburn area. Both ICP and invasive blood pressure were monitored continuously; CPP values were calculated directly by the monitoring calculator. Abnormal ICP and CPP values were treated, respectively, with infusions of thiopentone and dopamine. Survivor and nonsurvivor groups were compared for control of ICP and CPP.

Results.—Thirty-two patients with a mean age of 37 years were studied. Initial ICP measurements were achieved within a mean of 13.3 hours after thermal injury. Fourteen patients died, including 3 between days 4 and 5 of multiple organ failure and 11 after day 10 of septic and/or cardiopulmonary complications. All patients had abnormal cerebral pressure values in the first 3 days post injury. During the first week post injury, ICP values were always higher and mean arterial pressure and CPP values lower in nonsurvivors than in survivors. During the first 5 days post injury, all patients had received at least 1 catecholamine to improve the hemodynamic profile. Despite therapy to treat CPP and ICP, intracranial pressure was incompletely controlled in nonsurvivors.

Discussion.—Cerebral edema capable of inducing abnormal intracranial pressure appears to develop in severely burned patients. During massive fluid resuscitation administered in the early postburn period, cerebral hypoperfusion may occur and cause adverse outcomes. Treatment of cerebral edema combined with catecholamines may help to limit cerebral perfusion after thermal injury. In this series of patients, survivors' ICP and CPP values were always closer to normal than those of nonsurvivors.

▶ To me, this is a fascinating study. I have always wondered why so many severely burned patients have acute changes in their sensorium. This clinical study—by documenting the fact that intracranial pressure is increased and blood flow to the brain is likely to be decreased after a major thermal injury—provides a potential answer to that question. Because we know that maintaining the ICP at values at less than 20 mm Hg and the CPP at more than 65–70 mm Hg improves functional outcome in patients with head injury, one must wonder whether burn patients with increased ICP values and decreased CPP values would benefit from treatment as well.

Although the authors treated their patients (thiopentone to lower ICP and inotropic agents to increase CPP), the series was not controlled and the number of patients was too small to draw any conclusions. Nonetheless, the observation that significant deleterious changes in cerebral perfusion seem to be occurring in these patients is of major importance. Hopefully, as other investigators begin to examine this phenomenon, its true clinical importance will be determined.

E.A. Deitch, M.D.

Anti-Interleukin-10 Antibody Restores Burn-induced Defects in T-Cell Function

Kelly JL, Lyons A, Soberg CC, et al (Harvard Med School/Brigham and Women's Hosp, Boston)

Surgery 122:146–152, 1997 3–11

Introduction.—The decreased resistance to infection that occurs after major trauma or burns may be the result of changes in both natural and adaptive immunity. Injured patients exhibit diminished production of interleukin-2 (IL-2) and interferon-γ (IFN-γ) (cytokines made by T-helper 1 [Th1] cells) and increased production of IL-4 and IL-10 (cytokines made by Th2 cells). A T-dependent antigen was used to study the effect of burn injury on antigen-specific Th functions in vivo and the effect of anti–IL-10 antibody on these functions.

Methods.—The experimental study used male A/J mice. Groups of 10 animals underwent full-thickness burn or sham burn injury, followed by immunization with 100 μg trinitrobenzene sulfonic acid (TNP) haptenated ovalbumin (TNP-OVA) in complete Freund's adjuvant. The animals received either 250 μg monoclonal rat antimurine IL-10 antibody (anti–IL-10 MAB) or control rat IgG on day 0; 100 μg anti–IL-10 MAB or IgG was given on day 2. The mice were killed 10 days later and serum and spleen cells prepared for analysis.

Results.—Levels of the TNP-specific IgG2a antibody isotype (Th1 dependent) were depressed in the animals with burn injury, but TNP-specific IgG1 and IgE (Th2 dependent) levels were not depressed in either sham burn or burn groups. The IgG2a response was restored by anti–IL-10 MAB, but not by IgG. Animals with burn injury also had reduced TNP-OVA–specific proliferation of splenocytes. Sham and burn groups had equivalent anti-CD3 proliferation. Both TNP-OVA–specific IL-2 and IFN-γ production were significantly reduced by burn injury. Treatment with anti–IL-10 MAB restored IL-2 production by splenocytes from burn mice.

Conclusion.—The effects of treatment with anti–IL-10 antibody indicate that IL-10 acts as a trigger for the abnormalities in Th function that occur after burn injury. The source of IL-10 after burn injury has yet to be determined, as does the potential role of anti–IL-10 as a therapeutic agent.

► This study was chosen because it deals with an important and recently understood biological concept in host defense. That concept is that there are 2 distinct populations of helper T cells (thymus-derived), which serve different functions. Specifically, Th1-type T cells are involved in cell-mediated immunity, and these T cells are characterized by the production of specific cytokines, such as IL-2, which facilitate the cellular immune response. In contrast, Th2-type T cells are involved in aspects of humoral immunity and the cytokines they produce (IL-4, IL-5, IL-10, etc) promote B-cell proliferation and the production of certain classes of antibody.

These facts may be nice and interesting, but as clinicians, you might rightly ask "So what?" The "what" is the recent recognition that once Th2 lymphocytes are turned on, the same cytokines (IL-4 and IL-10) that induce a humoral immune response also turn off the cell-mediated immune response by inhibiting Th1 cellular proliferation. Because Th1 cells are important in antibacterial host defense as well as in the cellular immune response after burns or trauma, this suppression of their activity may lead to infectious complications. Recognition of the potential deleterious consequences of the increased production of these antiinflammatory cytokines produced by Th2 cells has led individuals to investigate the potential clinical benefits of neutralizing IL-10 and other Th2-produced cytokines. The study chosen here is an example of such a new therapeutic strategy.

E.A. Deitch, M.D.

A Novel Model to Study the Effects of Burn Lymph on Pulmonary Vascular Hemodynamic Variables

Hao Q, Hyman AL, Choe EU, et al (Tulane Univ, New Orleans, La)

J Trauma: Injury Infect Crit Care 43:453–457, 1997 3–12

Introduction.—There is a high incidence of respiratory failure in patients with a large–body-surface-area burn injury, and the presence of respiratory failure is associated with a significantly higher death rate. One proposed mechanism for respiratory failure in this setting is the generation of inflammatory mediators at the site of burn injury. An animal study examined the effects of burn lymph on pulmonary hemodynamic variables.

Methods.—Male Sprague-Dawley rats had a balloon-tipped catheter fluoroscopically passed from a jugular vein into the right lower lobe (RLL) pulmonary artery. The distal lumen of the catheter was used to measure pulmonary artery pressure. Brief inflation of the balloon occluded blood flow to the RLL and allowed measurement of RLL wedge pressure, representing pulmonary venous pressure. The RLL then underwent constant flow pump-perfusion with carotid artery blood. Lymph was obtained from dogs that were undergoing experiments on burn injury. For 50 minutes,

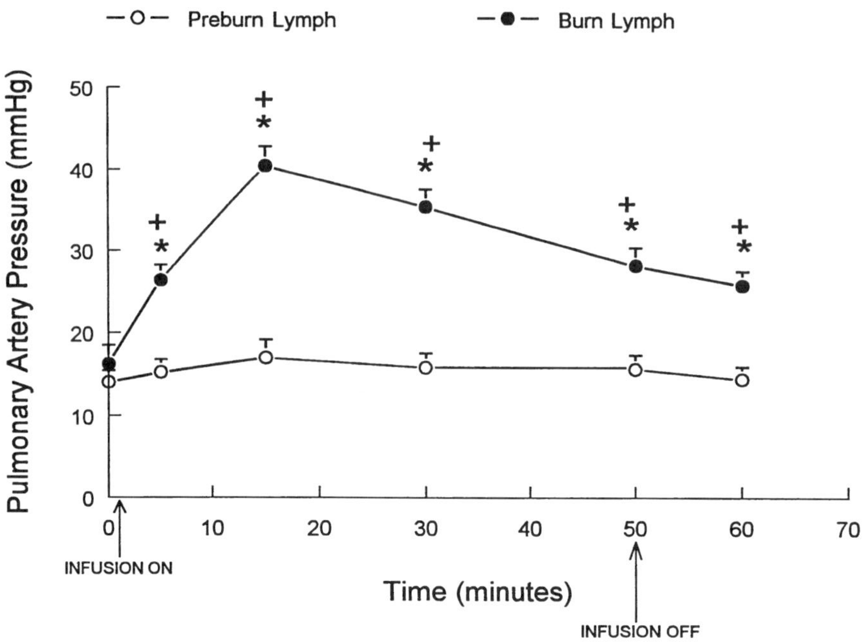

FIGURE 1.—Time-course analysis of the effect of preburn lymph (control) and burn lymph on pulmonary artery pressure. Although preburn lymph produced no effect on pulmonary artery pressure, administration of postburn lymph produced a marked, persistent increase in pulmonary artery pressure that persisted beyond discontinuation of the lymph infusion. *Asterisk* indicates *P* less than 0.01 vs. baseline. *Plus sign* indicates *P* less than 0.001 vs. preburn lymph. (Courtesy of Hao Q, Hyman AL, Choe EU, et al: A novel model to study the effects of burn lymph on pulmonary vascular hemodynamic variables. *J Trauma: Injury Infect Crit Care* 43[3]:453–457, 1997.)

preburn (5 rats) or postburn (6 rats) lymph was infused into the RLL. Variables monitored were mean aortic blood pressure, RLL pulmonary artery pressure, and pulmonary wedge pressure.

Results.—Baseline mean pulmonary artery pressures were similar in the 2 groups of rats at baseline, and an intrapulmonary artery infusion of preburn lymph produced no change. Postburn lymph, however, produced an immediate and significant increase from baseline pulmonary artery pressure that continued despite interruption of the infusion. A comparison of the 2 groups in time-course fashion revealed significantly higher mean pulmonary artery pressure in the postburn lymph group at all observation points (Fig 1). Mean calculated pulmonary vascular resistance was similarly affected by preburn vs. postburn lymph.

Conclusion.—Even without smoke inhalation injury, patients with severe thermal injury have a high incidence of respiratory failure. It is possible that toxic mediators arising from the burn site itself induce alterations in pulmonary hemodynamics.

► The concept that a number of the systemic consequences of a burn injury—including the development of respiratory distress—are related to factors produced in the burn wound has been generally accepted. However, although it is true that respiratory dysfunction and even respiratory failure are commonly observed after a major thermal injury, and it has been speculated that burn-related factors are involved in the pathophysiology of pulmonary injury, direct evidence supporting this potential relationship is largely lacking. Thus, the value of this clever experimental study documenting the fact that postburn lymph causes pulmonary vascular changes characteristic of adult respiratory distress syndrome. In fact, not only does this study directly indicate that pulmonary dysfunction after thermal injury can be induced by factors liberated from the burn wound, it also provides a model system that can be used to determine what those factors are. Because clarification of the mechanisms by which a major thermal injury can lead to respiratory dysfunction is a necessary prelude to the development of new potential therapeutic agents and strategies, this article was selected for inclusion in this year's section on burns.

E.A. Deitch, M.D.

4 Trauma

Introduction

The best treatment of an injury is prevention. Thus, did you know that the use of a cellular telephone while driving is associated with a quadrupling of the risk of a motor vehicle collision or that passenger-side air bags kill more children than they save? The first article in this year's selection of trauma papers is an epidemiologic study that documents the dangers of using a cellular telephone while driving. The second study documents that, although passenger-side air bags reduce fatalities in adults after frontal crashes, passenger air bags are responsible for more children being killed than saved. Based on these two studies, it is clear that talking on the phone while driving can be dangerous and that young children should be in car seats placed in the rear rather than the front seat.

Because by no means is all trauma preventable, several articles on the diagnosis of injuries in patients with blunt trauma have been chosen. The first article in this group, by Branney et al., presents a clinical pathway outlining the use of abdominal US as the initial diagnostic test in a series of 1,000 blunt trauma victims. The value of this algorithm is that it recognizes the advantages and limitations of abdominal US and nicely integrates the use of this diagnostic modality with diagnostic peritoneal lavage and abdominal CT scans. Although highly accurate, the limitations of diagnostic US is highlighted by an article documenting the poor accuracy of abdominal US in pediatric patients with suspected splenic injuries. The bugaboo of both abdominal US or abdominal CT scans is hollow viscus injuries. Thus, the study by Nance et al. showing that the risk of a hollow viscus injury is directly related to the member of solid organs injured was chosen. This study of over 3,000 blunt trauma patients undergoing CT scans documented that the incidence of hollow viscus injury was 15% and 34%, respectively, when two or three solid organs were injured. Lastly, a prospective study of thoracic CT scans showed that CT scans identify more injuries than plain chest X-rays in seriously injured patients. Since the most common significant thoracic injury missed by chest X-ray was an anterior pneumothorax, this study provides support for a policy of routine CT evaluation of the chest in stable multi-trauma patients undergoing diagnostic abdominal CT scans. Along the same lines, it is almost axiomatic to say that when one knows what organs or systems are likely to be injured, one is less likely to miss an injury. This point is well illustrated in an article on the pattern of injuries in patients sustaining urban free falls, which documents the relatively high incidence of intra-abdominal and spinal cord injuries. In the field of diagnosis, an area of controversy has been the approach to the hemodynamically stable patient with a stab wound to the back or flank. The algorithm presented in the article by Kirton et al. showing the utility of contrast-enhanced abdominal CT in this subgroup of patients should prove helpful in dealing with this problem.

Several therapeutically based articles were chosen. The first of which was a prospective randomized clinical trial (PRCT) indicating that the administration of hypertonic saline/dextran in the emergency department to patients with hemorrhage-based hypotension improved survival. The treatment of patients with head injuries continues to be an area of active study. The article by Jaicks et al. raises the warning that early fracture fixation in patients with significant head injuries may worsen the ultimate neurologic outcome by contributing to cerebral edema and by increasing the risk of hypoxemia. On the other hand, the results of a PRCT indicates that a 24- to 36-hour period of moderate hypothermia (32°C to 33°C) significantly improves functional outcome in patients with severe head injuries. Two other therapeutically related articles chosen include a PRCT documenting that patients receiving intravenous fat emulsions during the early postinjury phase have an increased susceptibility to infection and that removing bullets that traverse the colon reduces the incidence of soft-tissue sepsis.

Three trauma-oriented basic science articles dealing with immunology and inflammatory mediators were chosen. The first is a study by Hauser et al., who is the first to investigate the immune microenvironment of human fracture fluids and their relationship to the systemic trauma response. The take-home message of this study is that locally generated immunoinflammatory factors generated in the fracture wound may be contributing to the hyperdynamic response observed after trauma. The second paper illustrates the effects of hemorrhage alone or hemorrhage and tibial fracture on immune regulation of T-cells in the thymus. The third paper, investigating the benefits of platelet-activating factor (PAF) blockade in a model of sepsis and in a trauma model, provides important insights into the complexity of the host response to injury. This article reminds us that the response of an injured patient is complex and that optimistic results obtained from agents tested in simplistic and clinically irrelevant models may not hold up in real-life models.

The last article chosen is a study of the long-term sequelae of trauma patients who survived severe multiple organ failure. The optimistic results observed in this survival are encouraging.

Edwin A. Deitch, M.D.

Association Between Cellular-Telephone Calls and Motor Vehicle Collisions

Redelmeier DA, Tibshirani RJ (Univ of Toronto; Sunnybrook Health Science Centre, North York, Ont, Canada)

N Engl J Med 336:453–458, 1997 4–1

Background.—The use of cellular telephones while driving seems to many observers to be distracting to the driver, and intuitively it seems likely that the risk of motor vehicle collisions would be increased. However, 2 industry-sponsored surveys have found no increased risk. This study investigated the risk of motor vehicle collision while using a cellular telephone was examined by using a case-crossover design, a technique that assesses the brief change in risk associated with a transient exposure, and in which research subjects serve as his or her own control.

Methods.—Consenting subjects were enrolled if they came to a collision reporting center in Toronto during peak hours between July 1, 1994 and August 31, 1995; their collision had involved substantial property damage as judged by police (collisions involving injuries are not reported to the center); they reported owning a cellular phone; and their cellular phone bills could be obtained. Subjects answered a brief questionnaire about themselves and the collision, and the time of the collision was estimated from subject reports, police records, and telephone records of calls to emergency services. Telephone bills were examined to determine telephone use during the 10 minutes before the collision and during the comparable period on the day preceding the collision. If more calls were made immediately before the collision than would be expected as a result of chance, that was interpreted as an increase in risk. Supplemental analyses were made to evaluate alternative comparison days and shorter and longer times before the collision. In addition, the data were adjusted to account for intermittent driving (i.e., not all participants had driven on the previous day).

Results.—Of 5,890 eligible drivers, 1,064 acknowledged owning a cellular phone, 742 agreed to participate, and billing records were obtained for 699. After adjusting for intermittent driving, analysis indicated that cellular telephone activity in the 10 minutes immediately before the collision was associated with a 4.3-fold increase in relative risk of a motor vehicle collision (95% confidence interval, 3.0–6.5). The results were not significantly different for drivers using hands-free telephones.

Conclusions.—In this population, use of a cellular telephone while driving was associated with a risk of motor vehicle collision that was 4 times higher than that for the same drivers when they did not use their cellular telephones. This association does not prove a causal relationship. However, individual drivers who use cellular telephones are at greater risk and should act accordingly. Physicians have a responsibility to identify patients who may be at risk and advise them about safety precautions.

► The message of this interesting epidemiologic study is quite clear and is well captured by the title of the article. There is an association between cellular-telephone calls and motor vehicle collisions. It is not surprising that anything which diverts a driver's attention from driving can lead to an accident, because driver error or inattention plays a major role in the majority of automobile collisions. Because most physicians have car phones and frequently use them, this article may be a wake-up call for us as well as the patients we treat in our emergency departments.

E.A. Deitch, M.D.

Reductions in Deaths in Frontal Crashes Among Right Front Passengers in Vehicles Equipped With Passenger Air Bags

Braver ER, Ferguson SA, Greene MA, et al (Insurance Inst for Highway Safety, Arlington, Va)

JAMA 278:1437–1439, 1997 4–2

Introduction.—Although cars equipped with driver air bags have reduced driver death in frontal crashes, passenger air bags had caused the deaths of 45 children and infants and 3 adults as of September 1, 1997. Almost all of the children were unbelted and the infants had been placed in rear-facing child seats with their heads close to air bag modules. Using data from the Fatality Analysis Reporting System, investigators sought to assess the effectiveness of passenger air bags.

Methods.—The study population consisted of individuals killed from 1992 to 1995 by crashes in which they were right front passengers in 1992 to 1995 model year cars with air bags (dual or driver-only). Excluded were crashes involving more than 2 vehicles and single-vehicle noncollision events. The odds of right front passengers dying in frontal vs. nonfrontal crashes with dual or driver-only air bags were calculated and the percentage reductions in right front passenger deaths in dual–air-bag vehicles estimated. Various occupant age groups were considered because of the reported increased risk to children and the elderly.

Results.—During the 4-year study, 336 right front passengers in dual–air-bag-cars (model years 1992 through 1995) died in frontal crashes; 288 died in nonfrontal crashes. In cars with driver-only air bags, 688 right front passengers died in frontal crashes and 470 died in nonfrontal crashes. It is estimated that 73 fewer than expected right front passengers died in cars with dual air bags. In frontal crashes of cars with dual air bags, right front passenger fatalities were 18% fewer than expected. When frontal and nonfrontal crashes were considered, deaths were 11% lower among right front passengers in cars with dual air bags. In contrast, fatalities were 34% higher than expected among children younger than 10 years who were right front passengers in cars with dual air bags involved in frontal crashes. Many of these crashes were of low severity and should not have caused serious injury. The reduction in deaths among passengers aged 65 years and older was only 6%.

Discussion.—Initial estimates of the benefits of passenger air bags suggest that fatalities have been substantially reduced in frontal crashes.

Findings are quite different when children are analyzed separately, however, for children have a 34% increased risk of dying in frontal crashes when passengers in a vehicle with dual air bags. Shorter adults, unbelted adults, and children are at highest risk of air-bag–related injuries. The enforcement of correct restraint use is recommended, together with modifications in air bag technology.

► It is well recognized that the institution of any policy or intervention has its own set of advantages and risks. This appears to be the case for the institution of front passenger seat air bags. One of the most conceptually attractive features of air bags is that active participation of the occupants of the car is not required for this device to be operational. This is in contrast to passenger restraint (i.e., seat belt) devices, which necessitate active cooperation of the occupant for them to be effective.

Although air bags are conceptually attractive and appear to be effective and save lives, as of late 1997, 45 deaths in infants and children have been attributed to the deployment of passenger-side air bags in low severity crashes that should have been survivable. Because of this concern over safety, data were needed to better quantitate the risk-benefit ratio of passenger-side air bags. This article has met that need and provides reasonably convincing evidence that passenger-side air bags *save* lives of adults but *cost* lives of children.

The importance of this article is several fold. First, at the level of individuals and families, it highlights the fact that lives can be saved by ensuring that children in car seats are placed in the rear seat rather than the front seat. Secondly, it provides information that can be used as an impetus for instituting policies and making technical changes in the construction of air bags that will improve their safety.

E.A. Deitch, M.D

Ultrasound Based Key Clinical Pathway Reduces the Use of Hospital Resources for the Evaluation of Blunt Abdominal Trauma

Branney SW, Moore EE, Cantrill SV, et al (Univ of Colorado, Denver)

J Trauma: Injury Infect Crit Care 42:1086–1090, 1997 4–3

Introduction.—One of the most resource intensive aspects of acute trauma management is examining patients who sustained blunt abdominal trauma. Traditional methods have included diagnostic peritoneal lavage and hospitalization for serial physical examinations and laboratory tests. Computed tomography has been shown to be a sensitive test in the last decade, and US has emerged as an alternative method more recently. For the evaluation of patients with blunt abdominal trauma, a key clinical pathway was developed to test the hypothesis that emergency department US would reduce the need for invasive diagnostic peritoneal lavage and costly CT scans.

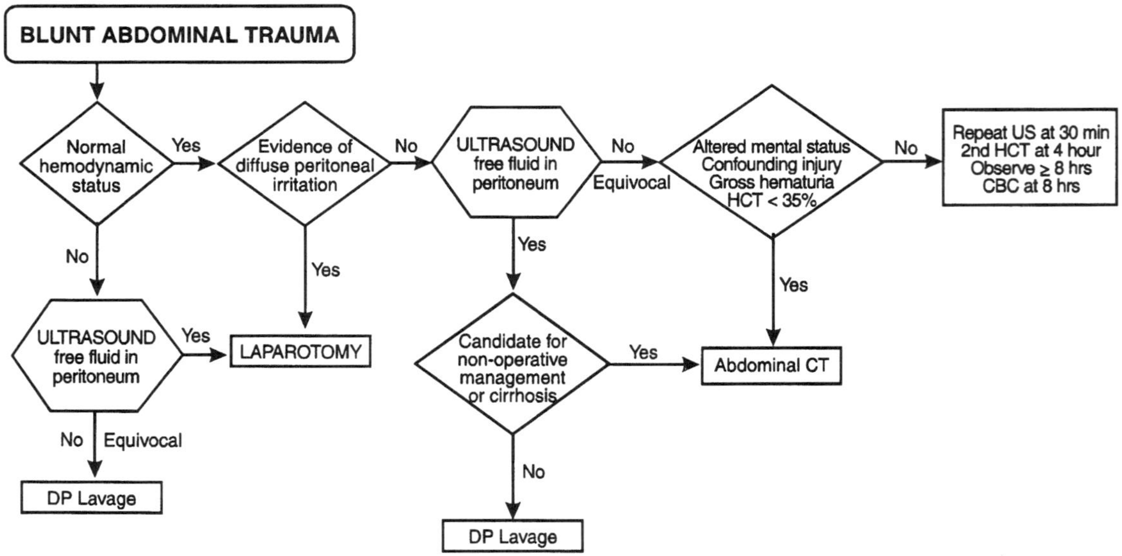

FIGURE 1.—Key clinical pathway for the evaluation of blunt abdominal trauma. *Abbreviations: HCT*, hematocrit; *CBC*, complete blood cell count; *DP*, diagnostic peritoneal. (Courtesy of Branney SW, Moore EE, Cantrill SV, et al: Ultrasound based key clinical pathway reduces the use of hospital resources for the evaluation of blunt abdominal trauma. *J Trauma: Injury Infect Crit Care* 42(6):1086–1090, 1997.)

Methods.—Using the key clinical pathway, a prospective analysis was conducted on 486 patients evaluated for blunt abdominal trauma during a 3-month period, and this was compared with a 3-month historical cohort of 516 patients. The pathway involves the use of the initial US examination serving as the first level of triage to laparotomy or additional diagnostic testing (Fig 1). Diagnostic peritoneal lavage, CT scanning and serial US examinations were the other diagnostic modalities. Laparoscopy was not found to be useful for evaluating acute blunt abdominal trauma.

Results.—Regarding demographics, the number of laparotomies, or the type of injuries, no differences were found between the 2 groups. Diagnostic peritoneal lavage was reduced from 17% to 4% using the key clinical pathway, and CT was reduced from 56% to 26%. For patients undergoing diagnostic peritoneal lavage, the injury severity score increased from 11.6 to 21.5. For patients undergoing CT, the injury severity score increased from 4.6 to 8.3. In 65% of patients, US examinations were used exclusively.

Conclusion.—Significant reductions in the use of invasive diagnostic peritoneal lavage and costly CT scanning were found with the use of the US-based key clinical pathway in evaluating blunt abdominal trauma. There was no risk to the patient.

▶ Based on an ever-enlarging number of clinical studies, US evaluation of the abdomen in patients with blunt trauma appears to accurately identify the majority of adult patients who require operative repair of intra-abdominal injuries. Thus, abdominal US is an excellent screening test in this patient population, although it is not perfect and lacks some of the advantages of diagnostic peritoneal lavage and abdominal tomography. Based on the advantages of US as a screening test, the question is not whether US should be used in the emergency department but how it should be integrated with other currently available diagnostic modalities. It is for this reason that the study by Branney et al. was chosen. It provides a well-conceived algorithm for the use of US in adult patients with blunt abdominal trauma.

E.A. Deitch, M.D.

Use of Abdominal Ultrasonography to Assess Pediatric Splenic Trauma: Potential Pitfalls in the Diagnosis

Krupnick AS, Teitelbaum DH, Geiger JD, et al (Univ of Michigan, Ann Arbor; CS Mott Children's Hosp, Ann Arbor, Mich)

Ann Surg 225:408–414, 1997 4–4

Background.—Splenic injury is common in children with blunt abdominal trauma. The most accurate method for evaluating these injuries is CT. Ultrasound (US) is increasingly used as a screening study for splenic injury, yet there are few data on its accuracy. This prospective study evaluated the accuracy of abdominal US in screening and grading splenic injury in children.

Methods.—The study included 32 children with blunt abdominal trauma and splenic injury identified by CT. Both CT and US were used to assess the degree of splenic injury. The study analyzed the initial US reading, as well as further readings made with and without knowledge of the CT findings.

Results.—The initial US report missed 38% of the CT-confirmed splenic injuries. In 22% of patients with splenic fractures, no free intraperitoneal fluid was shown on CT. Ultrasound's sensitivity in detecting splenic injury was only 62% to 78%, and it tended to downgrade the severity of the injuries.

Conclusion.—On its own, US is inadequate for the evaluation of splenic trauma in children. The US finding of free intraperitoneal fluid cannot be used to detect splenic injuries, because not all patients have free intra-abdominal fluid. Ultrasound appears to be of low value for initial assessment, management, and follow-up of children with splenic trauma.

▶ New clinical techniques and approaches tend to go through several stages. In the first stage, a large number of clinicians are resistant to accepting the new idea for any number of reasons, including the fear that it will not stand the test of time. As more positive information is generated, a stage of over-enthusiasm may occur, during which the new technique is used beyond its limitations. Lastly, a stage of re-evaluation occurs, and here the test or technique is put into its proper clinical context.

This may be the case for emergency room diagnostic ultrasound in patients with blunt trauma. It is clear that abdominal ultrasound is a sensitive diagnostic test in adults with blunt trauma and aids in decision making, especially in those patients with nonabdominal injuries that require rapid operative intervention. However, this article indicates that this test may not be as reliable in pediatric patients with splenic injuries. This does not mean that abdominal sonography is not a good screening test; it just means that the results of the test must be used with caution and in conjunction with other clinically relevant information.

E.A. Deitch, M.D.

Solid Viscus Injury Predicts Major Hollow Viscus Injury in Blunt Abdominal Trauma

Nance ML, Peden GW, Shapiro MB, et al (Children's Hosp of Philadelphia; Lankenau Hosp, Wynnewood, Pa; Univ of Pennsylvania, Philadephia)
J Trauma: Injury Infect Crit Care 43:618–623, 1997 4–5

Introduction.—The nonoperative management of blunt abdominal trauma has become more acceptable with widespread availability of CT. Reliable models for predicting the likelihood of a concomitant hollow viscus injury (HVI) in the hemodynamically stable patient with a solid viscus injury are of increasing importance. The rate of HVI in hemody-

TABLE 4.—Ranking of Injury Type by Odds of HVI Compared With Kidney Injury Only

Organs Injured	Odds of HVI*
Spleen only	4.36
Liver only	5.05
KID/LIV	5.78
KID/SPL	6.01
LIV/SPL	12.11
KID/LIV/PNC/SPL	14.61
Pancreas only	18.14
KID/LIV/SPL	19.95
LIV/PNC	20.45
KID/PNC/SPL	25.56
PNC/SPL	26.78
KID/LIV/PNC	40.90
LIV/PNC/SPL	46.47

*All $P < 0.05$ compared with kidney only.

Abbreviations: KID, kidney; *LIV*, liver; *PNC*, pancreas; *SPL*, spleen; *HVI*, hollow viscus injury.

(Courtesy of Nance ML, Peden GW, Shapiro MB, et al: Solid viscus injury predicts major hollow viscus injury in blunt abdominal trauma. *J Trauma: Injury Infect Crit Care* 43(4):618–623, 1997.)

namically stable patients with either single or multiple solid viscus injuries from blunt abdominal trauma was assessed.

Methods.—Data from all patients age 12 years and older with blunt trauma and an Abbreviated Injury Scale score of 2 or more for solid viscus injuries in the Pennsylvania Trauma Systems Foundation registry for a 4-year period from January 1992 to December 1995 were reviewed. Patients were not included if they had an initial systolic blood pressure less than 90 mm Hg.

Results.—Of 3,089 patients with solid viscus injuries, 296 (9.6%) had HVIs. In 2,437 patients with single solid viscus injuries, 177 (7.3%) had HVIs. The rate of HVIs increased with the number of solid organs injured. Concomitant HVIs were observed in 15.4% (547) of patients with 2 solid viscus injuries and in 34.4% (96) of patients with 3 solid viscus injuries. Compared with a solitary solid viscus injury, 2 solid viscus injuries were 2.3 times more likely to be associated with an HVI and 3 solid viscus injuries were 6.7 times more likely to be associated with an HVI. The incidence of an HVI was related more to the number of solid visceral injuries than to the severity of individual organ injuries. Pancreatic injuries (33.3%) in combination with any other organ injury were most likely to have associated HVIs, compared with other organ combinations. Kidney injuries in combination with another organ injury were least likely (14.1%) to be associated with an HVI. Because a kidney injury was not a significant predictor of an HVI, the odds of an HVI for a particular injury combination in comparison with a kidney-only injury was predicted. The most likely injury combination to have an associated HVI was the liver–pancreas–spleen combination (Table 4).

Conclusion.—The HVI rate increases with the number of solid organs injured in patients with blunt trauma to the abdomen. Pancreatic injuries with any combination of solid viscus injuries and a Solid Viscus Score of 6 or greater are predictive of an increased risk for an HVI.

▶ In observing patients with blunt trauma, it is the risk of a missed injury requiring surgery that concerns us all. As illustrated by the overall 10% incidence of HVIs in these 3,089 patients, this is a real concern. As stated by the authors, a continuing nemesis of CT-based nonoperative management of patients with blunt trauma and solid organ injuries is the risk of an unrecognized, associated HVI. Although missed HVIs in patients treated nonoperatively for injuries to the liver, spleen, or pancreas are not common, neither are they rare. All of us have had the unsettling experience of having signs of peritonitis or sepsis develop in a patient while observing them for a solid organ injury, only to find an initially unsuspected HVI at surgery.

By providing information on the relative risk of an HVI (based on the spectrum and number of solid organs injured), the authors have given us useful information that can be used to fine-tune our clinical judgment.

E.A. Deitch, M.D.

Value of Thoracic Computed Tomography in the First Assessment of Severely Injured Patients With Blunt Chest Trauma: Results of a Prospective Study

Trupka A, Waydhas C, Hallfeldt KKJ, et al (Ludwig-Maximilian-Univ Munich, Germany)

J Trauma: Injury Infect Crit Care 43:405–411, 1997 4–6

Background.—Blunt chest trauma is present in two thirds of patients with multiple injuries. Lung contusion is a particularly serious finding for it may lead to respiratory failure and is associated with an increased incidence of multiple organ failure. Early and exact diagnosis of lung contusion is important in identifying patients at high risk for these complications. A prospective study compared the value of early thoracic CT and routine chest x-ray in the diagnostic work-up of blunt thoracic trauma.

Methods.—Study participants were 103 consecutive patients admitted to the emergency department of a level I trauma center with clinical or radiologic signs of chest trauma. Nine had isolated chest trauma and 94 had multiple injuries. The patients had an average Injury Severity Score of 30 and an average Abbreviated Injury Scale thorax score of 3. Seventy-eight patients underwent early thoracic CT because of signs of thoracic injury or equivocal findings on the initial chest x-ray study. All imaging findings and therapeutic consequences were recorded and analyzed.

Results.—Compared with the diagnosis after the initial chest x-ray study, thoracic CT yielded important additional information about chest trauma in 65% of patients. The diagnostic accuracy of thoracic CT was significantly better than that of plain x-ray film for lung contusion, pneumothorax, and hemothorax (Table 3). Overall, the additional diagnostic

TABLE 3.—Accuracy of Routine X-Ray Studies and Thoracic CT in Early Diagnosis of Intrathoracic Injuries

	CXR	TCT	*p* Value
Lung contusion	25	61	<0.001
Pneumothorax	17	44	<0.005
Hemothorax	23	44	0.05
Rupture of diaphragm	2	2	
Myocardial rupture		1	

Note: Table gives injured hemothoraces in a total of 103 patients, χ^2 test with Yates' correction.

Abbreviations: CXR, initial chest x-ray after arrival of patient in the emergency room; *TCT*, early thoracic CT.

(Courtesy of Trupka A, Waydhas C, Hallfeldt KKJ, et al: Value of thoracic computed tomography in the first assessment of severely injured patients with blunt chest trauma: Results of a prospective study. *J Trauma: Injury Infect Crit Care* 43(3):405–411, 1997.)

information provided by thoracic CT had direct consequences in early trauma management for 42% of the total study population. Therapy changes frequently used because of thoracic CT included chest tube placement, changes in the mode of ventilation and respiratory care, and management of fracture stabilization. Compared with a historical control group, patients evaluated with thoracic CT experienced significant reductions in both the rate of adult respiratory distress syndrome and mortality.

Discussion.—The clinical value of CT in blunt chest trauma has been controversial, but findings of this and other studies confirm that thoracic CT is superior to plain x-ray film in visualizing intrathoracic injuries and complications. Early and exact diagnosis of lung contusion is particularly crucial in patients with multiple injuries, because blunt chest trauma negatively affects outcome in such cases.

► This prospective study of severely injured trauma patients clearly shows that CT scans of the chest identify more injuries (contusions, hemothoraces, pneumothoraces) than conventional chest x-ray studies. Although some of the injuries, especially the hemothoraces, do not require therapy, many of the other injuries identified changed required therapy. According to the authors, the results of the CT scans altered therapy in 42 of the 103 patients (40%). In fact, the most common finding diagnosed by CT that modified therapy was the presence of an anterior pneumothorax not suspected on the initial x-ray film.

The authors also attempted to determine whether the changes in therapy based on the CT-diagnosed injuries improved outcome. To assess this, the authors compared the outcomes of these prospectively studied patients with a comparably injured group of patients treated earlier who did not have CT scans of the thorax performed. Although the authors used historical controls in this analysis, the fact that the mortality rate of the patients given CT scans was half that of the patients having only plain x-ray studies (10% vs. 21%) is impressive and warrents attention. The explanation for how and why the information obtained by the CT scans may have improved survival is well covered by the authors in their discussion, which I commend for your reading.

With the advent of the helical CT scanner, both the quality of the image and the time required to perform a CT examination have improved. To these facts is now added data suggesting that routine CT scanning of multiple trauma patients with thoracic trauma both aids in the diagnosis of thoracic injuries and improves outcome. For these reasons, it seems prudent to adopt a liberal policy of chest CT scanning in this patient population.

E.A. Deitch, M.D.

Patterns of Injury in Victims of Urban Free-Falls

Velmahos GC, Demetriades D, Theodorou D, et al (Univ of Southern California, Los Angeles)

World J Surg 21:816–821, 1997 4–7

Introduction.—A prospective study was conducted to analyze patterns of injury after fall from a height in an urban setting. Most previous studies have been retrospective reviews or autopsy series, and none have been stratified for height of the fall, which is the most significant determinant of survival.

Methods.—Enrolled in the study were all patients who entered the emergency department of an academic level I trauma center with a diagnosis of a fall from a height from September 1994 to June 1995. Excluded were patients who sustained simple falls at ground level and those with lethal penetrating injuries. The patients, paramedics, and any witnesses were interviewed regarding details of the injury. Patients were followed for diagnostic and therapeutic interventions, hospital course, and final outcome.

Results.—The mean age of the 187 consecutive fall victims was 31.6 years, and the mean fall height was 19.5 ft. Only 3 patients fell from a height of more than 40 ft. Toxic screens, obtained in 109 cases, were positive in 71 (65.1%). The fall was judged intentional in 11 cases. Nine patients arrived in shock with significant visceral, skeletal, and head injuries; 5 died of their injuries. Five patients with severe head injuries arrived intubated; 1 died. Significant injuries were present in approximately two thirds of the group (Table 1), with skeletal injuries accounting for 76.2% of all injuries. Three patients had spinal cord injury resulting in paraplegia. Even falls from 10 ft resulted in spinal fractures. Eleven patients, all but 1 of whom fell from a height of more than 20 ft, had intra-abdominal injuries; 2 of these patients died.

Overall, 60 major surgical procedures were performed in 45 patients (24%). Adult respiratory distress syndrome developed in 9 patients, all of whom had fallen from a height of more than 20 ft. Twenty-six fall victims required ICU admission. Greater fall height was directly correlated with the frequency of intoxication, significant injuries, need for operation, duration of hospitalization, and death.

TABLE 1.—Incidence of Various Injuries in 187 Fall Victims

Site	No. of patients with specific injuries	Percent of patients (n = 187)	Percent of injured patients (n = 122)
Extremity	70	37.4	57.4
Craniofacial fractures	15	8.0	12.3
Spinal fractures	37	19.8	30.3
Head injuries	27	14.4	22.1
Intra-abdominal organ injuries	11	5.9	9.0
Pelvic fracture	17	9.1	13.9
Retroperitoneal injuries	2	1.1	1.6

(Courtesy of Velmahos GC, Demetriades D, Theodorou D, et al: Patterns of injury in victims of urban free-falls. *World J Surg* 21:816–821, copyright 1997, Springer-Verlag.)

Conclusion.—In the urban setting, falls from height are frequently associated with intoxication. The height of the fall is a good predictor of injury severity and outcome. Few survive a free-fall of more than 40 ft, but falls from moderate heights can result in death or significant disability. Although fractures are the most common type of injury, spinal trauma should be suspected in all fall victims. Intra-abdominal injuries were found to be far more common than retroperitoneal injuries.

► The take-home message of this prospective study of 187 patients is very clear. It is that one must carefully search for spinal column fractures and intra-abdominal injuries in patients with falls. This is true even if the fall is from a height of less than 20 ft, because 30% of the spinal fractures occurred in this subpopulation of patients. A diligent search for these potentially occult injuries is very important in patients with urban falls, as many of these patients are intoxicated at the time of the fall or have concomitant head injuries, making it difficult for the examining physician to get a reliable history and compromising the physical examination. Because of the high incidence of spinal column injury, an aggressive protocol of clinical and radiographic evaluation of the entire spinal column is mandatory to avoid missing injuries.

E.A. Deitch, M.D.

Stab Wounds to the Back and Flank in the Hemodynamically Stable Patient: A Decision Algorithm Based on Contrast-enhanced Computed Tomography With Colonic Opacification

Kirton OC, Wint D, Thrasher B, et al (Univ of Miami, Fla)

Am J Surg 173:189–193, 1997 4–8

Objective.—Surgery is rarely required for wounds of the back and flank. However, signs of peritoneal inflammation can sometimes be missed in

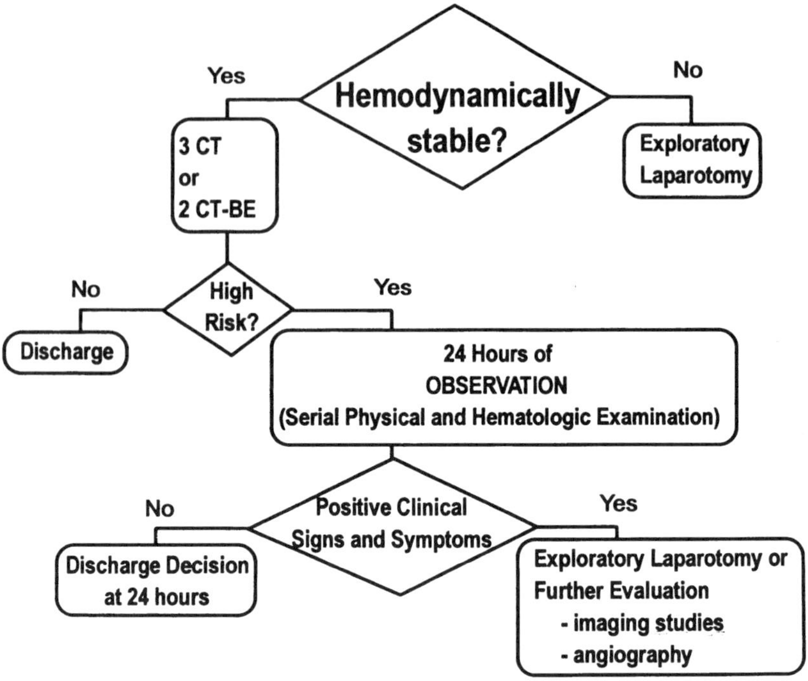

FIGURE.—Algorithm depicting the evaluation of the hemodynamically stable patient. *Abbreviations*: *3 CT*, triple-contrast CT; *CT-BE*, double-contrast CT with immediate barium enema. (Reprinted by permission of the publisher from Stab wounds to the back and flank in the hemodynamically stable patient: A decision algorithm based on contrast-enhanced CT with colonic opacification, by Kirton OC, Wint D, Thrasher B, et al: *Am J Surg*, Vol. 173, pp 189–193, Copyright 1997 by Excerpta Medica Inc.)

patients with these posterior injuries. The effectiveness of contrast-enhanced CT with colonic opacification (CE-CT) in triage of hemodynamically stable patients with stab wounds to the flank and back was investigated.

Methods.—The retrospective study included 145 patients with stab wounds to the flank and/or back. All were hemodynamically stable on admission to the emergency department, with no signs of acute abdomen or ongoing blood loss. Each patient underwent retroperitoneal CE-CT evaluation. Double-contrast scans, followed immediately with a barium enema examination, were performed from October 1991 to February 1993. From March 1993 to April 1994, intravenous, oral, and rectal administered contrast, or 3CT, was the only diagnostic procedure performed. Wounds that penetrated superficially to the deep fascia were categorized as *low risk*, whereas those that penetrated beyond the deep fascia were regarded as *high risk*.

Results.—Based on CE-CT results, 92 patients were classified as low risk and 53 as high risk. The 2 groups were similar in terms of characteristics at admission, including vital signs, Glasgow Coma Scale score, and complete blood count. No patient in the low-risk group required surgery or experienced any sequelae. Six patients from the high-risk group (6.5%) underwent surgery—5 for exploratory laparotomy and 1 for local exploration because of persistent wound bleeding. Two patients were sent to surgery on the basis of CE-CT findings—a filling defect in the abdominal aorta of 1 patient and a suspected major diaphragmatic injury in the other. The other patients went to surgery based on evolving clinical findings. The clinical findings of all 6 patients were correctly predicted by CE-CT.

Conclusions.—Contrast-enhanced CT is a useful tool for triage of hemodynamically stable patients with stab wounds to the back and/or flank. Patients with wound penetration superficial to the deep fascia are considered low risk and can be discharged immediately. Those with wound penetration beyond the deep fascia are considered high risk and should be evaluated for discharge after 24 hours of observation. Decisions about surgery in this group depend on physical examination, diagnostic tests, and clinical judgment (Figure).

▶ This clinical study deals with a controversial and potentially difficult problem: how best to treat an asymptomatic or intoxicated patient with a stab wound to the back or flank. Historically, patients with posterior wounds that were thought to penetrate the deep fascia underwent laparotomy to be sure that injuries to the colon and retroperitoneal structures were not missed. However, because of the high incidence (greater than 80% to 85% in most series) of nontherapeutic laparotomies, most trauma centers have abandoned this policy of mandatory exploration in favor of a selective operative approach. Although most trauma centers utilize a selective approach, this approach varies widely between centers. Consequently, the goal of this study was to evaluate a CT scan–based triage protocol using triple contrast in this patient population. The approach outlined in the author's algorithm is the result of this study. This algorithm seems quite reasonable and is highly likely to be effective as long as a few critical points are kept in mind. First, the patients studied did *not* have evidence of an acute abdomen or ongoing blood loss on presentation and the development of positive physical findings overruled a "negative" CT scan. Lastly, all patients had triple contrast studies that included rectal contrast. The need for rectal contrast is very important, because without rectal contrast, subtle colonic injuries may be missed.

E.A. Deitch, M.D.

Prognostic Factors to Predict Outcome Following the Administration of Hypertonic/Hyperoncotic Solution in Hypovolemic Patients

Younes RN, Aun F, Ching CT, et al (Univ of São Paulo, Brazil; Hosp AC Camargo, São Paulo, Brazil)

Shock 7:79–83, 1997 4–9

Purpose.—The hemodynamic condition of patients admitted to the emergency department (ED) can be significantly improved by administration of hypertonic fluids. However, clinical studies generally do not show

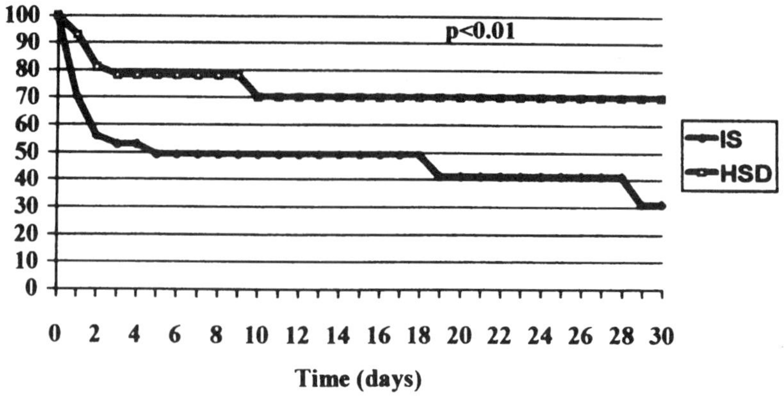

FIGURE 6.—Overall survival in the 2 groups during the 30-day period for patients admitted with mean arterial pressure less than 70 mm Hg. *Abbreviations: HSD*, hypertonic solution: *IS*, isotonic solution. (Courtesy of Younes RN, Aun F, Ching CT, et al: Prognostic factors to predict outcome following the administration of hypertonic/hyperoncotic solution in hypovolemic patients. *Shock* 7:79–84, 1997.)

that hypertonic fluids lead to any improvement in long-term survival or complication rates, compared with standard isotonic treatment. Factors associated with a beneficial effect of hypertonic solutions in patients admitted to the ED with hemorrhagic hypovolemia were identified in a randomized, double-blind trial.

Methods.—The study included 212 patients seen in the ED with hemorrhagic hypovolemia who required blood volume expansion. On admission, they were randomly assigned to receive either hypertonic saline with dextran (HSD) (a 250 mL IV bolus of hypertonic 7.5% NaCl + 6% dextran) or an isotonic solution (IS) (0.9% NaCl). This initial treatment was followed by standard resuscitation. The patients' sex, age, cause of hypovolemia, Revised Trauma Score (RTS), Glasgow index, and mean arterial pressure (MAP) were assessed on admission. Survival at 24 hours and 30 days was compared between groups. The groups were also compared for infused volumes.

Results.—In patients who received HSD, MAP was significantly increased and IV crystalloid infusions to maintain hemodynamic status were significantly reduced. The 2 groups were similar in number of blood transfusions and complication rates, about 24% in each group. Overall 30-day survival was 73% in the HSD group and 64% in the IS group, a significant difference. Survival at 24 hours was 87% with HSD vs. 72% with IS. On univariate analysis, factors predictive of 24–hour survival in patients receiving HSD were an RTS less than 14, MAP less than 70 mm Hg, and Glasgow index less than 12. On multivariate analysis, RTS and MAP were independent predictors. For long-term survival, HSD conferred a significant advantage only for patients with an admission MAP of less than 70 mm Hg (Fig 6).

Conclusions.—This prospective, randomized clinical trial shows a significant survival benefit of hypertonic fluid administration for patients with hypovolemia admitted to the ED. However, long-term survival is improved only for patients with an admission MAP of less than 70 mm Hg. Further study is needed to validate the prognostic factors identified in this study and to assess the survival benefits of hypertonic solutions in the prehospital setting.

► The debate concerning the role of HSD in the acute resuscitation of hypotensive trauma patients centers on whether HSD improves patient outcome. What do we know so far about HSD? We know that in most animal studies, the use of HSD was associated with an improved hemodynamic response, although its effect on survival is variable. We know from clinical trials that HSD appears to be safe, and in none of the trials did the patient groups receiving HSD vs. isotonic saline have worse outcomes. In fact, most of the previously published clinical trials have shown that HSD is associated with a more rapid improvement in the hemodynamic response than isotonic saline and, although survival of the HSD groups was not significantly improved, there was a trend toward better survival in the patients receiving HSD. On a practical level, we also know that HSD is easy to use and convenient to store and is relatively inexpensive. Putting this information into perspective with the positive results of the current study, it appears likely that HSD will be found ultimately to have a role in the early resuscitation of the hypotensive trauma patient.

E.A. Deitch, M.D.

Early Fracture Fixation May Be Deleterious After Head Injury

Jaicks RR, Cohn SM, Moller BA (Yale Univ, New Haven, Conn)

J Trauma: Injury Infect Crit Care 42:1–5, 1997 4–10

Introduction.—Early fracture fixation (FF) is generally regarded as useful in minimizing morbidity in trauma patients. However, some authors have questioned whether early FF should be performed in certain subsets of patients with multitrauma. They worry that performing early FF after severe head trauma could expose a vulnerable patient to a risk of secondary brain injury. Two major determinants of secondary brain injury are hypotension and hypoxemia. The neurologic risks of early FF in patients with multitrauma with head injury were retrospectively assessed.

Methods.—The review included 33 patients with blunt trauma and significant closed head injuries who required operative FF. The Abbreviated Injury Scale (AIS) score was 2 or greater in each patient. Fracture fixation was performed within 24 hours in 19 patients and after 24 hours in 14. These early and late FF groups were comparable in terms of age, admission Glasgow Coma Scale score, Injury Severity score, and neurologic and orthopedic injury scores. The 2 groups were compared for volume of fluid resuscitation, neurologic complications, and clinical outcomes.

Results.—Patients undergoing early FF received significantly more fluids within the first 48 hours. They were also somewhat more likely to have intraoperative hypotension, with 16% having a systolic blood pressure of less than 90 mm Hg, compared to 7% in the delayed FF group. Rates of intraoperative hypoxia, with an oxygen saturation of 90% or less, were 11% and 7%, respectively. Sixteen percent of patients in the early FF group and 21% of those in the late FF group had neurologic complications, a similar rate. However, patients in the early FF group had a lower average Glasgow Coma Scale score at discharge, 13.5 vs. 15.0.

Conclusions.—For patients with multitrauma with head injuries, early FF is associated with significantly greater fluid administration. These patients tend to have a higher risk of hypoxemia and hypotension, which could contribute to a poor neurologic outcome. The authors call for prospective studies to determine how the timing of FF affects outcomes in patients with head injury.

► The data continue to accrue that a policy of early fracture fixation of long bones is not always safe. This article suggests that patients with head injuries may need to be added to the list of multitrauma patients for whom delayed fracture fixation is superior to immediate fracture fixation. The other group in whom early fracture fixation has been shown to lead to a worse outcome is patients with severe chest injuries. Although most agree that early fracture fixation decreases pulmonary complications and improves outcome, it is becoming clear that clinical judgment is important to identify the subgroups of patients in whom this policy does not work.

The current study is retrospective and has some weaknesses, but it does make sense. To quote the authors, "In the head-injured patient, the avoidance of secondary brain injury is of paramount importance. Hypotension and hypoxemia are the two most significant determinants of secondary brain injury." Because hypotension and hypoxia seem to occur more often with early than with late fracture fixation, I believe the warning raised in this article should be taken seriously.

E.A. Deitch, M.D.

Treatment of Traumatic Brain Injury With Moderate Hypothermia
Marion DW, Penrod LE, Kelsey SF, et al (Univ of Pittsburgh, Pa)
N Engl J Med 336:540–546, 1997 4–11

Objective.—In patients with traumatic brain injury, several metabolic processes are initiated that can worsen the severity of injury. Recent evidence suggests that some of these harmful metabolic responses may be reduced by hypothermia. A randomized, controlled trial of moderate hypothermia for patients with traumatic brain injury is reported.

Methods.—The study included 82 patients with severe closed-head injuries, each with a Glasgow Coma Scale (GCS) score of 3–7. Patients were randomized to a hypothermia or normothermia group. Those assigned to the hypothermia group were cooled to 33°C immediately after enrollment, a mean of 10 hours after injury. Their temperature was maintained at 32°C

TABLE 2.—Glasgow Outcome Scores in the Hypothermia and Normothermia Groups at 3, 6, and 12 Months*

Glasgow Outcome Score	At 3 Months		At 6 Months		At 12 Months	
	Hypothermia	Normothermia	Hypothermia	Normothermia	Hypothermia†	Normothermia
	number of patients (percent)					
All patients						
1 (Death)	8 (20)	9 (21)	8 (20)	10 (24)	9 (23)	10 (24)
2 (Vegetative state)	6 (15)	11 (26)	3 (8)	7 (17)	3 (8)	8 (19)
3 (Severe disability)	11 (28)	15 (36)	7 (18)	11 (26)	3 (8)	8 (19)
4 (Moderate disability)	8 (20)	4 (10)	7 (18)	8 (19)	9 (23)	5 (12)
5 (Mild or no disability)	7 (18)	3 (7)	15 (38)	6 (14)	15 (38)	11 (26)
Total	40	42	40	42	39	42
P value‡	0.12		0.05		0.18	
Patients with coma score of 5 to 7						
1 (Death)	2 (9)	5 (19)	2 (9)	6 (23)	2 (9)	6 (23)
2 (Vegetative state)	2 (9)	7 (27)	1 (5)	3 (12)	1 (5)	4 (15)
3 (Severe disability)	6 (27)	9 (35)	3 (14)	8 (31)	3 (14)	6 (23)
4 (Moderate disability)	6 (27)	3 (12)	4 (18)	6 (23)	5 (23)	2 (8)
5 (Mild or no disability)	6 (27)	2 (8)	12 (55)	3 (12)	11 (50)	8 (31)
Total	22	26	22	26	22	26
P value‡	0.01		0.01		0.04	

*Percentages may not add up to 100 because of rounding.

†One patient was lost to follow-up.

‡*P* values are for comparison of all 5 outcomes in the hypothermia and normothermia groups.

(Reprinted by permission of *The New England Journal of Medicine*, from Marion DW, Penrod LE, Kelsey SF, et al: Treatment of traumatic brain injury with moderate hypothermia. *N Engl J Med* 336:540–546, 1997.)

to 33°C for 24 hours, after which they were rewarmed. The GCS was used to assess patient outcomes after 3, 6, and 12 months.

Results.—The 2 groups were similar in their demographic characteristics and in the causes and severity of their injuries. The 12-month evaluations found moderate, mild, or no disabilities in 62% of the hypothermia group versus 38% of the normothermia group. When the GCS score was 3 or 4 at admission, patient outcomes were unaffected by hypothermia. However, when the admission GCS score was 5–7, outcomes at 3 and 6 months were significantly improved (adjusted risk ratio for a poor outcome, 0.2). However, hypothermia made no significant difference in 12-month outcomes for this group (risk ratio, 0.3) (Table 2).

Conclusions.—Moderate hypothermia appears to improve outcomes for some patients with traumatic brain injury, for example, those with admission GCS scores of 5–7. For patients managed with hypothermia, outcomes are significantly better at 3–6 months and tend to be better at 12 months.

▶ Improving the long-term clinical outcome of patients with traumatic brain injury is one of the major challenges of modern trauma care. While prevention of secondary brain injuries through the avoidance of hypoxia and hypotension has been shown to improve long-term neurologic outcome, more is needed, especially in those patients with the most severe neurologic injuries (GCS < 7). Therefore, this promising randomized, controlled clinical trial, showing that a 24- to 36-hour period of hypothermia (32°C to 33°C) initiated shortly after injury resulted in a significant improvement in functional outcome, was chosen for inclusion in this year's articles.

E.A. Deitch, M.D.

A Prospective, Randomized Trial of Intravenous Fat Emulsion Administration in Trauma Victims Requiring Total Parenteral Nutrition

Battistella FD, Widergren JT, Anderson JT, et al (Univ of California, Sacramento)

J Trauma: Injury Infect Crit Care 43:52–57, 1997 4–12

Introduction.—Several recent studies report an increased incidence of infectious complications in surgically stressed patients administered total parenteral nutrition (TPN). In more recent trials, patients received 20% to 30% of nonprotein calories as an IV fat emulsion (IVFE). In contrast, smaller amounts or no IV lipids were given in previous trials. In a study of 60 polytrauma patients, the effects of withholding fat infusions from TPN were examined.

Methods.—Patients were randomly allocated to a standard fat emulsion dose (L) or to have fat infusions withheld (NL) for the first 10 days of TPN. With the exception of fat emulsion, the TPN regimen was similar in the 2 groups. Clinical outcome parameters, including infectious complications and clinical signs of fatty acid deficiency, were measured; T-cell

TABLE 3.—Clinical Outcome Parameters for Patients Randomized to Receive or Not Receive Lipid Emulsion as Part of the Total Parental Nutrition Regimen

	Lipid	No Lipid	p
Hospital length of stay (days)	39 ± 24	27 ± 16	0.03
ICU length of stay (days)	29 ± 22	18 ± 12	0.02
Days requiring mechanical ventilation	27 ± 21	15 ± 12	0.01

Abbreviation: TPN, total parenteral nutrition.
(Courtesy of Battistella FD, Widergren JT, Anderson JT, et al: A prospective, randomized trial of intravenous fat emulsion administration in trauma victims requiring total parenteral nutrition. *J Trauma: Injury, Infection, and Critical Care* 43(1):52–57, 1997.)

function was assessed by measuring lymphokine activated killer cell activity and natural killer cell activity.

Results.—Outcome data were available for 57 patients, 30 in the L group and 27 in the NL group. The 2 groups were similar in demographics, including Injury Severity Score and APACHE II scores. No patient was underweight at admission or showed clinical signs of fatty acid deficiency. The hospital courses of the 2 groups differed significantly in a number of measures (Table 3). The lipid group required a longer period of mechanical ventilation, had a longer ICU stay, and had a longer hospital stay. There were more infectious complications in the L group (72 overall, average 2.4 per patient) than in the NL group (39 overall, average 1.4 per patient). Whereas T-cell function (both activated killer cell and natural killer cell activities) improved from baseline values during the first 5 days of TPN in the NL group, the L group showed deterioration of T-cell function. None of the patients exhibited clinical signs of fatty acid deficiency during hospitalization.

Conclusion.—In this group of trauma patients, the inclusion of IV lipids in TPN increased susceptibility to infection, prolonged pulmonary failure, and delayed recovery in the early postinjury period. Improved outcome in the NL group may be directly related to withholding IV lipids or to the underfeeding that resulted.

► The take-home message of this prospective randomized trial is that IV fat should not be part of the TPN formula administered to trauma patients, because its administration is associated with an increased incidence of infectious complications and a prolonged ICU stay. Although one can quibble with the study design, I liked this study, because it fits a large body of somewhat ignored information documenting that IV fats are immunosuppressive and may have deleterious pulmonary effects. In fact, the authors' justification for carrying out this study was their impression from the literature that the recent addition of fat to TPN feeding regimens explains the increase in infectious complications observed in patients receiving TPN. That is, in earlier TPN studies, when fat was not routinely administered, the incidence of infectious complications was much lower than that observed in more recent studies in which TPN-fed patients received IV fat.

It is also important to stress that the population of trauma patients studied was limited to those patients who could not tolerate enteral feeding by the fifth postinjury day and thus required parenteral nutrition to meet their nutritional needs. Consequently, the results of the study should not be interpreted to indicate that enteral alimentation is not superior to parenteral nutrition.

E.A. Deitch, M.D.

Bullets and Their Role in Sepsis After Colon Wounds

Sarmiento JM, Yugueros P, Garcia AF, et al (Universidad del Valle, Cali, Colombia; Mayo Clinic, Rochester, Minn)

World J Surg 21:648–652, 1997 4–13

Objective.—Studies disagree as to whether the presence of a retained bullet after colonic wounds increases the risk of abdominal sepsis. The authors have observed a high incidence of infectious complications among patients with bullets left in place. They studied the association between the presence of a retained bullet after gunshot wounds to the colon and the incidence of sepsis in the bullet track and in the soft tissue in which it is retained.

Methods.—The investigators reviewed the records of 185 consecutive patients hospitalized with abdominal gunshot wounds and laparotomy-confirmed colonic injury. The patients were divided into 3 groups. The 21 patients in group 1 had the bullet removed at surgery, together with additional cleansing and debridement. The 81 patients in group 2 had the bullet left in place. In the case of the 83 patients in group 3, the bullet exited spontaneously; these patients underwent only debridement of the skin. The 3 groups were compared for their incidence of sepsis.

Results.—Patients in group 3 had a higher incidence of shock than the other 2 groups. The incidence of sepsis was 5% in group 1, compared with 25% in group 2 and 37% in group 3. In group 3, there were 46 cases of soft tissue abscess, 3 of osteomyelitis, and 6 of necrotizing fasciitis. Some patients had more than 1 infectious complication.

Conclusion.—For patients with gunshot wounds causing injury to the colon, the presence of a retained bullet increases the risk of sepsis. Patients with such injuries should undergo removal of the bullet, if possible, and local tissue debridement. Those in whom the bullet has exited spontaneously should undergo debridement of the bullet track with extensive lavage.

► In general, bullets have been considered to be sterile because of their high velocity and the resultant friction generated. However, the subgroup of patients in whom the bullet passes through the colon appear to be at high risk of development of an infection within the bullet tract. Based on this study and other information in the literature, it appears wise to remove the bullet and debride bullet tracts when the bullet has traversed the colon, as the belief that bullets are always sterile is clearly not true. As a corollary, should signs of an occult infection develop in a patient with a gunshot wound of the colon, one should remember not to overlook the bullet tract as a potential source of infection.

E.A. Deitch, M.D.

Adult Respiratory Distress Syndrome, Pneumonia, and Mortality Following Thoracic Injury and a Femoral Fracture Treated Either With Intramedullary Nailing With Reaming or With a Plate: A Comparative Study

Bosse MJ, MacKenzie EJ, Reimer BL, et al (Carolinas Med Ctr, Charlotte, NC; Allegheny Gen Hosp, Pittsburgh, Pa; Johns Hopkins Univ, Baltimore, Md; et al)

J Bone Joint Surg Am 79-A:799–809, 1997 4–14

Introduction.—The well-established practice of delaying early fixation of femoral fractures with intramedullary nailing and reaming in multiply injured patients because of concern about pulmonary outcomes has been questioned. The rate of adult respiratory distress syndrome (ARDS) was retrospectively assessed in multiply injured patients with fractures of the femoral shaft and thoracic injuries admitted to 1 of 2 level I regional trauma centers.

Methods.—The centers were similar in patient populations and protocols for treatment of trauma. Center 1 used intramedullary nailing with reaming in 217 of 229 patients (95%), and center 2 used a plate in 206 of 224 patients (92%). The rate of ARDS at the 2 centers was compared in multiply injured patients with chest injuries. Medical records were reviewed to determine duration of intubation, duration of hospitalizations, and occurrence of adverse outcomes. Patients were stratified into subgroups according to the presence or absence of thoracic injuries and according to Injury Severity Scores. Three groups of patients were followed up: those with fractures of the femur and thoracic injuries, those with fractures of the femur and no thoracic injuries, and those with thoracic injuries and no fractures of the femur or tibia. The third group at each center was evaluated to determine whether there was a difference between institutions regarding ARDS rates.

Results.—The ARDS rates were 6% (8 patients) for 129 patients at center 1 with thoracic injuries and no femoral fractures compared with 8% (10 patients) for 125 patients at center 2. The rate of ARDS was similar for patients at both centers with femoral fractures and no thoracic injuries. Rates of ARDS, pneumonia, pulmonary embolisms, failure of multiple organs, and death were similar at both institutions for patients with thoracic injuries and femoral fractures, regardless of whether nailing with reaming (117 patients) or plates (104 patients) were used.

Conclusion.—These findings do not support the practice of delaying fixation of femoral fractures with nailing and reaming in patients with thoracic injuries. Patient outcomes were similar when nailing with reaming or plates were used.

▶ During the last few years, the following concept has been suggested: that immediate long-bone fracture fixation in patients with trauma and concomitant thoracic injuries is associated with an increased incidence of pulmonary complications. This concept was based on clinical data first presented by Pape et al.[1] and supported by experimental studies indicating that femoral canal reaming in preparation for femoral nailing resulted in the liberation of bone marrow contents, which accentuated the degree of pulmonary dysfunction in patients with significant thoracic injuries. Proposed solutions to this problem were to delay femoral fracture fixation for 2–3 days or, if immediate fracture fixation were to take place, to use alternative operative strategies (i.e., femoral nailing without reaming of the bone or the use of plate fixation). However, not all trauma teams accepted this notion that early fracture fixation using intramedullary nailing with reaming was deleterious. Consequently, the authors of this paper tested this concept by comparing the clinical course of 2 large cohorts of patients who had fracture fixation either by intramedullary nailing with reaming or with a plate.

Although the study was retrospective, this study of more than 600 patients was well done, and all the necessary controls were included. Thus, their observation that both methods of immediate fracture fixation were equivalent and appeared safe in patients with thoracic injuries is compelling. After reading this and similarly published papers, I am beginning to wonder whether the fear of immediate fracture fixation in patients with thoracic injuries might just be an example of crying wolf. This is not to say that in some patients with severe pulmonary contusions delaying fracture fixation for 2–3 days may not be prudent. However, it does indicate that the majority of patients with thoracic injuries can safely undergo immediate fracture fixation. As more data are generated, it should be possible to resolve this clinically important controversy.

E.A. Deitch, M.D.

Reference

1. Pape HC, Auf'm'Kolk M, Paffrath T, et al: Primary intramedullary femur fixation in multiple trauma patients with associated lung contusion—a cause of posttraumatic ARDS? *J Trauma* 34:540–547, 1993.

Influence of Continuous Hemofiltration on the Hemodynamics of Trauma Patients

S-Izquierdo Riera JA, Alted E, Lozano MJ, et al (12 De Octubre Univ, Madrid)
Surgery 122:902–908, 1997 4–15

Introduction.—The prognosis of patients with multiple organ dysfunction syndrome (MODS) remains poor, despite improvements in hemodynamic and respiratory support. Continuous renal replacement therapies

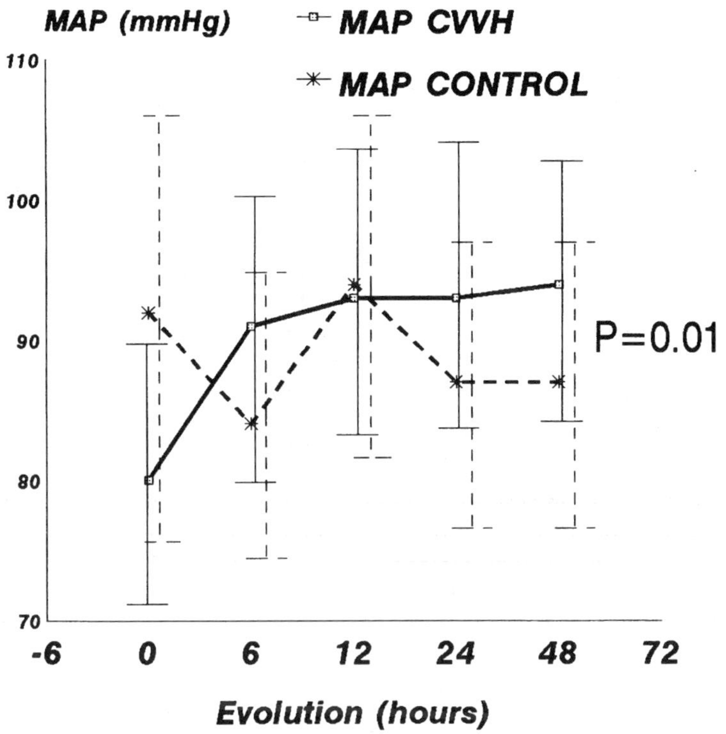

FIGURE 1.—Mean arterial pressure (MAP) evolution in study patients (mean plus or minus standard error of the mean). Significant improvements in continuous venovenous hemofiltration (CVVH) group was found. (Courtesy of S-Izquierdo Riera JA, Alted E, Lozano MJ, et al: Influence of continuous hemofiltration on the hemodynamics of trauma patients. *Surgery* 122:902–208, 1997.)

CVVH

have the potential to remove circulating low molecular weight toxins and mediators from the intravascular space that may be responsible for adult respiratory distress syndrome and MODS. Few trials have examined the hemodynamic and respiratory response to continuous venovenous hemofiltration (CVVH) in critically ill patients. The effect of CVVH on the hemodynamics and respiratory function of critically ill trauma patients with MODS was evaluated.

Methods.—Thirty consecutive patients with severe trauma and incipient traumatic MODS without kidney failure were randomized to treatment with or without CVVH. Mean Injury Severity Score of each group was 30–32. Hemodynamic profiles were recorded before hemofiltration started and at 6, 12, and 48 hours after its initiation. Ventilatory support parameters remained the same throughout.

Results.—Patients who received CVVH had significant improvements in mean arterial pressure and the partial pressure of oxygen in arterial blood–inspiratory oxygen supply index (Fig 1). There were no significant between-group differences in any other variables.

Conclusion.—Significant improvements in hemodynamic and respiratory variables were observed in critically ill patients with severe trauma and MODS who underwent CVVH. This invasive technique needs further study to determine whether it can decrease the high mortality in this patient cohort.

► As stated by the authors, this is the first prospective, randomized, controlled trial of CVVH in trauma patients with acute respiratory failure and MODS without renal failure to test whether CVVH would improve oxygenation and the hemodynamic response. As illustrated in Figure 1, it appears that the institution of CVVH improves oxygenation and raises the mean arterial pressure. Although the mortality rate of the patients receiving CVVH was less than that of the control group (47% vs. 27%), this improvement in the survival rate did not reach statistical significance, perhaps because of the small size of the study populations.

Because CVVH appears to improve outcome in patients with trauma and MODS without renal failure, the obvious next question is how does it do this. One putative mechanism is that CVVH improves the patient's physiologic response by the removal of potential toxins or proinflammatory factors, such as cytokines, from the circulation. This notion is supported by several uncontrolled clinical studies documenting that plasma cytokines can be removed from the plasma by CVVH. In a second paper describing this patient population,[1] the authors report that approximately 100–150 µg/day of tumor necrosis factor (TNF) and 2,000 µg per day of interleukin-6 (IL-6) were removed in the CVVH filtrate. These results support the concept that CVVH can remove proinflammatory cytokines. However, there is a problem. The plasma levels of TNF and IL-6 were similar between the patients treated with CVVH and the patients in the control group throughout the period of study, which indicates that the beneficial effects of CVVH were not directly related to a decrease in TNF or IL-6 plasma levels. Thus, the mechanism by which CVVH worked in these patients remain unknown.

The take-home message is that when the engine begins to malfunction, it may be time for an oil change.

E.A. Deitch, M.D.

Reference

1. Sanchez Izquierdo JA, Perez Vela JL, Lozano Quintana MJ, et al: Cytokines clearance during venovenous hemofiltration in the trauma patient. *Am J Kidney Dis* 30:483–488, 1997.

Prediction of Posttraumatic Adult Respiratory Distress Syndrome by Albumin Excretion Rate Eight Hours After Admission

Pallister I, Gosling P, Alpar K, et al (Univ Hosp Birmingham Natl Health Service Trust, England)

J Trauma: Injury Infect Crit Care 42:1056–1061, 1997 4–16

Introduction.—Increased capillary permeability develops early in the course of adult respiratory distress syndrome (ARDS) and can lead to interstitial edema. Increased microvascular permeability in the kidney gives rise to increased excretion of albumin, which can be detected by a sensitive immunoassay. The ability of excessive microalbuminuria to predict developing ARDS was studied.

Methods.—The study included 47 trauma patients, 32 with Injury Severity Scores of greater than 18. Thirteen of these patients had pulmonary dysfunction, including 8 patients with ARDS. The near patient urine albumin immunoassay was used to measure albumin excretion rate (AER) after admission. The results were compared with the severity of injury and the development of ARDS or pulmonary dysfunction.

Results.—Eight hours after admission of patients with an Injury Severity Score of greater than 18, the median AER was 63 μg/min for patients without pulmonary abnormality compared with 339 μg/min for those with pulmonary dysfunction or ARDS. For the range of values, the figures were 40 to 99 μg/min and 162 to 454 μg/min, respectively. An AER of greater than 130 μg/min had an 85% positive predictive value and a 95% negative predictive value for the development of ARDS or pulmonary dysfunction.

Conclusion.—In trauma patients, the AER at 8 hours after admission can identify capillary leak associated with the development of pulmonary dysfunction and ARDS. This provides a useful bedside test for early identification and management of patients at high risk of ARDS. A multicenter trial to confirm the predictive value of this test is underway.

► Although the results of this clinical study are limited by the small number of patients studied and must be verified in future studies, if it is true that it is possible, within 8 hours of injury, to identify patients who will develop pulmonary dysfunction by measuring urinary albumin levels, this approach will likely find widespread use. For example, by identifying high-risk patients early, it would be possible to selectively use specific approaches before the development of ARDS. It would, likewise, be possible to correctly identify appropriate patients for enrollment into clinical trials testing new therapeutic agents.

The physiologic concept behind measuring the urinary microalbumin excretion rate is that when microvascular permeability is increased, albumin will leak out of the renal microvasculature and, thus, be detectable in the urine. In this situation, increased urinary albumin will reflect a generalized state of increased capillary leak and, thus, mirror what is occurring in the pulmonary microcirculation. Future clinical trials will establish whether this prognostic test is too good to be true.

E.A. Deitch, M.D.

The Immune Microenviroment of Human Fracture/Soft-Tissue Hematomas and Its Relationship to Systemic Immunity

Hauser CJ, Zhou X, Joshi P, et al (Univ of Medicine and Dentistry of New Jersey, Newark; Univ of Mississippi, Jackson)

J Trauma: Injury Infect Crit Care 42:895–904, 1997 4–17

Purpose.—It is generally agreed that the development of sepsis after trauma can be related to either impaired immune responses to bacteria or to a nonbacterially mediated inflammatory response to injury. Little is known regarding the immune environment of soft tissue injuries in humans. This issue was addressed in a study of patients undergoing open reduction and internal fixation for major fractures.

Methods.—The study included 56 patients with fracture soft-tissue hematomas (FxSTHs) associated with a high-energy mechanism of injury. The immune environment of the injuries was studied by sampling FxSTH serum and mononuclear cells. Plasma and blood mononuclear cells from the fracture patients and from 20 uninjured controls were studied as well.

Findings.—Plasma specimens from control subjects rarely showed cytokines, and the FxSTH, serum, or plasma from fracture patients rarely showed tumor necrosis factor (TNF)-α, interleukin (IL)-1β, IL-2, or interferon-γ. However, The FxTSH sera showed high levels of IL-6, which peaked by 48 hours. Although IL-6 was usually not detected in plasma in the early stages after fracture, it increased after 48 hours. After 72 hours, circulating IL-8 was detected. There was a gradient in IL-6 and IL-8 levels between FxSTH serum and paired patient serum. In the first 48 hours, the only cytokine that was higher in fracture patient plasma than in FxSTH serum was IL-12, with concentrations of 1,279 and 591 pg/mL, respectively. The FxSTH monocytes showed greater upregulation of cell membrane TNF-α than did peripheral blood monocytes (3,202 vs. 584 sites/cell, respectively). Expression of human leukocyte antigen was far lower in fracture and peripheral blood monocytes than in control monocytes.

Conclusion.—The findings document the presence of an inflammatory local environment around major fractures. Because of the high local levels of IL-6, IL-8, and IL-10 in the fracture site, the wound presumably exported levels of cytokines to the plasma. In trauma patients, the FxSTH may be an important source of immunomodulatory cytokines.

▶ This study was chosen because it is the first human study to examine the local wound immuno-inflammatory microenvironment, as well as the potential relationship between the local wound and the systemic immune and inflammatory responses in trauma patients. This relationship between the wound and the systemic host response is of potential clinical importance, because locally generated wound factors (such as cytokines) could directly modulate the systemic immune response, as well as contribute to the hypermetabolic response observed after trauma. Although more work needs to be done to verify and expand the authors' findings, their conclusion that wound hematomas are potentially important sources of immunomodulatory cytokines is worthy of keeping in mind. It provides further impetus for the practice of good wound debridement and the evacuation of hematomas.

E.A. Deitch, M.D.

Trauma–Hemorrhage Induces Increased Thymic Apoptosis While Decreasing IL-3 Release and Increasing GM-CSF[1]

Xu YX, Wichmann MW, Ayala A, et al (Brown Univ, Providence, RI; Rhode Island Hosp, Providence)

J Surg Res 68:24–30, 1997 4–18

Background.—The thymus is known to play a key role in the ontogeny of T lymphocytes. However, we know little about how the thymus is affected by hemorrhage and/or trauma, which are known to produce a severe and prolonged state of immunodepression. The potential effects of trauma or hemorrhage on thymic apoptosis were experimentally assessed in mice, including an evaluation of which, if any, mediators are involved in this process.

Methods.—Male C3H/HeN mice were assigned to 1 of 4 groups. One group underwent a sham operation; one group was subjected to hemorrhagic shock, to produce a mean arterial blood pressure of 35 mm Hg for 90 minutes, followed by blood and fluid resuscitation; one group was subjected to fracture of the right tibia; and one was subjected to fracture plus hemorrhage. Three days later, the animals' total viable thymocyte yield was assessed. Thymocyte apoptosis was measured by flow cytometry, thymus-derived interleukin (IL)-3 by bioassay, and granulocyte-macrophage colony-stimulating factor (GM-CSF) by enzyme-linked immunosorbent assay. The goal was to see whether severe trauma and hemorrhage induced thymic atrophy via apoptosis, and whether changes in the release of hematopoietic factors played a role in this process.

Results.—None of the measured parameters changed significantly in response to fracture only. However, mice subjected to hemorrhage or fracture plus hemorrhage showed a significant reduction in total viable thymocyte yield. Animals in these same 2 groups also had a significant reduction in thymocyte IL-3 release. Animals undergoing fracture plus hemorrhage had a significant increase in thymus-derived GM-CSF. However, this parameter was unaffected by hemorrhage alone.

Conclusions.—In this animal model, severe hemorrhage—alone or accompanied by fracture—can lead to thymic atrophy by way of apoptosis. These conditions also reduce IL-3 release, suggesting that lack of growth factor support may cause apoptotic thymic involution. The resulting inappropriate or inadequate T-cell maturation could play a role in host immune suppression. The systemic inflammatory response observed in victims of trauma and hemorrhage could be partly related to an increase in thymus-derived GM-CSF.

▶ Because infection is a common consequence of injury and the development of infection can lead to death, the goal of understanding how immune suppression occurs after trauma has been intensely studied for more than 25 years. The idea is that, once one understands the mechanisms that cause a specific immune defect, one can develop therapeutic strategies aimed at reversing that defect. Thus, there is value in this basic science article on trauma and hemorrhage-induced thymic lymphocyte apoptosis.

The term *apoptosis* comes from the Greek and means "falling leaves." It was used to described a nonnecrotic form of cell death, where the cells basically shrivel up and die. A basic difference between apoptotic cell death and necrotic cell death is that in apoptotic cell death the cells die without causing an inflammatory response. Apoptosis also has been referred to as "programmed cell death." Over the past 5 years, it has become clear that apoptosis is a common mechanism used by all mammals to clear the body of senescent cells as well as to regulate growth and development. Likewise, studies such as the one selected indicate that apoptosis may play a significant role in the development of immune suppression observed after trauma. Because apoptosis is highly likely to be shown to be a major factor in the pathogenesis of the immune and inflammatory consequences of trauma and sepsis, it is important for clinicians to know about this process.

E.A. Deitch, M.D.

Unexpected Action of Platelet Activating Factor Antagonism After Fluid Resuscitation From Traumatic Shock

Schurr MJ, Fabian TC, Croce MA, et al (Univ of Tennessee, Memphis; Univ of Wisconsin, Madison)

Surgery 121:493–500, 1997 4–19

Introduction.—Previous research has suggested that blocking non–CD18-dependent polymorphonuclear neutrophil (PMN) adherence may reduce pulmonary dysfunction observed in response to trauma or lipopolysaccharide (LPS) challenge. If so, then blocking platelet-activating factor (PAF) with the receptor antagonist WEB-2086 could have benefits similar to those of anti-CD18 therapy. This hypothesis was examined in a study of pigs.

Methods.—Experiments were performed in anesthetized swine that underwent soft-tissue injury to the hind limb with 30% hemorrhage. They were resuscitated after 1 hour using shed blood and lactated Ringer's solution, plus either WEB-2086, 10 mg/kg/hr, or vehicle. At 72 hours, an LPS challenge was given. The same challenge was also administered to pigs that had not been traumatized and bled, but had been treated with WEB-

2086 or vehicle. A PAF dose-response curve was calculated by administering PAF before and after trauma.

Results.—Mortality 72 hours after trauma was increased in animals receiving PAF blockade—5 of 11 swine in the WEB-2086 group died, compared with 1 of 9 in the vehicle group. WEB-2086 administration was also associated with depressed cardiac index and oxygen delivery. Compared with vehicle-treated animals, those receiving WEB-2086 did not have the same hyperdynamic circulatory compensation in response to LPS challenge. In nontraumatized pigs, WEB-2086 treatment reduced mortality—4 of 5 animals in the WEB-2086 group survived for 5 hours, compared with 2 of 5 in the vehicle group. Blockade of PAF was also associated with improved arterial PO_2 and base excess at 1 hour after LPS challenge.

Conclusions.—These surprising experimental findings suggest that the PAF receptor antagonist WEB-2086 has opposite effects in the presence and absence of trauma. The results indicate a possible homeostatic role of PAF in the compensatory response to injury. Blockade of endogenous mediators—depending on the timing of administration and the subjects' underlying condition—may have a beneficial or harmful effect. Further research in relevant animal models is needed before the clinical application of endogenous mediator blockade in trauma patients.

▶ This article was chosen because it highlights an important and critical but often neglected point. That is, that results using one experimental model may not predict results in a different model. Let me illustrate. As would be predicted from the literature on sepsis, the authors found that blocking PAF protected animals challenged with endotoxin. This part of the study was consistent with other published reports indicating that elevated levels of PAF are bad and that by neutralizing this pro-inflammatory mediator, survival can be improved. In fact, based on this type of animal data, PAF antagonists are being used in clinical trials. Now comes the rub. When the authors tested PAF blockade in a more clinically-relevant model of trauma and hemorrhage, PAF blockade unexpectedly did not protect the animals but instead worsened survival.

This article serves to remind all of us that the response of an injured patient is complex and coordinated and that optimistic results obtained from agents tested in simplistic and clinically-irrelevant models may not hold up in a more real-life-type situation.

E.A. Deitch, M.D.

Rehabilitation Results of Patients With Multiple Injuries and Multiple Organ Failure and Long-term Intensive Care

Grotz M, Hohensee A, Remmers D, et al (Hannover Med School, Germany)

J Trauma 42:919–926, 1997 4–20

Objective.—For trauma patients in the ICU, the main complication is multiple organ failure (MOF). The incidence and mortality of this com-

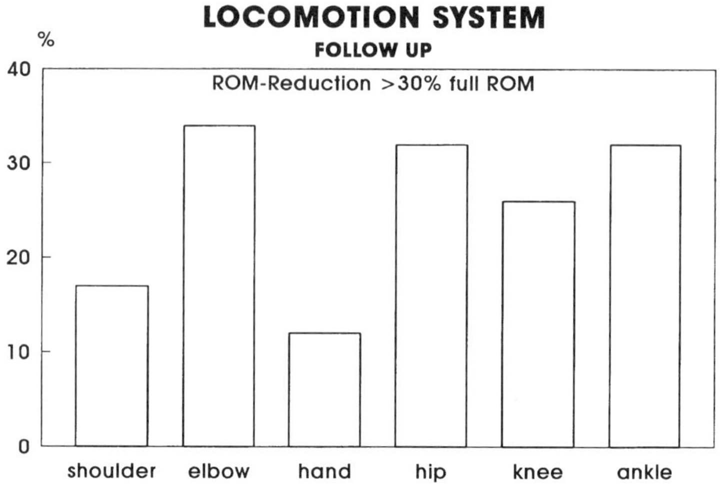

FIGURE 6.—Rehabilitation of the locomotive system. Limitations of range of motion (ROM) of more than 30% of the normal range of motion for different joints. (Courtesy of Grotz M, Hohensee A, Remmers D, et al: Rehabilitation results of patients with multiple injuries and multiple organ failure and long-term intensive care. *J Trauma: Injury Infect Crit Care* 42:919–926, 1997.)

plication have been little changed over the years. Thorough assessment of the functional outcomes of patients with MOF must include inquiry into the potential effects on social and occupational quality of life. Few studies have specifically examined the long-term results of rehabilitation for patients with MOF. Survivors of multiple trauma and MOF were studied to identify any permanent sequelae in the affected organs and to document the long-term functional and occupational rehabilitation results.

Methods.—The study included 50 patients with multiple injuries and MOF treated in 1 trauma department over a 10-year period. The patients had a mean injury severity score of 36.8 and a mean Glasgow Coma Scale score of 10.4. Mean ICU time was 30 days and average ventilator time was 25 days. Follow-up examinations were conducted a mean of 5 years after the trauma. Laboratory tests of lung, liver, kidney, and hematologic function were performed to assess possible organotropic aftereffects of MOF. The rehabilitation results were assessed in terms of function (i.e., locomotor and neurologic function) and occupational status.

Results.—The laboratory tests were mainly normal, with pathologic results noted only on pulmonary function tests. Nearly one fifth of patients had abnormalities on spirometric, body plethysmographic, or carbon monoxide diffusion capacity testing. Joint range of motion was permanently reduced—i.e., more than 30% limitation of elbow, hip, knee, or ankle motion—in more than one fourth of patients (Fig 6). About one fourth of patients did not attain the maximal Glasgow Outcome Score of 5. Forty percent of patients had permanent motor nerve lesions, while 50% had permanent sensory nerve lesions. Of patients who had been working full-time at the time of trauma, 60% had returned to work.

Conclusions.—For survivors of multiple trauma and MOF, no major organ function abnormalities are apparent at a mean 5 years' follow-up. The results of rehabilitation, in terms of function and occupation, are excellent. Many patients are left with permanent central or peripheral paralysis and decreased range of joint motion. However, most survivors are still able to return to work.

► A question often asked by families is what kind of long-term problems can the patient expect to have once they leave the hospital. Answering this question about trauma patients with MOF is difficult in the absence of long-term data. Thus, the value of this clinical study indicating that lung, kidney, and hepatic organ function tends to fully recover over time. As illustrated in the study, residual disability seems to be related to limitations in joint movement and polyneuropathies and to the fact that these limitations generally do not prevent employment. These optimistic findings should help all of us answer our patients' families' questions. In case one questions the severity of the organ failure in this study group, I point out that the mean time these patients were intubated was 26 days, their mean hospitalization period was 2 months, and the majority of patients spent an average of 5 months in a rehabilitation facility after discharge from the hospital.

E.A. Deitch, M.D.

5 Infection

Introduction

Surgical infections continue to affect the practice of every surgeon. At minimum, they lead to inconvenience for the patient (and surgeon). Infections can increase a patient's stay in the hospital, create discomfort, cause disfigurement, and lead to failure of the operation. At worst, they cause death. Therefore, infections always have been and most likely always will be of great concern for the surgeon. The first paper reviewed (Abstract 5–1) discusses the risk of HIV infection among surgeons and other health care workers. Although reviews are not usually included in the YEAR BOOK OF SURGERY, this was felt to be important enough to be included here. While HIV is of great concern to the surgeon, hepatitis B and hepatitis C are much more common infections in health care personnel. The transmission of hepatitis B to patients from infected surgeons is reported by Heptonstall (Abstract 5–2). Previously, surgeons without hepatitis B e antigen were thought to be at low risk for transmitting hepatitis B, but this report provides information on four surgeons who transmitted hepatitis to their patients. None of the surgeons had the hepatitis B e antigen.

Three other articles also deal with the epidemiology of infections. Abstracts 5–3 to 5–5 discuss the basis of surgical site infection and how to have an effective surgical site surveillance program. With so many outpatient operations being done or because hospital stays have been shortened, most surgical infections now occur after patients have been discharged from the hospital. Surveillance of these infections is increasingly difficult and expensive, especially because of the potential sanctions against surgeons whose patients are identified with postoperative infections. Abstract 5–3 discusses measures of intrinsic risk of postoperative infections in surgical patients by using two previous indices that came out of the Centers for Disease Control and Prevention. Both these indices were based on large population studies of postoperative wound infections (currently called *surgical site infections*), but they may also be used as risk indices of infections in other surgical sites. Another method is studied by Manian and Meyer (Abstract 5–4). They find that monthly physician questionnaires for surveillance can be useful in providing additional data about surgical site infection.

Bacterial translocation is an important potential source of infection in surgical patients. MacFie (Abstract 5–7) investigated the occurrence of bacterial translocation in patients having surgical procedures. While bacterial translocation can be demonstrated, its importance in clinical infection is less certain.

Two studies address the use of antibiotics in surgery. A study by Ho and Fry (Abstract 5–8) investigated the use of antibiotic prophylaxis in severe acute pancreatitis, something that has been previously investigated. The authors limited their subjects to those with severe acute pancreatitis. The use of prophylaxis significantly reduced the infection rate but did not significantly affect survival. Yet infection was the only thing antibiotic prophylaxis should affect. Many other factors also enter into whether the patient survives. Numerous antibiotic prophylaxis trials have been performed. Before a new antibiotic is marketed, randomized, controlled trials must be done. Very few have been reported in recent years in the YEAR BOOK OF SURGERY. One such study is reported this year, not only because it was a well-done trial but also because it reports on an antibiotic that appears to be as effective as, and possibly an improvement over, imipenem/cilistatin (Abstract 5–9). As in virtually all recent antibiotic trials, meropenem was as effective as the control antibiotics (clindamycin/tobramycin). Because existing antibiotics are so effective for the treatment of severe surgical infections, it is unlikely that any new antibiotic will ever be shown in a controlled trial to be more effective than what is currently available. Such a study will be too expensive for pharmaceutical companies to conduct because so many patients would have to be included to achieve statistical significance.

Poor outcome from peritonitis was found by Wickel (Abstract 5–10) to be due to the systemic effects of peritonitis rather than to recurrent peritoneal infection. We are getting better at controlling the local effects of infections, but the systemic effects continue to be responsible for much of the mortality. Sautner (Abstract 5–11) raises a question of whether reoperation for the treatment of abdominal sepsis enhances the systemic inflammatory response. If patients have recurrent or tertiary peritonitis, another operation is necessary if they are likely to survive. The authors find that reoperation may also cause substantial hypotension and harm. Percutaneous drainage of intra-abdominal abscess in patients with Crohn's disease was studied by Sahai and others (Abstract 5–12). They found that percutaneous drainage of abscess in patients with Crohn's disease can prevent the need for early operation and make later operation more successful and also can shorten hospital stay. Whedell et al. (Abstract 5–13) studied the surgical management of complicated diverticulitis. These authors found that, of the many procedures for complicated diverticulitis, resection with primary anastomosis was the safest and reduced cost—something that differs with classic teaching of first draining the abscess and performing a colostomy. A two-stage procedure superseded a three-stage procedure for complicated diverticulitis. Now the authors propose to treat this problem with a single-stage procedure.

Appendicitis is the focus of two studies. Recurrent appendicitis does exist and affects at least 6.5% of those who ultimately require appendectomy. Hallan et al. (Abstract 5–15) wrote a controversial paper discussing the value of biochemical tests in suspected acute appendicitis. Certainly, appendicitis is largely a clinical diagnosis. The authors found that biochemical tests contributed to their computer models and could provide important additional information. Many would disagree with this controversial paper. The attempts of many computer models at diagnosis have not been as successful as good clinicians. The hope is that eventually computers will be as good as, or better than, clinicians in making diagnoses, but this has not yet occurred.

Richard J. Howard, M.D., Ph.D.

The Surgeon's Database for AIDS: A Collective Review

Flum DR, Wallack MK (St Vincents Hosp and Med Ctr, New York)

J Am Coll Surg 184:403–412, 1997 5–1

Introduction.—Surgical practice has been greatly affected by the emergence of HIV and AIDS. Surgeons have been at the forefront in discussing such issues as the risks to surgeons operating on HIV-infected patients, the value of chemoprophylaxis after a needlestick, the chances that an infected surgeon will transmit HIV to a patient, and whether mandatory testing should be performed. The authors reviewed the literature to provide an accessible database for practicing surgeons with questions about HIV and AIDS.

Findings.—The review includes information on the epidemiology of HIV, surgeons' attitudes toward HIV infection, the risks of blood contact, how seroconversion occurs after HIV exposure, chemoprophylaxis after exposure, the risk posed to patients by HIV-infected surgeons, and the need for routine preoperative HIV screening. Infection with HIV has been reported in 1.3% of patients at sentinel hospitals and in 1.5/1,000 patients in lower-risk environments. Although estimates of seroprevalence vary widely, it seems clear that every surgeon will operate on patients with HIV infection. The surgeon may or may not be aware of this fact. The situation of surgeons operating on HIV-infected patients without knowledge of the infection seem more frequent than surgeons refusing to operate on such patients. It is increasingly difficult to predict which patients are infected with HIV. Surgeons are frequently exposed to patients' blood during surgery. Percutaneous injury during surgery occurs at a rate of 5% to 6%, whereas HIV transmission caused by percutaneous injury with a contaminated needle occurs at a rate of 0.3%.

There is confusion in the literature regarding the use of zidovudine (ZVD) therapy after occupational exposure to HIV. Current Public Health Service recommendations call for ZDV to be given after percutaneous exposures associated with the highest risk of transmission. These are exposures involving larger volumes of blood and blood containing a high titer of HIV. For lower-risk exposures, the potential benefits of chemoprophylaxis must be balanced against the uncertain efficacy and toxicity of the treatment. If the patient's HIV status is unknown, chemoprophylaxis decisions must be made on a case-by-case basis. Prophylaxis should start within 1 to 2 hours and continue for 4 weeks, with recommended doses of ZDV of 200 mg 3 times daily; lamivudine, 150 mg 2 times daily; and indinavir, 800 mg 3 times daily. Treatment should be given only with expert consultation and recommended monitoring for toxicity.

The risk that an infected surgeon will transmit HIV to a patient is very low—1 in 83,000 hours of surgery by a surgeon known to be HIV-positive. It is recommended that surgeons with HIV infection avoid performing interventions that carry a recognized risk of percutaneous injury. The possibility of HIV transmission in health care settings has led some to call for universal testing of both patients and physicians. However, there is no evidence that knowing a patient's HIV status would offer any protection to the surgeon. Also, knowing a patient's HIV status could negatively influence that patient's care.

Discussion.—Fear of AIDS has sometimes interfered with the usually rational decision-making process of the surgical community. The authors hope that their database will help surgeons in making decisions related to HIV and AIDS.

► Usually, review articles are not presented in the YEAR BOOK OF SURGERY. This article, however, is helpful to all surgeons interested in the risk of HIV infection to patients and the risk of contracting HIV as a result of operating on HIV-infected patients. The authors discuss the risk of an infected surgeon transmitting this infection to his patients. During the 1980s, concern among surgeons that they might become infected from caring for infected patients led many of them to find excuses or simply refuse to operate on HIV-infected patients. Because the risk of infection is so much lower than what was once feared, most surgeons are now willing to operate on such patients.

The risks cited in this paper are estimates. No one knows, with any degree of precision, what the risks are. They are based on assumptions and transmission rates that occur from needlesticks with hollow-bore needles. It is frequently assumed that the same risk occurs when a surgeon or a patient is contaminated with blood from any suture needle. It has been demonstrated[1] that the amount of blood transmitted by a suture needle is considerably less than that transmitted by a hollow-bore hypodermic needle. Furthermore, in most cases in which HIV transmission has occurred as a result of a needlestick injury, the needle was attached to a syringe containing blood and the person who became infected actually got an injection of contaminated blood. A review of the risk of hepatitis C infection and relevant data of concern to surgeons regarding hepatitis C also appeared in the Collective Reviews section of the same issue of the *Journal of the American College of Surgeons* in which the article abstracted here appeared.[2]

R.J. Howard, M.D., Ph.D.

References

1. Bennett NT, Howard RJ: Quantity of blood inoculated in a needlestick injury from suture needles. *J Am Coll Surg* 178:107–112, 1994.

2. Howard RJ, Fry DE, Davis JM, et al: Hepatitis C virus infection in healthcare workers. *J Am Coll Surg* 184:540–552, 1997.

Transmission of Hepatitis B to Patients From Four Infected Surgeons Without Hepatitis B e Antigen

Heptonstall J, and the Incident Investigation Teams and Others (Public Health Lab Service Communicable Disease Surveillance, London)

N Engl J Med 336:178–184, 1997 5–2

Introduction.—The transmission of hepatitis B virus (HBV) to patients from surgeons who carry hepatitis B e antigen (HBeAg) has been documented in numerous reports. Reported are 4 unconnected instances of transmission of HBV to patients by 4 infected surgeons whose serum did not show HBeAg.

Case Reports.—All 4 patients were female and were seen for acute onset of jaundice (Table 1). None of them received blood transfusions. Each patient had surgery within the past 6 months. An investigation was begun and members of each surgical team were tested for HBV carrier status. Three surgeons were positive for HBsAg and negative for anti-HBc IgM. One surgeon was known to be an HBeAg-negative carrier of HBV and continued to operate within existing guidelines. All other members of the 4 surgical teams were immune to HBV or uninfected. All patients recovered completely and no patients experienced fulminant hepatitis.

Methods.—Serum HBV DNA was amplified by a nested polymerase chain reaction from serum of the 4 infected surgeons and infected patients. Direct sequencing of the 2 regions of the HBV genome was executed. Patients who underwent surgeries by the infected surgeons were offered testing.

Results.—All 4 surgeons were carriers of HBV and none of them had detectable levels of HBeAg. It was not possible to distinguish the nucleotide sequences of HBV DNA from the surgeons and their corresponding infected patients. At least 2 other exposed patients who were offered screening probably acquired hepatitis B from their respective infected surgeon. All surgeons made career changes that did not put patients at risk of exposure to the virus.

Conclusion.—Surgeons who are carriers of HBV with no detectable serum HBeAg can transmit HBV to their patients. Surgeons in the United Kingdom are presently allowed to perform procedures within guidelines if their serum contains HBsAg, but not HBeAg.

► There have been many reported cases and clusters of transmission of hepatitis B from surgeons and dentists to their patients. Where investigated,

TABLE 1.—Characteristics of the Four Index Patients Whose HBV Infections Were Associated with Contact

Characteristic	Patient 1	Patient 2	Patient 3	Patient 4
Sex	F	F	F	F
Age group (yr)	30–39	30–39	60–69	70–79
Date of onset of jaundice	June 1988	October 1993	August 1994	January 1995
HBV subtype	ayw	adw	ayw	ayw
Type of procedure	Elective cholecystectomy	Elective cesarean section	Elective hysterectomy and removal of ovarian cyst	Elective cholecystectomy and nephrectomy
Interval between procedure and onset of jaundice (wk)	12	11	12	12
Blood transfusion	No	No	No	No
Sexual partner tested for HBV markers	Not tested	Anti-HBe-negative*	Anti-HBe-negative*	Not applicable
Other identified risk factors for HBV	None known	No	No	No
Identified source†	Surgeon 1	Surgeon 2	Surgeon 3	Surgeon 4
Role of infected surgeon in procedure	Main operator	Main operator	Assistant	Assistant

*Anti-HBe denotes antibodies against hepatitis B core antigen.
†All other members of the surgical teams were either immune to HBV or uninfected.
(Reprinted by permission of The New England Journal of Medicine from Heptonstall J, and the Incident Investigation Teams and Others: Transmission of hepatitis B to patients from four infected surgeons without hepatitis B e antigen. *N Engl J Med* 336:178–184, 1996.)

however, all these surgeons and dentists were HBeAg-positive. Hepatitis B antigen is associated with the DNA of the virus. Individuals who have e-antigen in their blood are thought to be approximately 1 million times more infectious than those without e-antigen. Hepatitis B infected cells can produce an excess of surface antigen so that it is possible that blood of the chronically infected patients may have surface antigen (the protein coat of virus) but not be infectious because they do not have nucleic acid.

This article from the United Kingdom reports 4 patients who were infected by their surgeons. A detailed investigation found that all the surgeons were surface-antigen positive and that none were e-antigen positive. The nucleotide sequences of HBV-DNA from the surgeons were the same as those of the patients.

Along with the AIDS epidemic in the 1980s came the concern about what to do with infected physicians—especially surgeons—and patients. Should they all be tested? Should infected surgeons be restricted from practice? This concern only came to public awareness with the rise of AIDS, although it had been known for years that hepatitis B could be transmitted from surgeons and dentists to patients. In the United Kingdom, there are no practice restrictions for carriers of hepatitis B surface antigen without detectable HBeAg unless transmission has been documented. The United States does not have any national policies. The Centers for Disease Control has put forth guidelines for health care workers to prevent transmission of infectious materials to patients. (MMWR 191;40(RR-8): 1–9).

R.J. Howard, M.D., Ph.D.

Nosocomial Infections in Surgical Patients: Comparison of Two Measures of Intrinsic Patient Risk

Delgado-Rodriguez M, Sillero-Arenas M, Medina-Cuadros M, et al (Univ of Cantabria, Santander, Spain; Provincial Office for Health, Jaén, Spain; Gen Hosp Cuidad de Jaén, Spain)

Infect Control Hosp Epidemiol 18:19–23, 1997 5–3

Objective.—A surgical patient's "intrinsic risk" for nosocomial infection refers to the baseline probability of such infection arising from conditions present at the start of care, and from the diagnostic tests and treatments performed for those conditions. Some means of measuring intrinsic risk to adjust for case mix is needed. This prospective study compared 2 measures of intrinsic risk for nosocomial infection: the Study on the Efficacy of Nosocomial Infection Control (SENIC) index and the National Nosocomial Infection Surveillance (NNIS) System index.

Methods.—One thousand four hundred eighty-three surgical patients (age range, 10 to 92 years) were prospectively studied and followed for 1 month after hospital discharge. Extensive preoperative and postoperative data were collected for use in computing the SENIC and NNIS indexes. The SENIC index was developed as a simplified multivariate risk index for surgical wound infection; the NNIS index, a modification of the SENIC, was not developed by multivariate modeling techniques. The 2 indices were compared for their ability to predict the occurrence of surgical site infection.

Results.—Nosocomial infections developed during follow-up in 155 patients, for a cumulative incidence of 10.5%. Analysis revealed a linear trend of the NNIS index with both the crude and SENIC-adjusted rates of surgical wound infection. In contrast, the SENIC index showed no linear trend with NNIS-adjusted rates of surgical wound infection. When each variable was regressed on the other, the residuals of the NNIS index added to the discriminating powers of the SENIC index, whereas the residuals of the SENIC index did not improve the predictive power of the NNIS index.

Conclusion.—For discrimination and prediction of the risk of nosocomial infection in surgical patients, the NNIS index shows better performance than the earlier SENIC index. The SENIC index provides no additional information for predicting surgical wound infection beyond that provided by the NNIS index.

▶ To further refine risk of surgical infections as part of the SENIC project, Haley[1] developed a risk index for wound infection based on 4 factors: the number of discharge diagnoses, the length of the operation, whether or not the operation was an abdominal operation, and classification of an operation as either contaminated or dirty-infected. Culver[2] refined this risk index in the NNIS study and included 3 factors in his index: the length of the operation, the American Society of Anesthesiologists score, and classification of an operation as either contaminated or dirty-infected.

Whereas Haley confirmed the validity of his risk index in a prospective study, Culver never did. The risk index categories—1–4 for SENIC and 1–3 for NNIS—were a better indicator of the risk of postoperative wound infection than was the traditional categorization of wounds into clean, clean-contaminated, contaminated, and dirty. This study evaluates both of these risk indices against each other and finds that the NNIS index is better able to predict surgical wound infection rate than is the SENIC index. The NNIS index did not use the term *wound infection* but the current term, *surgical-site infection*, which was developed by mutual collaboration of the Surgical Infection Society, The Society of Hospital Epidemiologists of America, and the Centers for Disease Control. The term "surgical site infection" is more inclusive than "surgical wound infection" and includes operative sites not in direct contact with the surgical wound.

Societies concerned with infection in surgical patients are continuing to refine terms and categories so that more discriminating ways of categorizing surgical patients for the risk of wound infection can be established. As Dr. James Lee points out in an editorial accompanying the article abstracted here, Haley previously tested the SENIC and NNIS schemes and came to a different conclusion.[3] Nevertheless, striving for valid risk indexes is important to allow different hospitals and different surgeons to reliably compare their data.

R.J. Howard, M.D., Ph.D.

References

1. Haley RW, Culver DH, White JW, et al: The efficacy of infection surveillance and control programs in preventing nonsocomial infections in US hospitals. *Am J Epidemiol* 121:182–205, 1985.
2. Culver DH, Horan TC, Gaynes RP, et al: Surgical wound infection rates by wound class, operative procedure, and patient risk index. *Am J Med* 91 (Suppl 3B):152S–157S, 1991.
3. Haley RW: Measuring the intrinsic risk of wound infection in surgical patients. *Probl Gen Surg* 10:396–417, 1993.

Adjunctive Use of Monthly Physician Questionnaires for Surveillance of Surgical Site Infections After Hospital Discharge and in Ambulatory Surgical Patients: Report of a Seven-Year Experience

Manian FA, Meyer L (St John's Mercy Med Ctr, St Louis)
Am J Infect Control 25:390–394, 1997 5–4

Introduction.—Surveillance of surgical site infections (SSIs) has been made more difficult by the growing trend toward outpatient surgery and shorter postoperative hospital stays. Monthly physician questionnaires have been used since 1988 at the study institution for surveillance of SSIs after hospital discharge. The results of this program, which is performed in conjunction with traditional in-house monitoring, are reported for the 7-year period from July 1988 through June 1995.

Methods.—At the tertiary care hospital in a suburb of St. Louis, more than 10,000 ambulatory surgical procedures are performed each year. This number represents more than half of all surgical procedures performed annually. The operating room computer provides a monthly questionnaire/printout for each surgeon, and surgeons are asked to check the appropriate SSI column ("Yes," "No," or "No Follow-up") for each surgical case. Additional information regarding the date of diagnosis and culture results are requested for cases associated with SSI. Survey participation is voluntary.

Results.—During the 7-year study period, 156,977 surgical procedures were performed at the study center; 43% involved inpatients, and 53% involved ambulatory surgical patients. The surveys had annual response rates of 71% to 75%. There was a significant increase in the percentage of survey-covered surgical procedures in both inpatients and ambulatory surgical patients. The total SSI rate for all procedures was 0.7% (1,051 of 156,977). Almost one fourth of the SSIs (22%) were identified solely by returned questionnaires. Nearly half (47%) of the 787 cases meeting the criteria for SSI on the basis of in-house surveillance and listed on returned questionnaires were not marked as SSIs by the responding surgeons. After inclusion of survey-identified cases, SSI rates were significantly higher than those reported previously in both inpatients and ambulatory surgical patients.

Discussion.—Traditional in-house surveillance fails to identify some SSIs in ambulatory patients and those with short postoperative hospital stays. Monthly physician surveys were found to significantly increase the identification of SSIs in the ambulatory setting.

► Using mailed surveys to detect SSIs has been suspect because it was felt that surgeons might be unlikely to comply with mailing back the surveys or to be less than completely honest because of the possible sanctions that might be taken on those with excessive SSI rates. This paper from a large, private hospital in a St. Louis suburb demonstrates that the return rate of the surveys was high (between 73% and 79%). Furthermore, 22% to 35% of the SSIs were diagnosed in patients having inpatient surgery, but did add significantly to SSIs in ambulatory surgical patients. Over the period of the study, 47% of patients having SSIs by traditional identification methods were unreported in the survey. Those data suggest that only slightly more than half of the SSIs are identified by using mailed surveys alone. Identifiying SSIs continues to be a challenge. It is costly to obtain reliable data. With current pressures for cost reduction by hospitals, obtaining valid hospital-acquired infection data of all types (of which SSI is one of the more common) will be increasingly difficult.

R.J. Howard, M.D., Ph.D.

Basics of Surgical-site Infection Surveillance

Roy M-C, Perl TM (Hôpital de L'Enfant-Jésus, Québec City; Johns Hopkins Univ, Baltimore, Md)

Infect Control Hosp Epidemiol 18:659–668, 1997 5–5

Objective.—Surgical-site infections (SSIs) account for 15% of all reported nosocomial infections. Because of the morbidity and excess costs of SSIs, investigators from the Study of the Efficacy of Nosocomial Infection Control (SENIC) concluded that an infection surveillance program be instituted to decrease SSI rates. Questions about which surveillance methods to use, which patients to surveil, and the value and methods of postdischarge surveillance are answered, and a summary of the basic steps required to implement an in-hospital surveillance program for SSIs is discussed.

Methods.—Control program objectives should be established to reduce SSI rates by determining baseline SSI rates and identifying situations that increase SSI rates over endemic rates. Control programs should include preventive plans and methods for measuring the success of those plans everywhere in the hospital and disseminating the information appropriately. SSIs must be defined objectively, and definitions must be applied consistently (Fig 1). Daily wound examination and chart review form the most sensitive way to perform SSI surveillance. Selective chart review with Kardex review, microbiology reports, and pharmacy files have limited sensitivity. The effectiveness of combined methods that rely on integrated

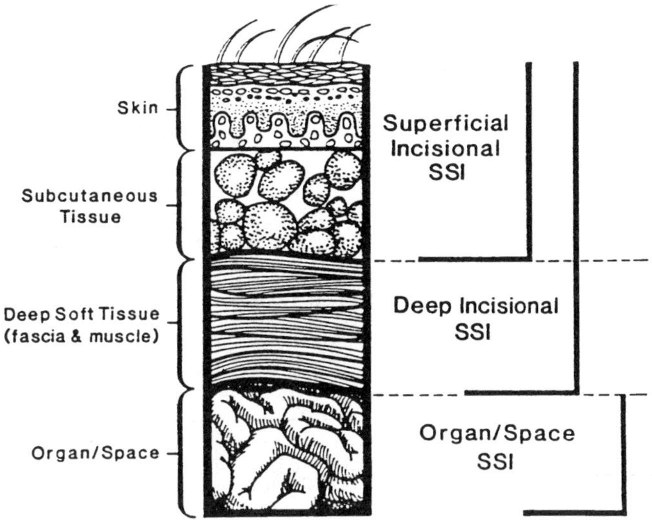

FIGURE 1.—Schematic of surgical-site infection (SSI) anatomy and appropriate classification. This figure depicts the cross-sectional anatomy of a surgical incision upon which is superimposed the most recent classification for SSI and the definition of an infection at each site.[10] (Courtesy of Roy M-C, Perl TM: Basics of surgical-site infection surveillance. *Infect Control Hosp Epidemiol* 18:659–668, 1997).

computer systems for data analysis has not been assessed. Data should be collected on host factors, surgical and environmental factors, and microbial factors. All categories of surgical procedures should be surveilled. Targeted surveillance can focus on stratifying patients according to their risk of SSI. Postdischarge surveillance is recommended because almost half of SSIs were identified after discharge. SSI rates can be calculated as service-specific, surgeon-specific, procedure-specific, risk-specific, for example. Interventions depend on the problems identified. The infection control practitioner must be able to work well with surgeons and surgical staff and be provided with training, feedback, and continuing education.

Conclusion.—An infection control program should be established and implemented with the same precision as any other continuous quality assurance program. More research needs to be conducted to determine how to adapt and adopt the specialized programs and techniques required to assure effectiveness.

▶ This articles reviews some of the present-day difficulties of conducting surgical site infection surveillance. Since more than half the operations in the United States are done as outpatient procedures and because of early discharge of patients who have inpatient operations, finding which patients develop infections in the postoperative period can be difficult and expensive. The least reliable way of finding out about postoperative wound infections is to rely on physicians themselves to report their surgical site infections. Reliable physician reporting may become less likely in the future because of the possible negative economic impact on physicians who have infection rates above the expected norm. Even hospitals, having to reduce personnel and expense as much as possible because of increasing price competition, are being forced to curtail their surveillance activities or to substitute less costly surrogate methods of surveillance that will be less costly in the future but also less reliable.

R.J. Howard, M.D., Ph.D.

Unopposed Interleukin-1 Is Necessary for Increased Plasma Cytokine and Eicosanoid Levels to Develop in Severe Sepsis

Slotman GJ, Quinn JV, Wry PC, et al (Robert Wood Johnson Med School at Camden, NJ)

Ann Surg 226:77–84, 1997 5–6

Introduction.—Although circulating prostaglandins, leukotrienes, and cytokines are implicated in the systemic inflammatory response syndrome caused by severe sepsis, little is known about the interactions between interleukin-1 (IL-1) and other cytokine and eicosanoid mediators of severe sepsis. A preliminary evaluation of 19 critically ill septic patients tested the hypothesis that IL-1 stimulates release of these and other inflammatory mediators and that inhibition of IL-1 would modify the circulating acute inflammatory mediator milieu and identify changes for which IL-1 is necessary.

Methods.—Two sequential multisite, prospective, double-blind clinical trials enrolled 37 adult patients with sepsis. Patients were randomized to receive IL-1 receptor antagonist (IL-1ra) or placebo. The 20 patients in the IL-1ra group were administered a 100 mg bolus followed by 2 mg/kg hr intraveneously for 72 hours. The remaining 17 patients received matching placebo. Each patient had 10 mL of blood drawn at baseline and at 24, 48, and 72 hours after the initiation of IL-1ra or placebo. Enzyme-linked immunosorbent assay was used to measure plasma thromboxane B_2; prostaglandin 6-keto-F1α (PGI); leukotriene B_4, $C_4D_4E_4$; interleukin-1 beta (IL-1β), interleukin-6 (IL-6); and tumor necrosis factor alpha (TNF-α).

Results.—Placebo and IL-1ra groups were similar in age, gender, clinical and laboratory findings, and mortality. Plasma leukotriene B_4 increased significantly from baseline among IL-1ra patients at 48 and 72 hours, but no changes were observed in the placebo group. Compared with the placebo group, plasma IL-1 increased significantly from baseline in the IL-1ra group. Significant decreases in patients receiving IL-1ra were recorded for plasma thromboxane B_2, PGI, TNF, IL-6, and leukotriene $C_4D_4E_4$.

Discussion.—Under conditions of severe sepsis and septic shock, IL-1 appears to be a necessary mediator of increased eicosanoid and cytokine release. Evidence was provided by the significantly reduced plasma levels of thromboxane B_2, PGI, TNF, IL-6, and leukotriene $C_4D_4E_4$, compared with the placebo group. Paradoxically, both plasma IL-1 and leukotriene B_4 are increased with infusion of IL-1ra.

► This study was done in conjunction with the clinical trial of IL-1ra, which failed to show clinical efficacy in patients with severe sepsis. It shows that useful information can be obtained even in clinical trials where efficacy of the agent studied is not found. It further defines changes that occur in plasma inflammatory mediators in patients with severe sepsis. The authors demonstrated that plasma IL-1 levels increased in patients receiving IL-1ra, compared with those receiving placebo. They hypothesize that it may be a necessary mediator for increasing other inflammatory mediators and cytokines. This and many other papers in the past several years have attempted to delineate the role of inflammatory mediators in sepsis and infection. The hope is that a better understanding of the process involved in sepsis and inflammation will allow intervention to ameliorate the septic response.

R.J. Howard, M.D., Ph.D.

Bacterial Translocation in Surgical Patients

MacFie J (Scarborough Hosp, England)

Ann R Coll Surg Engl 79:183–189, 1997 5–7

Purpose.—Bacterial translocation occurs when intestinal microflora cross the lamina propria to local mesenteric lymph nodes, and move on to other extraintestinal sites. Previous reports have suggested that this process may initiate a macrophage-mediated response that can predispose the host to sepsis and multiple organ failure. However, the clinical importance of bacterial translocation in surgical patients remains unclear. The authors recently conducted several studies of bacterial translocation in surgical patients.

Prevalence of Bacterial Translocation.—The first study confirmed the presence of bacterial translocation in 15% of a series of 448 consecutive patients undergoing laparotomy. *Escherichia coli* was involved in 54% of these cases. In 41% of patients with evidence of bacterial translocation, sepsis developed. This compared with 14% of patients in whom no organisms were cultured.

Intestinal Barrier Function.—Two studies examined the role of intestinal barrier function in bacterial translocation. One study found that short-villous morphology was unaffected by short courses of total parenteral nutrition (TPN), which deprives the intestinal tract on luminal nutrients; neither did TPN increase the risk of bacterial translocation. The incidence of sepsis was nonsignificantly higher in TPN patients than in normally fed controls, but the mechanism was not bacterial translocation. Another study examined the role of intestinal permeability. There was no apparent association between measurements of permeability and clinically significant bacterial translocation. These 2 studies found no correlation between measurements of villous morphology and intestinal permeability.

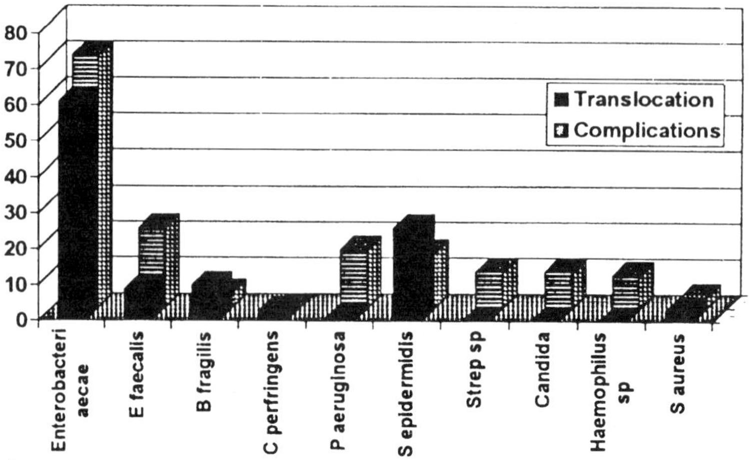

FIGURE 2.—Comparison of organisms from mesenteric lymph nodes and septic complications. (Courtesy of MacFie J: Bacterial translocation in surgical patients. *Ann R Coll Surg Engl* 79:183–189, 1997.)

Changes in Gastrointestinal Microflora.—Three studies looked at the effects of alterations in gastrointestinal (GI) microflora on the incidence of bacterial translocation and sepsis. Culture studies of mesenteric lymph nodes most commonly identified gram-negative facultative anaerobes, especially *E. coli*. The intraluminal population density of bacteria did not appear to be the main influence on bacterial translocation. In 45% of patients with bacterial translocation, a septic focus developed, compared with 19% of patients without bacterial sepsis. Enterobacteriaceae were the most common translocating organisms and the main organisms responsible for postoperative sepsis. The findings provide a rationale for the use of selective gut decontamination.

A study of the microbiology of the upper GI tract in surgical patients found that the stomach was rarely stable. It also found that overgrowth of the upper GI tract with multiple colonies predisposed to sepsis, especially when enteric organisms were present (Fig 2). The final study examined the associations between gastric microflora, bacterial translocations, and sepsis. The findings strongly suggested that bacteria translocating across the intestinal barrier to the local mesenteric lymph nodes do predispose to sepsis. Again, Enterobacteriaceae and enteric bacteria were the most frequently involved. There were no signs of candidal translocation.

Conclusion.—These studies demonstrate that bacterial translocation does occur in surgical patients and is linked to sepsis. The likelihood of bacterial translocation cannot be assessed by measures of intestinal barrier function in the form of villous morphology and permeability. In healthy subjects with a normal immune system, bacterial translocation probably occurs without causing clinically significant disease. In debilitated surgical patients, bacterial translocation may be a key early step in the development of sepsis but not the only initiating factor. The findings provide a rationale for the practice of selective gut decontamination to prevent sepsis.

► This study is one of the more complete attempts to define parameters associated with bacterial translocation, although the authors do not define terms as clearly as possible (they did not define what they meant by sepsis). It is unclear whether bacterial translocation was associated with any increased risk of infection. In this study, 69 of 448 patients (15.4%) having laparotomy had bacteria cultured from the serosal surface or mesenteric lymph nodes. The important finding was that of patients who had bacterial translocation, sepsis developed in 41% compared with only 14% in whom no organisms were cultured. The authors do not define sepsis, however, and no additional information is provided regarding infections that developed in these patients.

Alterations in villous morphology or intestinal permeability to sugars was not associated with bacterial translocation. In 32% (10/31) of patients with evidence of translocation at laparotomy, the same bacteria grew from both the operative node sample and the postoperative septic focus, suggesting that translocated bacteria may cause an actual infection. Therefore, translocation may not be just an interesting phenomenon but may actually be important in disease solving.

R.J. Howard, M.D., Ph.D.

The Role of Antibiotic Prophylaxis in Severe Acute Pancreatitis

Ho HS, Frey CF (Univ of California at Davis, Sacramento)

Arch Surg 132:487–493, 1997 5–8

Background.—Patients with infected necrotizing pancreatitis are difficult to manage, often requiring repeated surgical debridement and lengthy hospital stays. In patients with acute pancreatitis, death often results from bacterial infection and sepsis. There is clinical evidence that prophylactic antibiotics may reduce the infection rate and the need for surgery in patients with severe acute pancreatitis. An evolving experience with prophylactic IV antibiotics for patients with severe acute pancreatitis was reported.

Methods.—The study included 180 patients with severe acute pancreatitis. The 50 patients seen from 1982 to 1989 received no antibiotics. From 1990 to 1992, 55 patients received prophylactic antibiotics but not according to any protocol. From 1993 to 1996, 75 patients received a 4-week course of IV imipenem-cilastatin sodium, according to protocol. The study definition of severe acute pancreatitis was an Acute Physiology and Chronic Health Evaluation II score of greater than 6 plus pancreatic necrosis involving more than 15% of the gland, peripancreatic necrosis, or a peripancreatic infection. The 3 groups were compared for the incidence of pancreatic infection and for mortality.

Results.—Pancreatic infection developed in 76% of patients who received no antibiotics, 45% of those who received nonprotocol antibiotic prophylaxis, and 27% of those treated with the imipenem-cilastatin protocol. The mortality rate decreased from 16% to 7% to 5%, respectively, although the trend was nonsignificant. The overall mortality rate was 2% for patients with sterile severe acute pancreatitis vs. 17% for those with infection. The mortality rate was 19% to 40% for patients with infection developing within 4 weeks after the onset of illness, compared to 0% to 8% for those with later-developing infection. There were no deaths among patients with late infections who were treated on the imipenem-cilastatin protocol.

Conclusion.—For patients with severe acute pancreatitis, the risk of infection can be significantly reduced with IV antibiotic prophylaxis. There is a nonsignificant reduction in the risk of death as well. The authors call for a prospective, randomized, double-blind, multicenter trial to compare various approaches to antibiotic prophylaxis in patients with severe acute pancreatitis.

► Because of the high mortality rate (10% to 30%) caused by infection associated with pancreatitis, antibiotics are a tempting means of possibly preventing infections in these patients. Early randomized studies[1] did not demonstrate that antibiotics could prevent infection in patients with pancreatitis. The problem with these early studies, however, was that the antibiotic used (ampicillin) was not as effective as current antibiotics and, furthermore, ampicillin was not effective against the bacteria likely to be found associated with pancreatitis. Experts still disagree on whether antibiotics should be administered to patients with pancreatitis. Many surgeons would give antibiotics to patients with severe pancreatitis.

This study compares patients over a 15-year period. They divided these groups historically into those given no antibiotics, those to whom it was given on a nonprotocol basis, and recent patients from 1993 to 1996 who were given a full course of imipenem-cilastatin. Furthermore, the patients who received antibiotics were only those with severe pancreatitis. The authors found a decrease in the infection rate from 76% to 45% to 27% among the 3 groups. This paper suffers from all the problems that historical papers do. The treatment of severe pancreatitis itself has changed over this time, even without the use of antibiotics. Furthermore, the definition of severe pancreatitis has changed as CT scanning has refined the definition and its application to this group of patients.

The authors state that a randomized study should be done. In fact, a randomized study using imipenem-cilastatin for patients with acute necrotizing pancreatitis has already been done in Italy.[2] It seems advisable to administer antibiotics to patients with severe pancreatitis.

R.J. Howard, M.D., Ph.D.

References

1. Finch WT, Sawyers JL, Schenker S, et al: A prospective study to determine the efficacy of antibiotics in acute pancreatitis. *Ann Surg* 183:667–671, 1976.
2. Pederzolip C, Bassi C, Vesentini S, et al: A randomized multicenter clinical trial of antibiotic prophlaxis accepted complications in acute necrotizing pancreatitis with imipenem. *Surg Gynecol Obstet.* 176:480–483, 1993.

Results of a Randomized, Multicenter Trial of Meropenem Versus Clindamycin/Tobramycin for the Treatment of Intra-Abdominal Infections

Wilson SE (UCI Med Ctr, Orange, Calif)

Clin Infect Dis 24:S197–S206, 1997 5–9

Introduction.—A multicenter trial compared meropenem with a standard aminoglycoside regimen for treating anaerobic intra-abdominal infection. Meropenem is active against most gram-negative and gram-positive bacteria and has an in vitro spectrum activity similar to that of imipenem.

Methods.—The prospective trial was conducted at 13 sites in North America. In a randomized, double-blind design, 215 patients received meropenem (1,000 mg IV every 8 hours) and 212 were given a combination regimen of clindamycin (900 mg every 8 hours) and tobramycin (5 mg/kg/day in 3 divided doses). All patients had been hospitalized with intra-abdominal infection requiring surgical intervention and parenteral antibiotic therapy. Diagnostic categories eligible for inclusion were complicated appendicitis, gynecologic infection, hepatobiliary infection, pancreatic infection, intra-abdominal abscess, and perforation of the stomach or bowel. Investigators rated both clinical and bacteriologic responses to study treatments.

Results.—A total of 191 patients, 97 in the meropenem arm and 94 in the clindamycin–tobramycin arm, met all criteria for evaluation of efficacy. All treated patients were included in the safety analysis. Among the intent-to-treat patients, the cure rates did not differ significantly between the meropenem (91%) and clindamycin–tobramycin (86%) groups. Similarly, 92% of evaluable patients in the meropenem group and 86% of evaluable patients in the clindamycin–tobramycin groups were cured (Table 6). Bacteriologic response rates were also comparable for all evaluable patients—96% and 93%, respectively, for the meropenem and clindamycin–tobramycin groups. Neither group had treatment-related seizure or deaths, and other adverse events occurred at a similar frequency with each therapy. Diarrhea and nausea were the most common adverse clinical events in both groups.

Conclusion.—Meropenem appeared to be well tolerated and safe, and the antibiotic's clinical and bacterial response rates were quite similar to those obtained with a combination regimen of clindamycin plus tobramy-

TABLE 6.—Clinical Results of Therapy for Intra-Abdominal Infections With Meropenem or Clindamycin/Tobramycin Among Evaluable and Intent-to-Treat Patients

Result	No. receiving menoperem with indicated result		No. receiving clindamycin/ tobramycin with indicated result	
	Evaluable (n = 97)	Intent-to-treat (n = 215)	Evaluable (n = 94)	Intent-to-treat (n = 212)
Early follow-up				
Cured	89	120	81	115
Improved	4	7	6	11
Unchanged or worse	4	5	7	8
Total	97	132	94	134
Follow-up at 4–14 days				
Cured	65	112	51	113
Improved	0	2	1	4
Unchanged or worse	0	2	1	2
Relapse	1	5	3	3
Total	66	121	56	122
Follow-up at 28–42 days				
Cured	17	109	13	113
Improved	0	2	0	4
Unchanged or worse	0	0	0	1
Relapse	1	5	0	2
Total	18	116	13	120

(Courtesy of Wilson SE: Results of a randomized, multicenter trial of meropenem versus clindamycin/tobramycin for the treatment of intra-abdominal infections. *Clin Infect Dis* 24:S197–S206, 1997. Copyright 1997 by The University of Chicago.)

cin. Patients treated in the study had bacterial intraabdominal infections requiring surgery. Most cases involved complications of appendicitis.

▶ Meropenem is a new carbapenem β-lactamase antibiotic. It is in the same class as imipenem. This article is taken from a supplemental issue of *Clinical Infectious Disease* devoted to clinical trials of meropenem. The author, speaking for individuals who participated in a muticenter trial, found that meropenem was comparable to clindamycin and tobramycin in treating intra-abdominal infections. It is virtually impossible to conduct a trial of intra-abdominal infections showing that one antibiotic is better than another. Like so many in the past, this also shows that a new antibiotic, meropenem, is comparable to standard therapy, clindamycin or tobramycin, and surgical treatment. Yet this study shows some of the difficulties of conducting clinical trials of intra-abdominal infections. Over half the patients who were entered into the trial were nonevaluable because they didn't meet strict entry criteria. In addition, over 70% of the patients who were entered into the trial had perforative appendicitis. Certainly, most patients with perforative appendicitis and localized peritonitis can be treated by operation and a variety of antibiotic combinations. Because these patients generally are young and otherwise healthy, recovery can be expected in a majority of cases, no matter what antibiotic is used.

Today surgeons have a wide number of choices of antibiotics for treating intra-abdominal and other surgical infections. There are no clear data that one is necessarily better than another, yet newer antibiotics tend to be more expensive than many older and equally effective antibiotics.

R.J. Howard, M.D., Ph.D.

Poor Outcome From Peritonitis is Caused by Disease Acuity and Organ Failure, Not Recurrent Peritoneal Infection

Wickel DJ, Cheadle WG, Mercer-Jones MA, et al (Univ of Louisville, Ky)
Ann Surg 225:744–756, 1997 5–10

Background.—Although peritonitis generally responds to prompt surgical and systemic antibiotic treatments, in some cases it progresses to organ failure and death. The questions are whether organ failure develops despite control of peritoneal infection, and whether it is mediated by polymorphonuclear leukocytes (PMNLs).

Methods.—Clinical studies and a PMNL-deleted experimental model of peritonitis produced by cecal ligation and puncture (CLP) were used. Clinical studies were of 105 consecutive patients with peritonitis who underwent operation and had postoperative stays longer than 10 days. Experimentally, mice were injected with monoclonal anti-PMNL antibody 1 day before CLP for PMNL depletion.

Results.—Patients studied were 48 men and 57 women, whose mean age was 59 years (20–87 years); 38 died, and 77 had organ failure. Perforated hollow viscus was the most common cause of peritonitis. All but 1 of the patients who died had organ failure. Although 15 patients had recurrent or persistent intraperitoneal infection, only 1 had organ failure, and only 2 died. Fourteen recovered without organ failure. Seventy-seven patients had pulmonary failure. All but 1 had resolution of intraperitoneal infection. Nearly 61% of patients with multisystem organ failure eventually died, despite adequate treatment. The lungs, the most commonly affected of remote organ systems, were either first to fail or one of several organ systems to fail simultaneously. In the mouse study, acute lung injury was significantly increased in the control CLP group, compared with normal mice, and was 3 times higher than it was in the group treated with anti-PMNL antibody before CLP ($P < 0.05$). Normal mice and the antibody-treated CLP group did not differ. Cecal ligation and puncture significantly elevated serum liver enzymes, but less so (if not significantly) in PMNL-depleted animals. Lung injury, PMNL content, interleukin-1 messenger RNA, and liver injury were all reduced significantly by anti-PMNL treatment.

Conclusions.—Recurrent peritoneal infection is not a major cause of adverse outcome in peritonitis, but disease acuity and organ failure are. Organ injury, although complex and multifactorial, has some PMNL mediation. Therapeutic approaches could involve blocking PMNL endothelial adherence in remote organs and directing them instead to the peritoneal cavity.

► This clinical and experimental study suggests that patients who die with peritonitis die of multiple organ failure, and those patients who develop multiple organ failure are not necessarily those who have recurrent or persistent peritonitis. Thus, peritonitis appears to trigger a series of events that leads to multiple system organ failure and death. Treating peritonitis may stop the initiating event of the multiple system organ failure but does not treat the organ failure itself. Yet this hypothesis suggests that by the time the patients present for operation for peritonitis, the die is already cast. That is, when the patient initially presents for operation, whether he or she is going to develop multiple system organ failure has already been determined, and treating the peritonitis will not influence the development of multiple system organ failure. Thus, other interventions may be required to successfully treat multiple system organ failure, and treating the peritonitis only stops the initiating event. In the experimental part of the paper, the authors suggest that neutrophils are instrumental in promoting systemic effects of infection and that treating mice with antineutrophil antibodies can ameliorate these systemic effects. Because neutrophils are the cells responsible for phagocytosis of bacteria, one is reluctant to treat infected humans with antibodies that inactivate these cells.

R.J. Howard, M.D., Ph.D.

Does Reoperation for Abdominal Sepsis Enhance the Inflammatory Host Response?

Sautner T, Götzinger P, Redl-Wenzl E-M, et al (Univ of Vienna; Krankenanstalt Rudolfstiftung Vienna)

Arch Surg 132:250–255, 1997 5–11

Introduction.—Abdominal sepsis remains a life-threatening surgical complication, and reoperation for the purpose of reducing the contaminating inocula may actually escalate the ongoing inflammatory response. A study of 15 patients with severe peritonitis tested the hypothesis that manipulation of the infected peritoneal cavity leads to an increase of endotoxin and proinflammatory cytokine levels of the circulatory system.

Methods.—Patients had abdominal sepsis caused by small bowel or large bowel perforation, infected necrotizing pancreatitis, perforated appendicitis, or perforated duodenal ulcer. Nineteen reoperations were performed at a mean of 3.9 days after the initial operation. Repeated operative revision was undertaken when the patient's clinical status worsened. Plasma samples obtained immediately before and after reoperation and at 1, 3, 6, 12, and 24 hours postoperatively were analyzed for levels of endotoxin, tumor necrosis factor α (TNF-α), and interleukin-6 (IL-6). The courses of proinflammatory mediators were correlated with hemodynamic findings (mean arterial pressure, MAP; pulmonary capillary wedge pressure, PCWP; and vasopressor support).

Results.—Five (33%) patients died in-hospital of intractable organ failure resulting from underlying abdominal sepsis. Abdominal cavity exudates showed a growth of pathogens in all patients and multiple pathogens in 9 of 15 cases. Overall changes in MAP, PCWP, and vasopressor levels were significant. For MAP, the decrease was from 94 mm Hg postoperatively to 80 mm Hg at 3 hours and 81 mm Hg at 6 hours. From immediately after reoperation to 1 hour, mean PCWP fell from 13.8 to 12.0 mm Hg. Vasopressor support increased significantly from 6 to 24 hours postoperatively. Systemic endotoxin and TNF-α levels did not change significantly during the observation period, but IL-6 increased significantly at 1 and 3 hours. Overall IL-6 levels were inversely correlated with postoperative MAP.

Conclusion.—Substantial hypotension is a frequent aftermath of reoperation for abdominal sepsis, and levels of IL-6 may increase in the early postoperative period as a result of reoperative trauma. It is possible that a relationship exists between the kinetics of IL-6 and hemodynamic instability. The risk–benefit ratio of reoperation for abdominal sepsis must be considered on an individual basis.

▶ Numerous papers have examined plasma cytokine levels in a variety of clinical circumstances. The proinflammatory cytokines TNF-α, IL-1β, and IL-6 have been most often studied in order to predict mortality and morbidity in a variety of human diseases. With the possible exception of IL-6, this approach has not been fruitful. The current study measures endotoxin levels, TNF-α, and IL-6 in patients having reoperation for abdominal sepsis. It showed no change in endotoxin or TNF-α levels but a significant increase in IL-6 concentrations up to 3 hours after operation. Elevated IL-6 levels return to normal within 6 hours after operation. Because the increase in IL-6 concentrations occurred before the development of hypotension, the authors have hypothesized that these increases cause this observed hypotension.

It is extremely difficult to measure all the possible variables in these complicated patients. The ultimate hope is that by blocking the actions of these cytokines, either with antibodies against them or with molecules that compete for their receptors, the adverse biological affects can be decreased or eliminated. Unfortunately, despite the investment of much time, energy, and money, no clinical studies have shown efficacy of such an approach thus far. This and numerous other papers suggest that the inflammatory response and its clinical manifestations are much more complex than we realize and that there are many possible paths to the same biological effect, so that possibly blocking one cytokine does not eliminate the same biological effect by other routes.

R.J. Howard, M.D., Ph.D.

Percutaneous Drainage of Intra-Abdominal Abscesses in Crohn's Disease: Short and Long Term Outcome

Sahai A, Bélair M, Gianfelice D, et al (Université de Montréal)

Am J Gastroenterol 92:275–278, 1997 5–12

Introduction.—For patients with intra-abdominal abscesses, percutaneous drainage is usually the first treatment option, rather than surgery. In patients with Crohn's disease, these abscesses pose particular problems in the form of associated fistulas and active underlying inflammatory bowel disease. Although percutaneous drainage of abscesses in patients with Crohn's disease is feasible, it is unclear whether it is the best choice. This retrospective study sought to determine whether performing percutaneous drainage of abscesses in patients with Crohn's disease avoids the need for surgical drainage.

Methods.—The analysis included 27 percutaneous drainage procedures performed in 24 patients with Crohn's abscesses over a 5-year period. Cases in which no surgery was required within 30 days after catheter removal were classified as successes. The long-term maintenance of this benefit was analyzed, as were the factors associated with a favorable or unfavorable outcome.

Results.—The success rate was 56%. The patient's demographic and Crohn's disease characteristics did not influence the probability of success. Associated fistulas were present in 47% of patients whose abscesses were successfully drained, as opposed to 92% of those in whom drainage was unsuccessful. Successfully drained abscesses tended to be initial rather than recurrent, spontaneous vs. postoperative, located in the right lower quadrant, and of smaller size. Patients with successful drainage had longer durations with the catheter in place and underwent more imaging procedures.

The complication rate was 15%, including 2 cases of enterocutaneous fistula at the site of catheter insertion and 1 case of postprocedural fever. Patients with successful drainage stayed in the hospital a mean of 16 days, compared with 32 days for those with unsuccessful drainage. The patients were followed for a total of 543.5 patient-months. Just 3 patients required intra-abdominal surgery for Crohn's disease during this time: 2 with successful drainage and 1 with unsuccessful drainage.

Conclusion.—In about half of patients with Crohn's disease with intra-abdominal abscesses, percutaneous drainage avoids the need for early surgical drainage. The benefits of drainage are maintained on long-term follow-up. Percutaneous drainage can be successfully performed in single or multiple abscesses in various locations and with or without an associated fistula. However, drainage may be less likely to succeed if a fistula is present.

▶ Percutaneous drainage of intra-abdominal abscess has saved many patients from the need for surgical drainage. Success rates, according to reports by radiologists, are at least 75%. In reports of studies by surgeons, success rates seem to be somewhat less. The reasons for these differences is unclear. A concern regarding patients with Crohn's disease is that they might have accompanying fistulas that might not be amenable to radiologic drainage.

In this series, 5 of the 12 patients classified as failures were operated on for other reasons. If they had an operation within 30 days of catheter removal or while the catheter was in place, they were classified as failures. Realistically, these patients were probably successes, and if they had been grouped with the 15 successes, the success rate would have been 74%. It is significant that in 3 patients, an enterocutaneous fistula developed at the site of catheter insertion. Whether the fistula was created by the catheter insertion or already existed was not clearly stated.

Because of its proven safety, even with the only 56% success rate quoted in this article, percutaneous catheter drainage is probably worthwhile in most patients with intra-abdominal abscess. Patients are seldom harmed by an initial attempt at percutaneous drainage and, if needed, open drainage can be done later.

R.J. Howard, M.D., Ph.D.

Surgical Management of Complicated Colonic Diverticulitis

Wedell J, Banzhaf G, Chaoui R, et al (Academic Teaching Hosp Herford, Germany)

Br J Surg 84:380–383, 1997 5–13

Introduction.—Diverticulosis of the colon is a common condition among older patients, but only a few will have complications that require surgery. The classic 3-stage procedure was replaced by Hartmann's operation, which eliminates the septic focus and does not require an anastomosis. More recently, resection with primary anastomosis has been favored as an alternative to Hartmann's operation. A series of 224 patients treated surgically over a 22-year period was reviewed for outcome after the various operative procedures.

Methods.—Surgery was performed electively in 75% of cases and as an emergency in 25%. Clinical signs of peritonitis were present in all 56 patients who had emergency surgery. Complications at admission were acute phlegmon without pus formation in 92 patients, parabolic abscess and/or localized peritonitis in 99, diffuse purulent peritonitis in 33, complete obstruction of the sigmoid colon in 8, and parabolic abscess complicated by fistula in 27. Primary resection and primary anastomosis, the most frequent procedures, were performed in 148 patients; 35 had primary resection and primary anastomosis with protective colostomy, 31 underwent Hartmann's operation, and 10 had the 3-stage procedure of colostomy, resection, and anastomosis, and closure of colostomy.

Results.—There were 2 deaths among the 183 patients who had resection with primary anastomosis, with and without protective colostomy. Seven of 31 patients died after Hartmann's procedure, and 4 of 10 died after the 3-stage procedure. There was a higher incidence of complications after both Hartmann's operation and the delayed 3-stage procedure.

Discussion.—Based on these findings, the authors recommend that both the 3-stage operation and the drainage-only operation be abandoned. Mortality was high after Hartmann's operation, and restoration of continuity is difficult after this procedure. Greater use should be made of primary resection with primary anastomosis in all stages of diverticular disease. Planned sequential peritoneal lavage may allow primary resection with anastomosis to be performed more often in patients with diffuse peritonitis.

► Primary resection and anastomosis (with proximal colostomy) can be done safely even in patients with complicated diverticulitis (pericolonic abscess and diffuse peritonitis). Some patients with diffuse peritonitis underwent staged peritoneal lavage and planned relaparotomy. Only a small number of patients had either a Hartmann's procedure or a 3-stage procedure. This paper demonstrates that an aggressive approach, even in patients with complicated diverticulitis, can be done safely. Proximal diverting colostomy was done in all patients who had primary resection and anastomosis; thus, they had 2 procedures (the second procedure being closure of the colostomy).

It seems to me better to perform a primary resection of the involved colon with end-colostomy and mucous fistula or Hartmann's procedure rather than to perform a primary anastomosis in the face of peritonitis or abscess. With either procedure, the patient still needs 2 operations. If it is safe to do a primary resection and anastomosis, why does the patient need a proximal colostomy? There are techniques for removing stool from the unprepared colon intraoperatively.

R.J. Howard, M.D., Ph.D.

Recurrent Appendicitits

Barber MD, McLaren J, Rainey JB (St John's Hosp at Howden, UK)
Br J Surg 84:110–112, 1997 5–14

Introduction.—Despite doubts about the existence of recurrent and chronic appendicitis, several studies have reported cases in which symptoms of appendicitis resolved without surgical intervention. Data over a 10-year period on 1,084 patients who had an inflamed appendix removed at the study institution were studied in detail for evidence of recurrent appendiceal disease.

Methods.—In addition to the 1084 patients who had an inflamed appendix removed, 60 consecutive patients who had a normal appendix removed during the 10-year period were studied for comparison. Data examined included the clinical signs and symptoms of the Alvarado scoring system. Differences in signs and symptoms were compared for patients whose symptoms resolved, those with a normal appendix, and those with an inflamed appendix.

Results.—Of the 153 (14.1%) patients who had previously attended the hospital with abdominal pain, 71 (6.5%) appeared to have had a separate disease episode that resolved spontaneously. The median interval between presentations was 8 months. Fifty-one had come to the hospital once with similar symptoms, 14 had come twice, and 2 had come 3 times. On 63% of these occasions the patient was admitted. Significantly more women than men had a negative appendectomy (67% vs. 33%, respectively). Pathologic examination of the appendix revealed evidence of chronicity in 8 (11%) patients. The Alvarado scores did not differ significantly between patients with episodes that resolved and those that proceeded to appendectomy. Scores of patients having a negative appendectomy, however, differed significantly from both those with resolving episodes and those subsequently confirmed at surgery to have an inflamed appendix.

Discussion.—The diagnosis of chronic appendicitis fell into disrepute after many patients with nonspecific abdominal complaints continued to have symptoms after appendectomy. Findings in this large series of patients confirm the existence of recurrent appendicitis, which affects at least 6.5% of those who ultimately have an inflamed appendix removed after 1 or more episodes of symptoms compatible with appendicitis.

▶ I have no doubt that recurrent appendicitis can occur. The authors found the clinical suggestion that it does in 6.5% of over 1,000 patients with appendixes. Years ago, I took care of a physician who liked to hike in the wilderness and came in requesting an appendectomy. He said he had several episodes of right lower quadrant pain and tenderness that he thought might be appendicitis. He was concerned that he might be in the woods away from any medical help when an attack of appendicitis that did not resolve spontaneously might come. Somewhat uneasy, I admitted him (one could in those days) for an elective appendectomy. The night before the planned procedure he developed a typical attack, was operated on, and was found to have acute fulminating appendicitis. The paper should not be taken as an argument for waiting to operate on someone with the clinical presentation of appendicitis with the hopes that it may resolve spontaneously.

R.J. Howard, M.D., Ph.D.

Additional Value of Biochemical Tests in Suspected Acute Appendicitis

Hallan S, Åsberg A, Edna T-H (Innherred Hosp, Levanger, Norway)

Eur J Surg 163:533–538, 1997 5–15

Introduction.—The diagnosis of acute appendicitis is often a difficult one, even for experienced surgeons. Biochemical tests are widely used to improve diagnostic accuracy, but their value is controversial. An open prospective study analyzed the estmated probabilities of appendicitis in models using clinical variables alone or with additional data.

TABLE 5.—Mean (SD) Performance Rates of Various Ways of Discriminating Acute Appendicitis*

	Initial negative appendicectomy rate	Potential perforation rate	Missed appendicitis rate
Clinical variables alone	0.223 (0.0559)	0.265 (0.0753)	0.025 (0.0216)
Clinical variables + WBC	0.155 (0.0449)	0.211 (0.0580)	0.020 (0.0170)
Clinical variables + WBC + CRP + Neutrophil count	0.157 (0.0450)	0.152 (0.0561)	0.022 (0.0189)
Alvarado score	0.187 (0.0755)	0.370 (0.0436)	0.021 (0.0112)

*The initial negative appendicectomy rates and the missed appendicitis rates were sought adjusted to be not more than 0.15 and 0.05, respectively.
WBC, white blood cell; *CRP*, C-reactive protein.
(Courtesy of Hallan S, Åsberg A, Edna T-H: Additional value of biochemical tests in suspected acute appendicitis. *Eur J Surg* 163:533–538, 1997.)

Methods.—During the study period (March 1992 to January 1994), surgeons completed data collection sheets for 309 patients with a possible diagnosis of acute appendicitis. Blood was drawn for measurement of erythrocyte sedimentation rate (ESR), total white blood cell (WBC) count, neutrophil count, and C-reactive protein (CRP) concentration. Fifty-two patients were excluded for incomplete data, leaving 142 men and 115 women with a median age of 22 years and a median duration of symptoms of 22 hours. Final diagnosis was based on histologic diagnosis of the excised appendix. Logistic regression was used at completion of the study to estimate a function discriminating acute appendicitis from all other diseases. Repeated measures analysis of variance was used to compare the different models.

Results.—Acute appendicitis was the final diagnosis in 98 patients, nonspecific abdominal pain was diagnosed in 96, and gastroenteritis in 16. The remaining 47 cases represented a variety of disorders. Logistic regression analysis showed classic migration of the pain to be the most important clinical variable, followed by rebound tenderness in the right lower quadrant, male sex, tenderness in the right lower quadrant, aggravation of pain by coughing, and abdominal guarding. Inclusion of these variables in a computer model yielded a mean area under the receiver operating characteristic (ROC) curve of 0.854. Inclusion of WBC count in the calculations increased the mean area under the ROC curve to 0.901. The model improved to 0.920 by addition of CRP concentration and the neutrophil count, and this model showed the best performance rate (Table 5).

Conclusion.—After immediate determination of clinical variables, easily obtained biochemical tests can improve diagnostic accuracy in cases of suspected acute appendicitis. The potential perforation rate is significantly improved by adding total WBC count to clinical variables. Further significant improvement can be gained by inclusion of CPR concentration and a differential count.

► Virtually all surgeons agree that appendicitis can be diagnosed from a history and physical examination alone. Yet using only clinical criteria, most surgeons find that 10% to 15% of patients do not have appendicitis. To increase accuracy of the diagnosis, the authors add certain laboratory tests such as the total white blood cell count, the neutrophil count, and the C-reactive protein concentration. Using a computer model, they find that adding the white blood cell count, neutrophil count, and C-reactive protein determination can decrease the potential perforation rate and missed appendicitis rate. I would guess that virtually all patients with suspected appendicitis have a white blood cell count and neutrophil count determination. Thus, the real question from this paper is does the C-reactive protein determination increase the accuracy of the diagnosis of acute appendicitis? Unfortunately, the authors do not give the data. They only add the C-reactive protein determination and neutrophil count together and find a slight increase in accuracy. Thus, from a practical standpoint, adding the C-reactive protein to what is already done to the patients adds very little. I don't know many surgeons who would be dissuaded from operating on a patient with a history and physical examination consistent with acute appendicitis, even if the white blood cell count and neutrophil count were normal. Unfortunately, the authors use only a computer model to determine whether laboratory tests were helpful, and they didn't compare the value of these tests in patients who ultimately turned out to have appendicitis and those who did not. Thus, it seems that biochemical tests add little to the history and physical examination in deciding whether patients need to have an operation for appendicitis. The authors do not look at the value of x-ray studies of the abdomen, obtained in many hospitals, and, which according to studies we have done, are not at all valuable in diagnosing appendicitis.

R.J. Howard, M.D., Ph.D.

6 Transplantation

Introduction

The increasing disparity between the number of patients awaiting transplantation and the number of donors has led to the use of donors that might not have been previously considered for transplantation. Two papers (Abstracts 6–2 and 6–3) deal with these extended criteria donors. A study from Stanford University (Abstract 6–2) discusses the use of kidneys that were turned down by all other transplant centers in northern California because of donor age, hypotension, hypertension, and other issues that made them less than ideal. Actuarial graft survival in these donors was not significantly different from those of standard criteria donors. Another paper by Hoofnagle (Abstract 6–3) found that livers from older (50 years and above) donors had graft survival as good as those from younger donors. Terasaki et al. (Abstract 6–4) have a cautionary note in the use of older donors in kidney transplant recipients. This group found that kidneys from older donors have a lower graft survival than those from younger donors and that this decrement in graft survival begins at age 31. Nevertheless, because of the critical need for more organ donors, transplant surgeons will continue to use as many donors as possible and many that heretofore were considered inappropriate. Donor determinants of renal allograft rejection were studied by Cosio and Henry (Abstract 6–5). They found that some factors of the donors can influence long-term graft survival. A report by Shapiro et al. (Abstract 6–1) studied recipients of suboptimal kidneys from donors treated with tacrolimus. They found that kidney donors over 60 were associated with inferior outcomes, but other recipients were not.

Two studies investigated renal allograft biopsies. Seròn et al. (Abstract 6–6) performed early protocol biopsies in renal transplant recipients. The biopsies were done at 3 months. They found that early biopsies were useful in detecting patients at risk of losing their grafts. Kon et al. (Abstract 6–7) studied renal allograft biopsies at various times after transplantation. It was found that late renal allograft biopsies were only rarely helpful in treating patients, whereas early allograft biopsies could frequently assist their treatment.

Delayed graft function can lead to decreased graft survival. A study from the Netherlands (Abstract 6–8) discusses the risk factors for delayed graft function in renal transplant patients. Most articles about delayed graft function suggest that it leads to poor long-term graft survival. A study by

Lehtonen et al. (Abstract 6–9) found that long-term graft survival was not necessarily affected by delayed onset of graft function or by early acute rejection. This article is at odds with most previously reported studies. Alejandro et al. (Abstract 6–11) studied the long-term function or islet allograft in type I diabetes. Islet transplantation, after many initial failures, has enjoyed a resurgence and improved survival, as documented in this article.

While comparison trials with tacrolimus and cyclosporine have been done for liver transplantation, a study by Pirsch et al. (Abstract 6–12) compared these two drugs in patients having renal transplantation. This study is presented because it is a large multi-institutional study that has an adequate number of patients in each group with which to make conclusions.

Infection of the transplanted liver with hepatitis C is a common problem in patients having liver transplantation as a result of hepatitis C. A study (Abstract 6–13) from the University of California, Los Angeles discussed graft loss in patients with hepatitis C. Hepatitis C, in many centers, is the most common reason for liver transplantation, and recurrent infection and graft loss from that infection can be a major problem following transplantation.

Richard J. Howard, M.D., Ph.D.

"Suboptimal" Kidney Donors: The Experience With Tacrolimus-based Immunosuppression

Shapiro R, Vivas C, Scantlebury VP, et al (Univ of Pittsburgh, Pa; Montefiore Med Ctr, Bronx, NY)

Transplantation 62:1242–1246, 1996 6–1

Background.—Use of renal donors who are female, pediatric, or older than 60 years of age may lead to inferior graft survival.

Methods.—Grafts from these 3 donor subgroups were compared with those from other donors in 397 recipients.

Results.—At a mean follow-up of 33 ± 10 months, groups did not differ in recipient age, incidence of retransplantation, or percentage of sensitized patients. Female donors were associated with 1- and 3-year patient survivals, 1- and 3-year graft survivals, and renal function comparable to those for male donors. For pediatric en bloc kidneys, 1-year and 3-year actuarial patient survivals were similar to those for all other cadaveric kidneys (Fig 2), as were 1- and 3-year graft survivals and incidence of delayed graft function. In the en bloc recipients, renal function was significantly better and the incidence of rejection was significantly lower. Donors older than 60 years of age were associated with worse 1- and 3-year patient survivals, 1- and 3-year graft survivals, and renal function. Recipients of kidneys from donors older than 60 years of age had significantly worse outcomes than those with kidneys from younger donors (Fig 3). Delayed graft function was significantly more common with grafts

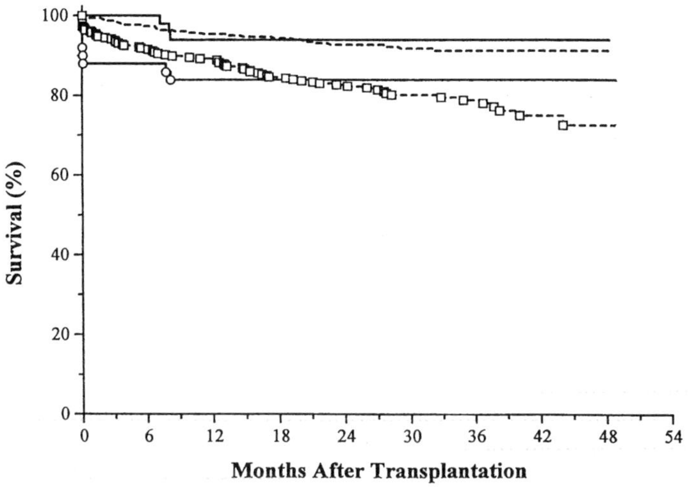

FIGURE 2.—Patient and graft survival rates in recipients of en bloc kidneys from pediatric donors versus other cadaveric donors. For patient survival, *solid line* represents en bloc (n = 50), and *dashed line* represents other cadaveric (n = 306), P =0.596 (log rank). For graft survival, *open circles* represent en bloc (n = 50), and *open squares* represent other cadaveric (n = 308), P = 0.440 (log rank). (Courtesy of Shapiro R, Vivas C, Scantlebury VP, et al. "Suboptimal" kidney donors: The experience with tacrolimus-based immunosuppression. *Transplantation* 62:1242–1246, 1996.)

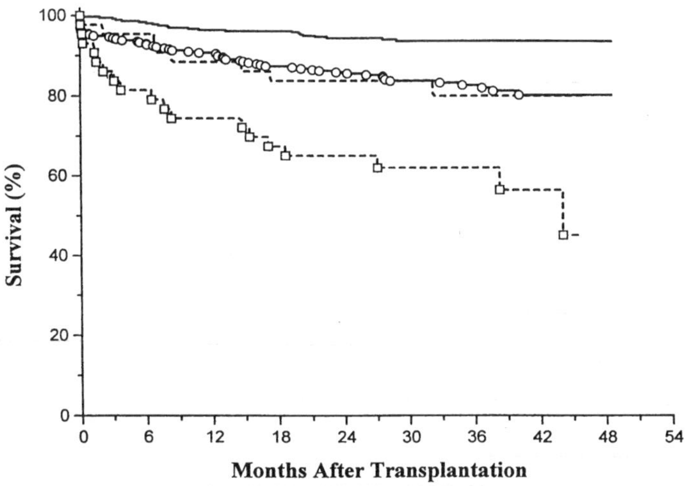

FIGURE 3.—Patient and graft survival rates in recipients of kidneys from donors older or younger than 60 years. For patient survival, *solid line* represents donors younger than 60 years (n = 352), and *dashed line* represents donors older than 60 years (n = 43), P = 0.003 (log rank). For graft survival, *open circles* represent donors younger than 60 years (n = 354), and *open squares* represent donors older than 60 years (n = 43), P = 0.0001 (log rank). (Courtesy of Shapiro R, Vivas C, Scantlebury VP, et al. "Suboptimal" kidney donors: The experience with tacrolimus-based immunosuppression. *Transplantation* 62:1242–1246, 1996.)

from donors older than 60 years, and the incidence of rejection was significantly higher.

Conclusions.—Kidneys from female or very young pediatric donors can be used without adverse outcomes, whereas those from donors older than 60 years cannot. With older donors, patient survival, graft survival, and renal function were inferior, with delayed graft function and rejection more common. Therefore, kidneys from donors older than 60 years of age should not be used.

The Kidneys That Nobody Wanted: Support for the Utilization of Expanded Criteria Donors

Lee CM, Scandling JD, Shen GK, et al (Stanford Univ, Calif)

Transplantation 62:1832–1841, 1996 6–2

Background.—Because of the shortage of cadaveric kidney donors, donor refusal criteria must be reappraised.

Methods.—Of 87 adult cadaveric renal transplants (CRTs), 31 were of kidneys declined by all other local transplant centers. These "kidneys that nobody wanted" (KNW) were compared with the other 56 CRTs

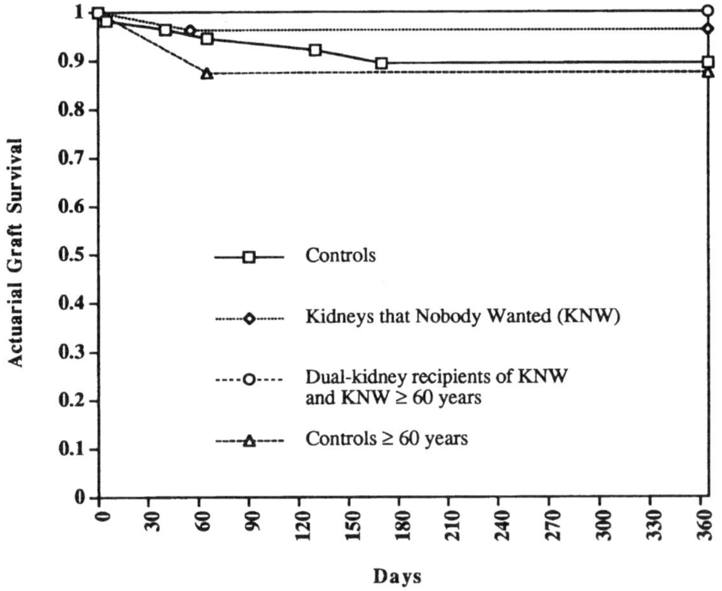

FIGURE 2.—Actuarial kidney graft survival is depicted for 5 groups: recipients of KNW, which other transplant centers declined; recipients of cadaveric kidney transplants performed during the same period, which other centers were willing to accept (*controls*); recipients of dual kidneys from KNW donors; recipients of kidneys from advanced-age (≥ 60 years) KNW donors (*KNW ≥ 60 years*), and recipients of kidneys from advanced-age control donors (*controls ≥ 60 years*). The 1-year actuarial graft survival was 100% for KNW, 91% for controls, 100% for dual-kidney recipients of KNWs, 97% for KNW ≥ 60 years, and 87.5% for controls ≥ 60 years. (Lee CM, Scandling JD, Shen GK, et al. The kidneys that nobody wanted: Support for the utilization of expanded criteria donors. *Transplantation* 62:1832–1841, 1996.)

(controls). Of the 31 KNW, 18 had been declined because of advanced age (also, 8 had a history of hypertension, 4 had more than 10% sclerosed glomeruli, and 3 had acute donor injury), 8 because of donor illness alone, 3 because of biopsy results alone, and 2 because of anatomical abnormalities (horseshoe kidney).

Results.—Twelve recipients of KNW had "dual transplantation" with both donor kidneys. Of 27 donor variables, only the lowest total 4 hour urinary output and donor age differed significantly between KNW and control groups ($P \leq 0.05$). Of 25 recipient variables, only serum creatinine 1 month after transplantation differed significantly, with no differences at 3 and 6 months. To date, KNW results are excellent, with no differences in recipient outcome variables between KNW and control groups for donors younger than 60 years (Fig 2).

Conclusions.—Through 31 transplantations of kidneys declined by other transplant centers, the total number of CRTs performed was increased by 55%. There were similar outcomes at 3 and 6 months after transplantation between KNW and control groups, predicting similar long-term outcomes. Use of kidneys declined by all other transplant centers allowed donors and recipients to be matched for age and size and both KNWs to be used in a single recipient. Donor selection criteria can, with age and size matching, be expanded, as long as adequate renal mass to provide 50 mL/min creatinine clearance is transplanted (possibly by using both kidneys in a single recipient). Decisions to use previously unacceptable kidneys must be made carefully on a case by case basis.

► Every year there is an increase in the number of patients waiting for organ transplants. And this increase far exceeds the small (5% to 10% per year) increase in cadaveric organ donors. Because of this ever-increasing disparity between potential recipients and available organs, transplant surgeons have been pushed to use organs that they might otherwise have discarded. These two papers review experience with kidney grafts from these less-than-ideal donors.

The paper by Lee et al. (Abstract 6–2) demonstrates that organs from donors turned down by other transplant centers function as well as organs that were not turned down by other transplant centers. The organs usually were turned down because of donor age, donor history, creatinine clearance, and other variables. No 2 centers are likely to have identical criteria for acceptable donor organs. Recipients of donors that were turned down by other centers had good graft survival, even donors older than 59 years.

Shapiro et al. (Abstract 6–1) studied "suboptimal" donors (female, pediatric, and older donors). They found that graft survival was as good with female as with male donors and with pediatric donors as with adult donors. They did find, in contrast to the study by Lee et al, that older donors (60 years or older) did have decreased graft survival. Some centers, including that of Lee et al., transplant both kidneys from older donors into 1 recipient if the donors are 60–65 years old. Using donors that heretofore were not used and kidneys from nonheartbeating donors are ways to increase the potential donor pool. Using these expanded-criteria donors will have a small but important effect on the number of transplants done in this country.

R.J. Howard, M.D., Ph.D.

Donor Age and Outcome of Liver Transplantation

Hoofnagle JH, Lombardero M, Zetterman RK, et al (NIH, Bethesda, Md; Univ of Pittsburgh, Pa; Univ of Nebraska, Omaha; et al)

Hepatology 24:89–96, 1996 6–3

Objective.—Although the upper age limit for liver donors has not been established, there are several reports of successful transplantation of older donor livers. The association between donor age and outcome of liver transplantation was evaluated prospectively in a large 7-year cohort study.

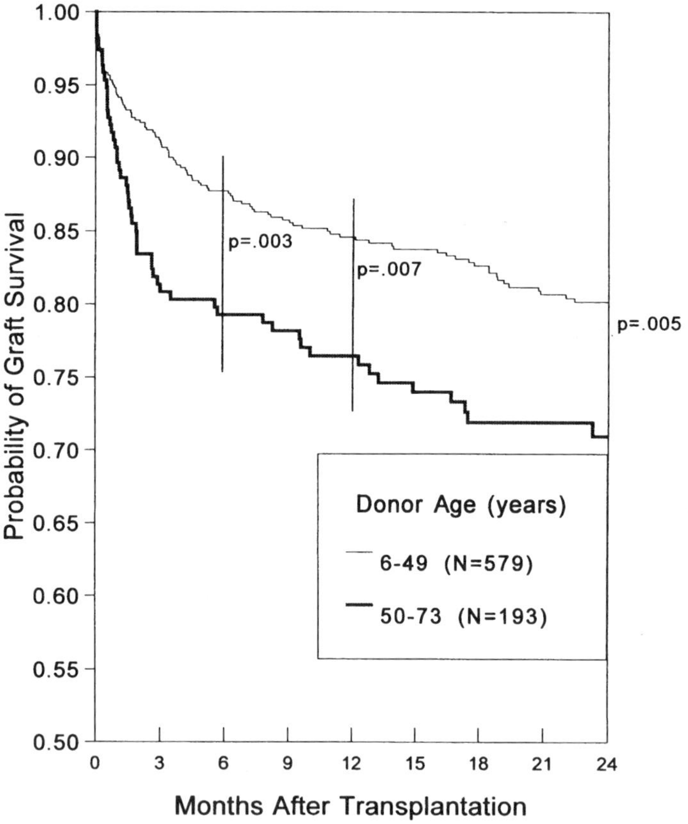

FIGURE 2.—Graft survival by donor age among 772 adults receiving a single-organ liver transplantation at three medical centers between April 15, 1990 and June 30, 1994. (Courtesy of Hoofnagle JH, Lombardero M, Zetterman RK, et al: Donor age and outcome of liver transplantation. *Hepatology* 24:89–96, 1996).

Methods.—Between April 1990 and June 1994, 772 adults underwent single-organ liver transplantation from donors aged 6 to 73 years with 25% (193) donors ≥50 years. All patients were followed for 3 months, 670 for 1 year, and 474 for 2 years. Graft and patient survival were determined at 6, 12, and 24 months.

Results.—Compared with younger donors, older donors were more likely to be women (59% vs. 33%), to have died from CNS causes (79% vs. 28%) as opposed to trauma (13% vs. 63%), to have had abdominal surgery, to have antibody to cytomegalovirus, and to be less likely to have acute alcoholism and chronic drug use. Compared with younger livers, older livers were significantly more likely to be termed "poor" or "fair" by both harvesting surgeon (17% vs. 4%) and transplantation surgeon (17% versus 10%), and to have "fair" or "poor" bile production at surgery (29% versus 18%). During the first week after transplantation, recipients of older livers had significantly higher alanine transaminase, aspartate transaminase, and bilirubin levels and longer prothrombin times than recipients of younger livers. Graft and patient survival were lower in recipients of older livers than in recipients of younger livers (Fig 2). In both univariate and bivariate analysis, donor age and "poor" to "fair" liver quality were associated with decreased patient and graft survival. Three-month graft survival for "good" quality older livers was similar to 3-month survival for younger livers (87% vs. 91%). Compared with "good" liver quality, factors associated with "poor" or "fair" liver quality were abnormal texture (48% vs. 2.5%), not being well perfused (21% vs. 1%), and not having been flushed well (10% vs. 5%). During the 3 months after transplantation, 52 patients died and 37 required retransplantation.

Conclusion.—It is not the donor age but the quality of the liver that determines patient and graft outcome after transplantation.

► While there is a price to be paid for using kidneys from older donors, such does not seem to be the case with liver donors. This study found that livers from older donors had the same draft survival as livers from younger donors. "Older" donors were those 50 years and older. Some livers that were judged to be a "poor" quality and were associated with poorer graft survival came mainly from older donors. The question is, do livers age the same way that kidneys age? Kidneys are made up of functioning units of glomeruli and nephrons. Nephrons decrease in number, and glomeruli, which are vascular structures, become sclerotic. Thus, the number of functioning units decreases with age. Do liver cells age? There is no indication that they do. Biopsies from older livers are difficult to differentiate from those of young individuals. Furthermore, good long-term graft survival has been reported with liver donors who are 70 to 85 years old. This issue is important because a great shortage of these organs is pushing the transplant community to use livers from older donors.

R.J. Howard, M.D., Ph.D.

Significance of the Donor Age Effect on Kidney Transplants

Terasaki PI, Gjertson DW, Cecka JM, et al (Univ of California, Los Angeles)
Clin Transplant 11:366–372, 1997 6–4

Introduction.—As a result of better immunosuppression, clinical kidney transplant success rates continue to improve. But transplants from older cadaver donors have continued to result in diminished transplants survival, which cannot be overcome by improvements in immunosuppression. With increasing donor age, progressively poorer graft survival and quality of function results because the reduction in nephrons in the aging kidney is profound. Kidneys from older donors continue to be used, however, because of the critical shortage of cadaveric organs. The consequences of donor age on kidney transplants was explored.

Methods.—The review included 43,172 cadaver donor transplants in an 8-year period. To assess the joint effects on graft survival of donor age and HLA mismatch, recipient sex, age, race, donor death cause, original disease, transplant year, and ischemia time, Cox regression analysis was used.

Results.—Even on the first day after transplantation, the donor age effect was apparent. With increasing donor age, there was increased first day anuria, dialysis requirement and discharge serum creatinine. A strikingly higher incidence of dialysis requirement was seen within the first week with increasing donor age. As donor age increased, long-term graft and patient survival diminished. When the donor was aged 21–30 years, the 5-year graft survival of zero HLA-A, B, DR mismatched kidneys was 81%, and it was 39% when the donor age was older than 60 years (Fig 4).

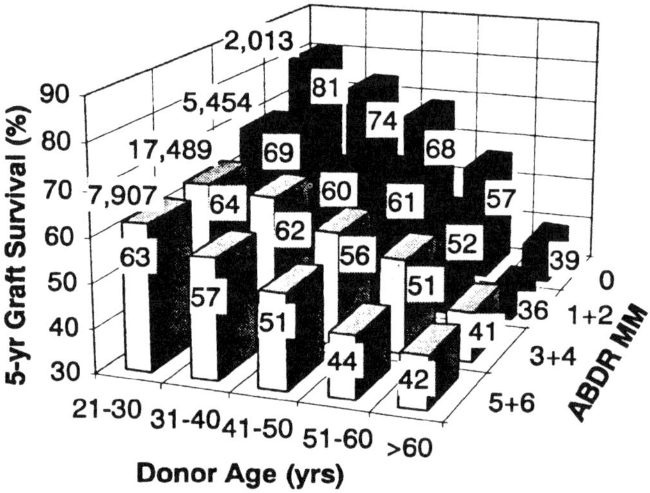

FIGURE 4.—Combined effects of donor age and number of HLA-A, B, DR antigens mismatched on 5-year graft survival. (Courtesy of Terasaki PI, Gjertson DW, Cecka JM, et al: Significance of the donor age effect on kidney transplants. *Clin Transplant* 11:366–372, 1997. Copyright 1997, Munksgaard International Publishers, Inc. Copenhagen, Denmark.)

With both old and young donors, the reported causes of kidney transplant failure were similar.

Conclusion.—Young donor transplants were the best with zero HLA-A, B, DR mismatched transplants. Older donor kidneys were responsible for the worst transplant results, regardless of HLA compatibility. Insufficient renal mass resulting from age was the cause of up to 21% of kidney failures, which were incorrectly attributed to chronic rejection. Treatment of rejection should improve with recognition of this source of kidney failure. New parameters for kidney allocation may be suggested by this information.

▶ This large collective study from the UNOS Scientific Renal Transplant Registry shows that graft survival is progressively decreased as the age of the donor increases, even when controlled for tissue typing. This decreased survival was attributed to the diminishing numbers of active nephrons with age. Johnson et al.[1] have proposed transplanting 2 kidneys instead of 1 in the case of donors older than 65 years to make up for the decrease in functioning nephrons. The study abstracted here is disturbing in that it shows progressively decreasing graft survival in the case of donors over the age of 30 years. Thus, an "older" donor may be far younger than many of us imagine.

R.J. Howard, M.D., Ph.D.

Reference

1. Johnson LB, Kno PC, Dafoe DC. et al: Double adult renal allografts: A technique for expansion of the cadaveric kidney donor pool. *Surgery* 120:580–583, 1996.

Factors Related to the Donor Organ Are Major Determinants of Renal Allograft Function and Survival

Cosio FG, Qiu W, Henry ML, et al (Ohio State Univ, Columbus)

Transplantation 62:1571–1576, 1996 6–5

Introduction.—Many different factors affect the survival of renal allografts: donor-related factors, recipient-related factors, donor-recipient relationships, and external factors. Of these, donor-related factors appear to be more important than recipient-related and donor-recipient factors. This study examined the relative importance of donor factors in terms of renal allograft survival, including which donor factors are correlated with graft survival.

Methods.—The study included a unique sample of 378 adult recipients of cadaveric renal allografts in which paired recipients each received an allograft from the same donor. Both transplants were done at the same institution. In 129 recipient pairs, both were white; in 60 pairs, 1 recipient was white and the other African-American. The functional behavior of the 2 grafts was analyzed by statistical methods developed to compare pairs of identical twins. Differences in renal function were compared within pairs

TABLE 4.—Comparison Between Transplant Recipients Who Lost Their Kidneys Anytime After Transplantation and Those Who Maintained Allograft Function Throughout the Follow-up Period

Variable	Allograft OK	Allograft lost	p*
Donor age	35 ± 16	35 ± 16	NS
Donor weight (kg)	62 ± 22	63 ± 24	NS
Donor gender (% male)	51	60	NS
Donor race (% Caucasian)	95	89	NS
Preservation time (hr)	18 ± 6	20 ± 8	NS
Recipient age	45 ± 13	40 ± 14	<0.0001
Recipient weight (kg)	73 ± 16	75 ± 19	NS
Recipient gender (% male)	62	60	NS
Recipient race (% African-American)	12	30	<0.0001†
PRA peak	13 ± 23	23 ± 33	<0.0001
PRA pre-Tx	9 ± 20	7 ± 20	ns
HLA matching	1.4 ± 1.2	1.3 ± 1.2	ns
SCr_{10d}	1.9 ± 1.2	2.6 ± 2.7	460.0001
SCr_{6mo}	1.9 ± .7	2.2 ± .8	0.02
AR first 6 months	0.6 ± 9	1 ± 1.7	<0.0001
Average MAP_{6mo}	102 ± 8	105 ± 7	0.02

*By Wilcoxon rank test, unless otherwise specified.
†P-value by chi-square (Fisher's exact text).
(Courtesy of Cosio FG, Qiu W, Henry ML, et al: Factors related to the donor organ are major determinants of renal allograft function and survival. *Transplantation* 62:1571–1576, 1996.)

of recipients who had received renal grafts from a single donor and among pairs of recipients. In this way, the contribution of donor factors to graft survival was analyzed. In addition, possible differences in the importance of donor factors between racial groups were assessed.

Results.—Allograft function at 6 months after survival—expressed in terms of serum creatinine at that time (SCr_{6mo})—was significantly related to donor variables. Donor factors accounted for 64% of the variability in SCr_{6mo}, whereas recipient factors accounted for 36%. Transplants with older donors, male recipients, and patients with acute rejection were likely to have a higher SCr_{6mo} (Table 4). There was also evidence of other, unidentified donor factors affecting allograft function. The SCr_{6mo} values of paired recipients were significantly related to each other.

Comparison of the white/African-American paired recipients found no significant differences in SCr_{6mo} or graft survival at 6 months. After 6 months, however, the African-American patients had poorer graft survival. Factors related to the worse outcomes of African-American recipients included poor blood pressure control; graft survival was decreased only for African-American recipients with mean arterial pressures of greater than 105 mm Hg.

Conclusion.—This study shows the importance of donor factors regarding renal allograft function, even when those factors are not readily identifiable or measurable. Donor factors have an important impact not only on early transplant function but also on long-term survival. Differences in graft survival between African-American and white patients cannot be attributed to donor factors. African-American recipients with poor blood pressure control have lower graft survival.

▶ In agreement with the article by Terasaki (Abstract 6–4), this study reports that donor age is a significant risk factor for elevated creatinine values 6 months after transplantation. In spite of the suggestion of the title that *factors* related to the donor organs are determinants of renal allograft survival, the authors show only that 1 factor—age of 30–40 years or more—significantly impacts renal function and survival. Unfortunately, with the increasing use of extended-criteria donors (see the articles by Lee and others reviewed in this section) other donor factors such as hypotension, hypertension, and donor creatinine level were not evaluated in this study. With the increasing use of extended-criteria donors, it is important to study how those parameters that lead to ones becoming an extended criteria donor affect graft function and survival.

R.J. Howard, M.D., Ph.D.

Early Protocol Renal Allograft Biopsies and Graft Outcome

Serón D, Moreso F, Bover J, et al (Ciutat Sanitària i Universitária de Bellvitge, Barcelona)

Kidney Int 51:310–316, 1997 6–6

Introduction.—Since the introduction of cyclosporine, the incidence of acute rejection of transplants and the proportion of grafts lost during the first year after transplantation have decreased, but the rate of grafts lost after the first year is unchanged. The most common cause of late graft failure is chronic transplant nephropathy. A sustained and irreversible decline of renal function in conjunction with hypertension and proteinuria causes graft failure to be suspected. Little is known about the clinical implications of the Banff classification of kidney transplant pathology, although it has contributed to uniformity in the evaluation of renal allograft biopsies. Renal damage in biopsies performed in stable renal allografts early after transplantation was characterized. It was determined whether these lesions could help predict graft loss caused by chronic transplant nephropathy.

Methods.—In 98 patients treated with antilymphocytic antibodies, cyclosporine and prednisone, a protocol biopsy was performed at 3 months. Patients were studied for 58 ± 16 months to determine whether there was a relationship between biopsy findings and graft failure. There were 41 patients who had normal histologic diagnosis results, 12 with borderline change, 30 with chronic transplant nephropathy, 11 with chronic transplant nephropathy associated with borderline change, and 4 with acute rejection. Biopsies were then grouped as those with chronic transplant nephropathy and those without.

Results.—An increased incidence of acute rejection before biopsy was found among patients displaying chronic transplant nephropathy (23.4% vs. 3.0%). Patients with chronic transplant nephropathy also had a higher mean cyclosporine level until biopsy when compared with those patients without chronic transplant nephropathy (242 ± 74 vs. 214 ± 59 ng/mL).

Patients with chronic transplant nephropathy also had a lower actuarial graft survival (80.5% vs. 94.5%).

Conclusion.—To detect patients at risk of losing their graft because of chronic transplant nephropathy, early protocol biopsies are useful.

► Protocol biopsy specimens can be useful in detecting rejection in liver allografts and heart allografts because elevated laboratory tests or symptoms may not occur until rejection has progressed further than the clinician would like. Protocol biopsies are usually done early after transplantation (within the first 5 to 10 days). This study investigates biopsies of renal allografts 3 months after transplantation, a time when early acute rejection is far less likely.

The authors found that 30 patients had chronic transplant nephropathy and that these patients had lower graft survival and frequently had had previous acute rejection. Although they conclude that early protocol biopsies are useful to protect patients at risk of losing their graft as the result of chronic transplant nephropathy, there is little one can do to alter the course of this nephropathy.

If that is so, why do the biopsy? Biopsies have risks and are expensive. What the transplant community needs is a study of early (within the first 14 days) renal allograft biopsy to look for histologic evidence of acute rejection in individuals with apparently normal or improving renal function. Patients who have rejection but have no biochemical abnormalities of their kidneys or improving creatinine levels should be randomized to be treated or not treated. One study previously reviewed in the YEAR BOOK OF SURGERY[1] did perform biopsies 14 days after transplantation but treated all individuals who were found to have histologic evidence of rejection.

R.J. Howard, M.D., Ph.D.

Reference

1. 1995 YEAR BOOK OF SURGERY, p 154.

Diagnostic Contribution of Renal Allograft Biopsies at Various Intervals After Transplantation

Kon SP, Templar J, Dodd SM, et al (Royal London Hosp)

Transplantation 63:547–550, 1997 6–7

Background.—The gold standard for assessing episodes of graft dysfunction in the early posttransplant period is renal allograft biopsy. However, later renal biopsies done for graft dysfunction or as part of routine care have not been critically evaluated.

Methods.—Two hundred sixty-three consecutive renal allograft biopsy specimens at 1 center were analyzed. One hundred seventeen were performed in the first 3 months (group 1); 60, between 4 and 12 months (group 2); and 86, more than 12 months after transplantation (group 3).

Findings.—A significant reduction in the frequency of acute rejection was noted in group 3 compared with groups 1 and 2. The frequency of chronic rejection was significantly greater in group 3 than in groups 1 and 2. Acute tubular necrosis occurred almost exclusively in group 1. In all 3 groups, cyclosporin A nephrotoxicity was an important cause of graft dysfunction, with no significant differences in incidence among the 3 groups. The biopsy report prompted management changes for 72% of patients in group 1, 75% of patients in group 2, and 19% of patients in group 3.

Conclusion.—Late renal allograft biopsies are usually not helpful in patient management. Thus, such biopsies should only be performed as a last resort.

► In contrast to the previous study by Serón (Abstract 6–6), these investigators found that biopsies performed late (3 months after transplantation) were rarely helpful in patient management. In this study, biopsies were performed to investigate the cause of allograft dysfunction or, occasionally, to investigate the failure of renal function to improve. These biopsies were not performed in a protocol fashion as they were in the study by Serón. As might be expected, the earlier the biopsy was performed, the more likely it was to change patient management. In this study, however, the authors do not correlate clinical suspicion with histologic diagnosis. If a patient has an elevated creatinine level and is thought to have acute rejection, and biopsy results confirm that diagnosis, then a case could be made that the biopsy was not helpful in patient management, because the patient would be treated for rejection anyway. On the other hand, if the patient is thought to have rejection and the biopsy results showed another cause of an elevated creatinine level, such as cyclosporine nephrotoxicity, then the biopsy findings would be helpful. In practice, the dilemma is frequently a patient with an elevated creatinine who might have rejection and another cause of the elevated creatinine. If the cause might be rejection, the physician is reluctant to delay treatment too long.

R.J. Howard, M.D., Ph.D.

Risk Factors for Delayed Graft Function in Cadaveric Kidney Transplantation: A Prospective Study of Renal Function and Graft Survival After Preservation With University of Wisconsin Solution in Multi-Organ Donors

Koning OHJ, for the European Multicenter Study Group (Univ Hosp Leiden, The Netherlands; Univ Hosp Groningen, The Netherlands; Univ Hosp Mannheim, Germany)

Transplantation 63:1620–1628, 1997 6–8

Objective.—Patients receiving cadaveric kidney grafts are at risk of delayed graft function (DGF), with most studies reporting an incidence of 25% to 35%. The causes of DGF are unknown. However, several associ-

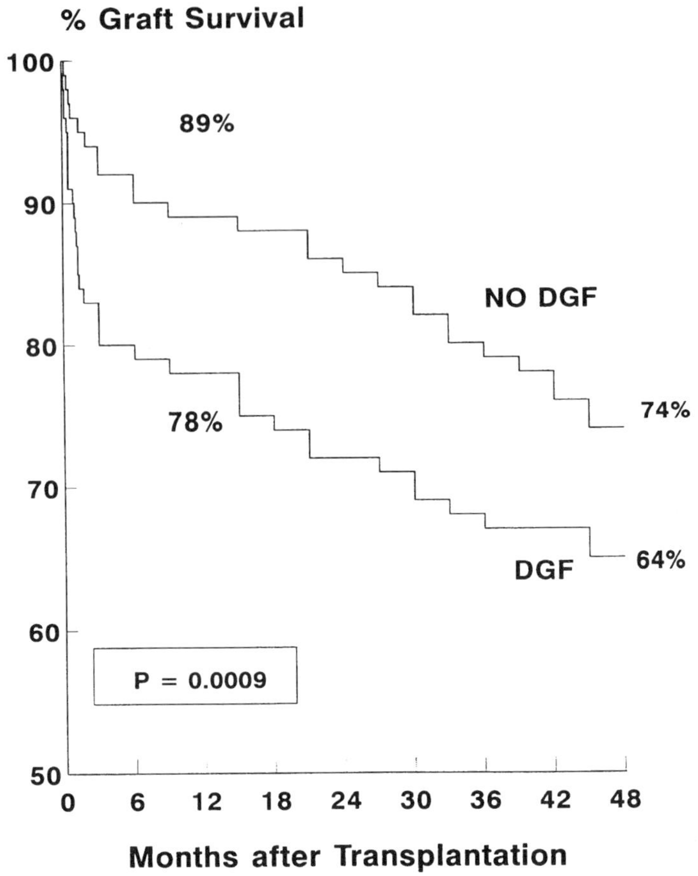

FIGURE 1.—Graft survival in relation to delayed graft function (*DGF*). Number of patients at risk at transplantation: with DGF, n = 129; without DGF, n = 418. The number of patients at risk at 1 year and at 4 years is given in *parentheses*. (Courtesy of Koning OHJ, for the European Multicenter Study Group: Risk factors for delayed graft function in cadaveric kidney transplantation: A prospective study of renal function and graft survival after preservation with University of Wisconsin solution in multi-organ donors. *Transplantation* 63(11):1620–1628, 1997.)

ated factors have been identified, including receiving kidneys from multiorgan donors. Donor and recipient factors affecting the occurrence of DGF were analyzed, along with the effects of DGF on long-term graft survival.

Methods.—A total of 547 kidney allografts transplanted from multiorgan donors were studied. The results of these transplants were compared with reported studies of kidney-only donors. Potential associated factors analyzed included many different aspects of the donor procedure, preservation quality, and posttransplant recipient-related factors.

Results.—Patients without graft failure were followed up for a median of 3.4 years. The incidence of DGF was 24%. On univariate analysis, donor factors associated with an increased risk of DGF were a mean creatinine level of greater than 120 μmol/L and prolonged cold ischemia time (CIT). Recipient factors were previous transplantation, no intraoperative mannitol use, poor reperfusion quality, absence of intraoperative diuresis, and pretransplant anuria and oliguria. Independent predictors after stepwise logistic regression were donor age, CIT, number of previous transplants in the recipient, and intraoperative diuresis. The posttransplant graft survival rate was 91% at 3 months, 87% at 1 year, and 72% at 4 years. Graft survival was about 10% lower for patients with DGF compared with those with immediate graft function (Fig 1). Compared with published data, the incidence of DGF was comparable for grafts from multiorgan and single-organ donors.

Conclusions.—The findings suggest that giving mannitol during transplantation can reduce the risk of DGF by minimizing CIT and optimizing donor management. The evidence links DGF to a 10% increase in the risk of graft failure.

► Virtually every study of the effect of DGF on long-term cadaveric kidney transplants shows a deleterious affect. This study also shows that kidneys with DGF have a 10% lower graft survival than those with immediate function. The incidence of DGF varies markedly among transplant centers from approximately 5% to 25% to 30%. Two papers (Abstracts 6–4 and 6–8) look at donor factors, and their importance determining DGF. Minimizing the incidence of DGF not only leads to better patient outcomes but greatly lowers the cost of kidney transplantation. Because of the shortage of organ donors, more use is being made of extended criteria cadaveric donors. As more donors in this category are used (such as older donors), it is not unexpected that DGF may even increase. By studying those factors that we can influence and optimizing conditions for both the donor and recipient as far as possible, we can at least minimize the incidence of DGF.

R.J. Howard, M.D., Ph.D.

Long-term Graft Outcome Is Not Necessarily Affected by Delayed Onset of Graft Function and Early Acute Rejection

Lehtonen SRK, Isoniemi HM, Salmela KT, et al (Helsinki Univ)

Transplantation 64:103–107, 1997 6–9

Objective.—The factors affecting risk of chronic transplant rejection are unknown. In studies of renal allograft survival, acute rejection and delayed graft function (DGF) have both been linked to reduced 1-year graft survival. The authors' center has been using cyclosporine-based triple-drug immunosuppressive therapy and has found it to reduce the incidence and intensity of acute rejection. The center has also found that, on its own, DGF does not adversely affect long-term graft survival. In this study, the authors analyzed the significance of an acute episode of rejection, together with DGF, as a risk factor for subsequent chronic rejection.

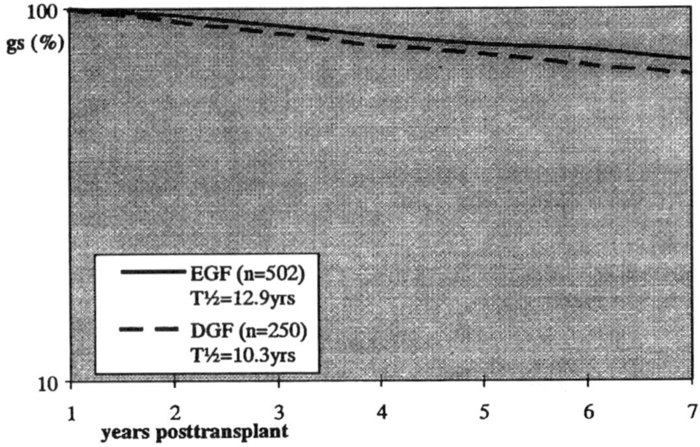

FIGURE 1.—First transplants: Graft survival (*gs*) and half-life (*T½*) for the grafts with early graft function (*EGF*) and the grafts with delayed graft function (*DGF*). (Courtesy of Lehtonen SRK, Isoniemi HM, Salmela KT, et al: Long-term graft outcome is not necessarily affected by delayed onset of graft function and early acute rejection. *Transplantation* 64:103–107, 1997.)

Methods.—The study included 862 first and 182 subsequent renal transplants; the mean patient ages were 45 and 40 years, respectively. All patients received initial triple-drug therapy with cyclosporine, azathioprine, and methylprednisone. The study definition of DGF was a requirement for dialysis in the first week after transplantation or the lack of a spontaneous drop in serum creatinine level. Episodes of acute rejection were diagnosed clinically and confirmed by fine-needle aspiration and/or core biopsy. The effects of acute rejection, together with DGF, on long-term outcome were analyzed. All patients were followed for at least 1 year.

Results.—Thirty-three percent of initial transplants and 44% of repeat transplants were followed by DGF. The incidences of acute rejection were 23% and 28%, respectively. For patients receiving their initial transplants, graft survival and half-life were similar for patients with and without DGF, in the presence or absence of acute rejection episodes (Fig 1). For repeat grafts, patients with early graft function and without acute rejection had better graft survival than those with DGF and acute rejection. Excluding all other causes except chronic rejection, graft half-life for the initial transplant group was 17.3 years for patients without DGF or acute rejection vs. 11.5 years for those with DGF plus acute rejection. For the repeat transplant group, half-life values were 12.3 and 6.1 years, respectively.

Conclusion.—In renal allograft recipients, the combination of acute rejection and DGF may lead to chronic graft failure. However, this effect was found only in patients undergoing repeat transplantations. Even when DGF is present, the influence of acute rejection on long-term graft survival is becoming less important. However, it is still important to detect and treat acute rejection as early as possible to prevent further damage to the graft.

► It is unclear why this study shows no adverse effect of DGF on early acute rejection. Virtually every study from the United States confirms that patients who have DGF have decreased graft survival 1 or 2 years after transplantation, compared with those who have immediate function. Many studies also show decrease survival for patients who have acute rejection episodes in the early posttransplant period. Except for retransplant, primary graft recipients in Finland do not seem to pay a price for these 2 events. The authors report higher rates of DGF survival than seen in the United States: 33% in first transplant recipients. This difference in the long-term effects of DGF between Finland and the United States is not clear.

R.J. Howard, M.D., Ph.D.

The Psychosocial Impact of Donating a Kidney: Long-term Followup From a Urology Based Center

Schover LR, Streem SB, Boparai N, et al (Cleveland Clinic Found, Ohio)

J Urol 157:1596–1601, 1997 6–10

Introduction.—About a quarter of the renal transplants in the United States are donated by first degree relatives of recipients. Previous surveys of kidney donors have shown that the great majority of kidney donors are satisfied with their decision. Negative psychological, health, or financial consequences were noted by a minority of kidney donors, but these surveys extended only to the early 1980s; newer surveys would provide more recent data. To evaluate the psychosocial outcome of kidney donation since the advent of improved surgical techniques, a standardized team approach, and improved patient and graft survival, donors were again surveyed.

Methods.—There were 167 donors who completed a new questionnaire regarding donor satisfaction and the Medical Outcomes Study Short-Form Health Survey, a standardized measure of health-related quality of life. There was a 67% response rate. Donors answered questions on demography, judgment of the medical status of the kidney recipient, perceptions of the ease of deciding to donate, perceptions about the emotional and physical recovery from surgery, the impact of donating on finances and insurance eligibility, and whether the donor would make the same decision again.

Results.—Of the respondents, 83% would strongly encourage others to donate and 90% would make the same choice again. A negative impact on their health was reported by 15% of respondents and negative financial consequences were reported by 23%. There was no impairment of respondent health-related quality of life. A conflicted initial relationship with the recipient was the strongest correlate of donor dissatisfaction; donors believed that information given preoperative was inadequate, and there was a perceived damage to health or finances.

Conclusion.—Psychosocial morbidity is experienced by only a minority of living kidney donors. Negative outcomes could be further decreased by better psychological preparation for surgery and more consistent follow-up.

► Living kidney donation may be of great benefit to both the recipient and the donor. In addition, it can lead to an increase in family bonding. But not every donor has long-term satisfaction with kidney donation. Years ago, Dr. Roberta Simmons[1] did extensive studies on the family dynamics of recipients and donors. She found that some donors were left psychologically less well off than before donation. This study also indicates that there can be negative psychosocial outcomes for some donors.

R.J. Howard, M.D., Ph.D.

Reference

1. Simmons RG: Related donors: Costs and gains. *Transplant Proc* 9:143–145, 1977.

Long-term Function (6 Years) of Islet Allografts in Type 1 Diabetes

Alejandro R, Lehmann R, Ricordi C, et al (Diabetes Research Inst, Miami, Fla; Univ of Miami, Fla; VA Med Ctr, Miami, Fla)

Diabetes 46:1983–1989, 1997 6–11

Introduction.—Islet cell transplantation in patients with type I diabetes has achieved insulin independence in some cases, but most recipients still require some exogenous insulin. When grafts fulfill certain defined criteria, however, the rates of both graft survival and insulin independence at 1-year follow-up are considerably increased. Eight patients who had received islet transplants between September 1990 and November 1993 were observed for long-term (6 years) function of the allografts.

Methods.—Patients ranged in age from 29 to 41 years; duration of diabetes was 18–29 years. Seven patients had stable kidney allografts that had been placed 1 to 11 years before islet transplant, and 1 had a simultaneous islet-kidney transplant. Patients were selected for islet transplant on the basis of C-peptide negativity. One to 5 donors provided islets in each case. Islet allograft function was evaluated before and at different intervals after transplantation. Variables analyzed were basal and peak C-peptide response to 6 kcal/kg Sustacal and the calculated Sustacal stimulation index, loss of basal C-peptide response, and blood glucose and HbA_{1c} levels.

Results.—Two of the 8 patients rejected their islet grafts within the first month and were excluded from analysis. The 6 remaining patients, all of whom had persistent islet function for at least 60 days (range 125 to 2,353 days), had a significant reduction in HbA_{1c} and insulin requirement (from 9.3% to 6.4% and from 0.75 to 0.35 U/kg/day, respectively). In the absence of severe episodes of hypoglycemia, the 2 patients with the longest graft survival exhibited normalization or near-normalization of HbA_{1c} levels during follow-up. All 8 patients achieved normalization of HbA_{1c}

levels with adjuvant insulin therapy. Despite persistence of normal or near-normal HbA-$_{1c}$ levels, Sustacal challenge tests revealed diminution of islet allograft function over time.

Discussion.—Patients in this study received, on average, nearly 15,000 islet equivalents (IEQs)/kg body weight, far above the suggested 6,000 IEQ/kg body weight. Early graft loss still occurred, but some patients achieved long-term islet allograft function. When small dosages of exogenous insulin are taken, blood glucose levels can be close to normal and HbA$_{1c}$ significantly improved by islet transplantation.

► Although pancreas transplantation was tried for the first time in 1963 by Lillehei, it was associated with poor graft survival until the development of cyclosporine and refinement of surgical techniques. There were several early attempts at islet transplantation to eliminate the need to transplant the exocrine pancreas, but they were unsuccessful, in part, because enough islets could not be transplanted to render the patient normoglycemic. Therefore, efforts were switched back to whole pancreas transplantation. Whole pancreas transplantation required extra exocrine tissues to be transplanted that did not benefit the recipient and only caused complications. Currently there is a renewed effort and interest in islet transplantation because of the advances in the number and purity of islets that can be harvested from the human pancreas. An analysis of the islet transplant registry of 96 pretransplantation C-peptide–negative type 1 diabetes patients showed that 27% had a functional graft 1 year after transplantation but only 7% were insulin independent.[1] The present study investigates long-term (up to 6 years) function in 8 recipients of islets recovered from 1 to 5 donors. Two of the first 3 patients achieved insulin independence. Two rejected their islets within one month, but insulin was still required in 6 patients. The number of patients is extremely small, even in this center devoted to islet transplantation. While islet (and pancreas) transplantation can greatly reduce or eliminate the need for insulin, thus far the promise of decreasing or halting the progression of diabetic complication has not been realized.

R.J. Howard, M.D., Ph.D.

Reference

1. Hering BJ, Brendel MD, Schultz AO, et al: Newsletter No. 7. International Islet Transplant Registry 6:1–20, 1996.

A Comparison of Tacrolimus (FK506) and Cyclosporine for Immunosuppression After Cadaveric Renal Transplantation

Pirsch JD, Miller J, Deierhoi MH, et al (Univ of Wisconsin, Madison; Univ of Miami, Fla; Univ of Alabama, Birmingham; et al)

Transplantation 63:977–983, 1997 6–12

Background.—Tacrolimus is a potent inhibitor of interleukin-2 expression by T lymphocytes. In an open-label, randomized study, tacrolimus

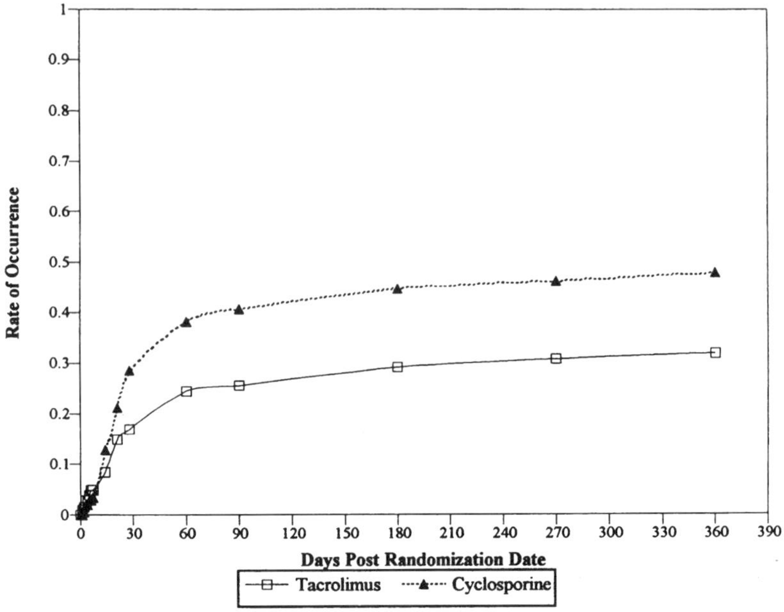

FIGURE 2.—Kaplan-Meier estimates of biopsy-verified acute rejection. (Courtesy of Pirsch JD, Miller J, Deierhoi MH, et al: A comparison of tacrolimus (FK506) and cyclosporine for immunosuppression after cadaveric renal transplantation. *Transplantation* 63:977–983, 1997.)

was compared with cyclosporine for cadaveric renal transplantation (CRT).

Methods.—In sum, 412 patients were randomly assigned to receive tacrolimus (n =205) or cyclosporine (n = 207) after CRT. They were monitored for 1 year for patient and graft survivals and other clinical data.

Results.—During the study, 16 patients (9 in the tacrolimus group and 7 in the cyclosporine group) died, most commonly of infection (overall infection rates were comparable). The tacrolimus group had nonsignificantly fewer graft failures (P = 0.098). Survival at 1 year for the tacrolimus group was 95.6% and for the cyclosporine group was 96.6% (P = 0.576). The tacrolimus group had significantly lower rates of biopsy-confirmed acute rejection (30.7% vs. 46.4%; P = 0.001; Fig 2) and of antilymphocyte therapy use (10.7% vs. 25.1%; $P < 0.001$). In both treatment groups, impaired renal function, gastrointestinal disorders, and neurologic complications were common, although tremor and paresthesia not requiring treatment or dosage change were more frequent in the tacrolimus group. Post-CRT diabetes mellitus, which occurred in 19.9% of the tacrolimus group and in 4% of the cyclosporine group ($P < 0.001$), was reversible in some cases. Hyperlipidemia and hypercholesterolemia were substantially decreased in the tacrolimus group. Although such well-documented side effects of cyclosporine as hirsutism, gingivitis, and gum hyperplasia were rarely seen in the tacrolimus group, alopecia and pruritus were more frequent.

Conclusions.—The dramatic reduction in biopsy-proven acute rejection, significantly reducing the need for antilymphocyte antibody treatment, has great clinical significance. Neurologic events were increased but were rarely treatment limiting, and post-CRT diabetes mellitus was increased but was reversible in some cases. Increasing clinical experience should foster better management. Tacrolimus is safe, effective, and superior to cyclosporine in CRT.

▶ Two large prospective randomized studies comparing cyclosporine with tacrolimus for immunosuppression in liver transplantation have been published previously (1995 YEAR BOOK OF SURGERY, pp 143–148). This year 2 large prospective, randomized studies compared these 2 agents in cadaveric kidney transplantation. This study is from the United States. A European study[1] found a decreased incidence of rejection in patients receiving tacrolimus. There was no difference in graft or patient survival. As was the case with liver transplant studies and the European study, this study found no differences in graft survival or patient survival at 1 year, but patients treated with cyclosporine had significantly more rejection episodes than those treated with tacrolimus. The down side is that patients treated with tacrolimus had more complications, especially more neurologic complications, and a higher incidence of diabetes mellitus. Unfortunately, the authors did not do a cost comparison. Because the agents are so expensive and graft survival at 1 year is comparable, there is some justification for making a therapeutic decision based on cost. Whether the decreased rejection episodes of the tacrolimus group will translate to greater graft survival after 1 year remains to be determined. Another author[2] has found that early rejection episodes were an important predictor of decreased long-term renal allograft survival.

R.J. Howard, M.D., Ph.D.

References

1. Mayer AD, for the European Tacrolimus Multicenter Renal Study Group: Multicenter randomized trial comparing tacrolimus (FK506) and cyclosporine in the prevention of renal allograft rejection. *Transplantation* 64:436–433, 1997.
2. Ferguson R: Acute rejection episodes—best predictor of long-term primary cadaveric renal transplant survival. *Clin Transplant* 8:328–331, 1994.

Graft Loss Following Liver Transplantation in Patients With Chronic Hepatitis C

Rosen HR, O'Reilly PM, Shackleton CR, et al (Univ of California, Los Angeles)
Transplantation 62:1773–1776, 1996 6–13

Background.—Hepatitis C (HCV)-induced liver disease is a frequent indication for orthotopic liver transplantation (OLT). To analyze the reasons for graft loss following OLT for chronic HCV and the outcome after

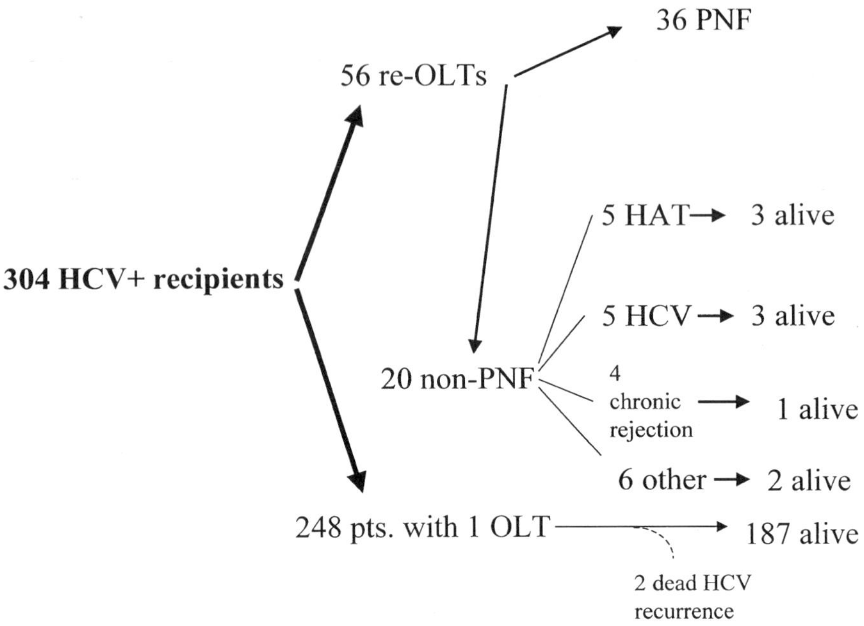

FIGURE 1.—Clinical course of 304 hepatitis C (HCV)-positive patients undergoing orthotopic liver transplantation. Five patients were retransplanted for severe, recurrent HCV. *Abbreviations: re-OLT*, repeat liver transplantation; *HAT*, hepatic artery thrombosis; *PNF*, primary nonfunction. (Courtesy of Rosen HR, O'Reilly PM, Shackleton CR, et al: Graft loss following liver transplantation in patients with chronic hepatitis C. *Transplantation* 62:1773–1776, 1996.)

retransplantation, a retrospective study of 304 consecutive HCV-positive liver transplant recipients was performed.

Study Design.—Between 1990 and 1995, 1,183 OLTs were performed at the UCLA Medical Center. Among these 1,183 OLTs, HCV was diagnosed by ELISA or polymerase chain reaction (PCR) in 304 patients before transplantation. Of these 304 patients, 56 underwent retransplantation. The 36 patients who underwent retransplantation for primary nonfunction (PNF) were excluded from this analysis.

Findings.—The cumulative 1-year survival rate for the 248 patients who had only 1 OLT was 84%. The 3-year survival rate for this group was 75%. The cumulative 1-year survival rate for the 20 non-PNF patients who had a second OLT was 60%. The 3-year survival rate in this group was 43%. The differences in survival between these 2 groups were highly significant (Fig 1). Logistic regression analysis confirmed that the retransplanted patients had a mortality rate more than 4 times higher than the patients in the single OLT group. This higher mortality rate was associated with a high rate of serious infections. Two patients died while awaiting liver donations. Of the 304 patients in this study group transplanted for chronic HCV, 8 developed graft failure secondary to HCV recurrence, and 6 were retransplanted. Of these 6 patients, 3 are alive without evidence of recurrence.

Conclusions.—This review of a large group of patients undergoing OLT for chronic HCV-related liver disease indicated that although recurrence of HCV was common, graft loss resulting from HCV recurrence was not common. Retransplantation itself, for any cause, was an important risk factor for fatal outcome. Monitoring over a follow-up period longer than 2 years will be necessary to determine the true rate of graft loss caused by recurrence of HCV.

► Hepatitis C is the most common cause of liver transplantation (with or without alcohol abuse) in many liver transplant centers. A concern is that hepatitis C will recur in the transplanted liver and will inevitably lead to recurrent end-stage liver disease. This large series of patients with liver transplantation for hepatitis C from a single center demonstrates that the recurrence rate of hepatitis C after primary liver transplantation was only 70% at 3 years and that graft loss attributable to hepatitis C was infrequent. The method of diagnostic testing for hepatitis C is important. The authors used either the ELISA and/or the polymerase chain reaction for detection of HCV-RNA. Polymerase chain reaction testing is more sensitive than ELISA testing in these patients. For instance, using PCR testing, recurrence of hepatitis C after liver transplantation is well over 90%. Because of the long course of hepatitis C infection, it may still take several years before the manifestations of these infections are known, and infected patients may again reach end-stage disease.

R.J. Howard, M.D., Ph.D.

7 Endocrinology

Introduction

The papers reviewed in this section further refine and extend the field of endocrine surgery. The paper by Samson et al. (Abstract 7–1) from the Philippines discussed outpatient thyroidectomy. The authors concluded that outpatient thyroidectomy is appropriate for certain selected patients. Their large series indicated that outpatient thyroidectomy is indeed safe. Nevertheless, many surgeons in this country would still be reluctant to perform outpatient surgery in these patients because of the drastic consequences of possible postoperative hemorrhage. In the 1997 YEAR BOOK OF SURGERY (page 166), we reviewed a series of outpatient operations for primary hyperthyroidism. That paper was followed by a discussion, and many of the commentators objected to the outpatient procedure.

Survival of differentiated thyroid carcinoma in 500 patients was studied by Lurch et al. (Abstract 7–2). An excellent 5-year survival rate (92%) was documented, and none of the patients died of thyroid cancer. Patients with medullary carcinoma have a lower survival rate (Abstract 7–3). This cancer is not as common as other forms of thyroid cancer, and the survival rate was 69.2% at 5 years in 247 patients and 64.7% at 10 years. There was still an excess mortality 10 years or longer after the diagnosis of medullary carcinoma. Thyroid scans are usually obtained for patients with thyroid nodules. A study from Chicago (Abstract 7–4) investigated whether thyroid scanning adds information regarding which nodules should be excised. The authors concluded that scanning is no longer indicated because it does not provide useful information about which nodules should be excised.

Computed tomography (CT) is the main modality used to locate adrenal tumors in patients with primary aldosteronism. Adrenal vein sampling can be helpful in determining the functional significance of a lesion seen on CT (Abstract 7–5). Finding a unilateral source of aldosterone in patients with adrenal glands that appear normal or show only a minimally expanded adrenal gland on CT scan can help determine which side should be operated. While surgery is the primary treatment for adrenal removal, catheter ablation with alcohol can be used in some patients. A study by Inoue et al. (Abstract 7–6) had a success rate of 83% in 18 patients, obviating the need for a surgical procedure. Linos et al. (Abstract 7–7) compared anterior, posterior, and laparoscopic approaches to the management of adrenal disease. They concluded that the laparoscopic approach promises to be safest and least painful, with the shortest hospital stay and the best long-term results.

Parathyroid surgery was the subject of four papers reviewed this year. Ditkoff et al. (Abstract 7–8) studied parathyroid surgery with monitored anesthesia care instead of general anesthesia. They were successful and were able to discharge 47 of the 49 patients within 6 hours of operation. Surgeons disagree whether bilateral or unilateral exploration should be done in patients with hyperparathyroidism. Ryan et al. (Abstract 7–9) studied unilateral exploration in 94 patients with solitary adenomas, 43 of whom had unilateral explorations. All of the 43 had single adenomas and no cases of multiple-gland disease were found. How do patients do when fewer than four diseased glands are identified at operation? This was the subject of a study by Donckier (Abstract 7–10), who performed bilateral exploration, in contrast to the previous paper. While the subjects of their study differed from that of the previous paper, it highlighted the disagreement among surgeons. It described 23 cases among 157 surgical patients in whom fewer than four parathyroid glands were identified.

Parathyroid disease is common in patients with renal failure and in those undergoing a renal transplantation. The hope for some patients with renal failure and secondary hyperparathyroidism is that after the reestablishment of normal renal function with kidney transplantation, the hyperparathyroidism will resolve. A study by Dumonulin (Abstract 7–11) found that there was no evidence of spontaneous improvement of either persistent hyperparathyroidism or the high bone turnover in normocalcemic long-term transplant patients. Thus, an expectation of a return to normal parathyroid function after transplantation seems to be unjustified.

Richard J. Howard, M.D., Ph.D.

Outpatient Thyroidectomy

Samson PS, Reyes FR, Saludares WN, et al (East Avenue Med Ctr, Quezon City, Philippines)

Am J Surg 173:499–503, 1997 7–1

Objective.—Outpatient thyroidectomy (OPT) is practical, safe, and effective. The validity and practicality of OPT versus standard thyroidectomy (ST) are reassessed.

Methods.—Between 1982 and 1994, 1,178 thyroidectomies (809 OPT and 369 ST), including a controlled trial of 309 patients (154 OPT and 155 ST), were performed at the East Avenue Medical Center, Quezon City, Philippines. Indications for OPT included unsightly, bulky goiter (n = 679), pressure symptoms (n = 352), nodule (n = 101), failed medications (n = 26), and controlled toxic goiter (n = 20). Patients who were elderly or weak or who had comorbid conditions, malignancies, or hypertoxicity were excluded.

Results.—Patients, aged 18 to 65 years, were predominantly female (9.8:1). All patients survived. The mean operating time, including anes-

TABLE 5.—Thyroidectomy: Comparison of Overall Results in 1,178 Cases (1982–1994)

	OPT (n = 809)	ST (n = 369)	*P* Value
Complications (no.)			
Intraoperative bleed	1	0	NS
Hoarseness (temporary)	19	7	NS
Hypocalcemia (mild)	16	8	NS
Mortality (no.)	1	0	NS
Operation/anesthesia time (average, minutes)	95.45	134.48	<0.001
Duration of hospitalization (average, hours)	19.81	84.00	<0.001
Cost of treatment per capita (pesos, average)	P2, 124.34	P4, 538.92	<0.001
Patient satisfaction/acceptance			
Very pleased	798	25	
Pleased	11	344	<0.001
Not pleased	0	0	

OPT = outpatient thyroidectomy; ST = standard thyroidectomy; NS = not significant; P = Philippine peso ($1 = P26).

(Reprinted by permission of the publisher from Samson PS, Reyes FR, Saludares WN, et al: Outpatient thyroidectomy. *American Journal of Surgery* 173:499–503, Copyright 1997 by Excerpta Medica Inc.)

thesia time for OPT, was 97 minutes. The cost of OPT was significantly less than for ST. Patients' satisfaction after OPT was high. Complication and mortality rates were similar (Table 5).

Conclusion.—OPT is the treatment of choice for selected patients, particularly those in rural areas.

► This large series reports the results of outpatient thyroidectomy and the great patient satisfaction with the outpatient procedure. The 1997 YEAR BOOK OF SURGERY discusses a paper that described outpatient parathyroidectomy. There were some objections to that paper because of the possibility of early hypocalcemia and/or bleeding that might only be recognized in the postoperative period. In this very large series of 809 outpatient thyroidectomies, 16 patients developed mild hypocalcemia and 1 patient had a major intraoperative hemorrhage when a tie slipped from a superior thyroid vessel. No patients developed hemorrhage after they went home from the hospital, but 1 patient died after outpatient thyroidectomy as a result of postoperative "toxic crisis." This patient had a clinically undetected toxic goiter. Thus, like outpatient parathyroidectomy, outpatient thyroidectomy appears to be a safe procedure. Some might say that even 1 death out of 809 patients having outpatient thyroidectomy is too many and that all thyroidectomies should be done as inpatient procedures. But I don't believe that 1 untoward event among such a large number of patients should be enough to condemn outpatient thyroidectomy.

R.J. Howard, M.D., Ph.D.

Survival of Differentiated Thyroid Carcinoma Studied in 500 Patients

Lerch H, Schober O, Kuwert T, et al (Univ of Münster, Germany)

J Clin Oncol 15:2067–2075, 1997 7–2

Introduction.—Modern strategies of surgery and postoperative management, including high-dose radioiodine therapy, have improved the therapeutic potential of patients with differentiated thyroid carcinoma. There is still controversy over the dose management of radioiodine therapy, the usefulness of routine external radiotherapy of the neck, and the influence of the extent of initial surgery. Survival rates were reviewed in patients with differentiated thyroid carcinoma in whom the therapeutic strategy consisted of almost complete surgical thyroidectomy, early surgical rein-

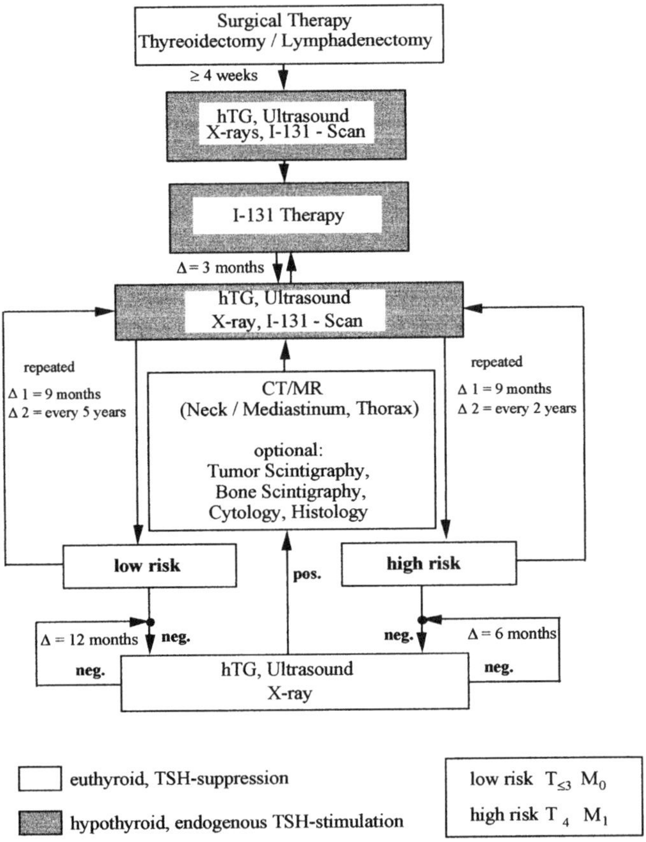

FIGURE 1.—Therapeutic protocol and follow-up evaluation in differentiated thyroid carcinoma. *Abbreviation*: *hTG*, serum-thyroglobulin. (Courtesy of Lerch H, Schober O, Kuwert T, et al: Survival of differentiated thyroid carcinoma studied in 500 patients. *J Clin Oncol* 15:2067–2075, 1997.)

tervention, and high-dose radiodine therapy with no routine external radiotherapy of the neck.

Methods.—A retrospective review included 500 patients. There were 199 patients with follicular thyroid carcinoma and 301 with papillary carcinoma. At presentation, the mean age of the 120 men and 380 women was 46.8 ± 16.4 years. Surgical thyroidectomy was performed on all patients, as well as treatment with high-dose radioactive iodine, and early surgical reintervention with compartment-oriented lymphadenectomy in the patients who had locoregional recurence. There was no routine adjuvant external radiotherapy of the neck. The median follow-up was 5.6 years, with some patients being followed for up to 23 years (Fig 1).

Results.—Of 500 patients, 29 died and 19 of these died of thyroid cancer. There was 0.92 corrected overall 5-year survival rate. None of the patients with a low-risk tumor died of thyroid carcinoma, and their 5-year survival rate was 0.97, whereas patients with a high-risk tumor had a 5-year survival rate of 0.83. In 8 patients, the cause of death was locoregional recurrence, and in 11 patients, the cause of death was metastatic disease. Local invasion, metastatic disease, and age were risk factors that significantly influenced survival, according to multivariate analysis.

Conclusion.—High survival rates from differentiated thyroid carcinoma were produced with the use of total surgical thyroidectomy followed by high-dose radioiodine therapy and early surgical reintervention in cases of locoregional recurrence, even without adjuvant external radiotherapy of the neck.

▶ Long-term survival of differentiated thyroid carcinoma is good. Only 19 of 500 patients died of thyroid cancer and the 5-year survival rate was 92%. As might be expected, the lowest survival rate was among those who had extensive local disease (pT4 and/or M1). The cause of death was locoregional recurrence or metastatic disease. The authors use the aggressive approach that is used by most surgeons; it includes surgical thyroidectomy followed by radioactive iodine and early surgical reintervention for any indication of recurrence.

It is difficult to know whether any changes in therapy have occurred over a long period. The 500 patients in this study were seen between 1972 and 1994, and there is no indication that there was any change in therapy during that period. Because the survival rate is so good and because it takes such an extended period to follow these patients and to see enough patients, it is unlikely that any new therapy could be statistically evaluated in any reasonable period, unless some large-scale cooperative trial were carried out.

R.J. Howard, M.D., Ph.D.

Long Term Follow-up of Patients With Medullary Carcinoma of the Thyroid

Bergholm U, Bergström R, Ekbom A (Univ Hosp, Uppsala, Sweden)
Cancer 79:132–138, 1997 7–3

Objective.—The authors have previously reported on the survival and prognostic factors of medullary carcinoma of the thyroid (MCT) in Sweden. Factors associated with survival included familial vs. sporadic MCT, patient age, tumor size, and disease stage at diagnosis. The analysis covered only the first 10 years after diagnosis. The longer-term survival of MCT and the relevant prognostic factors were analyzed.

Methods.—The analysis included all patients with MCT diagnosed in Sweden from 1959 through 1981. One hundred thirty-four were female and 113 were male (mean age, 52 years). Another 5 years of follow-up was analyzed, for a total of 11 to 32 years. Variables identified in previous studies were evaluated to see whether they continued to be independent prognostic factors.

Results.—The relative survival rate was 69% at 10 years after diagnosis and 65% at 15 years. After exclusion of patients with familial MCT, survival dropped to 61% at 10 years and 54% at 15 years. Independent prognostic factors on multivariate analysis were age, tumor size, disease stage at diagnosis, tumor amyloid content, and euploid DNA pattern. However, the only independent prognostic factors for survival at 10 years or longer after diagnosis were stage, tumor size, and age.

Conclusion.—Overall, patients who survive 10 years or longer after a diagnosis of MCT continue to have excess mortality rates. However, there are some groups of patients with MCT for whom survival is no different than that of the general population: patients with familial MCT detected by screening, patients with tumors smaller than 1 cm, and patients with early-stage disease at diagnosis. For patients with stage III or IV disease or tumors larger than 1 cm at diagnosis, surgery alone is unlikely to be sufficient therapy. More study is needed to identify effective forms of adjuvant therapy for this group of patients.

► A cell of origin of MCT, the perifollicular C-cell, is different from the cell of origin of papillary, follicular, and anaplastic carcinoma. The latter types originate from the follicular cells. Thus, MCT is a distinctly different tumor from other thyroid neoplasms. Because they all arise in the thyroid gland, however, survival of patients with MCT is frequently compared with survival of those with other thyroid neoplasms. Generally, the survival rate of MCT is not as good as that of papillary and follicular tumors. An extensive statistical study in this paper determines which factors lead to prolonged (10–15 year) survival.

R.J. Howard, M.D., Ph.D.

Effectiveness of the Thyroid Scan in Evaluation of the Solitary Thyroid Nodule

Sabel MS, Staren ED, Gianakakis LM, et al (Rush-Presbyterian-St Luke's Med Ctr, Chicago)

Am Surg 63:660–664, 1997 7–4

Background.—There is debate over how to manage the common finding of solitary thyroid nodules. Only a small percentage of nodules are cancerous. Of the 10 million thyroid nodules diagnosed each year in the United States, only 12,000 will turn out to be new thyroid cancers. With the emergence of fine needle aspiration biopsy (FNAB), the role of thyroid scanning needs to be reevaluated. A 20-year experience with radionuclide scanning in patients with a solitary thyroid nodule was reviewed.

Methods.—Thyroidectomy was performed in 770 patients with solitary palpable thyroid nodules between 1974 and 1994. Before surgery, 471 of these patients underwent thyroid scanning and 149 underwent FNAB. On thyroid scanning, nodules that were "cold"—i.e., showed less uptake than the surrounding thyroid tissue—were interpreted as suspicious for malignancy. The findings of thyroid scanning were compared with those of FNAB.

Results.—On thyroid scanning, 23% of "cold" nodules, 36% of indeterminate nodules, and 23% of "hot" nodules proved to be malignant. Just 23% of nodules excised on the basis of thyroid scanning were malignant, compared with 37% for FNAB. The prediction of malignancy was much better with FNAB than with thyroid scanning. In addition, FNAB led to a smaller percentage of patients undergoing excision for benign nodules. Thyroid scanning provided little information beyond that provided by FNAB.

Conclusion.—In patients with solitary thyroid nodules, thyroid scanning does not add significant information regarding which nodules should be excised. Thus, thyroid scanning is no longer indicated as a routine part of the diagnostic workup. Surgeons and primary care physicians alike should understand that surgical excision is the only reliable approach to ruling out cancer in patients with inconclusive results on repeat FNAB.

► The results of this study led the authors to conclude that FNAB has greater predictive power than thyroid scanning for patients with solitary thyroid nodules and, therefore, only FNAB should be done. However, the rationale for obtaining a thyroid scan was both to determine whether the thyroid had hyperfunction or hypofunction and to determine whether, indeed, the module was solitary because not all thyroid nodules are palpable. The final reading was based on the thyroidectomy specimen. The authors argue against obtaining a routine thyroid scan because it does not affect decision making. Yet, of the 83 patients who had both FNAB and scans and for whom they give the results, 12 had cancer on FNAB, so they would undergo thyroidectomy, of course. Forty-four patients who had inconclusive biopsy results would also most likely undergo thyroidectomy. That leaves 27 biopsy specimens that were read as benign; yet, it seems to me that a rate of 7% malignancies in this last group is too high to justify relying on a negative FNAB reading. Perhaps the FNAB results are not yet reliable enough to justify sole use of this technique. Thus, it seems to me, one could conclude 1 of 2 things: Either scans should be relied on or all patients with a solitary nodule should have thyroidectomy, thus ruling out both scans and FNAB. Although, it seems that the authors conclude that because the incidence of thyroid cancer was higher in those who had FNAB than in those who had scans, merely the act of having an FNAB led to a higher incidence of cancer. This ridiculous conclusion can be drawn because the authors do not give any indication of the criteria used to select a scan vs. an FNAB. For those who had both FNABs and scans, not enough data are given to provide any meaningful comparison.

R.J. Howard, M.D., Ph.D.

Primary Aldosteronism: Adrenal Venous Sampling

Young WF Jr, Stanson AW, Grant CS, et al (Mayo Clinic and Mayo Found, Rochester, Minn)

Surgery 120:913–920, 1996 7–5

Introduction.—One of the first tests used to distinguish an aldosterone-producing adenoma (APA) of the adrenal gland from idiopathic hyperaldosteronism (IHA) was selective adrenal venous sampling for aldosterone. This technique is invasive, however, and requires that both adrenal veins be sampled. A prospective study reviewed outcome of adrenal venous sampling in 34 patients with primary aldosteronism who had CT findings that were normal or indicated unilateral microadenoma, bilateral adrenal nodules, or atypical unilateral adrenal macroadenoma (15, 6, 9, and 4 patients, respectively).

Methods.—Patients were selected from among 184 individuals who were diagnosed with primary aldosteronism at the Mayo Clinic from 1990 to 1995. Eligibility criteria included hypertension, hypokalemia, a plasma aldosterone concentration (PAC) to plasma renin activity (PRA) ratio of greater than 15, unsuppressible 24-hour urinary aldosterone secretion of more than 10 μg during a high-sodium diet, and no typical solitary unilateral adrenal macroadenoma larger than 1 cm on CT scan. Blood obtained from both adrenal veins and the inferior vena cava (IVC) below the renal veins was assayed for aldosterone and cortisol concentrations. Sampling was considered successful if the plasma cortisol level in the adrenal vein was more than 5 times higher than that in the IVC.

Results.—Patients were 28 men and 6 women with a mean age of 54 years. The random ambulatory PRA was undetectable in all but 3 patients, and the mean PAC–PRA ratio was 60. Both adrenal glands were catheterized successfully in all but 1 case. Six (40%) patients with normal or minimal adrenal limb thickening on CT had a unilateral source of aldosterone. Ipsilateral aldosterone-producing adenomas were present in all 6

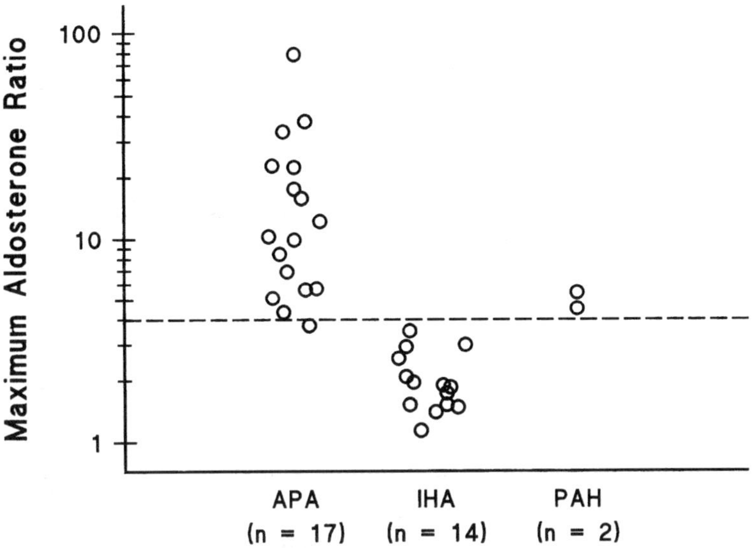

FIGURE 4.—Adrenal vein aldosterone ratios for patients with unilateral APAs, unilateral PAH, and bilateral IHA. Aldosterone levels were corrected for dilutional effects by dividing aldosterone concentration by simultaneously obtained adrenal cortisol concentration. *Abbreviations: APAs,* aldosterone-producing adenomas; *PAH,* primary adrenal hyperplasia; *IHA,* idiopathic hyperaldosteronism. (Courtesy of Young WF Jr, Stanson AW, Grant CS, et al: Primary aldosteronism: Adrenal venous sampling. *Surgery* 120:913–920, 1996.)

patients with a CT finding of unilateral microadenoma. Of those with bilateral adrenal masses, 4 (44%) had a unilateral source of aldosterone secretion, and 3 of 4 patients with unilateral atypical adrenal macroadenomas had ipsilateral aldosterone-producing adenomas. For the 17 patients with APAs, the mean cortisol-corrected aldosterone ratio was 17.7:1 (APA–normal adrenal). The 2 patients with a diagnosis of primary adrenal hyperplasia (PAH) had cortisol-corrected aldosterone ratios of 5.4 and 4.5, and the 14 (42%) patients with IHA (Fig 4) had a mean ratio of 2.0 ± 0.7.

Conclusion.—Although younger age and some laboratory findings are associated with a high probability of APA, these factors are not absolute predictors of unilateral versus bilateral disease. Some patients with adrenal glands that appear normal at CT or show a minimally extended adrenal limb may exhibit a unilateral source of aldosterone excess. Adrenal venous sampling is required to determine the source of aldosterone excess in those with bilateral adrenal masses or atypical-appearing macroadenomas.

► Aldosterone-secreting tumors of the adrenal gland are usually diagnosed in patients with hypertension who have hypokalemia and adenoma detected by CT scanning. Some patients have hypertension and biochemical evidence of an aldosterone-secreting tumor, yet no localization can be detected by CT scan. Adrenal venous sampling can be useful in certain patients in whom no mass is identified in the adrenal gland or in those who have small tumors, bilateral adrenal nodules, and other atypical findings. This study of venous sampling in 34 patients found the test to be helpful in the 33 patients for whom both adrenal veins were successfully cannulated. This invasive procedure is not needed for the majority of patients with aldosterone-secreting tumors of the adrenal gland. The authors do not tell us what the results were in the patient in whom both adrenal veins could not be cannulated. Because the authors' calculations required both adrenal veins to be cannulated, presumably the study was not helpful to patients in whom bilateral adrenal vein cannulation could not be accomplished.

R.J. Howard, M.D., Ph.D.

Transcatheter Arterial Ablation of Aldosteronomas With High-Concentration Ethanol: Preliminary and Long-term Results

Inoue H, Nakajo M, Miyazono N, et al (Kagoshima Univ, Japan)

AJR 168:1241–1245, 1997 7–6

Purpose.—For adrenal tumors of various types, embolization may be performed to reduce tumor bulk or vascularity, suppress hormone secretion, or reduce pain. However, the authors' institution has been the only 1 to report the use of high-concentration ethanol (HCE) for transcatheter arterial ablation (TAA) of aldosteronomas. The long-term follow-up results of this technique in 18 patients were reported.

Methods.—The patients were 15 women and 3 men treated over a 3-year period. Using coaxial technique with a microcatheter, the authors selectively infused a single, 0.2 to 7.0 mL dose of HCE into the feeding arterial branches of the aldosteronoma. A total of 31 such procedures were performed, with ablation monitored by measuring plasma aldosterone levels.

Results.—The aldosteronoma was successfully ablated in 83% of patients. Surgery was required because of insufficient response to TAA in 3 patients. In 14 patients, the destructive effects of TAA were maintained for a mean of 20 months. One patient had recurrent symptoms after 15 months; TAA was repeated, again normalizing plasma aldosterone levels. There were no severe complications. However, in the first week after the procedure, all patients had back pain, half had slight fever, 2 had pleural effusion, and 1 had labile changes in blood pressure.

Conclusion.—In most patients, TAA with HCE is a successful treatment for aldosteronoma. The results suggest that superselective infusion of HCE is a useful alternative to adrenalectomy, particularly for patients who refuse or are not candidates for surgery.

▶ Adrenal embolization has been used to suppress tumor secretion or to relieve pain in patients with functioning adrenal tumors and in patients with adrenal cortical or metastatic tumors. These authors add transcatheter embolization with alcohol to treat aldosterone-secreting tumors of the adrenal gland. They were successful in 15 (83%) of the 18 patients in whom the technique was tried. Minor side effects were noted in some patients, but there were no major complications. Of the 18 patients, 11 required 2 treatments and 2 required a third treatment because of the lack of response or partial efficacy.

Arterial embolization has infrequently been used to treat adrenal tumors. Some adrenal tumors have been treated by the retrograde venous route, using contrast agent. It is surprising that more patients did not require multiple treatments, because adrenal tumors frequently have more than 1 arterial blood supply. Thus, in skilled hands, arterial embolization is an effective means of treating unilateral aldosterone-secreting tumors of the adrenal gland and is in keeping with the general movement toward less invasive surgical procedures for treating disorders of the adrenal gland.

R.J. Howard, M.D., Ph.D.

Anterior, Posterior, or Laparoscopic Approach for the Management of Adrenal Diseases?

Linos DA, Stylopoulos N, Boukis M, et al (Athens Med School Hosp, Greece; Evangelismos Gen Hosp, Athens, Greece; Univ of Iraklion, Greece)

Am J Surg 173:120–125, 1997 7–7

Introduction.—With the expansion of laparoscopic surgery to the retroperitoneal region of the adrenal glands, surgeons can now choose from 3 approaches for the management of adrenal diseases: anterior, posterior, or laparoscopic. The selection of surgical approach was considered in a

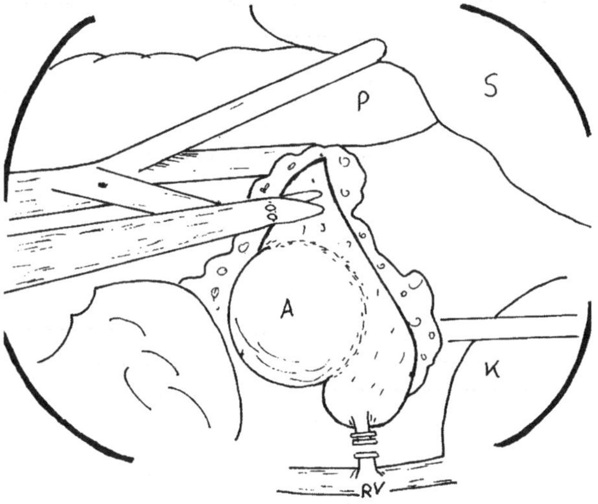

FIGURE 3.—Left laparoscopic adrenalectomy. The tail of the pancreas and the spleen are retracted superomedially. The adrenal tumor is recognized and the adrenal vein is clipped and divided at its junction with the renal vein. P = pancreas, S = spleen, A = adrenal tumor, K = kidney, RV = renal vein. (Reprinted from Linos DA, Stylopoulos N, Boukis M, et al: Anterior, posterior, or laparoscopic approach for the management of adrenal diseases? *Am J Surg* 173:120–125, 1997. Copyright 1997, with permission from Excerpta Medica Inc.)

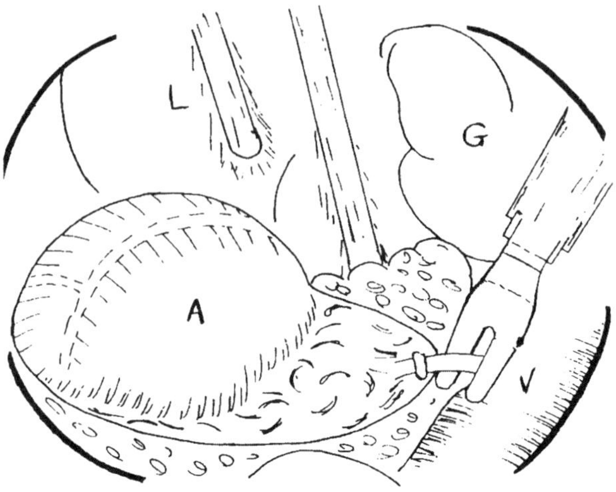

FIGURE 4.—Right laparoscopic adrenalectomy. Using a laparoscopic retractor the liver is drawn upward. Following the lateral border of IVC, the adrenal vein is identified, ligated with endoclips, and divided. *Abbreviation: IVC,* inferior vena cava. L = liver, A = adrenal tumor, V = inferior vena cava (IVC), G = gallbladder. (Reprinted from Linos DA, Stylopoulos N, Boukis M, et al: Anterior, posterior, or laparoscopic approach for the management of adrenal diseases? *Am J Surg* 173:120–125, 1997. Copyright 1997, with permission from Excerpta Medica Inc.)

review of 165 patients operated by a single surgeon between 1984 and 1995.

Methods.—The most common diagnoses were pheochromocytoma (22.4%), adrenal carcinoma (17.5%), and Cushing's syndrome (17.5%). Eighty-six patients underwent adrenalectomy by the anterior transperitoneal approach and 61 by the posterior retroperitoneal approach; 18 had a transperitoneal laparoscopic adrenalectomy. After the first few years of the study period, use of the posterior approach increased sharply when its advantages were recognized. The anterior approach was then reserved for adrenal carcinomas and very large adrenal tumors. The laparoscopic approach, first used in October 1993, has replaced the other surgical approaches for every adrenal pathologic condition except tumors larger than 6 cm (Figs 3 and 4). The 3 approaches were compared for morbidity and mortality rates, operating time, tumor size, duration of hospital stay, and postoperative analgesia requirements.

Results.—There were no operative deaths, and morbidity was low overall: 13.9% in the anterior approach, 9.8% in the posterior approach, and 0% in the laparoscopic approach. For unilateral adrenalectomy, mean operating time was significantly longer for the anterior (155.3 minutes) than for the posterior (108.6 minutes) and laparoscopic (116.1 minutes) approaches. Mean operative time for bilateral adrenalectomy was 165 minutes for the anterior and 178 minutes for the posterior approach, a difference that was not statistically significant. Tumor diameter averaged 8.07 cm for those resected anteriorly, 5.25 cm for those resected posteriorly, and 4.03 cm laparoscopically. Mean length of postoperative hospitalization was significantly shorter with laparoscopy (2.2 days) than with the anterior (8 days) and posterior (4.5 days) approaches to unilateral adrenalectomy. The laparoscopic group also required fewer days of analgesia than did the anterior and posterior groups (mean: 1.08, 3.4, and 2.3 days, respectively).

Conclusion.—The laparoscopic approach offers significant advantages for patients undergoing adrenalectomy: improved safety, less pain, shorter in-hospital stay, and best cosmetic and long-term results. Although the anterior approach is inferior to the posterior approach, it is preferred for removing very large adrenal tumors and when certain concomitant intraabdominal procedures are required.

► The laparoscopic approach to the treatment of adrenal masses is largely replacing open methods. The authors compared the open anterior and posterior approaches to laparoscopic adrenalectomy. The laparoscopic approach seemed to be the safest in their hands and was associated with the shortest hospital stay, best cosmetic results, and least pain. Even though open methods were somewhat faster, pressures from patients will continue to push surgeons to use laparoscopic techniques as long as they can be done safely and as long as the immediate and long-term results are as good as, or better than, open methods.

R.J. Howard, M.D., Ph.D.

Parathyroid Surgery Using Monitored Anesthesia Care as an Alternative to General Anesthesia

Ditkoff BA, Chabot J, Feind C, et al (Columbia Univ, New York)

Am J Surg 172:698–700, 1996 7–8

Introduction.—The few published reports of parathyroid surgery performed using local anesthesia (LA) suggest that LA may be safely and effectively used as an alternative to general anesthesia (GA). This retrospective review of 49 cases is the largest series in the literature reporting outcome of parathyroid surgery using regional anesthesia techniques.

Methods.—The patients were treated at a single institution between February 1987 and June 1996. All parathyroid operations were performed by the same surgeon, and the indication for LA was patient request in all cases. The senior surgeon administered a bilateral cervical block (C2-3) using lidocaine and bupivacaine. Postoperative follow-up evaluation was obtained by office visit and telephone survey. A control group consisted of age- and sex-matched patients who had parathyroid surgery performed under GA.

Results.—Patients in the LA group were 39 women and 10 men, with an average age of 62 years. Preoperative localization studies, ordered for 11 patients, were successful in 9. Forty-eight patients underwent primary neck exploration for parathyroid disease, and 1 underwent secondary neck exploration. Surgery was curative in all cases. Results of final pathology

TABLE 2.—Average Duration and Range of Time (in Minutes) of Operative Procedures Based on Operation Performed

	Average Time (Range)	
	Local Anesthesia	General Anesthesia
Single gland parathyroidectomy	56 (18–100)	59 (30–130)
Single gland parathyroidectomy and thyroidectomy	74 (35–140)	90 (45–135)
Multiple gland parathyroidectomy	65 (45–85)	66 (45–105)
Multiple gland parathyroidectomy and thyroidectomy	63 (55–80)	69 (55–85)

(Courtesy of Ditkoff BA, Chabot J, Feind C, et al: Parathyroid surgery using monitored anesthesia care as an alternative to general anesthesia. *Am J Surg* 172:698–700, 1996. Reprinted by permission of the publisher. Copyright 1996 by Excerpta Medica Inc.)

were parathyroid adenoma in 46 cases and parathyroid hyperplasia in 3. Overall, durations of the various operative procedures were similar for the LA and GA groups (Table 2). More procedures were performed on an outpatient basis in the LA group (47%) than in the GA group (27%). Average length of hospital stay was similar for the remaining patients (1.4 days for the LA group and 1.6 days for the GA group). Only 1 patient was converted from LA to GA. Most (87%) LA patients who were able to be contacted for a patient satisfaction survey found the procedure to be no more painful than a routine dental visit to have a cavity filled.

Conclusion.—Carefully screened patients who require parathroid surgery but who do not want GA can be safely and successfully treated using a regional block. Compared with GA, LA allows more operations to be performed on an outpatient basis and reduces the period of convalescence.

► This study demonstrates that parathyroid and thyroid surgery can be safely performed using local anesthesia with an anesthesiologist providing sedation and monitoring the patient. The 49 patients represented only 7% of the total number of individuals having parathyroid surgery. In all instances, the sole indication for local anesthesia seemed to be the patient's request. Even the senior surgeon in this study seemed to prefer general anesthesia unless the patient objected. Almost half the patients were able to leave the medical center 6 hours after the operation, something that has been criticized by some experts as being unsafe because the manifestations of hypocalcemia may not be present for several hours postoperatively. One of their patients did have postoperative hemorrhage, which was treated by immediate reoperation. Serious consequences could ensue if this hemorrhage did not manifest itself until the patient was already home. Nevertheless, in certain patients outpatient parathyroid surgery using local anesthesia can be done safely. With trends the way they are for increasing the frequency of outpatient surgery, outpatient parathyroid surgery will be used more in the future.

R.J. Howard, M.D., Ph.D.

Efficacy of Selective Unilateral Exploration in Hyperparathyroidism Based on Localization Tests

Ryan JA Jr, Eisenberg B, Pado KM, et al (Virginia Mason Med Ctr, Seattle)
Arch Surg 132:886–891, 1997 7–9

Background.—There is controversy regarding unilateral versus bilateral exploration in primary hyperparathyroidism. Unilateral exploration saves operating time and costs, is associated with lower morbidity, and decreases potential for hypoparathyroidism and recurrent laryngeal nerve damage. Preoperative localization could influence choice of approach.

Methods.—In a case–control study, 100 consecutive patients underwent surgical exploration for primary hyperparathyroidism (43 unilateral and 57 bilateral) with US examination of the neck and thallium–technetium scintigraphy before the operation. Unilateral exploration, at first uncommon, was eventually the standard approach with correct localization.

Results.—Solitary adenoma was demonstrated by US scan in 66%, thallium–technetium scintigraphy in 83%, and either test in 87% of 94 patients. Six patients had multiple gland hyperplasia, with a total of 15 abnormal glands. Identification was correct in 2 patients, and localization tests showed 9 abnormal glands of 15. Localization or intraoperative findings led to bilateral neck exploration in all 6 cases. In 43 unilateral explorations, 43 solitary adenomas and no multiple gland involvements were found. In 57 bilateral explorations, 51 solitary adenomas and 6 multiple gland involvements were found. Average operative times were 105 minutes for the unilateral procedure and 184 minutes for the bilateral. No complications occurred in either group. Hypercalcemia was persistent in 3 patients in the bilateral group and 1 patient per group had recurrent hypercalcemia.

Conclusions.—Anatomical location, relationship to thyroid, size, and shape of enlarged parathyroid glands are seen in successful localization images, making these tests helpful during exploration. Preoperative localization was completely correct for 73% of solitary adenomas, allowing confident unilateral exploration. Exploration of the contralateral side may cause scarring and may impede later operations. With appropriate imaging, unilateral versus bilateral exploration saved in operating room charges an amount equivalent to the cost of both US and thallium–technetium scan and produced results similar to those of bilateral exploration.

▶ The authors claim that using preoperative localization with US and technetium–thallium scintigraphy may eliminate the need for bilateral neck exploration in patients with hyperparathyroidism. They do not use technetium Tc 99m sestamibi scanning, which has been adopted by most centers for localization of parathyroid glands. The surgeons did not base their decision to operate unilaterally or bilaterally on these test results. Less than 50% of the patients had unilateral neck exploration. Furthermore, only 2 of 6 patients with multiple adenomas had both adenomas identified by preoperative localization techniques. Even experienced surgeons differ with each other on whether both sides of the neck should be explored. They also differ on whether an attempt should be made to identify all 4 parathyroid glands. Because preoperative localization techniques are less successful than localization done by an experienced surgeon, the argument has always been that the only localization technique that's needed is to locate an experienced parathyroid surgeon. Localization tests add to the cost of parathyroid surgery, and if both sides of the neck are going to be explored anyway, they may add little to shorten the operative time and thus, operative costs. Preoperative localization studies can be very helpful in re-explorations or where a gland has been missed during the initial procedure.

R.J. Howard, M.D., Ph.D.

Long-term Reults After Surgical Treatment of Renal Hyperparathyroidism When Fewer Than Four Glands Are Identified at Operation

Donckier V, Decoster-Gervy C, Kinnaert P (Université Libre de Bruxelles, Belgium)

J Am Coll Surg 184:70–74, 1997 7–10

Introduction.—A study published in 1987 recommended that patients with renal hyperparathyroidism who are found to have fewer than 4 parathyroid glands during cervical exploration not undergo autografting as part of their surgical treatment. Because long-term follow-up has not been reported for this strategy, investigators examined outcome in 16 cases.

Methods.—Between September 1979 and July 1995, 157 patients with renal hyperparathyroidism underwent parathyroidectomy at the study institution. Fewer than 4 parathyroid glands were found at operation in 23 patients, 16 of whom did not receive grafts. Follow-up for these patients ranged from 12 to 100 months. Immediate preoperative and postoperative values of intact parathyroid hormone (PTH) were available in 12 cases. Patients were divided into the following 4 groups, according to parathyroid function: (1) normal intact PTH blood levels, (2) persistently undetectable intact PTH blood levels, (3) elevated intact PTH blood concentrations without a need for surgery, and (4) elevated intact PTH requiring surgery.

Results.—Three parathyroid glands were excised in 12 patients and 2 glands in 4 patients. In 3 of the latter 4 cases, intact PTH blood levels were normalized on the first postoperative day. All patients showed a postoperative decrease in blood calcium concentration without a concomitant increase in phosphorus levels. Of the 12 patients whose intact PTH levels were known, 11 had a significant decrease in this parameter on the first postoperative day (Fig 2). Four patients had normal blood levels of intact PTH at a median of 60 months after parathyroidectomy, and PTH was undetectable in 2 patients at 16 and 76 months postoperatively. Although levels were elevated in the remaining 10 patients, 7 required either no

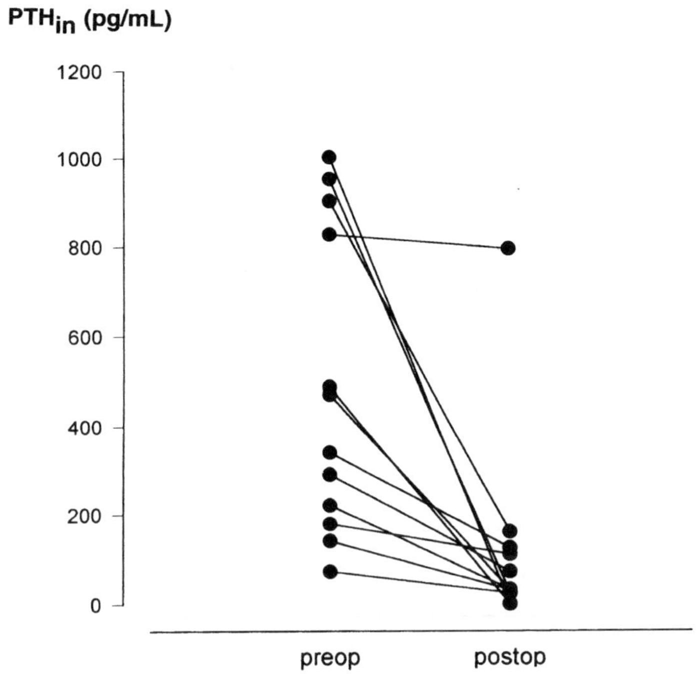

FIGURE 2.—Blood levels of intact parathyroid hormone (PTHin) preoperatively and on the first postoperative day in 12 patients. *Abbreviations: preop,* preoperative; *postop,* postoperative. (Courtesy of Donckier V, Decoster-Gervy C, Kinnaert P: Long-term results after surgical treatment of renal hyperparathyroidism when fewer than four glands are identified at operation. *J Am Coll Surg* 184:70–74, 1997. Reprinted by permission of the *Journal of the American College of Surgeons.*)

therapy or medical treatment. Two patients underwent reoperation, and a third died after refusing further surgical treatment.

Conclusion.—Autotransplantation of parathyroid tissue should not be required in most cases when fewer than 4 glands are identified at cervical exploration. Of the 16 patients in this series, 14 had normal or elevated blood levels of intact PTH at a median of 45 months after parathyroidectomy. Some glandular tissue should be cryopreserved, however, in the event that autotransplantation is eventually needed.

▶ Hyperparathyroidism is common in patients with end-stage renal disease. Many of these patients require surgical treatment for hyperparathyroidism. Virtually all of these patients have hyperplasia. The usual treatment is to remove all 4 glands and to reimplant part of 1 gland into the muscles of the forearm or into the sternocleidomastoid muscle. An alternative treatment is to remove 3½ glands. Most patients have 4 parathyroid glands. What does the surgeon do when only 3 glands are identified? This paper suggests that it is safe to remove all 3 glands and to not reimplant 1 of them, with the expectation that the fourth unidentified gland is still in the patient. One is reluctant to do that because of the slight possibility that the patient only has

3 parathyroid glands. The strategy used in this paper might leave the patient aparathyroid. That did happen in 2 of the 16 patients in this study, leaving the authors to suggest that parathyroid tissue should be cryopreserved for delayed autotransplantation if needed. Most medical centers do not have the capability for cryopreservation of tissue. Only certain centers that can cryopreserve tissue should consider excision of 3 parathyroid glands without reimplantation. Otherwise, as was the case in this paper, a small number of patients will be left aparathyroid.

R.J. Howard, M.D., Ph.D.

No Trend Toward a Spontaneous Improvement of Hyperparathyroidism and High Bone Turnover in Normocalcemic Long-term Renal Transplant Recipients

Dumoulin G, Hory B, Nguyen NU, et al (Centre Hospitalier Universitaire, Besançon, France)

Am J Kidney Dis 29:746–753, 1997 7–11

Introduction.—It is not known how the parathyroid gland adapts to graft restoration of renal function. Excessive parathyroid hormone (PTH) secretion remains common in renal transplant recipients, even those with normal renal function. Calcium-regulating hormones, calcium-phosphate metabolism, and serum osteocalcin were evaluated as markers of bone remodeling in 82 normocalcemic renal transplant recipients (6–73 months previously) with good renal function.

Methods.—Recipients and 82 well-matched healthy control subjects underwent fasting serum samples for the following: PTH, 1,25-$(OH)_2D$, 25(OH)D, osteocalcin, total and ionized calcium, phosphate, creatinine, and albumin, and 24-hour urinary phosphate and creatinine. Subgroups consisting of 25 members each underwent matching of serum creatinine and creatinine clearance.

Results.—Excessive PTH secretion was observed in transplant recipients, compared with controls (6.9 pmol/L vs 3.0 pmol/L). The recipient group had significantly higher bone turnover than controls (osteocalcin 16.6 µg/L vs 8.0 µg/L). An inappropriate PTH secretion was observed in recipients, as demonstrated by a slightly higher ionized calcium than that found in control. Creatinine clearance and serum creatinine were similar in the subgroups of 25 control subjects and recipients matched for creatinine clearance. There was no correlation between the time elapsed since transplantation and PTH concentrations and serum osteocalcin positively correlated with serum PTH (Fig 1). In the subgroup of recipients, serum PTH, osteocalcin, ionized calcium, and serum 1,25-$(OH)_2D$ were significantly higher, compared with controls. Serum phosphate, TRP, and Tmp/GFR were significantly lower in recipients than they were in controls.

Conclusion.—Compared with controls, renal transplant recipients had excessive secretion of PTH, renal phosphate wasting, and high bone turnover. Recipients had an adequate 1,25-$(OH)_2D$ synthesis. There was no

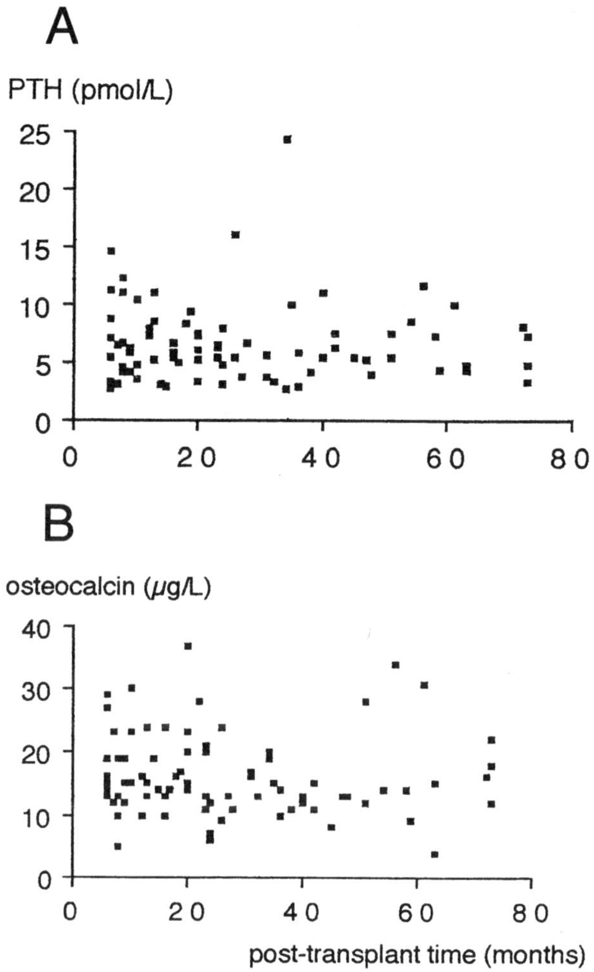

FIGURE 1.—Neither the serum PTH concentration (**A**) nor the serum osteocalcin concentration (**B**) were correlated with posttransplant time in 82 renal transplant recipients. (Courtesy of Dumoulin G. Hory B, Nguyen NU, et al: No trend toward a spontaneous improvement of hyperparathyroidism and high bone turnover in normocalcemic long-term renal transplant recipients. *Am J Kidney Dis* 29:746–753, 1997.)

biological evidence of a spontaneous improvement of these bone mineral disturbances after renal transplantation. The positive association between PTH levels and serum osteocalcin emphasizes the contribution of PTH to high bone turnover in long-term renal transplant recipients.

► Parathyroid disease is common in patients with renal disease. Dialysis patients frequency have hyperparathyroidism caused by hyperplasia, requiring parathyroidectomy. Patients who anticipate transplantation and who do not have severe hyperparathyroidism are frequently not operated on until after their transplants to determine whether the hyperparathyroidism will relent with return of normal renal function. Many surgeons will wait 2–6 months after transplantation before considering parathyroidectomy. This analysis provides no evidence for spontaneous improvement of either persistent hyperparathyroidism or high bone turnover in normocalcemic, long-term renal transplant recipients, suggesting that in most cases the wait for return to normal parathyroid function after transplantation is futile. This study indicates that changes that develop during the pretransplant phase of renal failure are persistent for up to 73 months after transplantation.

R.J. Howard, M.D., Ph.D.

8 Nutrition and Metabolism

Introduction

Nutritional support continues to be an important component in the care of the surgical patient. While its routine use in the healthy elective surgical patient is rarely necessary in the preoperative setting, nutrition support is indicated in severely catabolic patients or in the individual who cannot eat for long periods. As the shift from inpatient to outpatient care continues, the use of enteral nutrition in the home will grow. Because the costs associated with the use of specialized nutritional regimens can be high, there will be continued emphasis on documenting efficacy. Some HMOs are beginning to deny payment. In some hospitals, traditional nutrition support teams have been disbanded.

The optimal timing and the composition of nutritional regimens remain subjects of a considerable number of publications in the nutrition literature, as evidenced by numerous studies that endorse the use of specific nutrients. Is outcome improved by nutritional intervention? A meaningful impact on outcome (improved survival, fewer complications, reduced length of hospital stay) has been difficult to prove. Despite these uncertainties, it remains clear that enteral nutrition is the preferred route of feeding, both from a cost perspective and from an immunological viewpoint. Recent studies indicate that enteral nutrition confers systemic, as well as local (intestinal), benefits on the immune system.

The relationship between nutrients and mediators of the catabolic response continues to be studied from two broad perspectives. The first focuses on the notion that specific nutrients might be able to modify the production of inflammatory mediators in ways that are beneficial to the host. For example, cytokine elaboration by immune cells may reflect cell membrane lipid composition, which might be modulated by the type and amount of fat in the diet. Second, if stress mediators alter body metabolism, leading to nutrient depletion, can this depletion be corrected by the provision of exogenous nutrients? If so, does correction of metabolic deficits translate into functional improvements that are measureable?

For several reasons, it is imperative that surgeons continue to push these frontiers of discovery. First, surgeons care for patients who sustain pronounced catabolic insults and who undergo major operative procedures. Such individuals generally require vigorous metabolic monitoring. Second, as surgeons, we are uniquely equipped to study nutritional derangements and interventions because of our access to tissues and regional organ beds. These opportunities position surgeons to continue to advance this particular field of medicine.

The clinical use of parenteral nutrition is now entering its fourth decade, and its development has important implications. John Rombeau, M.D., professor of surgery at the University of Pennsylvania, has summarized the offshoots of its evolution.[1] First, its discovery has increased the awareness among physicians and surgeons of the importance of nutrition in the clinical care of hospitalized and home patients. It has also given a new identity to the hospital-based dietician. A further outcome is the recognition that more extensive nutritional education is needed in medical school curricula than in the past. In addition, the discovery of parenteral nutrition has led to the birth of a new clinical science, *nutritional pharmacotherapy*, defined as the use of nutrients that have more pharmacological effects than nutrient effects per se. Finally, the introduction of nutritional support regimens has led to the emergence of a multibillion dollar industry.

This chapter of the YEAR BOOK OF SURGERY on nutrition and metabolism divides the overview into papers that focus on research in the field and those that address clinical aspects of nutrition support. While some overlap exists, in the first section I have attempted to cover some of the newer areas of investigation that relate to metabolic regulation and derangements in stress states, the impact of nutrition on organ and cellular function, and mechanisms of nutrient utilization. The second section reviews some of the practical aspects of clinical nutrition support by including an overview of the indications for nutritional support in patients, an assessment of the efficacy of several new formulas, and quality of life and cost issues.

Wiley W. Souba, M.D., Sc.D.

Reference

1. Rombeau J, Muldoon D: *Jonathan Rhoads, M.D., Quaker Sense and Sensibility in the World of Surgery*. Philadelphia, Hanley & Belfus, 1997.

Basic and Clinical Research in Nutrition and Metabolism

Association Between Preoperative Acute Phase Response and Postoperative Complications

Haupt W, Hohenberger W, Mueller R, et al (Univ Hosp, Erlangen, Germany; FU Berlin; McGill Univ, Montreal)
Eur J Surg 163:39–44, 1997 8–1

Introduction.—It would be useful to identify patients at risk of postoperative complications so that treatment could be modified to reduce surgical risk. The inflammatory response and surgical infections play a major

TABLE 3.—Acute Phase Reactants in All Patients (n = 229) and in Patients With No Complications (n = 204) Compared With Those Who Developed Type II (Infective) Complications (n = 9)

	CRP (mg/L)	Prealbumin (mg/L)	Albumin (g/L)	α-1-antitrypsin (g/L)	Monocytes ($\times 10^8$/L)	IL-6 (pg/ml)	Acute phase response
Reference range	<50	≥100	≥34	<3.5	1–7	<4	none
No (%) outside reference range	19 (8)	11 (5)	22 (10)	31 (14)	33 (14)	26 (11)	28 (12)
Mean (SD) values							
All patients	13 (22)	267 (91)	39.7 (5.1)	2.7 (1.0)	4.3 (2.4)	—	—
No complications	12 (21)	272 (90)	39.9 (5.0)	2.7 (0.8)	4.3 (2.4)	—	—
Type II (infective) complications	37 (33)	182 (94)	35.6 (6.3)	3.4 (0.9)	4.5 (3.7)	—	—
No (%) wth no complications	—	—	—	—	—	19 (9)	21 (10)
No (%) with Type II (infective) complications	—	—	—	—	—	6 (67)	7 (78)
p values	0.049	0.004	0.02	0.02	0.9	<0.001	<0.001

(Courtesy of Haupt W, Hohenberger W, Mueller R, et al: Association between preoperative acute phase response and postoperative complications. *Eur J Surg* 163:39–44, 1997.)

role in morbidity and outcome in surgical patients. There is a suggestion that priming of the immune system may result in an inappropriate injury, and such patients might not tolerate minor contamination during elective surgery. Preoperative priming of the host response, as detected by an increased acute-phase response, may be associated with the development of postoperative infective complications.

Methods.—There were 229 patients having major abdominal operations in the prospective open study. Measurements were taken of the serum concentrations of C-reactive protein, albumin, prealbumin, interleukin-6, and α-1-antitrypsin. If interleukin-6 was detected in the serum or if 3 of the 4 serum acute-phase reacting proteins were found in concentrations outside their predefined reference ranges, a patient was defined as having mounted an acute-phase response (Table 3).

Results.—Serum levels of interleukin-6, α-1-antitrypsin, and C-reactive protein were increased, and serum concentrations levels of albumin and prealbumin were decreased in 5% to 14% of patients. Major complications developed in 25 patients (11%), and 9 patients (4%) died. Severe systemic inflammatory response caused by infective complications that did not result from technical failure of the operative technique occurred in 9 patients. Before the operation, 7 of the 9 patients (78%) had an increased acute-phase response, and this significantly differed from the incidence among the patients who recovered without complications.

Conclusions.—The patient's response to operation and infection during the postoperative period may be adversely affected when there are signs of an acute-phase response preoperatively.

► The authors studied 229 patients undergoing elective major abdominal surgery and demonstrated that outcome was worse when there were signs of an acute-phase response preoperatively. This raises the question of whether some form of preoperative intervention would benefit such patients. For example, if the immune system could be primed in such individuals, this might lead to an enhanced host response resulting in irradication of contaminating bacteria in the postoperative period. On the other hand, a primed immune system could result in a dysregulated, excessive response that could lead to hemodynamic instability. Despite a growing understanding of the metabolic response to sepsis, effective therapeutic strategies, be they preoperative administration of cytokine receptor antagonists or the administration of immunomodulatory agents, require further study.

W.W. Souba, M.D., Sc.D.

Effect of Bombesin on Impairment of Upper Respiratory Tract Immunity Induced by Total Parenteral Nutrition

Janu PG, Kudsk KA, Li J, et al (Univ of Tennessee, Memphis)

Arch Surg 132:89–93, 1997 8–2

Introduction.—The gastrointestinal tract serves as an important barrier function against potential pathogens, and more than 50% of the body's immunoglobulin production is secreted at the mucosal surface in the form of secretory IgA. There seems to be a breakdown of the mucosal protective barrier in critically ill patients who are susceptible to septic complications. To reduce susceptibility to invasive infection, specialized nutritional support is used. Bombesin is a tetradecaneuropeptide that stimulates the release of several gastrointestinal tract hormones, prevents total parenteral nutrition–associated mucosal atrophy of the gastrointestinal tract, increases levels of intestinal IgA, improves mortality in a lethal enterocolitis model, and reduces bacterial translocation. The effect of bombesin on total parenteral nutrition–induced impairment of upper respiratory tract immunity was determined.

Methods.—Mice were innoculated with H1N1 virus administered intranasally. The mice were randomly assigned to 1 of 3 groups at 3 weeks: 12 received chow and intravenous saline; 12 received intravenous total parenteral nutrition; and 12 received intravenous total parenteral nutrition and bombesin, 15 µg/kg administered 3 times daily. Mice were rechallenged after 5 days and after they were killed at 40 hours, viral shedding from the respiratory tract was measured. Virus is not shed by normal convalescent mice because of intact IgA-mediated mechanisms.

Results.—The total parenteral nutrition and bombesin groups had similar body weight, but both were significantly lower than the chow group. Compared with 6 mice (50%) in the total parenteral nutrition group who shed virus after 6 days of feeding, no mice in the chow group shed virus. Only 1 of the mice in the bombesin group was positive for viral shedding. Compared with the chow group and the bombesin group, the total parenteral nutrition group showed increased viral shedding.

Conclusions.—The total parenteral nutrition–associated impairment of upper respiratory tract immunity to an IgA-mediated infectious challenge was reversed with exogenous administration of bombesin. Because neuropeptides are endogenous to the gastrointestinal and respiratory tracts, the concept of a common mucosal immune system is supported. For patients who require total parenteral nutrition, hormonal modulation of immunity is a promising avenue of treatment.

Recovery of Gut-associated Lymphoid Tissue and Upper Respiratory Tract Immunity After Parenteral Nutrition

Janu P, Li J, Renegar KB, et al (Univ of Tennessee, Memphis)

Ann Surg 225:707–717, 1997 8–3

Introduction.—In maintaining nutritional status of critically ill patients, total parenteral nutrition can play a vital role. The immunologic defenses may not all be supported by this form of nutrition, particularly the mucosal immune system. Previous studies have shown that total parenteral nutrition administered to animals has resulted in fewer lamina propia, reduced levels of intestinal IgA, and impairs immunity to influenza virus when compared with chow-fed animals or those fed complex enteral diets.

TABLE 3.—T Cell Subsets (×10[6])

	Chow	Days of Chow Refeeding After Total Parenteral Nutrition Day 0	Day 1	Day 2	Day 3	Day 4
Peyer's patch						
CD4	2.8 ± 0.4	0.9 ± 0.3*	2.1 ± 0.4†	3.2 ± 0.4†‡	2.7 ± 0.3†	2.9 ± 0.4†
CD8	0.9 ± 0.1	0.2 ± 0.1*	0.5 ± 0.1	0.7 ± 0.1†	0.7 ± 0.1†	0.8 ± 0.1†
Lamina propria						
CD4	2.0 ± 0.2	0.7 ± 0.2*	1.0 ± 0.1*	1.5 ± 0.2†	1.3 ± 0.2*	1.9 ± 0.3†‡
CD8	0.9 ± 0.1	0.5 ± 0.1*	0.7 ± 0.1	0.9 ± 0.1†	0.6 ± 0.1	0.9 ± 0.1†

*$P < 0.05$ vs. chow.
†$p < 0.05$ vs. day 0.
‡$P < 0.05$ vs. day 1.
(Courtesy of Janu P, Li J, Renegar KB, et al: Recovery of gut-associated lymphoid tissue and upper respiratory tract immunity after parenteral nutrition. *Ann Surg* 225:707–717, 1997.)

The recovery of gut-associated lymphoid tissue and upper respiratory tract immunity was studied with an enteral diet administered after total parenteral nutrition.

Methods.—Total parenteral nutrition was administered to mice for 5 days, followed by up to 4 days of chow. Flow cytometry was used to measure small intestinal gut-associated lymphoid tissue. Mouse-adapted influenza virus was used to immunize the mice intranasally. One group of mice was administered total parenteral nutrition for 5 days, followed by enteral refeeding for 5 days. Another group of mice received only total parenteral nutrition. They were then all challenged with intranasal virus and after they were killed, viral shedding was determined.

Results.—Compared with the chow-fed controls, the animals fed only total parenteral nutrition had significantly fewer gut-associated lymphoid tissue lymphocytes. After a single day of refeeding, Peyer's patch counts increased and returned to normal levels by 48 hours. After 24 hours of refeeding, lamina propia counts remained significantly depressed, but after 2 days of refeeding, they returned to normal. Total cell patterns were mimicked by the T-cell and B-cell populations. After 72 hours of refeedings, the lamina propia CD4+/CD8+ ratio returned to normal (Table 3). Eight of 12 total parenteral nutrition–fed mice were positive for viral shedding after 5 days, whereas none of the mice refed enterally were positive for viral shedding.

Conclusions.—Rapid repletion of gut-associated lymphoid tissue is associated with enteral refeeding after total parenteral nutrition, initially within Peyer's patches and subsequently within the lamina propria. Impairment of IgA-mediated upper respiratory tract antiviral immunity that occurs with total parenteral nutrition administration is corrected with refeeding.

Postoperative Enteral Feeding Does Not Prevent Intestinal Bacterial Translocation, but Reduces the Rate of Pulmonary Infections in Pigs Undergoing Total Orthotopic Small Bowel Transplantation

Biffi R, Privitera G, Pozzi S, et al (Università di Milano, Milan, Italy)

Eur J Surg 163:703–709, 1997 8–4

Introduction.—Many infective complications can occur to recipients of experimental and clinical small bowel transplants. Previous studies have shown that enteral nutrition increases resistance to infection in hypercatabolic states such as burns, sepsis, peritonitis, and major trauma The effects of a nonelemental liquid diet were assessed in pigs who had orthotopic small bowel transplantation with cyclosporin A immunosuppression. Assessments were made of changes in the microflora of the small bowel, the rate of translocation to mesenteric lymph nodes and parenchymal organs, and the incidence of pneumonia.

Methods.—There were 32 white pigs divided into 5 groups: 6 had small bowel transplanted and were treated with immunosuppression and fed on chow; 6 had immunosuppression and were fed with an enteral feed through a tube gastrostomy beginning on the fourth day after small bowel transplantation; 6 had no immunosuppression and were fed on chow; 6 had orthotopic small bowel autotransplantation; and 8 were controls with a sham operation. The pigs were examined for graft-vs.-host-disease, bacterial translocation, luminal bacterial overgrowth, signs of rejection, pneumonia, and nutritional state.

Results.—Acute rejection occurred in the pigs who had no immunosuppression. After allotransplantation, there was appreciable overgrowth of aerobic and anaerobic bacteria in the experimental groups compared with the controls (Table 2). In the enterally fed animals, the counts of anaerobic bacteria were significantly lower compared with those given free access to commercial chow. After autografts and allografts, bacterial translocation developed to a similar degree in all the groups. One of 6 pigs given enteral feeding had pneumonia vs. 5 of 6 pigs fed conventionally, but this difference was not considered significant. There was less weight loss with enterally fed animals compared with the others.

Conclusions.—The rate of pneumonia was slightly reduced with enteral feeding for up to a month, and a better nutritional state resulted in the pigs after small bowel transplantation. Luminal bacterial overgrowth or translocation was not affected.

► These 3 studies (Abstracts 8–2 to 8–4) focus on the role of luminal nutrition and growth factors in maintaining the integrity of mucosal immunity. Although the majority of studies have focused on the gut immune system, there are now convincing data demonstrating that derangements in respiratory tract immunity occur with parenteral nutrition. The observation that both enteral feedings and exogenous gut-derived hormones can improve upper respiratory tract immunity suggests a common pathway that involves the gastrointestinal tract. These studies lend further credence to

TABLE 2.—Mean (SD) Counts of Total Aerobic and Anaerobic Bacteria Cultured From the Proximal Graft (log CFU/cm^2) and Mesenteric Lymph Nodes (log CFU/g) in the Experimental Groups

Group	No. of pigs	Proximal graft		Lymph nodes	
		Aerobes	Anaerobes	Aerobes	Anaerobes
Sham	8	1.51 (1.50)	0.99 (1.39)	not detected	not detected
1 (Transplantation, immunosuppression, commercial chow)	6	4.30 (1.18)	4.80 (1.65)*	0.71 (1.03)	0.64 (1.44)
2 (Transplantation, immunosuppression, enteral feeding)	6	2.88 (1.48)	2.81 (1.39)*	1.90 (2.00)	2.23 (2.46)
3 (Transplantation + commercial chow only)	6	6.14 (0.53)	5.54 (1.25)	1.19 (0.26)	1.06 (0.4)
4 (Autotransplantation + commercial chow only)	6	3.74 (2.18)	3.88 (2.04)	2.46 (1.86)	2.10 (2.23)

*$P = 0.047$.

(Courtesy of Biffi R, Privitera G, Pozzi S, et al: Postoperative enteral feeding does not prevent intestinal bacterial translocation, but reduces the rate of pulmonary infections in pigs undergoing total orthotopic small bowel transplantation. *Eur J Surg* 163:703–709, 1997.)

the notion that enteral nutrition not only has beneficial effects for the gut but is likely to improve the immune function of distant organs.

W.W. Souba, M.D. Sc.D.

Parenteral Nutrition Modifies Glucose and Glutamine Metabolism in Rat Isolated Enterocytes

Colomb V, Darcy-Vrillon B, Jobert A, et al (Institut Natl de la Recherche Agronomique, Jouy-en-Josas, France; Hôpital Necker-Enfants Malades, Paris)

Gastroenterology 112:429–436, 1997 8–5

Introduction.—Patients with extensive small bowel resection or functional intestinal diseases may have impaired nutritional status. Parenteral nutrition is an essential component of treatment because partial or total bowel rest is sometimes necessary for short or prolonged periods. The effects of parenteral and enteral delivery of the same glutamine-free formula on the ability of enterocytes to metabolize glutamine and glucose substrates in the fed state were compared.

Methods.—A continuous infusion of an all-in-one glutamine-free formula was given intravenously or intragastrically to rats. The third group served as the controls who were fed orally and received the same protein-caloric supplies. Blood samples were collected and the jejunoileum was removed after the rats were killed on the seventh day. The enterocytes were

TABLE 3.—Effects of Artificial Nutrition on Metabolite Production From Glucose and Glutamine in Rat Isolated Enterocytes

	OC	IG	IV
Endogenous metabolite production (*nmol · min^{-1} · 10^{6} viable cells^{-1}*)			
Lactate + pyruvate	0.03 ± 0.01	0.05 ± 0.01	0.03 ± 0.01
Alanine	0.01 ± 0.01	0.02 ± 0.01	0.01 ± 0.01
Ammonia	0.08 ± 0.06	0.08 ± 0.04	0.12 ± 0.06
Glutamate	0.01 ± 000	0.02 ± 0.01	0.01 ± 0.01
Metabolite production from glucose (*nmol · min^{-1} · 10^{6} viable cells^{-1}*)			
Lactate + pyruvate	1.28 ± 0.20	1.26 ± 0.14	0.76 ± 0.07*,†
Alanine	0.06 ± 0.02	0.06 ± 0.01	0.06 ± 0.02
Metabolite production from glutamine (*nmol · min^{-1} · 10^{6} viable cells^{-1}*)			
Glutamate	1.06 ± 0.16	0.86 ± 0.06	1.49 ± 0.13*,†
Ammonia	1.89 ± 0.23	1.52 ± 0.09	2.97 ± 0.05*,†
Alanine	0.28 ± 0.05	0.25 ± 0.02	0.15 ± 0.05

NOTE: Enterocytes were incubated (30 minutes at 37°C) in the absence or presence of 2 mmol/L glucose or 2 mmol/L glutamine. Values are means ± SEM of 6–10 different cell preparations per group.

*Significantly different from OC ($P < 0.05$).

†Significantly different from IG ($P < 0.05$).

Abbreviations: OC, orally fed control rats; *IG*, intragastric fed rats.

(Courtesy of Colomb V, Darcy-Vrillon B, Jobert A, et al: Parenteral nutrition modifies glucose and glutamine metabolism in rat isolated enterocytes. *Gastroenterology* 112:429–436, 1997.)

isolated. In the presence of ^{14}C-glucose and ^{14}C-glutamine, aliquots of cell suspensions were incubated for 30 minutes at 37°C.

Results.—Mild hyperglycemia and marked hyperinsulinemia were seen in the intravenously fed rats. The 3 groups had similar plasma glutamine levels. Compared with intragastrically fed and control rats, the intravenously fed rats showed a simultaneous increase in glutamine utilization and a decrease in glucose utilization (Table 3). There were no parallel changes in glutaminase and hexokinase activities. In intravenously fed rat enterocytes, the basolateral glucose transporter protein concentration was reduced.

Conclusions.—Fuel utilization is influenced by enterocytes in the route of nutrient delivery. High levels of counterregulatory hormones may cause the increase in glutamine utilization and decrease in glucose utilization in the intravenously fed rats. To investigate the underlying mechanisms, further studies are necessary.

Basal Nutrition Promotes Human Intestinal Epithelial (Caco-2) Proliferation, Brush Border Enzyme Activity, and Motility

Perdikis DA, Basson MD (Yale Univ, New Haven, Conn; VA Connecticut Health Care System, West Haven)

Crit Care Med 25:159–165, 1997 8–6

Introduction.—In the management of critically ill patients, nutrition plays an important role. Recovery from hypermetabolic states depends on maintaining gut mucosal biology, including absorptive capacity, proliferative renewal, and the ability to heal mucosal defects. The hypothesis that nutrients delivered to the basal aspect of an intestinal epithelial cell can modulate intestinal epithelial biology, as well as provide metabolic fuels, is fundamental to parenteral nutritional manipulation. The effects of supplemental basal nutrient delivery on intestinal epithelial cell biology are still unknown. One hypothesis is that intestinal epithelial differentiation, proliferation, and sheet migration may vary with the direction of nutrient delivery. This hypothesis was tested using the well-differentiated human intestinal epithelial Caco-2 cell line as a model.

Methods.—Experiments were performed on a well-differentiated subclone of cells derived from the established human Caco-2 colonic epithelial cell line. Type I collagen substrate was used to compare the brush border enzyme activity, proliferation, and motility of human intestinal epithelial (Caco-2) cells with culture inserts on 0.45-µ semipermeable membranes with culture medium beneath the monolayers as well as above them or with culture medium above the apical side of the cell monolayer. During a 13-day period, proliferation was assessed by serial hematocytometric counts. In protein-matched aliquots of cell lysates, the specific activity of the brush border enzymes, dipeptidyl dipeptidase and alkaline phosphatase, was assayed by the digestion of synthetic chromogenic substrates. By blocking proliferation with mitomycin C, motility was dissociated from the proliferative component of monolayer expansion.

Results.—Caco-2 proliferation, brush border enzyme activity, monolayer expansion, and cell activity were promoted with basal nutrient delivery. In cells nourished apically and basally, proliferation was increased by 694%, whereas cells receiving only apical nutrition increased by 314%. There was also a difference in sheet migration between cells receiving either single-mode, or apical delivery or dual-mode, or apical and basal, nutrient delivery. In the apically and basally nourished monolayers, motility increased by 389%. (Fig 4). Alkaline phosphatase activity was augmented by 116% with the addition of basal nutrient delivery to the cell culture system, and dipeptidyl dipeptidase specific activity was augmented by 256%. For alkaline phosphatase and dipeptidyl dipeptidase, the effects of basal nutrient delivery were maintained after mitomycin blockade of proliferation was performed. This suggested that differentiation was reflected by the increased digestive enzyme-specific activity rather than a slowing of proliferation. Compared with apical nutrient delivery only, proliferation-blocked cell motility increased by 76.5% and epithelial sheet migration increased by 389%.

Conclusions.—Nutrient delivery to the basal surface of intestinal epithelial cell membranes may promote intestinal epithelial differentiation,

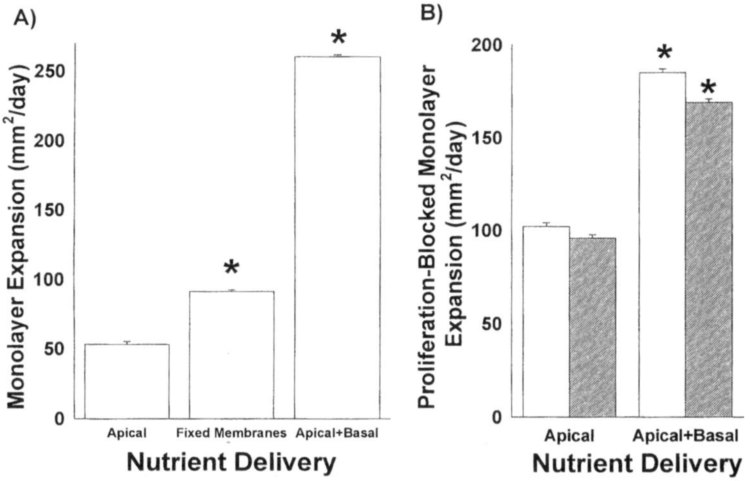

FIGURE 4.—A, effect of dual-mode nutrient delivery on Caco-2 sheet migration. Sheet migration was compared in cells cultivated on plastic dishes to cells cultivated either on semipermeable membranes affixed to plastic dishes or on cell culture inserts. Cells grown on inserts showed a greater sheet migration area per day, increasing by 389 ± 8.8% (n = 12, $P < 0.0005$). B, effect of dual-mode nutrient delivery on proliferation-blocked Caco-2 monolayer expansion. Sheet migration was compared in cells cultivated on plastic dishes to cells cultivated on cell culture inserts with (*shaded bars*) and without (*open bars*) mitomycin C pretreatment to inhibit cell proliferation. Proliferation-blocked cells grown on inserts showed a greater sheet migration area per day, increasing by 76.5 ± 1.6% (n = 12, $P < 0.0005$). *Asterisk* indicates $P < 0.001$. (Courtesy of Perdikis DA, Basson MD: Basal nutrition promotes human intestinal epithelial (Caco-2) proliferation, brush border enzyme activity, and motility. *Crit Care Med* 25(1):159–165, 1997.)

mucosal healing, and epithelial proliferation, although apical nutrition may be critical for intestinal epithelial cell biology.

Dietary Modulation of Amino Acid Transport in Rat and Human Liver

Espat NJ, Watkins KT, Lind DS, et al (Univ of Florida, Gainesville; Abbott Labs, Columbus, Ohio; Harvard Med School, Boston)

J Surg Res 63:263–268, 1996 8–7

Introduction.—Organ function and overall rates of complications can be affected by aggressive nutritional support. A balanced amino acid mixture is generally provided with a nutritional formula, but recent studies have suggested that the addition of glutamine and arginine would be helpful. During stress states, the liver's requirement for glutamine and arginine is increased; thus a diet enriched in arginine and glutamine may increase the activity of their respective transport proteins. It would be helpful to know which diet could alter transport at the cellular level and which could serve as a biochemical rationale for a diet in the future. The effects of 3 different diets containing varying amounts of arginine and glutamine on amino acid transport by the liver were studied.

Methods.—Eight surgical patients and 6 rats were fed a regular diet, an enteral liquid diet containing arginine and glutamine, or an enteral diet supplemented with pharmacologic amounts of arginine and glutamine. Administered for 3 days, diets were isocaloric. Rat liver and human wedge biopsy specimens obtained at laparotomy were used to prepare hepatic plasma membrane vesicles. Assays were taken of the transport of glutamine and arginine by rat and human vesicles. Osmolarity plots, enzyme marker enrichments, and time courses were used to verify vesicle integrity and functionality.

Results.—Compared with a control diet, the activities of Systems N (glutamine) and y^+(arginine) were increased with a standard enteral liquid diet and one enriched with glutamine and arginine in rat and human liver. The most effective diet in increasing transport activity was the diet supplemented with glutamine and arginine.

Conclusions.—Diets enriched with specific amino acids will cause the liver to respond by increasing membrane transport activity. Hepatic synthetic functions may be enhanced during catabolic states with this adaptive response that provides essential precursors for hepatocytes. Insights into mechanisms that regulate nutrient transport with enteral nutrition at the cellular level are provided. Formulas enriched with conditionally essential nutrients may have a biochemical rationale.

► These 3 papers (Abstracts 8–5 to 8–7) address the role of the route of nutrient administration on substrate utilization by the splanchnic bed. Specifically, the authors examine nutrient utilization by enterocytes and hepatocytes under different physiologic conditions. The key question raised by the studies is whether the differences in nutrient utilization that occur during enteral vs. parenteral feedings alter cellular function. Both animal and clinical studies have shown that under certain circumstances, the route of nutrient delivery can impact organ function. The impact of trophic agents and specific nutrients on cellular metabolism and function is currently an area of intense investigation.

W.W. Souba, M.D., Sc.D.

Dosage and Timing of Anti-TNF-α Antibody Treatment Determine Its Effect on Resistance to Sepsis After Injury

O'Riordain MG, O'Riordain DS, Molloy RG, et al (Harvard Med School, Boston; Brigham and Women's Hosp, Boston)

J Surg Res 64:95–101, 1996 8–8

Introduction.—In the pathogenesis of endotoxemia and septic shock, tumor necrosis factor-α (TNF-α) plays a central role. In humans with sepsis, elevated plasma TNF levels correlate with mortality. An animal burn sepsis model with a "two-hit" concept, a situation in which patients at risk for sepsis may be ill for some time before the sepsis supervenes, was developed to determine the effect of neutralizing antibody against TNF-α during this period.

Methods.—Mice were subjected to sham burns or full-thickness burns. At various time points, in vitro TNF-α production from cultured lipopolysaccharide-stimulated splenic adherent cells was determined by enzyme-

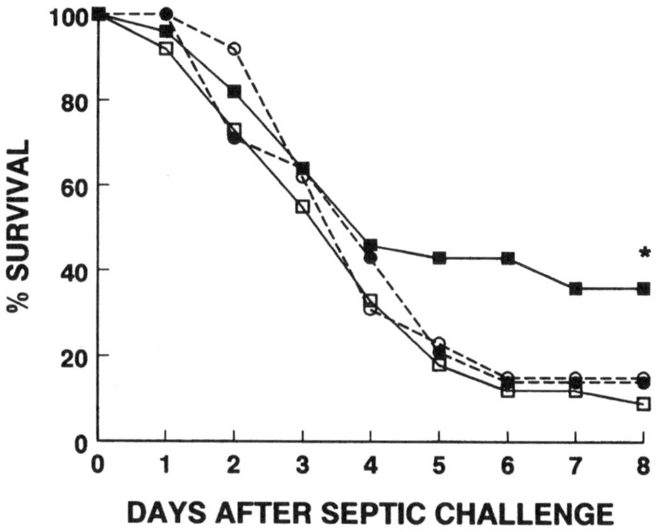

FIGURE 2.—Effect of administration of 1 × 10^4 neutralizing units (n.u.) kg^{-1} of anti–TNF-α antibody at the time of the burn (day 0), day 4, or day 7 after the burn on survival from septic challenge at day 10. *Black square*, antibody day 7; *white circle*, antibody day 4; *black circle*, antibody day 0; *white square*, vehicle control. *Asterisk* indicates $P = 0.01$ vs. control. (Courtesy of O'Riordain MG, O'Riordain DS, Molloy RG, et al: Dosage and timing of anti-TNF-α antibody treatment determine its effects on resistance to sepsis after injury. *J Surg Res* 64:95–101, 1996.)

linked immunosorbent assay. At different time points after the thermal injury, separate animals were treated with neutralizing antibody against TNF-α. On day 10 after the burn, survival was determined after septic challenge (cecal ligation and puncture).

Results.—In the early days after thermal injury, TNF-α production was not elevated. From day 6 onward, however, it was significantly enhanced when compared with sham-burned animals. There were 69% of the sham-burned control mice who survived the septic challenge compared with 9% of the burned mice. If given on day 7 after the burn when TNF-α production was elevated, therapy with anti–TNF-α at 1×10^4 neutralizing units kg^{-1} markedly improved outcome (Fig 2). When given on days 0 or 4 or at the time of the septic challenge on day 10, survival did not improve. There was no benefit to high doses of antibody at 3.2×10^5 neutralizing units kg^{-1}, and it may have been detrimental.

Conclusions.—The susceptibility to infection seen after thermal injury may be reduced with neutralizing antibody against TNF-α. The outcome is dependent upon the timing of administration of the antibody and the dose of antibody used. When neutralizing antibody against TNF is used in the clinical setting, this should be considered.

► The results of this study have important implications for clinical studies that have evaluated the role of biological response modifiers and cytokine antagonists in septic patients. Because bacterial invasion may be viewed as the "second hit" of a "two-hit" cascade in critically ill patients, both the timing of the administration of the antibody and the dose of the antibody are crucial in assessing outcome. These observations articulate the need for clinical studies that evaluate both dosing and kinetic response parameters.

W.W. Souba, M.D., Sc.D.

Prevention of Parenteral Nutrition–induced Gut Hypoplasia by Coinfusion of Glucagon-like Peptide-2

Chance WT, Foley-Nelson T, Thomas I, et al (Univ of Cincinnati, Ohio)
Am J Physiol 273:G559–G563, 1997 8–9

Introduction.—Total parenteral nutrition must be used to maintain adequate caloric intake in some catabolic diseases, major trauma, or gut intolerance to food. Total parenteral nutrition appeared to induce additional problems, however, such as immunosuppression and gut hypoplasia in rat studies. Prevention of these changes would simplify nutritional managing using total parenteral nutrition, although the clinical significance of these alterations in humans is still unknown. Intestinal growth-promoting effects were found in mice with a peptide fragment of the preproglucagon hormone, glucagon-like peptide-2. The hypoplasia normally observed with total parenteral nutrition may be prevented in rats with a coinfusion of glucagon-like peptide-2 and total parenteral nutrition.

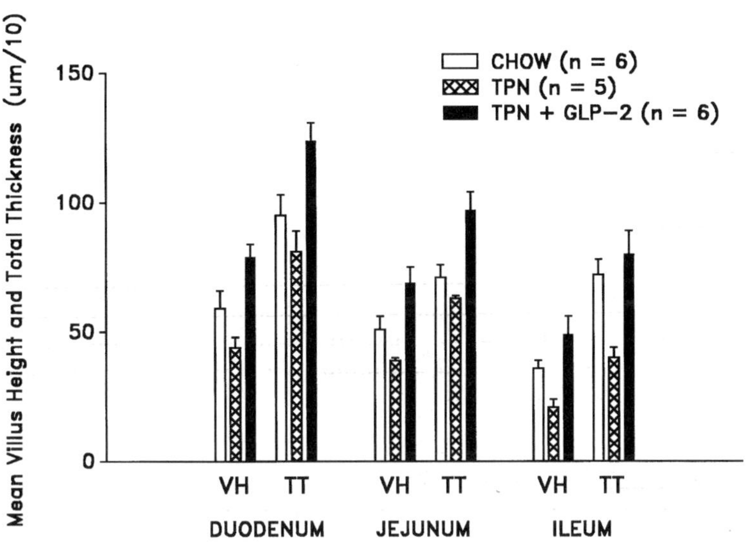

FIGURE 5.—Mean (±SE) villus height (*VH*) and total thickness (*TT*) of small intestinal histology sections taken from rats maintained on chow or total parenteral nutrition and treated with glucagon-like peptide-2. (Courtesy of Chance WT, Foley-Nelson T, Thomas I, et al: Prevention of parenteral nutrition–induced gut hypoplasia by coinfusion of glucagon-like peptide-2. *Am J Physiol* 273:G559–G563, 1997. Copyright The American Physiological Society.)

Methods.—Eleven rats had catheters implanted into their external jugular veins and 6 had sham operations. For the first 2 days after surgery, normal saline was infused, and this was followed with total parenteral solution. Six of the rats had glucose-like peptide-2 added to the total parenteral nutrition. After 6 days, the rats were killed by decapitation. The small intestine and colon were examined for morphologic changes. Determinations were made of protein and DNA content

Results.—There was a significant reduction in mass, protein, and DNA in the small intestine and colon when rats were maintained on total parenteral nutrition for 6 days. Each of these variables were normalized in the duodenum, jejunum, and ileum with coinfusion of glucagon-like peptide-2, but not in the colon. In the small intestine of rats treated with glucagon-like peptide-2, there was normal mucosa thickness and villus height, whereas villus shortening, by 30%, and thinning of mucosa by 23% occurred in nontreated rats maintained on total parenteral nutrition (Fig 5).

Conclusions.—An absence of luminal nutrition in total parenteral nutrition–associated mucosal changes may be less important than hormonal alterations. Accurate assessment of the influence of reversal of hypoplasia on gut barrier function is possible with glucagon-like peptide-2 normalization of gut mucosa.

Beneficial Effects of Growth Hormone Combined With Parenteral Nutrition in the Management of Inflammatory Bowel Disease: An Experimental Study

Chen K, Nezu R, Inoue M, et al (Osaka Univ, Japan)

Surgery 14:212–218, 1997 8–10

Introduction.—Nutritional therapy is one of the primary treatments for inflammatory bowel diseases, such as Crohn's disease. Because of the presence of hypermetabolism or alterations in the hormonal regulation of metabolism, anabolic and therapeutic responses to enteral and parenteral nutrition are often suboptimal. Protein synthesis is enhanced, intestinal growth is stimulated, and wound healing is promoted with growth hormone. In an experimental model of inflammatory bowel disease in rats, the effects of exogenous growth hormone co-infused with parenteral nutrition were evaluated.

Methods.—Central venous cannulation was performed on the rats who were then divided into 2 groups after induction of small intestinal ulceration with indomethacin. The same parenteral nutrition formula was administered to both groups. Ten rats received injections of normal saline solution, while 10 rats received subcutaneous injection of human growth hormone, 1.0 IU/kg daily for 4 days. Determinations were made of macroscopic inflammation score, nitrogen balance, intestinal myeloperoxidase activity, DNA content, and mucosal permeability. Reverse transcription and polymerase chain reaction were used for detection of insulin-like growth factor-I (IGF-I) mRNA.

Results.—The cumulative nitrogen balance was significantly improved with the administration of growth hormone. In the growth hormone group, the gross inflammation score was ameliorated (Table 2) and the intestinal myeloperoxidase activity was decreased. In the growth hormone group, intestinal permeability was also significantly decreased when compared with the control group. Increased plasma concentrations of IGF-I and IGF-I mRNA expressions resulted with growth hormone treatment in the liver and the small intestine when compared with the controls.

TABLE 2.—Inflammation Parameters

	Inflammation score	*Myeloperoxidase activity units/gm*	*Wet-to-dry ratio*
GH	2.0 ± 1.3	1.9 ± 0.6	3.8 ± 0.3
Control	4.2 ± 2.7*	5.1 ± 1.9†	4.1 ± 0.3

Note: data are mean ± SD.
**P* < 0.05.
†*P* < 0.01.
(Courtesy of Chen K, Nezu R, Inoue M, et al: Beneficial effects of growth hormone combined with parenteral nutrition in the management of inflammatory bowel disease: An experimental study. *Surgery* 14:212–218, 1997.)

Conclusions.—In an experimental model of small bowel ulceration in rats, exogenous growth hormone played an important role in accelerating intestinal healing. Stimulated IGF-I may be one of the mechanisms that augments intestinal epithelial cell growth.

▶ These 2 papers (Abstracts 8–9 and 8–10) add to the growing body of the literature that addresses means by which the intestinal mucosa can be supported when enteral nutrition is not feasible. It is important to emphasize that preventing or reversing gut atrophy may not translate into restoration of gut function. Relevant clinical measurements should focus on gut barrier function, gut immune function, and outcome rather than biochemical or morphologic indices. Thus, while clinical studies evaluating the effectiveness of exogenous growth hormone have demonstrated improvements in intestinal nutrient uptake and nitrogen balance, clear-cut beneficial effects in terms of outcome have been more difficult to demonstrate.

W.W. Souba, M.D., Sc.D.

Effects of Endotoxin on Zinc Metabolism in Human Volunteers

Gaetke LM, McClain CJ, Talwalkar RT, et al (Univ of Kentucky, Lexington; Lexington VA Med Ctr, Ky)

Am J Physiol 272:E952–E956, 1997 8–11

Introduction.—Normal growth, protein metabolism, membrane integrity, wound healing, and immune function are all dependent upon zinc, an essential trace mineral. A prominent decrease in the serum zinc concentration has been observed in the acute-phase host response to stress, trauma, inflammation, and infection. The mechanisms that cause hypozincemia in humans are still unknown. Some proposed mechanisms include increased urinary zinc excretion, decreased serum albumin concentration, and changes in serum albumin–zinc binding. Profound decreases in serum zinc levels have been induced with administration of lipopolysaccharide in animal models. Possible mechanisms for stress-related hypozincemia in men and women were evaluated using safe doses of lipopolysaccharide.

Methods.—In 12 healthy volunteers, 2 doses of endotoxin (lipopolysaccharide) were administered on consecutive mornings. The volunteers were also studied after saline injection. Evaluations of blood were conducted for cytokines (tumor necrosis factor-α, interleukin-6), zinc, albumin, albumin-zinc binding, and C-reactive protein. An analysis for zinc was done with serial 24-hour urine collections.

Results.—Plasma cytokine concentrations were briefly increased and serum zinc concentrations were decreased with each lipopolysaccharide dose (Fig 4) No decrease was observed in serum albumin, the major zinc-binding protein, but there was a progressive increase in C-reactive protein. Zinc-binding affinity to serum albumin was not affected by lipopolysaccharide. There was no increase of urine zinc loss.

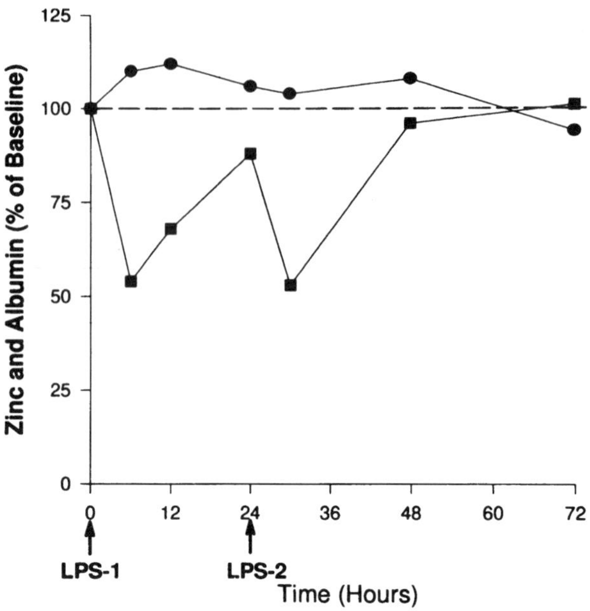

FIGURE 4.—Serum albumin (*black circles*) response compared with serum zinc (*black squares*) concentration over course of endotoxin (*LPS*) administration part of study from baseline to 72 hours in normal volunteers (n = 12). (Courtesy of Gaetke LM, McClain CJ, Talwalkar RT, et al: Effects of endotoxin on zinc metabolism in human volunteers. *Am J Physiol* 272:E952–E956, 1997. Copyright The American Physiological Society.)

Conclusions.—Decreased serum albumin, changes in serum albumin–zinc binding, or increased urinary zinc excretion could not explain hypozincemia in this model. A cytokine-directed internal redistribution of zinc may mediate lipopolysaccharide-stimulated hypozincemia because hypozincemia was transient and followed cytokine peaks.

▶ The authors used a human endotoxemia model to evaluate the possible mechanisms by which hypozincemia develops during sepsis. The profound drop in serum zinc that occurs as part of the acute-phase response is designed to withhold important minerals such as zinc, which is necessary for bacterial growth into the bloodstream and to reprioritize hepatic protein synthesis, in times of stress. The authors were unable to explain the endotoxin-induced hypozincemia on the basis of reductions in serum albumin, changes in zinc-albumin binding kinetics, or increases in urinary zinc excretion. Thus, it appears that cytokines may have direct or indirect effects on the transport of zinc across the hepatocyte plasma membrane.

W.W. Souba, M.D., Sc.D.

Clinical Aspects of Nutrition Support

Nutritional Support

Souba WW (Harvard Med School, Boston)

N Engl J Med 336:41–49, 1997 8–12

Introduction.—The efficacy of nutritional support has not been substantiated for many conditions. Parenteral and enteral formulations can provide all essential nutrients and prevent or reverse the wasting of host tissue. It is difficult to determine the risk of malnutrition because its causes are multiple and interrelated and include the patient's previous nutritional status, the disease process, and the magnitude and anticipated duration of associated catabolic stresses. The indications for nutritional support were discussed.

Indications for Nutritional Support.—Nutritional support is given to prevent the effects of starvation and to favorably alter the natural history or treatment of a specific disease. It is indicated for patients unable to eat or absorb nutrients for an indefinite period; well-nourished patients unable to eat for more than 10–14 days; severely malnourished patients who undergo major elective surgical procedures; patients with major trauma; and bone marrow–transplant recipients who undergo intensive anticancer therapy (Table 1).

Unproved Benefits of Nutritional Support.—Patients for whom nutritional support is not clearly defined because of its inability to affect the natural history or treatment of the disease include patients with AIDS, gastrointestinal tract dysfunction, liver failure, renal failure, and patients receiving chemotherapy and radiation therapy for cancer.

Conclusions.—The lack of evidence of nutritional support favorably affecting outcome should not prevent its use. The 2 groups of patients in whom nutritional support has a proven benefit are those who are severely injured and bone marrow–transplant recipients. When nutritional support is initiated, the enteral route should always be preferred. Additional groups of patients who can benefit from nutritional support can be identified with carefully constructed clinical trials.

► The author reviews the indications for nutritional support in the clinical setting, emphasizing the importance of establishing reliable criteria for identifying malnourished patients at risk. Although many studies have shown that nutritional intervention can alter biochemical and metabolic indices, few have documented improvements in outcome. Based on the existing literature, several conclusions can be drawn. First, most patients do not require formal nutritional support; short-term treatment (10–14 days) with isotonic glucose solutions does not affect the outcome negatively after major elective operations or other therapy. Second, to prevent starvation-induced complications, nutrition support should be initiated in most patients who are unable to eat for more than 10–14 days. Stressed patients tolerate starvation for shorter periods, but it is debatable how long nutritional support can be

TABLE 1.—Established and Unproved Indications for the Use of Nutritional Support

Established Indication	Benefit
Patients unable to eat or absorb nutrients for an indefinite period (permanent neurologic impairment, prematurity in an infant, oropharyngeal dysfunction short-gut syndrome)	Preserves nutritional status; lifesaving
Well-nourished, minimally stressed patients unable to eat for more than 10–14 days	Preserves nutritional status; prevents starvation-induced complications
Severely malnourished patients who undergo major elective surgical procedures	Preoperative nutrition decreases the incidence of major septic complications
Patients with major trauma (major blunt or penetrating trauma, head injury, burn injury)	Enteral nutrition is superior to parenteral nutrition in decreasing the incidence of septic complications; nutritional support improves outcome in patients with head injuries
Bone marrow-transplant recipients undergoing intensive anticancer therapy	Improves outcome

Condition	Unproved Indications for or Effects of Nutritional Support	Matters Requiring Further Study
Cancer	Is indicated in patients with severe, treatment-associated gastrointestinal toxic effects in whom oral intake is precluded for more than 10 days, and in patients with a reasonable life expectancy whose inability to eat is the principal impediment to normal functioning	Can specific nutritional formulas improve the efficacy of anticancer therapy?
Acquired immunodeficiency syndrome	Preserves nutritional status	Effect of nutritional support on treatment tolerance, quality of life, number of hospitalizations, and survival
Gastrointestinal tract dysfunction	Preserves nutritional status; can induce disease remission in patients with Crohn's disease; can increase the rate of closure of enterocutaneous fistulas	Effect of nutritional support on flare-ups and long-term outcome in patients with inflammatory bowel disease
Liver failure	Formulas with branched-chain amino acids relieve encephalopathy	Effect of nutritional support on survival
Renal failure	Treatment with glucose and essential amino acids may improve outcome and renal function in patients with acute renal failure	Effect of nutritional support on outcome and dialysis requirements in patients with chronic renal failure
Critically ill (intensive care unit) patients (excluding patients with trauma)	Nutritional support is indicated to prevent starvation-induced complications in patients in whom oral intake is precluded for 7–10 days	How long is too long to go without nutrition? Does nutritional support improve outcome in patients in intensive care units?

(Courtesy of Souba WW: Nutritional support. *N Engl J Med* 336:41–49.

withheld from critically ill patients. Lastly, in severely traumatized patients, early enteral nutritional intervention has been shown to be beneficial.

W.W. Souba, M.D., Sc.D.

Site of Insulin Resistance After Surgery: The Contribution of Hypocaloric Nutrition and Bed Rest

Nygren J, Thorell A, Efendic S, et al (Karolinska Hosp, Stockholm; Mayo Clinic and Found, Rochester, Minn)

Clin Sci (Colch) 93:137–146, 1997 8–13

Introduction.—One of the major features of the catabolic response is impaired glucose tolerance and diminished insulin sensitivity. Lowered insulin resistance after surgery is related to several important derangements in protein and fat metabolism. The mechanisms of impaired glucose tolerance after surgery are not adequately understood. The relative roles of insulin action and whole-body glucose disposal (WGD) in the impairment of glucose tolerance after surgery were assessed, along with the possible contribution of 24 hours of bed rest and hypocaloric nutrition.

Methods.—Insulin sensitivity and glucose kinetics were evaluated before and after elective surgery (surgery group) using two-step hyperinsulinemic (0.3 and 0.8 mU kg^{-1} min^{-1}), normoglycemic (4.5 mmol/L) clamps. The same experimental design was used for healthy research subjects before and after a similar period of bed rest and hypocaloric nutrition (fast/bed rest group) to determine the effects of surgery. Volunteers in the fast/bed rest group also received 2,000 mL of glucose intravenously.

Results.—Basal endogenous glucose production and WGD were significantly higher after surgery, compared with no change in the fast/bed rest group. The glucose infusion rates needed to maintain normoglycemic and WGD were significantly decreased after surgery during glucose clamps, while endogenous glucose production increased significantly. Levels of endogenous glucose production stayed the same in the control group after fast/bed rest. The glucose infusion rates and WGD during glucose clamps were significantly diminished after fast/bed rest. The relative reduction in both parameters was significantly higher after surgery than after fast/bed rest. There was a significant energy expenditure and increase in fat oxidation, a decrease in glucose oxidation, and no change in glucose utilization after surgery. There was no change in energy expenditure after fast/bed rest, but fat oxidation increased significantly and glucose oxidation and glucose utilization was reduced.

Conclusions.—Impaired glucose tolerance is observed on the first postoperative day as a result of reduced insulin-stimulated WGD and increased endogenous glucose release. The decrease in endogenous glucose production with each elevation of insulin was not affected by surgery, despite increases in endogenous glucose. Perioperative bed rest and fasting contribute to a reduction in insulin-stimulated WGD in the postoperative state but have no effects on endogenous glucose production.

▶ The authors have demonstrated that the impaired glucose tolerance that develops after elective surgery is caused by both a decrease in insulin-mediated WGD and an increase in endogenous glucose production. The bed rest and hypocaloric feedings that are characteristic of the postoperative period contribute to the decrease in insulin-stimulated WGD, but these factors have no effect on endogenous glucose production. These findings suggest that early mobilization and/or nutrition may minimize postsurgical derangements in glucose metabolism.

W.W. Souba, M.D., Sc.D.

Randomization to Nutritional Intervention at Home Did Not Improve Postoperative Function, Fatigue or Well-Being

Jensen MB, Hessov I (Univ Hosp of Aarhus, Denmark)
Br J Surg 84:113–118, 1997 8–14

Introduction.—Postoperative fatigue has been correlated with loss of body weight and fat mass, and deterioration of muscle performance and cardiovascular function after surgery. Patients were given nutritional support from the day of discharge from the hospital for 110 days to determine whether nutritional intervention could improve postoperative fatigue, functional capacity, or well-being.

Methods.—Thirty-two patients admitted for elective colorectal surgery and 21 patients who underwent surgery for acute obstruction or peritonitis were randomly assigned at discharge to standard management or dietary advice and protein-rich supplements for 4 months. Fatigue, quality of life, and subjective feelings of well-being and stress were assessed by questionnaires. Work capacity, pulmonary function, hand grip strength, and pinching strength were measured.

Results.—Patients in the nutrition intervention group had substantial increases in protein intake, body weight, and lean body capacity, compared with controls. There were no between-group differences in hand grip, pinching strength, fatigue, or quality of life; these measures returned to preoperative values 1–2 months after surgery in both groups (Fig 2). Fatigue scores remained high for 2–3 months after surgery in both groups.

Conclusions.—Nutritional intervention markedly enhanced restoration of weight and lean body mass, but did not improve functional measurements, fatigue, or well-being in patients with small-to-moderate weight losses. The changes in weight and lean body mass did not improve function of fatigue. Changes in body composition and fatigue depend on different mechanisms in patients recovering from surgery.

▶ The authors studied patients undergoing gastrointestinal surgery who were randomly assigned to receive a regular diet or a more aggressive nu-

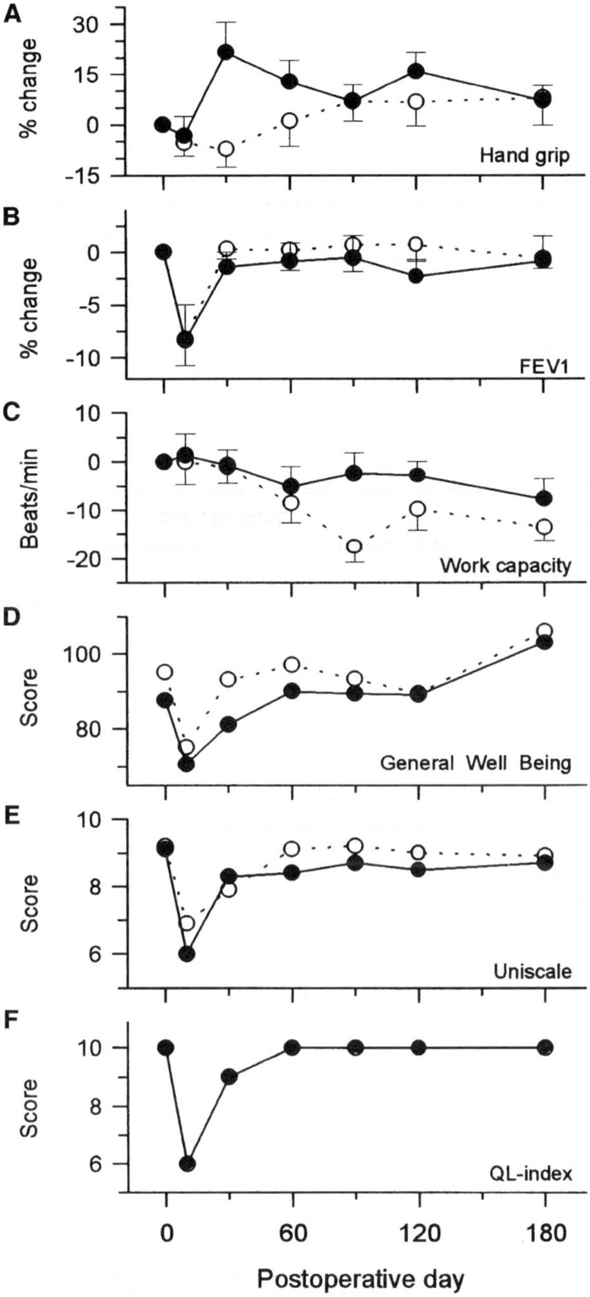

FIGURE 2.—Mean (S.E.M.) changes in (**A**) hand-grip strength, (**B**) forced expiratory volume in 1 second and (**C**) heart rate, compared with preoperative values in patients having elective surgery. The falling heart rate indicates improved work capacity. *Open circles*, controls; *dark circles*, intervention group. Median scores of quality of life: (**D**) General Well Being, (**E**) Uniscale, and (**F**) Quality of Life Index. (Courtesy of Jensen MB, Hessov I: Randomization to nutrition intervention at home did not improve postoperative function, fatigue, or well-being. *Br J Surg* 84:113–118. Copyright 1997, Blackwell Science Ltd.)

tritional support regimen after hospital discharge. Patients who received the nutritional invention arm of the study had an enhanced protein intake and gain in weight and lean body mass compared with controls. However, despite differences in nutritional intake and changes in body composition, postoperative fatigue and physical performance in both groups were similar. Thus, the study does not support the hypothesis that changes in weight and changes in lean body mass cause the postoperative changes in fatigue or function. Thus, other factors, independent of nutrient intake, are likely to determine the rate at which convalescence and full recovery occur.

W.W. Souba, M.D., Sc.D.

Assessing the Quality of Life of Patients With Intestinal Failure on Home Parenteral Nutrition

Richards DM, Irving MH (Univ of Manchester, England)
Gut 40:218–222, 1997 8–15

Introduction.—The technology involved in home parenteral nutrition (HPN) is complex and expensive, and requires the patient to depend on a machine for nutritional support. Quality of life is an important measure of the effectiveness of health technologies but has rarely been assessed in patients receiving HPN. Quality of life was measured to describe a profile of health status and examine which factors moderate outcomes in patients receiving HPN.

Methods.—The SF 36 and EuroQol questionnaires were mailed to 64 patients with intestinal failure who had benign disease. Thirty-five of 51 patients who completed the questionnaires had Crohn's disease. The SF 36 questionnaire measured 8 aspects of life: physical functioning, role functioning—physical, body pain, general health, vitality, social functioning, role functioning—emotional, mental health, and reported health transition. The EuroQol rated health status in the areas of mobility, self care, activity, pain, and mental status. Scores for this patient cohort were compared with those for the general population.

Results.—Compared with general population controls, patients receiving HPN had worse SF 36 scores for 6 of the 8 domains. Patients younger than 45 years scored significantly higher than patients older than 55 years. Very low scores were observed in patients addicted to narcotic substances. The SF questionnaire results were confirmed by the EuroQol utility scores. Of the 51 patients, 41 indicated they felt too ill to work. Only 5 patients were engaged in full-time work or education.

Conclusions.—Compared with the general population, the health status profile of younger patients receiving HPN was good. Poor scores were observed in patients who were older and patients dependent on narcotic substances. Outcomes of older patients receiving HPN must be considered but should not limit the use of HPN if there are other favorable factors involved.

► The authors studied the health status profile of patients receiving HPN. They observed that older patients have significantly lower quality-of-life scores compared with younger patients. These lower scores were most notable in the areas of physical, social, and emotional functionality. The patients who were addicted to narcotics had substantially lower scores than other patients receiving HPN. Treatment of catheter sepsis was more difficult for older patients, and they had a higher incidence of catheter infections.

W.W. Souba, M.D., Sc.D.

Influence of Postoperative Enteral Nutrition on Postsurgical Infections

Beier-Holgersen R, Boesby S (Dept of Surgical Gastroenterology, Glostrup, Denmark)

Gut 39:833–835, 1996 8–16

Introduction.—High-risk surgical patients receiving enteral nutrition have a lower incidence of septic complications, according to non–placebo-controlled trials from a recent meta-analysis evaluating the effect of enteral vs. parenteral nutrition. The effect of early postoperative enteral nutrition vs. no nutrition (placebo) on the postoperative course of patients after major abdominal surgery was evaluated in a randomized, double-blind prospective trial.

Methods.—Sixty patients were randomly assigned to receive enteral feedings of either Nutridrink or placebo. On the day of surgery, both groups received 600 mL of solution at 60 mL/hr. On the first postoperative day, both groups received 1,000 mL (median) of nutrition or placebo. On postoperative day 2, 1,200 mL (median) of nutrition and 1,400 mL of placebo were given. On day 3, 1,000 mL (median) nutrition and 1,150 mL of placebo were administered. On day 4, patients received either 1,000 mL (median) nutrition or 800 mL placebo. Patients were followed up for 30 days.

Results.—There were significantly fewer postoperative infectious complications in patients who received nutrition, compared with patients in the placebo group (2 of 30 patients vs. 14 of 30 patients).

Conclusions.—A considerable reduction in postoperative infectious complications was observed in patients who received enteral nutrition after major abdominal surgery, compared with patients who received placebo. Patients who received enteral nutrition had a 25% reduction in the cost of hospital stay, compared with patients who did not receive enteral nutrition.

Endotoxemia Following Enteral Refeeding in Children

Ravindranath T, Yoshioka T, Goto M, et al (Loyola Univ Chicago)
Clin Pediatr (Phila) 36:523–528, 1997 8–17

Introduction.—Enteral feedings can cause endotoxin translocation in neonates. Because the gastrointestinal (GI) tract is more permeable in the newborn than in the adult, it seems the endotoxin translocation is the result of an immature GI tract. Immaturity cannot totally explain the mechanism of endotoxin translocation. The increased plasma endotoxin concentration after enteral feeding is only temporary, suggesting the onset of enteral feeding, not immaturity of the GI tract, is important in endotoxin translocation. If this is so, translocation could be induced in children and adults by initiating feeding after food and water deprivation. Because endotoxin is a stimulus for the release of tumor necrosis factor α (TNFα), plasma TNFα may increase if enteral feedings cause endotoxin translocation. Plasma endotoxin-like activity and TNFα concentrations were determined after enteral feeding in 9 children.

Methods.—Nine children (age range 9 months to 10 years) who had been deprived of their enteral feeding for 5 days because of illness underwent measurements of plasma endotoxin-like activity, TNFα concentrations, core body temperature, and liver function before and after enteral feedings.

Results.—Transient endotoxemia and increased plasma TNFα concentrations were observed. Patients with elevated plasma endotoxin-like ac-

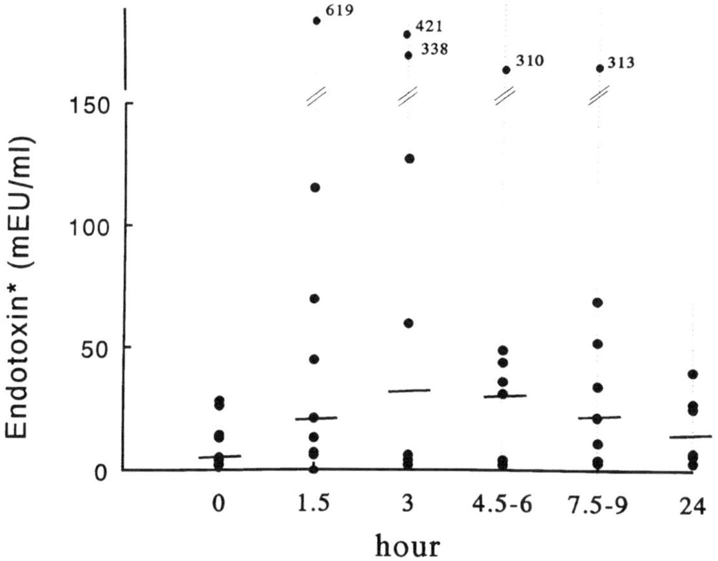

FIGURE 1.—Plasma endotoxin-like activity levels. Endotoxin* indicates plasma endotoxin-like activity; *solid horizontal lines*, median values. (Courtesy of Ravindranath T, Yoshioka T, Goto M, et al: Endotoxemia following enteral refeeding in children. *Clin Pediatr* 36:523–528, 1997.)

tivity (Fig 1) had normal measurements of core body temperature, aspartate aminotransferase, alanine aminotransferase, and bilirubin concentrations.

Conclusions.—Endotoxemia may occur in children after enteral feeding. Transient endotoxemia can result after prolonged fasting without any consequences.

Enteral or Parenteral Feeding After Total Gastrectomy: Prospective Randomised Pilot Study

Sand J, Luostarinen M, Matikainen M (Tampere Univ, Finland)

Eur J Surg 163:761–766, 1997 8–18

Introduction.—Patients who undergo total gastrectomy usually receive postoperative feeding parenterally until the esophagojejunal anastomosis has healed. Early enteral feedings are usually not used in these patients because of fear of complications at the esophagojejunal anastomosis. The safety, tolerability, and cost of enteral feedings, compared with parenteral feedings, were determined after total gastrectomy for gastric cancer in a prospective, randomized, open pilot investigation.

Methods.—Twenty-nine patients with gastric carcinoma who underwent macroscopically curative total gastrectomy were randomly assigned to receive either early enteral feedings by nasojejunal tube or parenteral nutrition by central venous catheter (13 and 16 patients, respectively). Patients were followed up for postoperative complications, duration of hospital stay, serum CRP and albumin concentrations, cost, and postoperative abdominal complications.

Results.—One patient in each group had an esophagojejunal leak develop. One patient in the enteral group was dropped from the trial before initial feeding on day 1 when she had mild postoperative pancreatitis. Three patients (23%) in the enteral group and 5 (31%) in the parenteral group had infectious complications. Serum CRP concentrations were significantly lower in the enteral group than in the parenteral group on day 6. Feedings in the enteral group were well tolerated. Sixteen patients (55%) had postoperative diarrhea. Patients in the enteral feeding group usually had diarrhea between days 3 and 5, and patients in the parenteral group usually had diarrhea between days 5 and 7. Patients in the parenteral group were at increased risk for diarrhea. The cost of parenteral feedings was 4 times greater than that of enteral feedings.

Conclusions.—Early enteral feedings are safe and well tolerated after total gastrectomy. Diarrhea occurred earlier and less frequently in the early enteral feeding group than in the parenteral feeding group. Parenteral feedings were about 4 times more expensive than early enteral feedings.

Early Postoperative Enteral Immunonutrition: Clinical Outcome and Cost-Comparison Analysis in Surgical Patients

Senkal M, Mumme A, Eickhoff U, et al (Ruhr-Univ Bochum, Germany; Univ Hosp Bonn, Germany; HealthEcon, Basel, Switzerland)

Crit Care Med 25:1489–1496, 1997 8–19

Introduction.—There is much interest in preventing postoperative infectious and septic complications by improving host defenses. Recent findings suggest that the immune system may be modulated by nutritional support. The clinical outcome of patients who received early enteral nutrition with a supplemented enteral diet or an isocaloric and isonitrogenous placebo diet were compared in a prospective, randomized, placebo-controlled, double-blind, multicenter trial. A cost-comparison analysis was performed retrospectively.

Methods.—One-hundred fifty-four patients admitted to the surgical ICU after upper gastrointestinal surgery for cancer were randomly assigned to receive either a supplemented enteral diet or placebo diet via needle catheter jejunostomy at 12–24 hours after surgery. The enteral diet was supplemented with arginine, dietary nucleotides, and ω-3 fatty acids. Complication events were considered to be early (postoperative days 1–5) or late (after the fifth postoperative day). Treatment costs of each complication were assessed and compared.

Results.—The enteral feedings were well tolerated, and tube feeding–related complications were few in both groups. Seventeen and 24 complications occurred in the immunonutrition and control groups, respectively. Early complications were similar in both groups (12 in the immunonutri-

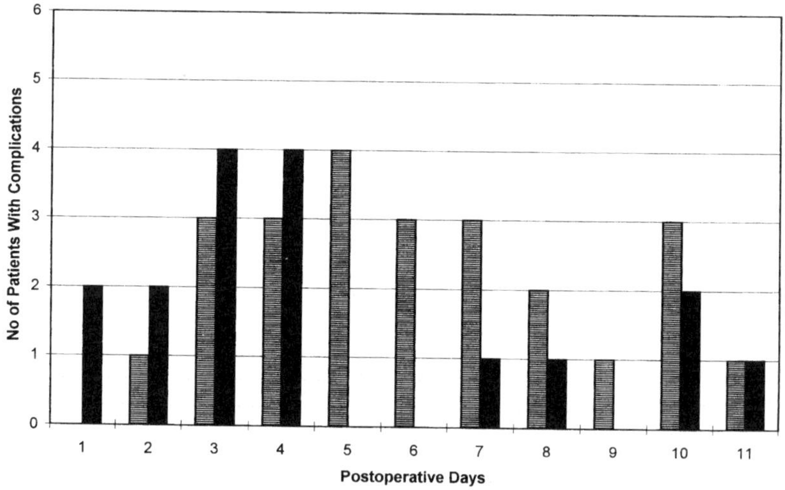

FIGURE 1.—Onset of complications and number of patients with complications in the postoperative period. Immunonutrition (*solid bars*) and control diet group (*lined bars*). (Courtesy of Senkal M, Mumme A, Eickhoff U, et al: Early postoperative enteral immunonutrition: Clinical outcome and cost-comparison analysis in surgical patients. *Crit Care Med* 25(9):1489–1496, 1997.)

TABLE 4.—Costs for the Treatment of Postoperative Complications in German Marks (*GM*)

	Immuno-nutrition	Placebo	Difference
Costs for each patient with complication (GM)	4,610	5,239	629
Costs for early complications (GM)	52,630	47,800	4,830
Costs for late complications (GM)	31,024	74,633	43,609
Total (GM)	83,654	122,433	38,779

(Courtesy of Senkal M, Mumme A, Eickhoff U, et al: Early postoperative enteral immunonutrition: Clinical outcome and cost-comparison analysis in surgical patients. *Crit Care Med* 25(9):1489–1496, 1997.)

tion and 11 in the control group). Five and 13 patients had late complications in the immunonutrition and control groups, respectively (a significant difference) (Fig 1). There were 22 and 32 complicating events in the immunonutrition and control groups, respectively. Late complicating events were significantly fewer in the immunonutrition group, compared with the control group (8 vs. 17 events). The total costs for treating complications were 83,563 and 122,430 German marks for the immunonutrition and control groups, respectively (Table 4). The difference in costs was 38,867 German marks (the conversion rate from German marks to U.S. dollars at time of calculation was 1.4365 German marks to $1.00).

Conclusions.—Patients who received early enteral feedings supplemented with arginine, dietary nucleotides, and ω-3 fatty acids had a significant decrease in the rate of late postoperative infectious and wound complications, compared with controls. Treatment costs were notably decreased in the immunonutrition group because of the lower rates of complications and complicating events.

► Collectively, these 4 studies (Abstracts 8–6 to 8–19) address the role of enteral nutrition in several different patient groups. I was struck by the high rate of wound infections in the control group in the study by Beier-Holgersen and Boesby which, in my opinion, places their conclusions on shaky ground. Meta-analyses have shown that nutritional support is not necessary in most patients after elective surgical procedures. The observation by Ravindranath et al. that transient endotoxemia occurs after enteral feeding in children that have been deprived of luminal nutrition appears to be without consequence. The study by Sand et al.showing the feasibility of enteral nutrition after total gastrectomy is not novel, nor is their observation that parenteral feeding was considerably more expensive than enteral feeding. What is absent from the study is any documentation of outcome. Finally, the study by Senkal et al. demonstrated a reduction in late postoperative complications in surgical patients who received a diet enriched in arginine, ω-3 fatty acids, and nucleotides. Previous studies have demonstrated similar benefits, suggesting that specific nutrients may improve outcome in selected groups of patients.

W.W. Souba, M.D., Sc.D.

The Choleretic Effect of Nonsteroidal Anti-inflammatory Drugs in Total Parenteral Nutrition-associated Cholestasis

Nussinovitch M, Zahavi I, Marcus H, et al (Tel Aviv Univ, Israel; Schneider Children's Med Ctr of Israel, Petah Tikva)

Isr J Med Sci 32:1262–1264, 1996 8–20

Introduction.—Cholestasis is a common problem in pediatric and sometimes adult patients receiving total parenteral nutrition (TPN). Nonsteroidal anti-inflammatory drugs, particularly acetylsalicylic acid (aspirin), produce choleresis in animals. The action of aspirin on bile flow and bile salt secretion rate was examined in rats receiving TPN to determine the choleretic effect of aspirin in TPN-associated cholestasis.

Methods.—Four groups of 6–10 male Wistar rats each received either 154 mmol/L NaCl (saline) or 2.5% amino acid solution and 10% glucose intravenously at a rate of 10 μmol/min/kg to avoid bile salt pool depletion. Aspirin was infused during the last 12 hours into groups of rats receiving saline and TPN treatment at a rate of 100 mg/kg. Bile was collected from the common bile duct during the next 3 hours.

Results.—Rats who received TPN had a significant decrease in bile flow and bile salt secretion rate, compared with saline controls. Aspirin caused a significant choleretic effect and was able to overcome the TPN-caused decrease in bile flow and bile salt secretion rate.

Conclusions.—Aspirin generated a marked choleretic effect that overcame the bile flow decrease caused by TPN treatment. Aspirin acted on both the bile salt–independent and dependent bile flow. Findings indicate that aspirin may help prevent TPN-induced cholestasis.

► The authors examined the choleretic effect of aspirin in TPN-associated cholestasis by measuring bile flow and bile salt secretion rate in rats receiving parenteral nutrition. Total parenteral nutrition–induced cholestasis develops in a short period, an effect that aspirin was able to overcome. Under certain circumstances, the use of aspirin for prevention of TPN-associated cholestasis may be appropriate. However, in view of the fact that TPN-induced cholestasis is most common in children, the use of aspirin as a choleretic agent will require further studies.

W.W. Souba, M.D., Sc.D.

Randomized, Double-blind Study of Intravenous Human Albumin in Hypoalbuminemic Patients Receiving Total Parenteral Nutrition

Rubin H, Carlson S, DeMeo M, et al (Northwestern Univ, Chicago)

Crit Care Med 25:249–252, 1997 8–21

Purpose.—Whether because of increased catabolism, decreased synthesis, or both, serum albumin concentrations decrease in patients who have acute illness or who have undergone major surgery. In hospitalized patients, serum albumin concentration is a useful predictor of mortality.

However, it is uncertain whether serum albumin concentration is a useful marker of nutrition. Most previous studies have shown no reduction in morbidity with the administration of human serum albumin to patients receiving total parenteral nutrition (TPN). The effects of IV albumin administration were investigated in hospitalized patients with hypoalbuminemia.

Methods.—The randomized, blind, placebo-controlled trial included 31 patients with a serum albumin concentration of less than 2.5 g/dL who were receiving at least 6 days of TPN. All were adults and free of metastatic cancer, cirrhosis, and nephrotic syndrome. Each patient received 6 or more days of therapy with either albumin or placebo. All were followed up through discharge or death. Albumin kinetics were evaluated as well.

Results.—The 2 groups were comparable in terms of hospital days on TPN and days on their assigned drug. Death occurred within 30 days for 1 patient in the placebo group and 2 in the albumin group. Sepsis or bacteremia occurred in 1 and 3 patients, respectively. Pneumonia occurred in 4 patients in the placebo group and 7 in the albumin group; none of these differences were significant. All patients in the albumin group had an increase in serum albumin concentration, including 1 patient who received albumin for only 6 days. The mean increase in serum albumin was 1.42 g/dL in the albumin group vs. 0.29 g/dL in the placebo group. Albumin metabolism increased from 17.4 to 20.5 g/day during the study. Overall, the results suggested that albumin was causing more harm than good, and the study was discontinued.

Conclusions.—Giving IV albumin to hospitalized patients with hypoalbuminemia does not appear to have any benefit, despite the fact that serum albumin concentration increases during such treatment. Given the high cost of human serum albumin, a reduction in its use for patients receiving TPN is recommended.

► Human serum albumin administration is very costly and infused albumin is rapidly catabolized. I agree with the following highlighted statement on page 251 of this article: "The current investigation does not show any benefit from administering intravenous albumin to hospitalized hypoalbuminemic patients receiving intravenous hyperalimentation, despite the increase in serum albumin concentrations."

W.W. Souba, M.D., Sc.D.

9 Growth Factors and Wound Healing

Introduction

The following chapter of the YEAR BOOK OF SURGERY on growth factors and wound healing has grouped the articles reviewed into those that are scientifically oriented and those that emphasize clinical issues. The two sections are meant to be complementary and integrative rather than disjointed. In the first segment, I have attempted to expose the reader to several of the newer areas of basic and clinical research. This includes the continued interest in the molecular mechanisms of action of growth factors. The second part of the chapter reviews some of the pragmatic aspects of wound healing in the clinical practice of surgery.

Wound healing continues to be a problem in surgical patients with specific underlying diseases, the most common of which is diabetes. Recent studies have demonstrated the importance of blood glucose control in the wound healing process and the role of the insulin-like growth factors in proper wound repair. While abnormalities in glucose homeostasis contribute to healing problems, derangements in blood flow can be implicated as well. The link between these two factors may be related, in part, to the deficient production of growth factors locally, which raises compelling questions about the use of exogenous therapies.

A major area of wound healing research has addressed the role of nitric oxide. It is now apparent that locally invading white blood cells, essential for wound healing, produce nitric oxide as part of the repair process. Factors such as severe malnutrition and steroid treatment may diminish nitric oxide production by local inflammatory cells. The clinical extension of this observation is uncertain, but it does provide a biochemical link with those studies that have implicated arginine-enriched diets in wound healing.

Recent studies have also improved our understanding of the similarities and differences between wound healing in the very young and the very old. Interestingly, wounds of the aged may contain a subpopulation of fibroblasts that are phenotypically similar to fetal fibroblasts. This may explain the often-observed high quality of scarring in the aged.

The potential clinical applicability of new growth-enhancing agents has resulted in the promotion of wound care as a commercial business. One website (http://members.aol.com/woundnet/trend.htm) reads as follows:

> Dedicated wound care programs are increasingly caring for Americans with chronic wounds and could offer the potential to produce enhanced outcomes at reduced costs for payers and consumers of healthcare services. A report by Frost and Sullivan indicates the U.S. wound management products market is now $1.74 billion and should grow to $2.57 billion by 2002. The cost of treating the chronic wound is estimated at $5 to $7 billion, and these wounds are increasing at a rate of 10% per year, according to the report. The development of the American Academy of Wound Management (AAWM), a national, non-profit certifying board is another indication that wound care is coming into its own as an industry. Board Certification is now available for physicians, nurses, therapists, researchers, and other healthcare professionals involved in wound care. Over 1,000 wound care professionals have requested applications for board certification through AAWM. Cerrtification up to December 1998 is via submission of a portfolio documenting professional experience in wound care. After December 1998, certification will be available only by achieving a passing score on an examination.

Wiley W. Souba, M.D., Sc.D.

Basic Research With Clinical Applicability

Complete Prevention of Impaired Anastomotic Healing in Diabetic Rats Requires Preoperative Blood Glucose Control

Verhofstad MHJ, Hendriks T (Univ Hosp Nijmegen, The Netherlands)
Br J Surg 83:1717–1721, 1996 9–1

Introduction.—Patients with diabetes mellitus frequently have impaired wound healing after surgery. Most clinical and experimental evidence for poor wound healing is based on data from skin wounds. It is only assumed that diabetes impairs intestinal healing. The potential beneficial effect of insulin administration, initiated before or immediately after surgery, was evaluated in 90 male Wistar rats.

Methods.—Rats were randomly assigned to 1 of 4 groups: nondiabetic control group, uncontrolled diabetic group, diabetic group treated before and after operation, and diabetic group treated with insulin after operation only. Rats in the diabetic group treated before and after surgery received twice-daily subcutaneous injections of insulin 4 days before operation (insulin-1 group). Rats in the diabetic group treated after surgery only began insulin injection on the day of surgery (insulin-2 group). All animals underwent anastomosis in both the ileum and colon. Half of the animals were sacrificed 3 days after surgery and remaining rats were killed

TABLE 2.—Anastomotic Bursting Pressure

Group		Bursting pressure (kPa)		
	n	Ileum	*n*	Colon
Day 3				
Control	10	8·1(2·9)	10	18·1(5·8)
Diabetic	10	1·0(1·4)*	11	4·9(4·7)†‡
Insulin-1	10	9·9(4·5)	10	20·7(7·9)
Insulin-2	7	10·9(7·5)	7	10·2(6·4)‡
Day 7				
Control	9	44·9(8·7)	10	30·7(3·0)
Diabetic	9	13·6(16·3)†‡	8	20·5(8·6)†‡
Insulin-1	10	43·8(7·6)	10	34·2(4·2)
Insulin-2	9	30·1(13·3)†‡	9	24·7(3·4)†‡

Note: Bursting pressure values are mean (SD).
*$P < 0.017$ vs. all other groups.
†$P < 0.017$ vs. control group.
‡$P < 0.017$ vs. insulin-1 group (Wilcoxon rank sum test).
(Courtesy of Verhofstad MHJ, Hendriks T: Complete prevention of impaired anastomotic healing in diabetic rats requires preoperative blood glucose control. *Br J Surg* 83:1717–1721. Copyright 1996, Blackwell Science Ltd.)

at 7 days. The anastomotic segment was tested for bursting pressure in each rat.

Results.—Ten rats from the diabetic group died prematurely. At 3 days after surgery, the mean bursting pressures in both the ileum and colon in the diabetic group were severely decreased, compared with nondiabetic controls. The ileal anastomosis values for the 2 groups of animals receiving insulin were similar to those of control animals. The mean bursting pressure for the colonic anastomosis of the insulin-2 group was significantly below that of the insulin-1 group. At 7 days, the mean bursting pressures for the ileum and colon anastomoses were restored to control levels for the insulin-1 group, but not the insulin-2 group (Table 2). Anastomotic abscess formation at 3 days occurred significantly more frequently in the diabetic and insulin-2 group, compared with the insulin-1 and control groups.

Conclusions.—Early anastomotic strength is severely decreased in uncontrolled diabetes in rats. This effect may be prevented with administration of insulin from 4 days before surgery onwards. Postoperative diabetic control alone is not sufficient to completely restore adequate healing.

Differential Expression and Localization of Insulin-like Growth Factors I and II in Cutaneous Wounds of Diabetic and Nondiabetic Mice

Brown DL, Kane CD, Chernausek SD, et al (Univ of Cincinnati, Ohio)

Am J Pathol 151:715–724, 1997 9–2

Background.—Whereas insulinlike growth factor (IGF)–I has major effects on tissue repair, IGF-II is thought to act mainly during fetal development. Topical application of platelet-derived growth factor and IGF-II, but not IGF-I, reverses the delay in healing of diabetic wounds. This study examined the localization and expression of IGF-I and IGF-II mRNA

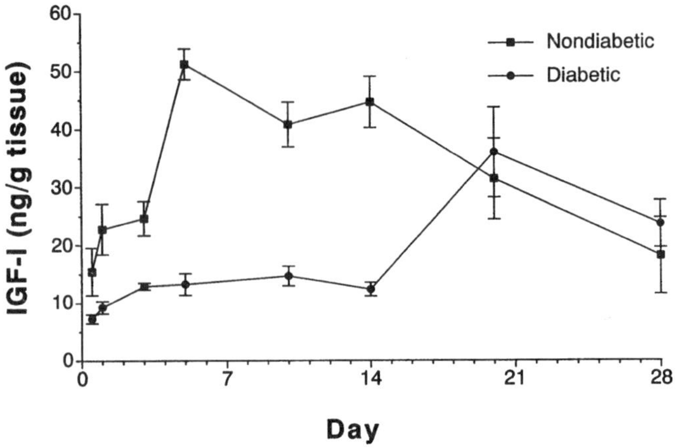

FIGURE 2.—IGF-I protein levels in diabetic and nondiabetic wounds over time, as determined by RIA (values expressed as mean ± SEM). The protein levels paralleled findings for IGF-I mRNA expression, again revealing a delay in diabetic animals. (Courtesy of Brown DL, Kane CD, Chernausek SD, et al: Differential expression and localization of insulin-like growth factors I and II in cutaneous wounds of diabetic and nondiabetic mice. *Am J Pathol* 151:715–724, 1997. Permission granted: Copyright, American Society for Investigative Pathology.)

and protein during early wound healing in diabetic and nondiabetic animals.

Methods.—The experimental model consisted of full-thickness cutaneous wounds in diabetic C57BL/KsJ-db/db mice and their nondiabetic littermates. Immunohistochemistry and in situ hybridization were performed in half of each wound at various intervals. In the other half of the wounds, IGF mRNA was measured by competitive reverse transcriptase–polymerase chain reaction and IGF protein by radioimmunoassay. The researchers hypothesized that IGF expression would be inhibited in diabetic animals and upregulated in healing wounds.

Results.—By day 3 after wounding, the nondiabetic wounds showed a sharp increase in IGF-I mRNA. This finding was delayed to day 14 in diabetic wounds, with peak levels 50% lower than in the nondiabetic wounds. The nondiabetic wounds also showed an increase in IGF-II mRNA, with a peak at day 3. Again, IGF-II mRNA expression was delayed in diabetic wounds, with the peak not reached until day 10. However, peak IGF-II mRNA levels were 4 times higher in diabetic than in nondiabetic wounds.

Expression of IGF-I protein was as expected from the findings of IGF-I mRNA expression (Fig 2). In the nondiabetic wounds, levels of IGF-I were initially twice as high as in the diabetic group, with a peak at 5 days. In diabetic wounds, IGF-I concentrations peaked at 21 days, reaching the same levels as in the nondiabetic group. Further studies localized both IGF proteins to the advancing epithelial edge, the epithelial cells of adjacent hair follicles, and the wound granulation tissue. The findings of IGF mRNA expression followed the same pattern.

Conclusions.—In this animal model, healing full-thickness wounds show upregulation of both IGF-I and IGF-II. However, both factors are delayed in wounds of diabetic animals. This could at least partly explain the deficient healing of diabetic wounds. The IGFs are linked to migrating epithelium, suggesting that the epithelium plays a major role in wound healing.

► These are 2 interesting papers that focus on regulation of wound healing in diabetic rodents. The paper by Verhofstad (Abstract 9–1) shows that uncontrolled diabetes reduces the strength of an experimental intestinal anastamosis by impairing healing. Postoperative blood glucose control did not completely prevent the detrimental effects of uncontrolled diabetes on anastomotic strength, indicating that other factors contribute to altered healing in diabetes. It is likely that the chronic nature of the disease induces local derangements that contribute to impaired healing independent of the blood sugar level. Brown et al. (Abstract 9–2) showed that the impairment in tissue repair in diabetic animals is, at least partially, due to a deficiency in the production of IGFs. This is an interesting observation, given the role of the IGFs in regulating glucose metabolism. The decreased expression of the IGFs in chronic diabetic wounds suggests that exogenous growth factors are a viable treatment option for some chronic, nonhealing wounds.

W.W. Souba, M.D., Sc.D.

Ischemia and Reperfusion Reduce the Endogenous Basic Fibroblast Growth Factor in Rat Skeletal Muscles: An Immunohistochemical Study

Fu X, Cuevas P, Gimenez-Gallego G, et al (304th Hosp, Beijing, China; Hosp Ramon y Cajal, Madrid)

Wound Rep Reg 4:381–385, 1996 9–3

Introduction.—Basic fibroblast growth factor (bFGF) is believed to stimulate proliferation of neuroectodermal and mesodermal tissues, such as endothelial cells and fibroblasts. It has been suggested that muscle myoblasts and satellite cells respond to bFGF and that various muscles store bFGF-like activity. However, there have been no studies of the distribution of bFGF in wounded muscle. This growth factor could play an important role in muscle injury and regeneration. Changes in endogenous bFGF in response to ischemia and reperfusion of rat skeletal muscle were investigated.

Methods.—The study used a Wistar rat model of ischemia and reperfusion injury. Immunohistochemical studies with polyclonal antibodies against human recombinant bFGF were used to localize bFGF in normal and wound rat skeletal muscle. Based on the intensity of staining, strongly, moderately, and weakly stained fibers were identified. Changes in the distribution and concentration of bFGF after ischemia and reperfusion injury were analyzed, along with the possible mechanisms involved.

TABLE 1.—Relative Intensity of bFGF Immunohistochemical Staining in Normal, Ischemic, and Ischemic and Reperfused Rat Skeletal Muscles

Groups*	Relative staining intensity Strong	Moderate	Weak	Negative
I	15/30	6/30	4/30	5/30
II	8/30	5/30	6/30	11/30
III	2/30	4/30	6/30	18/30

*Groups: I, normal muscle; II, muscle with ischemia; III, muscle with ischemia and reperfusion. Three levels of bFGF immunohistochemical staining were identified and designated: strong, moderate, and weak positive stain. The percentage of bFGF immunohistochemical stained fibers was estimated after counting all the fibers in 10 different fields randomly chosen from the preparation (n = 3). One preparation from each animal was studied.

(Courtesy of Fu X, Cuevas P, Gimenez-Gallego G, et al: Ischemia and reperfusion reduce the endogenous basic fibroblast growth factor in rat skeletal muscles: An immunohistochemical study. *Wound Rep Reg* 4:381–385, 1996.)

Results.—The major location of bFGF immunoreactivity was the extracellular matrix. bFGF activity was strongest in the endomysium, where the heparin-containing basal lamina is located, and in the capillary basal membrane of normal and wounded muscle. Normal muscle showed a stronger signal intensity, however (Table 1). In wounded muscle, bFGF distribution was considerably more heterogeneous and sparser. Four hours of ischemia led to loss of bFGF immunoreactivity in about 40% of skeletal muscle fibers. Ischemia followed by 24 hr of reperfusion showed only diminishment of bFGF immunoreactivity. Pathologic examination of ischemic/reperfused muscles suggested destroyed cell connections and fiber necrosis.

Conclusions.—Endogenous levels of bFGF in skeletal muscle are reduced by ischemia and reperfusion. Possible mechanisms of this process include oxygen radical activation, a generalized effect of the inflammatory response, or reduced bFGF secretion. Whatever the mechanism, reduced bFGF could play a role in delayed wound healing.

Elevated Levels of Basic Fibroblast Growth Factor in Patients With Limb Ischemia

Rohovsky S, Kearney M, Pieczek A, et al (Harvard Med School, Boston; Tufts Univ, Boston)

Am Heart J 132:1015–1019, 1996 9–4

Background.—The heparin-binding growth factor basic fibroblast growth factor (bFGF) has angiogenic activity both in vitro and in vivo. It has been linked to a broad range of conditions, such as atherosclerosis, wound healing, carcinoma, and Duchenne muscular dystrophy. This study sought to determine whether peripheral vascular insufficiency, particularly critical limb ischemia, might also be associated with upregulation of bFGF.

Methods.—The study included 40 patients with symptomatic peripheral vascular disease undergoing 46 percutaneous revascularization procedures. Serum samples were obtained at the time of each procedure. In each specimen, bFGF was measured using a specific enzyme-linked immunoassay. The assay's limit of detection was 1 pg/mL; the normal range for bFGF was 0 to 5 pg/mL.

Results.—Seventy-eight percent of serum samples showed circulating bFGF levels of ≥10 pg/mL. The mean value was 62 pg/mL, with a range of 10 to 310 pg/mL. There were 18 patients with rest pain and nonhealing ischemic ulcers. All but 2 of these patients had elevated serum bFGF values, with levels reaching up to 30 times normal.

Conclusions.—Patients with peripheral vascular insufficiency have elevated serum levels of bFGF. Upregulation of bFGF could be a physiologic response to limb ischemia. Elevation of bFGF occurs even in patients without overt loss of tissue integrity; thus it cannot be explained by grossly apparent wounds alone.

Double-blind Randomized Placebo-controlled Trial of the Use of Granulocyte-Macrophage Colony-stimulating Factor in Chronic Leg Ulcers

da Costa RM, Jesus FM, Aniceto C, et al (Hosp Distrital de Leiria, Portugal)

Am J Surg 173:165–168, 1997 9–5

Objective.—As the population ages, chronic wound care becomes an increasingly important health issue. Granulocyte-macrophage colony-stimulating factor (GM-CSF) is an important growth factor involved in wound repair, leading to studies of exogenous GM-CSF to improve impaired wound healing. Animal experiments and preliminary studies in humans have given promising results. A double-blind, randomized controlled trial of perilesional GM-CSF for the treatment of chronic leg ulcers was performed.

Methods.—The study sample comprised 40 patients with chronic leg ulcers of varicose or ischemic causes. They were assigned to receive a single perilesional injection of recombinant human GM-CSF, 400 μg, or placebo. Average wound size was about 10 cm² in both groups. The injections were made in 4 equal doses in the 4 quadrants of the wound. The wounds were assessed at 8, 15, and 29 days, then weekly for 3 months. Healing was compared in the 2 groups.

Results.—The results were so much better in the GM-CSF group that the study was ended early—16 patients were treated in the GM-CSF group and 9 in the placebo group. By day 8, ulcer size had decreased to 7 cm² in the GM-CSF group compared with a slight increase in the placebo group. In the GM-CSF group, ulcer healing occurred by 1 week in 19% of patients and by 8 weeks in 50%. In contrast, just 1 of 9 patients in the control group had ulcer healing at 1 week. That was the only ulcer that healed in the control group. Treatment with GM-CSF had no significant side effects and caused no alterations in hematologic or biochemical parameters.

Conclusions.—Recombinant human GM-CSF seems to be an effective treatment for chronic leg ulcers. Good results are achieved in both venous and ischemic ulcers with a single perilesional treatment. More research is needed to optimize the indications for treatment, the drug dose, and the dosing regimen. The histologic changes in the ulcer and the perilesional skin must be described as well.

▶ These papers provide additional evidence for the role of growth factors in modulating wound repair. Fu and colleagues (Abstract 9–3) demonstrated that nearly half of skeletal muscle fibers lost their basic fibroblast growth factor (bFGF) immunoreactivity after 4 hours of ischemia. Rohovsky et al. (Abstract 9–4) showed that circulating levels of bFGF were elevated in patients with vascular insufficiency and suggested that this might reflect a physiologic response to limb ischemia. Local growth factor production may be decreased during ischemia, and the body responds by increasing production and release in other tissues. Complementing these studies was the paper by Marques da Costa and associates, (Abstract 9–5) who demonstrated the efficacy of perilesional injection of GM-CSF in the treatment of chronic leg ulcers. These and other studies raise several key questions: (1) what are the indications for the use of growth factors in treating chronic wounds?; (2) how should these growth factors be administered?; (3) what is the ideal dose of the drug?; (4) what is the ideal number of treatments and the time interval between each?; and (5) how should wound healing be assessed?.

W.W. Souba, M.D., Sc.D.

Nitric Oxide, an Autocrine Regulator of Wound Fibroblast Synthetic Function

Schäffer MR, Efron PA, Thornton FJ, et al (Johns Hospkins Med Insts, Baltimore, Md; Eberhard-Karls-Universität, Tübingen, Germany; Cornell Univ, New York)

J Immunol 158:2375–2381, 1997 9–6

Introduction.—Although nitric oxide (NO) synthesis occurs in wounds, its precise role and cellular source are unknown. Among the changes seen in activated wound fibroblasts (WF) are increased collagen synthesis and contractility. This study sought to determine whether WF could be phenotypically altered during wound healing to synthesize NO.

Methods.—Polyvinyl alcohol sponges implanted in male Lewis rats were recovered after 10 days to obtain WF. Incorporation of [^{3}H]thymidine in a microculture system was used to assess WF proliferation in response to 10% fetal bovine serum. Contractility was examined using a fibroblast-populated collagen lattice. To determine whether the WF were synthesizing collagen, the collagenase-sensitive fraction of protein-incorporated [^{3}H]proline was measured. The WF were incubated with or without 2 competitive inhibitors of NO synthase: *S*-methyl-isothio-uronium (MITU), or *N*-monomethyl-L-arginine, both in concentrations of 0.5 mmol/L.

Results.—The experiments showed spontaneous synthesis and release of NO by WF at a rate of 4.60 nmol nitrite/μg DNA/48 hr. Nitric oxide was

TABLE 1.—Synthesis of Total Protein ([^{3}H]proline Incorporation) and Collagen (Collagenase-sensitive Fraction of Protein-incorporated [^{3}H]proline by WF[a]

Wound Fibroblasts	Total Protein Synthesis (dpm/ng DNA)	Collagen Synthesis (dpm/ng DNA)	Relative Collagen Synthesis (%)
	225 ± 12	23.3 ± 2.1	2.20 ± 0.20
+ MITU	258 ± 17	12.6 ± 2.6†	1.00 ± 0.21**‡
+ LPS + IFN-γ	212 ± 14	33.9 ± 2.3*	3.55 ± 0.32**
+ LPS + IFN-γ + MITU	213 ± 21	12.7 ± 1.4*†	1.32 ± 0.27**‡

[a]Cells were cultured in media containing 10% FBS and 50 μg/mL ascorbic acid (controls) and in the presence of 0.5 mmol/L MITU, 1 mg/mL LPS plus 10 U/mL IFN-γ, or 1 mg/mL LPS plus 10 U/mL IFN-γ plus 0.5 mmol/L MITU. Mean ± SEM of three separate quadruplicate experiments are shown.
*$p < 0.05$ vs. control.
†$p < 0.01$ vs. LPS + IFN.
**$p < 0.01$ vs. control.
‡$p < 0.001$ vs LPN + IFN.
(Courtesy of Schäffer MR, Efron PA, Thornton FJ, et al: Nitric oxide, an autocrine regulator of wound fibroblast synthetic function. *J Immunol* 158:2375–2381, 1997. Copyright 1997. The American Association of Immunologists.)

not synthesized by normal dermal fibroblasts, however. Synthesis of NO by WF was noted only during the first and second passages after harvest, and was largely inhibited by both NO synthase inhibitors. In situ hybridization and immunohistochemical studies confirmed that WF expressed inducible NO synthase in vivo. Fibroblast proliferation was unaffected by NO synthesis. However, inhibition of NO synthase enhanced fibroblast-mediated collagen contraction and reduced collagen synthesis (Table 1).

Conclusions.—During the process of wound healing, WF undergo phenotypic changes to permit synthesis of NO. Nitric oxide then acts in autocrine fashion to regulate the synthesis and contraction of collagen by WF. The findings support in vivo studies suggesting that NO plays a key role in wound healing.

Acute Protein-Calorie Malnutrition Impairs Wound Healing: A Possible Role of Decreased Wound Nitric Oxide Synthesis

Schäffer MR, Tantry U, Ahrendt GM, et al (Eberhard-Karls-Universität, Tübingen, Germany; Johns Hopkins Med Insts, Baltimore, Md)

J Am Coll Surg 184:37–43, 1997 9–7

Objective.—Nitric oxide (NO) synthesis occurs in wounds, and inhibition of NO synthesis reduces collagen accumulation in and mechanical strength of wounds. However, the function of NO in the setting of impaired wound healing is unknown. A model of impaired wound healing in animals with acute protein-calorie malnutrition (PCM) was used to study the effects on wound NO synthesis.

Methods.—Acute malnourishment of a group of Sprague-Dawley rats was achieved by limiting their food intake to 50% of food intake in a control group of rats fed ad libitum for 7 days. Dorsal skin wounds were created, and polyvinyl alcohol sponges were subcutaneously implanted.

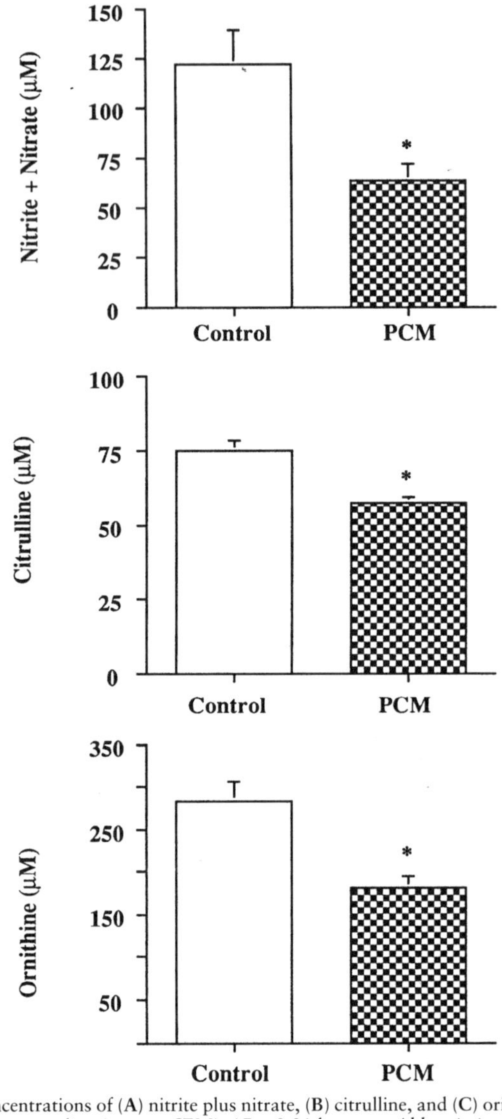

FIGURE 4.—Concentrations of (A) nitrite plus nitrate, (B) citrulline, and (C) orinithine in wound fluid harvested 10 days postwounding (mean ± SEM). *$P < 0.01$ by t test. *Abbreviation: PCM*, protein calorie malnutrition. (Courtesy of Schäffer MR, Tantry U, Ahrendt GM, et al: Acute protein-calorie malnutrition impairs wound healing: A possible role of decreased wound nitric oxide synthesis. *J Am Coll Surg* 184:37–43, 1997. By permission of the Journal of the American College of Surgeons.)

After 10 days, the sponges were removed for measurement of wound collagen accumulation and type I and III collagen gene expression. Measurements were made in wound fluid and wound cell culture supernatants to assess NO synthesis.

Results.—Body weight decreased by 10% for animals in the acute PCM group, compared with an 18% gain in the control group. Wound collagen accumulation was decreased in the PCM group, as evidenced by the finding of reduced sponge hydroxyproline contents: 995 μg/100 mg in the PCM group vs. 1,580 μg/100 mg in the control group. Wounds in the PCM group showed decreased gene expression of type III collagen but not type I collagen. Rats in the PCM group also had decreased concentrations of nitrite-nitrate and citrulline in wound fluid and wound cell supernatants, suggesting a net decline in NO production (Fig 4).

Conclusions.—In this animal model, impaired wound healing caused by acute PCM is associated with reduced wound collagen accumulation. This finding could reflect reduced synthesis of NO in the healing-impaired wound. Reduction of NO synthesis would result from a reduced number of cells in the wound or a change in metabolic activity secondary to reduced capacity to produce NO.

Differential Regulation of Macrophage Arginine Metabolism: A Proposed Role in Wound Healing

Shearer JD, Richards JR, Mills CD, et al (Univ of Minnesota, Minneapolis)
Am J Physiol 272:E181–E190, 1997 9–8

Purpose.—Nitric oxide (NO) is the product of NO synthase, and ornithine is the product of arginase. It is now thought that arginine metabolism, through increased arginase activity, may create an environment favoring cell growth and proliferation. Resident mouse peritoneal exudate cells (MPEC) were studied to determine the effects of factors mediating leukocyte activation and inhibition on arginine metabolism.

Findings.—In intact MPEC, the same factors that increased basal NO synthase activity, interferon (IFN)-γ, and lipopolysaccharide (LPS) also reduced arginase activity. Stimulation of NO synthase activity by IFN-γ was reduced by transforming growth factor (TGF)-β1, which also caused an increase in urea and ornithine release. In LPS-stimulated MPEC, TGF-β1 did not affect either of these enzymes; however, corticosterone (Cort), 100 ng/mL, decreased the basal activity of both. In MPEC exposed to either IFN-γ or LPS, Cort inhibited NO synthase activity and increased ornithine release. Arginase activity was different between intact cells and cell lysates, suggesting intracellular inhibition of arginase activity. NO and citrulline, both products of NO synthase, inhibited the activity of arginase in MPEC under maximal assay conditions. Exposure to LPS, IFN-γ, TGF-β1, or Cort had no effect on intracellular pH in MPEC.

Conclusions.—Factors that regulate arginine metabolism appear to influence cell function at the site of injury. In the early phase of wound healing, cells are signaled to metabolize arginine through NO synthase, leading to a cytotoxic environment. Arginine metabolism by arginase follows as the wound healing process continues and inflammatory cell cytolysis occurs. As a result, extracellular arginine decreases and ornithine

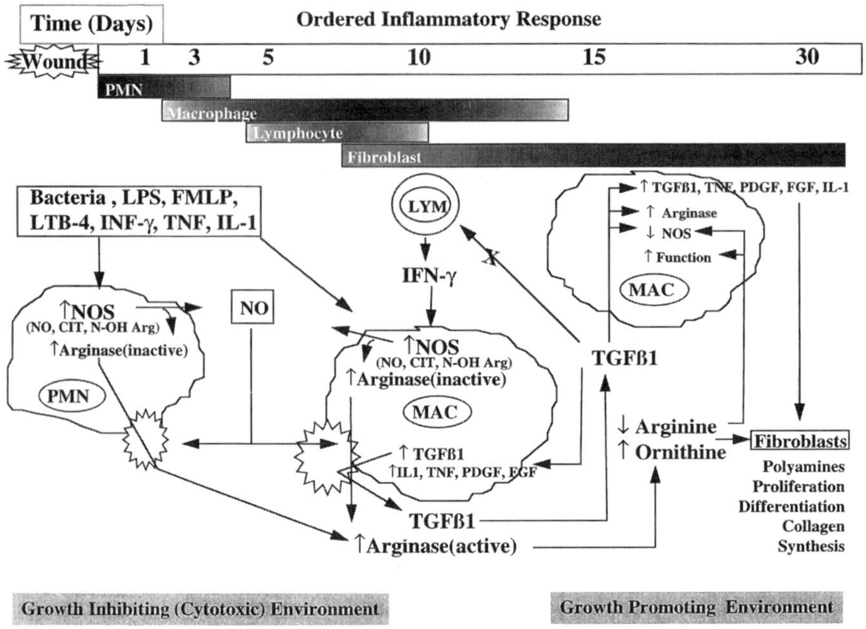

FIGURE 7.—Model for regulation of arginine metabolism during wound healing. Proposed importance of reciprocal regulation of NO synthase and arginase to wound healing is shown schematically. Cells present early in wound are signaled to metabolize arginine through NO synthase, creating a cytotoxic environment. As wound healing progresses and inflammatory cell cytolysis occurs, arginine is metabolized by arginase. Resulting decrease in extracellular arginine and increase in ornithine promote cell function and replication. TGF-β1 appears to play an important coregulatory role in this process. Abbreviations: *PMN*, polymorphonuclear leukocyte; *MAC*, macrophage; *FGF*, fibroblast growth factor; *FMLP*, formyl-Met-Leu-Phe; *IL-1*, interleukin-1; LTB_4, leukotriene B_4; *N*-OH Arg, N^G-hydroxy-L-arginine; *NOS*, nitric oxide synthase; *PDGF*, platelet-derived growth factor; *TNF*, tumor necrosis factor. (Courtesy of Shearer JD, Richards JR, Mills CD, et al: Differential regulation of macrophage arginine metabolism: A proposed role in wound healing. *Am J Physiol* 2723:E181–E190, 1997. Copyright, The American Physiological Society.)

increases, thus promoting cell function and replication. TGF-β1 appears to be an important coregulator of arginine metabolism during wound healing (Fig 7).

Nitric Oxide Metabolism in Wounds

Schäffer MR, Tantry U, van Wesep RA, et al (Eberhard-Karls-Universität, Tübingen, Germany; Johns Hopkins Med Insts, Baltimore, Md)
J Surg Res 71:25–31, 1997 9–9

Background.—In wounds, arginine can be metabolized to either nitric oxide (NO) and citrulline by NO synthase or to urea and ornithine by arginase. It is unknown whether NO acts as a mediator of nonspecific host defenses early in the healing process or as a control signal for successful completion of healing later on. The timing of NO expression and synthesis in wounds and wound cells was studied in mice.

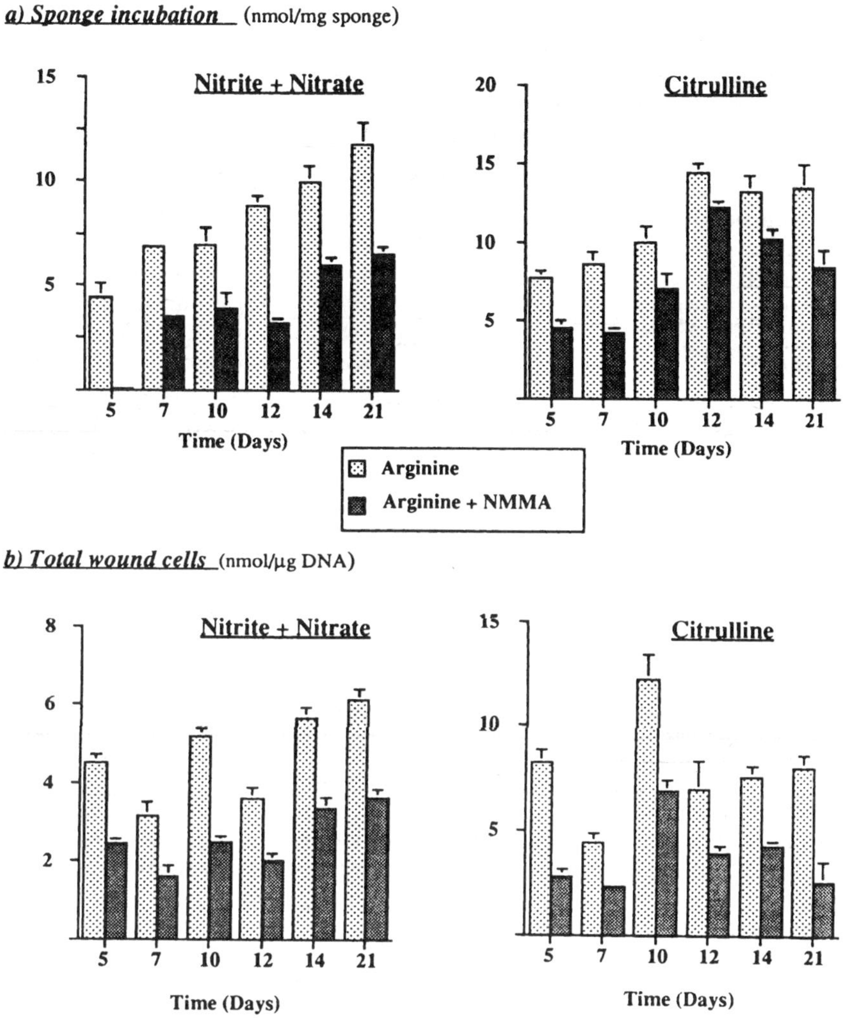

FIGURE 2.—In vitro nitrite plus nitrate and citrulline synthesis. Whole sponges and wound cells were harvested between 5 and 21 days post-wounding and incubated for 20 hr in the presence of 4 mmol/liter L-arginine, with or without 2 mmol/L N^G-L-monomethyl-arginine acetate (NMMA). (Courtesy of Schäffer MR, Tantry U, van Wesep RA, et al: Nitric oxide metabolism in wounds. *J Surg Res* 71:25–31, 1997.)

Methods.—In male Balb/C mice, the dorsal skin was incised, and polyvinyl alcohol sponges were implanted subcutaneously. At intervals from 12 hr to 21 days after wounding, the animals were killed and the sponges were recovered to obtain wound fluid and wound cells for study. The cells or sponges were incubated with L-[2,3-^{3}H]arginine, with or without the competitive NO synthase inhibitor N^G-L-monomethyl-arginine (NMMA). The wound fluid and wound cell culture supernatants were analyzed to determine levels of nitrite and nitrate, which are stable end-products of NO metabolism, and levels of amino acids.

Results.—In both wound fluid and whole sponge cultures, nitrite and nitrate concentrations increased until 2 weeks after wounding, suggesting prolonged NO synthesis. At no time was arginine detected in wound fluid, consistent with sustained arginine utilization. Citrulline levels in wound fluid peaked early, then gradually decreased, indicating possible recycling for continued NO production. Levels of ornithine in wound fluid increased up to day 10 and remained elevated thereafter, suggesting ongoing arginase activity. Incubation with NMMA inhibited nitrite-nitrate and citrulline production by cells and whole sponges (Fig 2). Immunoblotting demonstrated inducible NO synthase expression. Wound NO was found on immunohistochemical studies to arise largely from macrophages.

Conclusions.—This animal model demonstrates prolonged NO synthesis in wounds. Macrophages appear to be a major source of wound NO. The in vitro data support in vivo studies suggesting that NO plays a key role in wound healing.

Altered Wound Arginine Metabolism by Corticosterone and Retinoic Acid

Ulland AE, Shearer JD, Coulter C, et al (Univ of Minnesota, Minneapolis)
J Surg Res 70:84–88, 1997 9–10

Introduction.—Arginine metabolism is a key factor in inflammation and the wound healing process. It appears to be differentially regulated by steroids and retinoic acid. Arginine metabolism may thus be partly responsible for mediating the negative effects of steroid and retinoic acid on wound healing, which are improved by vitamin A. The effects of corticosterone and retinoic acid on wound metabolism were studied in vivo in rats.

Methods.—Male Sprague-Dawley rats underwent subcutaneous implantation of corticosterone pellets 2 days before full-thickness dorsal skin wounding. At the same time, and again 2 and 4 days later, the animals received intraperitoneal injections of all-*trans*-retinoic acid in peanut oil. Through the dorsal wounds, polyvinyl alcohol sponges were subcutaneously implanted. The sponges were recovered at intervals from 1 to 15 days after wounding to obtain wound fluid for study. Wound fluid levels of nitrite-nitrate, citrulline, arginine, and ornithine were measured, along with arginase activity.

Results-.—Arginine metabolism to nitric oxide (NO) in the early phase of wound healing was significantly reduced by corticosterone treatment. Retinoic acid treatment had no such effect. Later in the wound healing process, arginine metabolism to ornithine was reduced in steroid-treated rats. Concomitant retinoic acid treatment inhibited steroid-induced inhibition of ornithine.

Conclusions.—In this rat wound model, corticosterone and retinoic acid have differing effects on arginine metabolism. Early NO synthase activity is inhibited by corticosterone but is unaffected by retinoic acid. Corticosterone also inhibits the arginase pathway during later healing, which effect is reversed by retinoic acid. Given the importance of NO to host defense and of ornithine as a precursor to polyamine and proline synthesis, the results may provide a mechanism whereby vitamin A improves wound strength in steroid-treated animals without reducing infection rates.

► These 5 papers (Abstracts 9–6 to 9–10) build on the previous observation that wounds have been shown to synthesize NO and that NO is an important regulator of wound healing. The expression of NO synthase in wounds creates a local environment that appears to be important for wound healing. Macrophages are important sources of nitric oxide and physiologic derangements such as protein-calorie malnutrition may reduce NO production secondary to impaired macrophage function or decreased macrophage recruitment. In addition, steroid treatment can decrease the conversion of arginine to NO, which may contribute to an impairment in wound healing. Wound fibroblasts are phenotypically altered during the healing process and stimulated to synthesize NO, which in turn regulates collagen synthesis and contractile function. The role of exogenous arginine or NO in mediating wound healing has clinical implications.

W.W. Souba, M.D., Sc.D.

Direct Effects of Somatostatin Analog Octreotide on Insulin-like Growth Factor-I in the Arterial Wall

Yumi K, Fagin JA, Yamashita M, et al (Univ of California, Los Angeles; Karolinska Inst, Stockholm; Univ of Cincinnati, Ohio)

Lab Invest 76:329–338, 1997 9–11

Objective.—The authors have noted increased local expression of insulin-like growth factor I (IGF-I) in the vascular wall after balloon injury, and suggest that this growth factor may play a key role in the biologic events that follow arterial injury. The somatostatin analog octreotide is a powerful inhibitor of the growth hormone–IGF-I axis. The effects of octreotide treatment on IGF-I and the response to balloon injury in the rat arterial wall were studied.

Methods and Results.—Rats with balloon-induced arterial injury were treated with octreotide. Octreotide treatment was associated with a selective, 70% reduction in IGF-I mRNA expression in normal arteries. After balloon injury, it also prevented induction of the IGF-I gene. Octreotide had no affect on upregulation of the platelet-derived growth factor A gene or on plasma growth hormone, IGF-I, or glucagon levels. Thus, the effects of octreotide treatment were selective and locally mediated. Balloon injury was followed by modest upregulation of IGF binding protein 4, which was unaffected by octreotide treatment. Along with its effects on vascular IGF-I, octreotide decreased the number of proliferating cell nuclear antigen–positive cells. It also reduced the neointimal thickening response to balloon injury by as much as 90%, in dose-dependent fashion.

Conclusions.—Octreotide inhibits the neointimal proliferation response to vascular injury in rats. This effect seems to be at least partly mediated by local impairment of IGF-I gene expression. Treatments that modulate local IGF-I may be one way of inhibiting neointimal wall thickening after arterial wall injury.

The Adverse Effects of Octreotide on Wound Healing in Rats

Waddell BE, Calton WC Jr; Steinberg SR, et al (Dwight D Eisenhower Army Med Ctr, Fort Gordon; Med College of Georgia, Augusta)

Am Surg 63:446–449, 1997 9–12

Purpose.—The somatostatin analog octreotide has a wide variety of physiologic effects. As an inhibitory paracrine hormone, it is used to treat

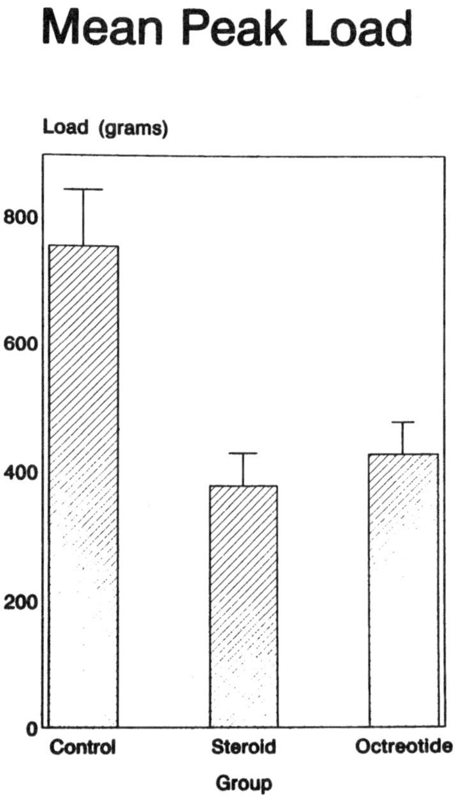

FIGURE 2.—Wound breaking strength for each experimental group, recorded as mean peak load (in grams). Control vs. steroid, $p < 0.015$; control vs. octreotide, $p < 0.030$. (Courtesy of Waddell BE, Calton WC Jr, Steinberg SR, et al: The adverse effects of octreotide on wound healing in rats. *Am Surg* 63:446–449, 1997.)

several different disorders, such as endocrine tumors and gastrointestinal hypersecretory states. Octreotide inhibits various trophic and anabolic hormones, raising the possibility of adverse effects on wound healing. Octreotide's effects on wound healing in rats were investigated in a randomized study.

Methods.—Sprague-Dawley rats were randomly assigned into an octreotide group; a control group; and, as a negative control, a steroid group. In each animal, a dorsal midline incision was made and closed primarily. After 7 days of healing, the animals were killed for measurements of wound breaking strength.

Results.—The mean peak load to wound breaking was 427 g in the octreotide group, 754 g in the control group, and 378 g in the steroid group. Wound breaking strength was significantly greater in the control group than in the other 2 groups (Fig 2).

Conclusions.—Octreotide treatment adversely affects wound healing in rats. The negative effect of octreotide is comparable in magnitude to that caused by steroids. The authors call for more research to determine the mechanism of this effect, and possible interventions.

▶ These 2 papers (Abstracts 9–11 and 9–12) focus on the somatostatin analog octreotide, which is often used as an inhibitory paracrine hormone to treat a variety of surgical disorders, such as gastrointestinal hypersecretory states. Waddell and colleagues speculate that octreotide adversely impacts wound healing by inhibiting the production of key trophic factors. The actions of octreotide could impair wound healing much as they might inhibit tumor growth. Yumi and colleagues demonstrated that octreotide selectively decreases IGF-I mRNA expression in normal rat arteries by 70%. Failure to produce growth factors such as insulin-like growth factor locally could have detrimental effects on wound healing.

W.W. Souba, M.D., Sc.D.

Effects of Growth Hormone and Insulin-like Growth Factor-I on Protein Metabolism, Gut Morphology, and Cell-mediated Immunity in Burned Rats

Shimoda N, Tashiro T, Yamamori H, et al (Chiba Univ, Japan)

Nutrition 13:540–546, 1997 9–13

Background.—In a previous study, the authors demonstrated strong anabolic effects of growth hormone (GH) and insulin-like growth factor I (IGF-I). They also found that IGF-I enhances intestinal mucosal proliferation. More information is needed on how these factors affect immune function and gut structure. The effects of GH and IGF-I were studied in burned rats.

Methods.—Twenty percent third-degree scald burns were induced in Sprague-Dawley rats that had been fed exclusively by total parenteral nutrition. One group was treated with GH at a dose of 1 IU/kg/day for 2 days; another group with IGF-I, 4 mg/kg/day; and control group of animals with saline solution. After measurement of total body protein turnover, the animals were killed. The effects on intestinal structure were assessed by histologic examination. The immune response was evaluated with a standard model of cell-mediated immunity.

Results.—Cumulative nitrogen balance was significantly increased over control values for the GH and IGF-I groups, with no significant difference between these groups. Compared with control animals, glucose was decreased in the IGF group and increased in the GH group. Both the GH and IGF-I groups showed significantly increased intestinal villus height and wall thickness. They also had enhanced delayed-type hypersensitivity, more so in the IGF-I group.

Conclusions.—In this rat burn model, GH and IGF-I improved protein metabolism and immune responsiveness while maintaining gut structure. These effects may make IGF-I and GH useful in the clinical management of sepsis, burns, multiple organ failure, and major surgery. The immune effect may be greater with IGF-I, although there is little difference in terms of nitrogen balance and whole body protein metabolism.

▶ Using a rat burn model, the authors have demonstrated that IGF-I and GH can improve protein synthesis, support cell-mediated immunity, maintain gut structure, and possibly reduce bacterial translocation. This study, like many others, focuses on biochemical and structural end points. However, what is lacking from clinical studies is the demonstration that such compounds can improve outcome, whether it be a reduction in morbidity or mortality.

W.W. Souba, M.D., Sc.D.

Myofibroblast Persistence in Fetal Sheep Wounds Is Associated With Scar Formation

Cass DL, Sylvester KG, Yang EY, et al (Univ of Pennsylvania, Philadelphia)
J Pediatr Surg 32:1017–1021, 1997 9–14

Introduction.—Some, but not all, skin wounds in fetuses heal without scarring. Factors that affect the potential for scarless repair include wound size and gestational age, small wounds will heal scarlessly, but large wounds in the same fetus will not. The small wounds may have a relative absence of myofibroblasts, specialized fibroblasts that express the contractile cytoskeletal protein α-smooth muscle actin (α-SMA). The authors studied this hypothesis in small and large wounds in midgestation fetal sheep.

Methods.—Wounds were created in the backs of sheep at 60 to 90 days' gestation, including an incisional wound and punch biopsy wounds 2, 4, 6, and 10 mm in diameter. After 14 days' healing, the wounds were classified as scarless, in a state of transitional repair, or scarred. Immunohistochemical studies were performed to measure α-SMA expression.

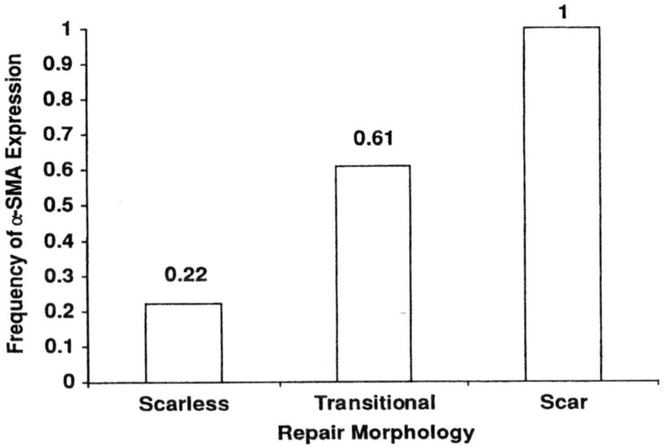

FIGURE 2.—Histogram showing the frequency of α-SMA expression in fetal sheep wounds showing scarless repair, transitional repair, or scar at 14 days (60 to 90 days' gestational age). α-SMA expression was seen in all (n = 18, 100%) wounds that healed with scar, and in only 10 of 46 (22%) wounds that healed scarlessly. (Courtesy of Cass DL, Sylvester KG, Yang EY, et al: Myofibroblast persistence in fetal sheep wounds is associated with scar formation. *J Pediatr Surg* 32:1017–1021, 1997.)

Wounds were also made in sheep at 70 days' gestation for determination of α-SMA expression at 1, 2, 3, and 7 days.

Results.—None of the incisional or 2 mm wounds that healed without scarring expressed α-SMA at 14 days. In contrast, all wounds that healed with scarring expressed α-SMA (Fig 2). As wound size increased, so did α-SMA expression. The temporal studies revealed the appearance of myofibroblasts as early as 24 hr. By 3 and 7 days, all wounds strongly expressed α-SMA.

Conclusions.—Induction of myofibroblasts is an early event in the fetal wound repair process. However, myofibroblast expression after healing is absent from scarless wounds but abundant in scarred wounds. More research is needed to determine the factors responsible for the disappearance of myofibroblasts in scarless fetal wounds.

Age-related Changes in the Temporal and Spatial Distributions of Fibrillin and Elastin mRNAs and Proteins in Acute Cutaneous Wounds of Healthy Humans

Ashcroft GS, Kielty CM, Horan MA, et al (Univ of Manchester, England; Hope Hosp, Salford, Manchester, England)

J Pathol 183:80–89, 1997 9–15

Background.—The elastin framework, with its microfibrillar scaffold made of fibrillin, is the major determinant of skin elasticity and resilience. Little is known about the patterns of elastin and fibrillin expression during wound healing. Fibrillin and elastin expression were studied at the protein and mRNA level in acute healing wounds in humans over time.

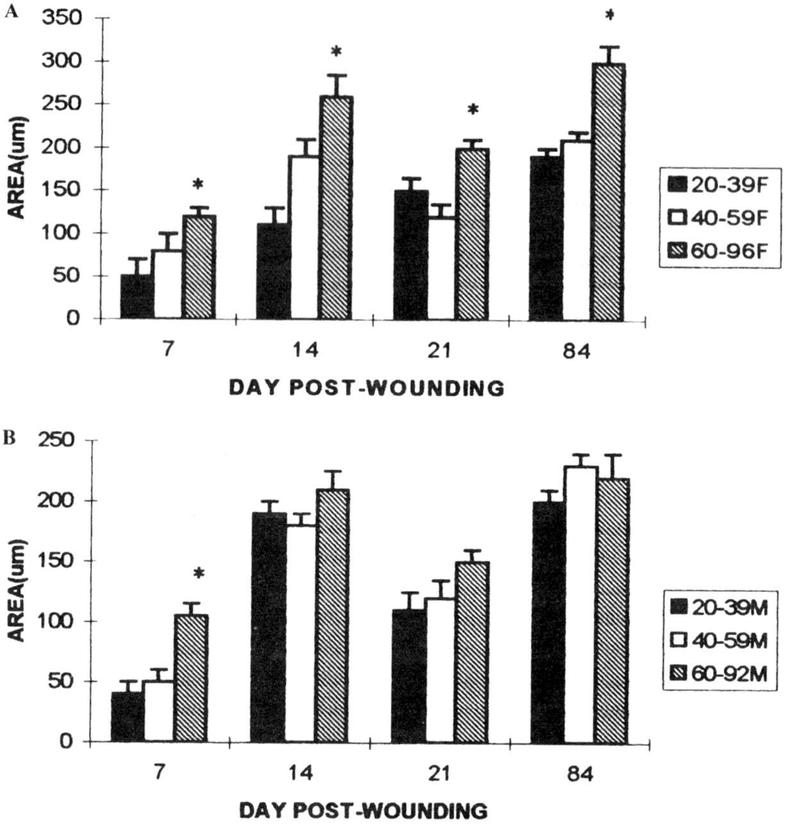

FIGURE 5.—The area of elastin staining within acute healing wounds increases with age. Using a fitted regression model, area values were significantly affected by day ($P < 0.0001$) with an increase in elastin area with age ($P = 0.001$), particularly in females. **A**, data from female subjects; **B**, data from male subjects. Data represent mean ± SD with n = 3. *Significant increase in staining in the aged group ($P < 0.05$, using Tukey's test). (Reprinted by permission of John Wiley & Sons, Ltd. from Ashcroft GS, Keilty CM, Horan MA, et al: Age-related changes in the temporal and spatial distributions of fibrillin and elastin mRNAs and proteins in acute cutaneous wounds of healthy humans. *J Pathol* 183:80–89, 1997. Copyright 1997, John Wiley & Sons, Ltd.)

Methods.—The study included 90 healthy white subjects, ages 19 to 96 years. Health status was known in each subject. Cutaneous punch biopsy wounds 4 mm in diameter were created on the upper inner arm of each subject. The wounds were then re-excised 3 days to 3 months after wounding. Immunocytochemical studies and in situ hybridization were performed to assess the temporal and spatial patterns of elastin and fibrillin expression during healing.

Results.—Messenger RNA levels of elastin, fibrillin-1, and fibrillin-2 did not change significantly with age. The wounds of elderly subjects, particularly women, expressed the greatest amounts of elastin and fibrillin (Fig 5). These wounds were marked by a regenerative pattern of elastin and fibrillin arcades at the dermoepidermal junction. In aged subjects, wound elastin mRNA expression peaked from day 3 to day 14. Fibrillin-1 expression had a comparable spatial and temporal pattern, suggesting that it played a key role in the formation of dermal elastic fibers during wound repair. Fibrillin-2 expression occurred only in the wounds of aged subjects and only near dermal blood vessels.

Conclusions.—Fibrillin and elastin expression are increased during acute wound healing in aged subjects. This leads to restoration of the papillary dermal architecture, with improved quality of scarring. Although healing may occur more slowly with aging, the quality of healing may be improved. The localization of fibrillin-1 and fibrillin-2 during wound healing is clearly distinct, suggesting that they have separate roles in normal skin and wound tissue.

► These 2 papers (Abstracts 9–14 and 9–15) focus on wound healing at 2 extremes: fetal wound healing and wound healing that occurs with aging. Cass and associates demonstrated that myofibroblasts participate in the early stages of fetal wound repair but that by 2 weeks they are relatively absent in wounds that heal scarlessly and abundant in wounds that scar. In contrast, Ashcroft and colleagues show that aging is associated with an increased expression of fibrillin and elastin during acute wound healing, which may contribute to an improved quality of scarring. The authors speculate that the wounds of the aged may contain a subpopulation of fibroblasts that have a fetal-like phenotype. It is of interest that, while aging may adversely affect the speed of wound healing, paradoxically it may improve the quality of wound healing.

W.W. Souba, M.D., Sc.D.

Wound Healing and Growth Factors in Clinical Practice

Vacuum-assisted Closure: A New Method for Wound Control and Treatment: Clinical Experience

Argenta LC, Morykwas MJ (Bowman Gray School of Medicine, Winston-Salem, NC)

Ann Plast Surg 38:563–577, 1997 9–16

Background.—Chronic, nonhealing wounds and wound complications pose difficult problems for patients and physicians alike. Even with various advances, these wounds continue to present treatment challenges. A new approach to wound treatment—vacuum-assisted closure (VAC)—was tested in patients with chronic, subacute, and acute wounds.

Methods.—In VAC, an open-cell foam is placed in the wound, the area is sealed with adhesive tape, and subatmospheric pressures 125 mm Hg below ambient pressure are applied. This technique was used in a series of 300 patients with wounds: 175 chronic wounds, such as pressure ulcers and stasis ulcers, that had not progressed toward healing for more than 1 week; 94 subacute wounds, such as infected and dehisced wounds and open amputations; and 31 acute wounds, such as acute avulsions, evacuated hematomas, and gunshot wounds. The initial patients were treated in the hospital by the senior author; later patients were managed as outpatients under the care of other practitioners. The VAC system was applied after thorough debridement and meticulous hemostasis. The results of patient follow-up and definitive treatment were reported.

Results.—Ninety-nine percent of the wounds showed increased granulation tissue formation in response to VAC. Subatmospheric pressure treatment continued until the wounds closed completely, split-thickness skin grafting was performed, or a flap was rotated into the granulating wound bed. In chronic wounds, the length of treatment ranged from less than 2 weeks to more than 16 weeks, depending on the size of the wound. There have been no pressure ulcer recurrences at the treated wound site. The subacute wounds showed a more rapid and uniform response than the chronic wounds. Successes in this category included many patients with exposed fixation hardware or bone. Healing was quicker still for patients with acute wounds. Except for 1 patient who died, all wounds were successfully closed. The few complications of VAC were mainly technical in nature.

Conclusions.—The VAC technique produces good results in patients with chronic or otherwise difficult wounds. The application of subatmospheric pressure eliminates chronic edema, thus increasing localized blood flow. The forces applied to the wound lead to enhanced granulation tissue formation. The article includes a discussion of the practical considerations involved in VAC. Further study of this new treatment modality is needed; a large, randomized trial is underway.

▶ The authors correctly point out that the VAC technique they have developed should be viewed as an adjunct to wound care. It is not meant to replace standard surgical procedures. They point out that in most cases the technique should be used to prepare the wound bed so that a lesser surgical procedure can be performed with a greater chance for successful wound closure, minimizing time to complete wound closure, and thus minimizing cost, hospitalization, and rehabilitation.

W.W. Souba, M.D., Sc.D.

Intravenous Insulin-like Growth Factor-I (IGF-I) in Moderate-to-Severe Head Injury: A Phase II Safety and Efficacy Trial

Hatton J, Rapp RP, Kudsk KA, et al (Univ of Kentucky, Lexington; Univ of Tennessee, Memphis; Genetech, San Francisco)

J Neurosurg 86:779–786, 1997 9–17

Introduction.—Moderate to severe traumatic brain injury is followed by a state of hypermetabolism and hypercatabolism, which can last for several months. Even with aggressive nutritional support, it can be difficult to achieve a positive calorie balance or positive nitrogen balance. Levels of insulin-like growth factor-I (IGF-I), which mediates many of the anabolic effects of growth hormone, are reduced after brain injury; patients with

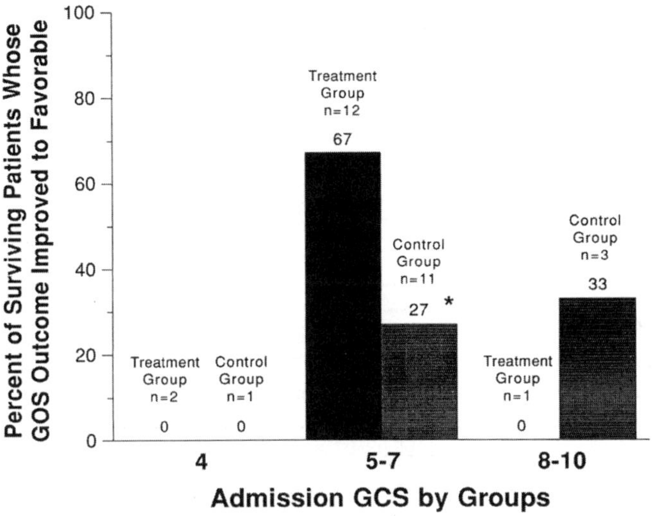

FIGURE 5.—Bar graph showing patient outcome as it relates to admission GCS score. All surviving patients admitted with a GCS score of 4 remained vegetative or severely disabled (according to GOS scores). For 8 patients in the treated group and 3 patients in the control group admitted with GCS scores of 5 through 7, GOS scores improved from poor outcome at day 15 to moderate disability or good recovery ($p = 0.06$). Patients with admission GCS scores of 8 through 10 had 15-day GOS scores of good, except for one of the control patients whose GOS score improved from vegetative to good recovery at 6 months. (Courtesy of Hatton J, Rapp RP, Kudsk KA, et al: Intravenous insulin-like growth factor [IGF-] in moderate-to-severe head injury: A phase II safety and efficacy trial. *J Neurosurg* 86:779–786, 1997.)

higher IGF-I concentrations have improved survival. The effects of recombinant human IGF-I on the catabolic state and clinical outcome of head-injured patients were studied.

Methods.—The phase II, open, randomized trial included 33 patients, 18 to 59 years old, with isolated traumatic head injury. All patients had Glasgow Coma Scale (GCS) scores of 4 to 10. Standard neurosurgical intensive care and aggressive nutritional support were provided in all patients. One group of patients also received IV therapy with continuous IGF-I, 0.01 mg/kg/hr for 14 days; the control group received no additional treatment. The safety and efficacy of IGF-I treatment were assessed.

Results.—The treated patients gained weight during IGF-I treatment, whereas the control patients lost weight. This was so even though the treated group had significantly higher energy expenditure and lower caloric intake. The control patients had higher daily glucose concentrations and nitrogen output. A positive nitrogen balance was achieved during the first week of treatment only in patients treated with IGF-I. Survival during the first week was 88% in the treated group and 81% in the control group; all patients who survived had a serum IGF-I concentration >350 ng/mL. Among patients with baseline GCS scores of 5 to 7, Glasgow Outcome Scale (GOS) score improved from poor to good for 67% of patients in the treated group versus 27% of those in the control group. In the treated group, 6-month outcomes were rated moderate to good in 73% of patients with serum IGF-I concentrations >350 ng/mL, compared with only 20% of patients with lower concentrations (Fig 5).

Conclusions.—For patients with moderate to severe head injury, treatment with recombinant human IGF-I may improve clinical outcomes and nitrogen balance. More research of this promising therapy is needed, including modified dosing strategies in larger numbers of head-injured patients. The optimal serum and CSF concentrations must be defined, and the dosing strategy needed to maintain those concentrations must be determined.

Growth Hormone Modulates Amino Acid Oxidation in the Surgical Patient: Leucine Kinetics During the Fasted and Fed State Using Moderate Nitrogenous and Caloric Diet and Recombinant Human Growth Hormone

Carli F, Webster JD, Halliday D (Northwick Park Hosp, Middlesex, England)
Metabolism 46:23–28, 1997 9–18

Objective.—Negative nitrogen balance is an important part of the metabolic response to major surgical trauma. Several studies have established the anabolic effects of recombinant human growth hormone (rGH), but there are conflicting reports as to the effects of growth hormone treatment of stressed patients in negative nitrogen balance. This study examined the effects of rGH administration on protein synthesis and leucine oxidation in previously healthy patients undergoing major surgery.

Methods.—The study included 12 patients scheduled for resection of localized, nonmetastatic adenocarcinoma of the rectosigmoid colon. After surgery, they were randomized to receive peripheral parenteral nutrition (PPN) alone or with rGH, 0.15 U/kg/day. Both groups received nutritional support in a regimen of 0.1 g nitrogen/kg/day and 20 kcal/kg/day, with nonprotein energy provided as 60% lipid and 40% carbohydrate. This regimen was started 6 days before surgery and continued for 6 days afterward. Before and 6 days after surgery, an 8 hr ^{13}C-leucine tracer infusion was used to study protein kinetics during the fasting and fed states. Each day, measurements of urinary nitrogen; gas exchange; and plasma insulin, GH, and insulin-like growth factor-I (IGF-I) were obtained. The effects of rGH supplementation on protein synthesis and leucine oxidation were analyzed, along with the acute effect of IV feeding on postoperative protein breakdown.

Results.—After surgery, there were significant increases in postabsorptive whole body protein flux and synthesis and leucine oxidation. Treatment with rGH significantly lessened the postoperative rise in leucine oxidation. Whole body protein synthesis was significantly increased, but protein breakdown was unchanged. Leucine oxidation was significantly increased in the fed state, with patients in the PPN-only group showing the greatest change. Both groups showed a significant reduction in whole body protein breakdown in association with feeding. The PPN plus rGH group had lower postoperative urinary nitrogen excretion than did the PPN-only group, but the difference was not significant.

Feeding and surgery caused significant increases in oxygen consumption and carbon dioxide production. Particularly after surgery, rGH treatment significantly reduced the respiratory quotient, suggesting a direct effect of rGH on fatty acid oxidation. Both groups had a significant increase in circulating plasma insulin after feeding. This response was greater after surgery, especially for patients receiving rGH. Though surgery was followed by a reduction in plasma GH in the PPN group, feeding was not responsible for this change. Before and after surgery, circulating GH levels increased after rGH administration. Postoperatively, plasma IGF-I was reduced in the PPN group. The PPN plus rGH group showed no changes in plasma IGF-I in association with feeding.

Conclusions.—In catabolic surgical patients receiving a moderate nitrogen and caloric intake via PPN, rGH has a significant and positive effect on protein synthesis, occurring through modulation of amino acid oxidation. During the catabolic phase of surgical stress, IV nutrient administration acutely reduces protein breakdown but has no effect on protein synthesis. The findings warrant further study of rGH therapy in the fasting and fed states for surgical patients who need nutritional support. Such studies will need to determine the rGH dose necessary to reverse protein catabolic effects and whether the anabolic effects continue over time.

▶ These two papers (Abstracts 9–17 and 9–18) look at the use of exogenous GH or IGF-I in treating 2 groups of surgical patients. The study by Carli and colleagues (Abstract 9–18) looked at a relatively small group of patients undergoing rectosigmoid colectomy. They demonstrated that rGH can increase protein synthesis in catabolic patients. This paper demonstrates that an anabolism can be achieved in surgical patients, but data on outcome are lacking. In contrast, Hatton and colleagues (Abstract 9–17) examined head-injury patients and demonstrated that patients with a Glasgow Coma Scale score of 5 to 7 who survived the initial week after injury and received GH had improved neurologic outcomes compared with similar patients in the control group. Growth hormone did not improve outcome in patients with severe head injuries. Future studies will be necessary to define the optimal serum and CSF concentrations of IGF-I in determining a dosage strategy for maintaining those concentrations.

W.W. Souba, M.D., Sc.D.

Effect of Prednisolone on the Systemic Response and Wound Healing After Colonic Surgery

Schulze S, Andersen J, Overgaard H, et al (Sundby Hosp, Copenhagen; Copenhagen Hosp Corp; Inst of Surgical Pathophysiology, Oslo, Norway, et al)

Arch Surg 132:129–135, 1997 9–19

Purpose.—Surgery causes profound systemic changes in neuroendocrine and immunologic function. Glucocorticoids play a key role in the humoral and immunologic responses to trauma, and previous studies have suggested that glucocorticoid administration may modify injury-induced humoral mediators. However, more information on the potential side effects, including impaired wound healing and immunosuppression, are needed. The effects of preoperative glucocorticoid administration in patients undergoing colonic surgery were evaluated in a randomized, double-blind trial.

Methods.—The study included 24 otherwise healthy patients undergoing elective open colonic resection. They were randomized to receive, 90 min before the induction of anesthesia and epidural analgesia, either methylprednisolone sodium succinate, 30 mg/kgIV, or placebo. The effects of the 2 treatments on systemic and immunologic responses, wound healing, and postoperative convalescence were compared. Assessments continued for 10 days after surgery.

Results.—Patients receiving methylprednisolone had a less-pronounced reduction in pulmonary function after surgery. They also had better mobilization. The methylprednisolone group had lesser increases in interleukin-6 and C-reactive protein, with abolition of delayed-type hypersensitivity. Activation of plasma cascade systems was also significantly less with methylprednisolone. Though collagen turnover was reduced in the methylprednisolone group, there were no adverse effects in terms of collagen accumulation. There were no significant differences in pain, fatigue, appetite, or wound complications.

Conclusions.—The effects of a single high dose of glucocorticoid before colonic surgery were studied. Preoperative methylprednisolone therapy appears to improve postoperative pulmonary function and mobilization while reducing plasma cascade system activation, inflammatory response, and immune function. Glucocorticoid administration does not seem to adversely affect wound healing, however. The clinical significance of preoperative glucocorticoid administration should be studied in high-risk patients (e.g., those with cardiopulmonary insufficiency), in whom the usual response to injury can have adverse effects.

► The major findings of this study are that a single preoperative dose of methylprednisolone improved pulmonary function, reduced the inflammatory response, and enhanced immune function without adversely impacting wound healing. The mechanism of action is unclear, and the clinical relevance of these findings remains to be determined.

W.W. Souba, M.D., Sc.D.

Effects of Electrical Stimulation on Wound Healing in Patients With Diabetic Ulcers

Baker LL, Chambers R, DeMuth SK, et al (Univ of Southern California, Los Angeles; Rancho Los Amigos Med Ctr, Downey, Calif)
Diabetes Care 20:405–412, 1997 9–20

Background.—Understanding which aspects of electric currents are most important to enhance healing effect would enable the development of better guidelines for the treatment of diabetic patients. The efficacy of neurally regulated regional effects of electric stimulation for enhanced wound healing, while minimizing the possible polar characteristics of the stimulation, was investigated.

Methods.—Eighty diabetic patients with open ulcers were enrolled in the prospective study. Stimulation was delivered with an asymmetric biphasic (A) or symmetric biphasic (B) square-wave pulse. The amplitudes used were designed to activate intact peripheral nerves in the skin. Another 2 groups of patients were given very low levels of stimulation current or no electric stimulation (combined and considered the control group). Daily

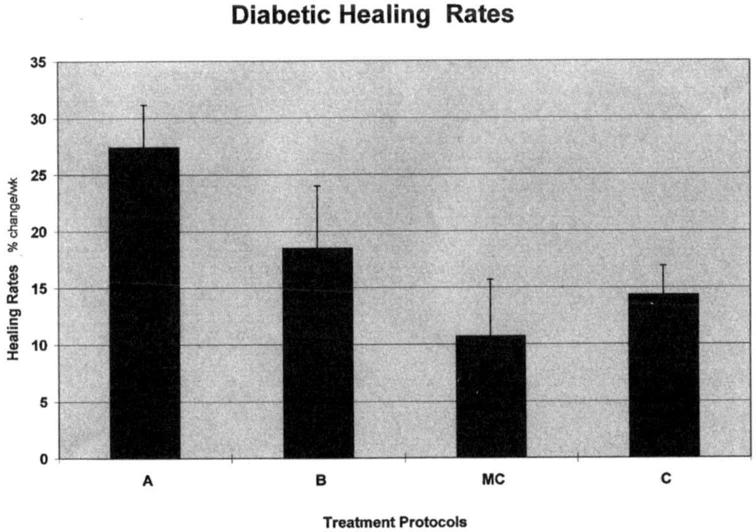

FIGURE 1.—Mean healing rates from each treatment protocol, including all wounds (n = 114). Although the healing rates appear different, statistical significance was not achieved. *Abbreviations: A*, asymmetric biphasic stimulation; *B*, symmetric biphasic stimulation; *MC*, microcurrent stimulation; *C*, control group—no current delivered to the patient. (Courtesy of Baker LL, Chambers R, DeMuth SK, et al: Effects of electrical stimulation on wound healing in patients with diabetic ulcers. *Diabetes Care* 20:405–412, 1997.)

treatments were delivered until the wound healed, the patient withdrew from the study, or the physician changed the overall management plan.

Outcomes.—Mean healing rates are compared among the 4 groups in Figure 1. Stimulation with the A protocol significantly increased the rate of healing compared with the control group. Healing was enhanced by almost 60% in the A group. Stimulation with the B protocol did not significantly increase the rate of healing compared to that in the control group.

Conclusions.—Electric stimulation with an asymmetric biphasic square waveform enhanced the healing rates in these diabetic patients with open ulcers. Further research is needed to determine the optimal choices for stimulus pulse duration and electrode placements in diabetic patients.

▶ This is an interesting study which shows that electrical stimulation given daily with a short-pulsed, asymmetric biphasic wayform, could enhance wound healing in patients with diabetic ulcers. The protocol requires patient compliance and requires a substantial amount of time. Nonetheless, the study demonstrates that the addition of electric stimulation is superior to healing without any stimulation. The definitive choice of stimulus waveform and pulse duration, and the physiologic mechanisms by which stimulation improves wound healing remain somewhat obscure.

W.W. Souba, M.D., Sc.D.

10 Gastrointestinal

Introduction

The many articles in medical and surgical journals attest to the formidable interest of our readers in surgical gastroenterology. Once again, the past year (1998–1999) has been unprecedented for basic and clinical science contributions to the YEAR BOOK OF SURGERY. For this 1998 edition, the editors have selected seminal contributions that bring together innovative basic appeal and science interests with clinical applications for the care of patients. We acknowledge that some important contributions may not be included due to space limitations. I continue to recognize contributions on the anatomical, pathophysiological, and technical issues for surgery and patient management; other articles in this section are contributions from basic science that may have an impact on the future practice of surgical science. Some selections highlight important clinical trials for the management of diseases of the gastrointestinal tract.

Kirby I. Bland, M.D.

Esophagus and Stomach

INTRODUCTION

In 1674, Thomas Willis was credited with the first successful management of achalasia. Forcible introduction of a bougie into the esophagus was the principal methodology to treat physiologic obstruction of the organ. In 1913, however, Heller devised the physiologic principles of esophagomyotomy for the treatment of achalasia. Zaaljer modified Heller's approach in 1923, applying a single esophageal incision for esophagomyotomy. In 1939, Browne and McHardy successfully treated achalasia by using pneumatic dilatation, applying the physiologic principle of lower esophageal sphincter disruption. Olsen and Harrington in 1951 introduced hydrostatic dilators that enhanced the results of Browne and McHardy. More recently, Ellis and colleagues developed transthoracic esophagomyotomy in the therapy of this benign disorder.

However, it was Lester R. Dragstedt, of the University of Chicago, who along with many of his students, advanced the modern treatment of esophageal and gastrointestinal disorders. Their significant influence began in the mid- to late 1940s with the application of sound physiologic principles to applied research. Pioneering efforts, led by the late Edward R.

Woodward and other North American and European surgeons, applied these physiologic approaches for the management of benign (ulceration, obstruction, hemorrhage, achalasia, fistula) and malignant diseases.

Esophageal carcinoma constitutes only 1% to 2% of all cancers in the United States but 99% of all esophageal neoplasms. The stomach is the organ most frequently used to restore gastrointestinal continuity following esophagogastrectomy. Gastric stasis from outlet obstruction may occur if a drainage procedure is not performed for the vagotomized stomach. This salient feature was first recognized in 1945 by Dragstedt, who observed that approximately half of all patients with duodenal ulcer treated by transthoracic vagotomy had gastric outlet obstruction develop. Law and associates (Abstract 10–1) completed a prospective, randomized, controlled trial of 92 patients with esophageal carcinoma; patients received either pyloroplasty or pyloromyotomy as a drainage procedure for the gastric conduit utilized for esophageal replacement. Both procedures were effective and provided safe drainage. The most significant differences in the techniques were identified regarding postoperative morbidity and mortality. Gastric outlet obstruction developed in only two patients undergoing pyloromyotomy, and both required reexploration. In long-term followup, the two groups of patients did not differ significantly in the quality or the quantity of food ingested or in other symptoms associated with eating after esophagectomy and replacement. The authors concluded in this important study that choice of therapy depends on the preference and experience of the operating surgeons.

Radiological and biochemical serum assays to evaluate intraabdominal tumor spread have been widely used to stage various neoplasms and to evaluate the current disease. In a recent report by Anderson et al.[1] on malignant tumors of the lower esophagus and esophagogastric junction, CT and transabdominal US correctly evaluated (staged) only two thirds of the primary tumors. Transesophageal US can be used to stage the primary tumor, but it is of little use to determine intra-abdominal extension of disease. A limited experience with staging of upper gastrointestinal tract malignancies has been reported by Bonavina and associates (Abstract 10–2), who compared the diagnostic value of laparoscopy to US and CT for detection of intraabdominal metastatic dissemination of disease. Laparoscopy changed the therapeutic approach in 10% of patients, and it yielded a higher sensitivity than US or CT to detect peritoneal metastases, macroscopic nodal metastases, and metastases to the liver. This safe, effective modality is a state-of-the-art approach for the evaluation of esophageal and gastric cardia lesions. Its application to these and other upper GI tract malignancies needs prospective studies to select the most cost-effective and efficacious therapy.

The stomach is also the organ most used to restore gastrointestinal continuity after esophagectomy. Despite improved suturing and anastomotic stapling devices, anastomotic dehiscence and resultant anastomotic stricture often cause major morbidity. Law and associates (Abstract 10–3) compared the hand-sewn and stapled methods for esophagogastric anastomosis. In 122 patients with squamous carcinoma of the thoracic esophagus undergoing Lewis-Tanner esophagectomy, no differences were evident in leakage rates, total operating time, or dissection margin leaks. Anastomotic strictures were observed less frequently in hand-sewn patients than in the stapled group (9.1% vs. 40%, $P = 0.0003$). The authors concluded that the one-layer continuous hand-sewn suturing method is safe and superior to stapling in preventing stricture.

Since its first use in 1991, laparoscopic Nissen fundoplication has become the principal surgical treatment for gastroesophageal reflux (GER). Formerly, surgeons preferred open fundoplication over the laparoscopic technique and argued that laparoscopy had unacceptably high complications and represented a laborious and technically difficult operative procedure. Postoperative side effects occurred with both open and laparoscopic Nissen fundoplication approaches. However, data accumulated this decade suggest that persistent, troublesome solid-food dysphagia is more common after laparoscopic Nissen approaches (range 4% to 24%) than was evident with the open "floppy" Nissen technique (less than 3%). The Rosetti-Nissen laparoscopic approach was observed to cause dysphagia more frequently than its antecedent laparoscopic technique, Toupet-Nissen fundoplication, which allows greater curvature mobilization. As a consequence, most international surgeons use the Toupet fundoplication approach, when a laparoscopic approach is preferred. These subjects appeared in the 1997 YEAR BOOK OF SURGERY and here are further addressed by Meehan and Georgeson (Abstract 10–4), who identified laparoscopic fundoplication as an effective treatment for GER in infants and children. These surgeons addressed the complication frequency and length of operation in a retrospective review of 160 consecutive pediatric patients undergoing laparoscopic fundoplication. The findings show the effect of the learning curve on average operating time, an average of 113 minutes (range 45–255 minutes) as the beginnning of the study and 90 minutes following the 75 cases.

Laparoscopic Nissen fundoplication has become increasingly popular for treating GER. Stimulated by the observation of periodic hypotension and hypoxia during the course of the dissection of the esophageal hiatus during laparoscopic surgery, Talamini and associates evaluated the hemodynamic effects and the additional consequences of hiatal dissection during laparoscopic Nissen fundoplication (Abstract 10–5). Using a porcine model, the authors concluded that surgical disruption of the hiatus during Nissen fundoplication increased both mediastinal and pleural pressure and reduced cardiac output significantly. However, these consequences were less evident in humans, because division of the phrenoesophageal ligament with an exposure of the esophagus does not induce a wide-open mediastinum and bilateral pneumothoraces. This study alerts surgeons to possible changes in cardiopulmonary physiology with this operation, as well as to the importance of position and capnothorax to induce hypoxia and hypotension.

Isolauri and colleagues (Abstract 10–6) looked at long-term symptomatic and endoscopic outcomes in gastroesophageal reflux disease with esophagitis, comparing conservative therapeutic measures to antireflux surgery. Of interest, patients in the surgical arm were selected from the failures of the medical therapy group. At followup, 84% of the operated patients had no, or only occasional, heartburn, 89% were free from erosive esophagitis, and only 5% required use of H-2 antagonists or omeprazole. This study verifies what others have confirmed, that surgical therapy provided results superior to conservative (medical) management of medication and lifestyle modification. The final outcome with conservative management is not yet known, as regular endoscopy for followup for individuals with Barrett's metaplasia in a nonsurgical group would often require esophagectomy after the transformation to carcinoma. The rarity of endoscopic and clinical healing in those patients who are treated conservatively provides objective evidence for the chronic nature and potential severity of reflux esophagitis.

The first diaphragmatic hernia repair was accomplished by Postempski in 1889. However, Akerlund in 1926 first described paraesophageal herniation, noting that this was an uncommon variant of hiatal hernia. Three types of hiatal hernia are recognized: *type 1*, a hiatal hernia in which the GE junction migrates cephalad via the esophageal hiatus; *type 2*, the rolling hernia (paraesophageal), in which the fundus herniates together with a normal position of the GE junction; and *type 3*, combination of type 1 and 2, in which both the GE junction and a large portion of the fundus herniate into the left chest. While type 2 hernias are rare, type 3 variant physiologically occurs and behaves like types 1 and 2, and is commonly classifed as paraesophageal. Ellis estimates that paraesophageal herniation overall accounts for 5% to 10% of all hiatal hernias. Perdikis and associates (Abstract 10–7) evaluated paraesophageal hiatal repair using laparoscopy. In this study of 64 patients with type 3 and type 2 hernias, 65% who underwent pH monitoring had a positive 24-hour pH score and 56% undergoing manometry had an incompetent lower esophageal sphincter. The authors concluded that most paraesophageal hernias are the type 3 variant, and they may be managed successfully by the laparoscopic approach.

Fredet in 1907 and Ramstedt in 1911 described the current application of pyloromyotomy for the therapy of infantile hypertrophic pyloric stenosis. This procedure is exceeded only by inguinal herniorrhaphy as the most common surgical procedure performed for infants. Predictably, the associated morbidity and mortality from the procedure is low.

Although gastric carcinoma and gastroduodenal ulcerations—seen with great frequency even 2 decades ago—are diminishing in industrialized societies, benign disorders of the stomach remain a challenge to physicians. Infantile hypertrophic pyloric stenosis continues to occur in 3 of every 1,000 live births, and it is a common underlying cause of emesis in infants. Theories on the pathogenesis of this disorder include abnormalities of hormonal influence on the gastric pylorus, reduction in nitric oxide, axonal degeneration in the myenteric plexus, and the loss of peptide-containing neural filaments in nerve fibers. Signal papers in last year's YEAR BOOK OF SURGERY emphasized the important role of the proto-oncogene c-*kit* in the development of a component of the pacemaker system that is required for the generation of autonomic gut motility. This protein may be responsible for the intestinal pacemaker activity as well. Yamataka and associates[2] have emphasized that the absence of *c-kit* expression in the hypertrophic pyloric smooth musculature may be an important etiologic factor in the pathogenesis of pyloric stenosis. The application of molecular biology to various benign and malignant diseases to outcomes in translational research will greatly aid clinical medicine.

Hulka and associates (Abstract 10–8) sought to determine the frequency of intraoperative and postoperative complications following pyloromyotomy. This retrospective review was completed for two pediatric surgery centers from community hospitals and for all infants referred from other institutions with postoperative complications following the procedure. Their purpose was to see if differences in the operative care and outcomes were evident between two groups. The authors emphasized that a single standard of care should be expected of all surgeons who perform this procedure.

Kirby I. Bland, M.D.

References

1. Anderson DN, Campbell S, Park KG: Accuracy of laparoscopic ultrasonography in the staging of upper gastrointestinal malignancies. *Br J Surg* 83:1424–1428, 1996.
2. Yamataka A, Fujiwara T, Kato Y, et al: Lack of intestinal pacemaker (C-KIT-positive) cells in infantile hypertrophic pyloric stenosis. *J Pediatr Surg* 31:96–98, 1996.

Pyloroplasty and Pyloromyotomy in Gastric Replacement of the Esophagus After Esophagectomy: A Randomized Controlled Trial

Law S, Cheung M-C, Fok M, et al (Univ of Hong Kong)

J Am Coll Surg 184:630–636, 1997 10–1

Introduction.—Disagreements abound regarding the advantages and disadvantages of pyloroplasty (PP) and pyloromyotomy (PM). A randomized trial was conducted to compare perioperative complications, long-term function of the gastric conduits, and symptoms after PP and PM.

Methods.—Ninety-two patients with esophageal carcinomas who underwent the Lewis–Tanner operation or esophagogastrectomy were randomized to undergo either PP or PM as a drainage procedure for the conduit used for esophageal replacement. All patients had normal pyloroduodenal regions.

Results.—The mean postoperative daily nasogastric output was similar for PP and PM (164 vs. 179 mL). No patients in either group experienced leakage at the pyloroduodenal region. For both groups, the anastomotic leakage rate was 2%, and the in-house mortality rate was 7%. There were no significant between-group differences in postoperative morbidity or mortality. Two patients who underwent PM experienced gastric outlet obstruction that required re-exploration. Of these, 1 patient died of malignant obstruction of the gastric outlet and aspiration pneumonia. At a 6-month follow-up evaluation, scintigraphy indicated that the median half-life for gastric emptying was 19 minutes for the PP group and 8 minutes for the PM group. At a 5-year follow-up evaluation, there were no significant between-group differences in the type or quantity of food consumed or incidence of symptoms such as regurgitation, diarrhea, bile reflux, and dumping.

Conclusion.—Pyloroplasty and PM may be considered safe and effective drainage procedures for the gastric conduit used for esophageal replacement. Surgeon preference and experience is important in deciding which procedure to use.

► In this paper, 92 patients with esophageal carcinomas were randomized to have PP or PM as a draining procedure for the gastric conduit used for esophageal replacement. This is an important issue because postoperative gastric outlet obstruction is associated with a high incidence of aspiration and subsequent pneumonia. The authors found that the mean postoperative daily nasal gastric tube output was not different between the 2 groups. No significant differences were found in postoperative morbidity; and mortality, importantly, gastric outlet obstruction developed in only 2 patients who underwent PM and both required re-exploration. The scintigraphy performed 6 months after the patients underwent their operations demonstrated that gastric emptying was 19 minutes in the PP group and 8 minutes in the PM group ($P = 0.04$). However, long-term follow-up to 5 years did not reveal significant differences between the 2 groups in the type and quantity of food consumed.

The authors have concluded that both PP and PM are effective and safe drainage procedures for the gastric conduit used for esophageal replacement. Our own experience would tend to confirm that although either procedure is applicable there remains the concern that in the performance of a PM a microperforation of the duodenum may occur; and thus many surgeons continue to believe that PP is the safer procedure.

At the current time, it would appear that surgical preference would be a key factor in dictating whether PP or PM is performed in gastric replacement of the esophagus after esophagectomy.

H.H. Simms, M.D.

Preoperative Laparoscopy in Management of Patients With Carcinoma of the Esophagus and of the Esophagogastric Junction

Bonavina L, Incarbone R, Lattuada E, et al (Univ of Milan, Italy; Ospedale Maggiore Policlinico IRCCS, Milan, Italy)

J Surg Oncol 65:171–174, 1997 10–2

Background.—CT or US are not very accurate in evaluating intra-abdominal tumor spread. A method that may prove more useful in this evaluation is laparoscopy. Results of laparoscopy were compared with those of CT and US in evaluating patients with cancers of the lower esophagus and esophagogastric junction.

Methods.—There were 36 patients with adenocarcinoma of the cardia and 14 patients with squamous cell carcinoma of the lower esophagus. Each of these 50 patients was evaluated preoperatively by US and CT. At surgery, laparoscopy was performed to explore the abdominal cavity. Operative time averaged 20 minutes (range, 15–55), with no deaths or morbidity associated with the laparoscopic procedure.

Findings.—Results of laparoscopy changed therapy in 3 patients with peritoneal carcinosis undetected by CT or US, in 1 patient with advanced liver cirrhosis who did not undergo resection, and in 1 patient who had a liver hemangioma that CT and US had mistakenly indicated to be a metastatic mass. Laparoscopy was substantially more sensitive than CT or US in detecting macroscopic nodal masses (78% vs. 55% vs. 11%, respectively) and peritoneal metastases (71% vs. 14% vs. 14%, respectively). Furthermore, the sensitivity of laparoscopy was equal to that of US (86%), and greater than that of CT (71%), in diagnosing liver metastases.

Conclusions.—Laparoscopy at the time of surgery offered increased sensitivity over CT or US in diagnosing macroscopic nodal metastases and peritoneal metastases in patients with esophageal carcinoma. This approach was safe and added important information from which to make treatment decisions. Laparoscopy at surgery should be considered part of the preoperative evaluation of patients with cancer of the cardia and distal esophagus.

► The use of diagnostic laparoscopy is well established in the management of pancreatic carcinoma. However, widespread use of diagnostic laparoscopy in other gastrointestinal malignancies is rare. Esophagogastric malignancy is an important area in which to consider diagnostic laparoscopy, since unresectable metastatic disease often can be missed by preoperative ultrasound and computed tomography. In this study by Bonavina and colleagues, therapeutic approaches were changed for 10% of the patients on the basis of the laparoscopic exam. Unfortunately, in all but 1 case, this was an adverse change, to no resection.

One area not explored by these authors is the routine use of laparoscopic ultrasound in the evaluation of metastatic disease. Van Delden and colleagues[1] have documented a significant advantage for laparoscopic ultrasound in detecting hepatic but not lymph node metastases, when compared to transabdominal ultrasound. Laparoscopic ultrasonography should be included in all diagnostic laparoscopies for malignant disease.

J.F. Amaral, M.D.

Reference

1. van Delden OM, Smits NJ, Bemelman WA, et al: Comparison of laparoscopic and transabdominal ultrasonography in staging of cancer of the pancreatic head region. *J Ultrasound Med* 15:207–212, 1996.

Comparison of Hand-Sewn and Stapled Esophagogastric Anastomosis After Esophageal Resection For Cancer: A Prospective Randomized Controlled Trial

Law S, Fok M, Chu K-M, et al (Univ of Hong Kong)
Ann Surg 226:169–173, 1997 10–3

Introduction.—Esophagogastric anastomosis after esophageal resection for cancer can be accomplished by hand-sewn or stapled methods. A prospective trial was undertaken to compare the relative merits of these methods, especially regarding leakage and stricture rates.

Methods.—The 122 patients included in the study had squamous cell carcinoma of the thoracic esophagus and underwent a Lewis-Tanner esophagectomy. After removal of the tumor, they were randomized to have an esophagogastric anastomosis constructed by the hand-sewn technique or by a circular stapler. A pyloric drainage procedure was performed in all cases, and the anastomosis was constructed at the apex of the right pleural cavity. Patients were stratified according to esophageal size, based on the diameter (less than 30 mm or 30 mm and larger) of the divided esophagus. The main outcome parameters of the study were perioperative morbidity and mortality, anastomotic leakage and recurrence, and benign stricture rates.

Results.—The 2 patient groups did not differ significantly in age, gender distribution, tumor stage, intent (curative or palliative) of the operation, mean total operating times, or median survival time. Forty patients in each group had a small esophagus. One patient in the hand-sewn group and 3 in the stapler group experienced anastomotic leakage. Four patients in each group died; 1 of the deaths, involving a patient in the hand-sewn group, was attributed to anastomotic leakage. Fifty patients in the stapled group and 55 in the hand-sewn group could be evaluated for benign stricture (mean follow-up time, 19 months and 20 months, respectively). Anastomotic stricture developed in 9.1% of the hand-sewn group vs. 40% of the stapled group. Esophageal size had no effect on stricture rate. Only 1 patient in each group had an anastomotic recurrence.

Conclusion.—Both the hand-sewn and the stapled methods of esophagogastric anastomosis were safe and had low leakage rates, but the development of anastomotic stricture was much more prevalent in the stapled group. The hand-sewn method is also less costly.

► The advent of improved adjuvant therapy for the treatment of patients with esophageal carcinoma, coupled with the continued decrease in morbidity and mortality after esophagectomy, increases the importance of this study's findings. The quality of life after either palliative or curative resection should be an important consideration in determining both surgical approach and technique. Dr. Wong and colleagues have demonstrated similar outcomes between hand-sewn and stapled anastomoses, with the exception of stricture rates.

The finding of a difference in stricture rates, favoring hand-sewn anastomosis regardless of the size of the esophagus, should make each surgeon revisit the use of stapling instruments. Although the authors rightfully point out that the rates of esophageal anastomotic leaks generally have been less with stapled anastomoses, in this series the leak rate was identical between the 2 techniques. Given the decreased cost of a hand-sewn anastomosis, in combination with lower stricture rates and decreased requirement for dilation, each surgeon should reconsider the use of stapling instruments in esophageal reconstruction.

W.G. Cioffi, M.D.

The Learning Curve Associated With Laparoscopic Antireflux Surgery in Infants and Children

Meehan JJ, Georgeson KE (Children's Hosp of Alabama, Birmingham; Univ of Alabama, Birmingham)

J Pediatr Surg 32:426–429, 1997 10–4

Introduction.—Gastroesophageal reflux may be treated successfully in infants and children using laparoscopic fundoplication. Many surgeons still prefer the open technique, arguing that the laparoscopic technique is too lengthy and is associated with a high complication rate. One-hundred sixty consecutive laparoscopic fundoplication procedures were reviewed to determine length of time and number of patients an experienced surgeon might expect to need before becoming proficient with the procedure.

Methods.—The average patient age was 6.5 years. All patients had gastroesophageal reflux and all had the same attending surgeon.

Results.—Twelve of 160 laparoscopic fundoplication procedures (7.5%) were converted to open procedures. The conversion rate improved from 30% with the first 20 patients to a cumulative rate of 7.5%. Four patients had to undergo open procedures because of equipment failure before having a backup system available. Operating time ranged from 45 to 255 minutes (average, 113 minutes). The average operating time for the first 25 patients was 170 minutes; it decreased to an average of 115 minutes for the next 25 patients and averaged 90 minutes for the last 25 patients (Fig 5). Complication rates declined rapidly in the early learning phase.

Conclusion.—Operative time and complication rates decreased quickly in the early learning phase in 148 patients who underwent laparoscopic fundoplication for gastroesophageal reflux. A surgeon can become proficient after treating 25 patients.

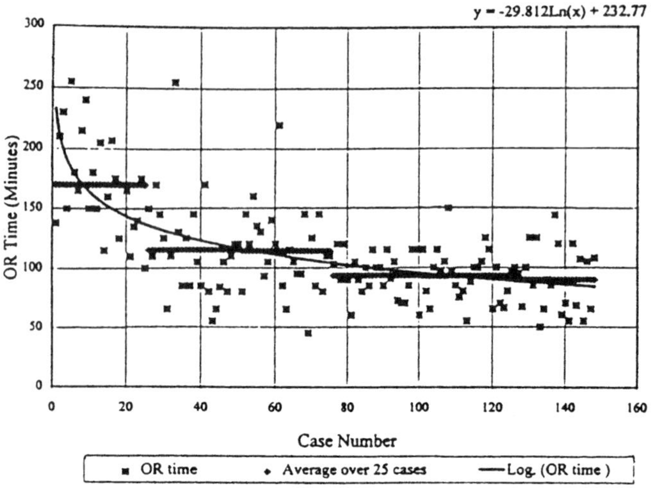

FIGURE 5.—Laparoscopic fundoplication learning curve-operating room (*OR*) time. (Courtesy of Meehan JJ, Georgeson KE: The learning curve associated with laparoscopic antireflux surgery in infants and children. *J Pediatr Surg* 32:426–429, 1997.)

▶ To talk about a learning curve in terms of operative time seems appropriate. Where this applies to technical skills, it is reasonable to assume that each surgeon will have to go through an apprenticeship which, according to these authors, will take an average of 25 cases. However, operating time depends on other factors as well, such as adequacy of the endoscopic equipment, familiarity of the operating room personnel, and degree of involvement of surgical residents—all of which will vary widely between institutions. As for the complication rate, we can hope that Dr. Georgeson's bad experiences (and the useful technical tips they have generated) will help shorten *our* learning curve.

F.I. Luks, M.D.

Increased Mediastinal Pressure and Decreased Cardiac Output During Laparoscopic Nissen Fundoplication

Talamini MA, Mendoza-Sagaon M, Gitzelmann CA, et al (Johns Hopkins Univ, Baltimore, Md)

Surgery 122:345–353, 1997 10–5

Introduction.—The physiologic insults associated with laparoscopic procedures are beginning to be recognized and reported, but findings have not been significant enough to question the advantages of procedures such as laparoscopic cholecystectomy over open surgery. Laparoscopic Nissen fundoplication (LNF), now gaining in popularity, has been associated with sporadic episodes of hypotension and hypoxia. An animal study was conducted to examine the specific hemodynamic and respiratory physiologic effects of LNF.

Methods.—Seven female pigs that had been anesthetized, intubated, and ventilated had hemodynamic and mechanical pressure monitoring devices placed for the experiments. Pressures were recorded every 15 minutes for 1 hour after each of 4 interventions: induction of anesthesia; carbon dioxided pneumoperitoneum (15 mm Hg); LNF; and release of pneumoperitoneum. Each animal served as its own control.

Results.—There was a significant increase in central venous pressure, inferior vena caval pressure, pulmonary artery pressure, and pulmonary capillary wedge pressure with the institution of pneumoperitoneum, but only a slight increase after LNF. All values except central venous pressure returned to near baseline after release of the pneumoperitoneum. No significant change in mean arterial pressure was observed during any experimental phase. Airway, pleural, and mediastinal pressures all showed significant increases after the institution of pneumoperitoneum, and pleural and mediastinal pressures further significantly increased after LNF. With release of the pneumoperitoneum, all 3 pressure values were significantly elevated over baseline.

Conclusion.—This porcine model showed a significant reduction in cardiac output after laparoscopic Nissen fundoplication. Both mediastinal and pleural pressure were increased. These effects could lead to complications in some patients, such as those in New York Heart Association class III or IV.

► Sporadic episodes of hypotension and hypoxia during LNF led Talamini and colleagues to evaluate the role of laparoscopic surgery of the gastroesophageal junction on cardiopulmonary parameters during the procedure. Unfortunately, the model they chose—the pig—is a poor one for this analysis, because division of the phrenoesophageal ligament and exposure of the esophagus leads to a wide open mediastinum with bilateral pneumothorax. Although a chest tube was present on the left side, none was present on the right. We cannot be sure, therefore, that some, if not all, of the changes seen for the fundoplication are not the result of the anatomical peculiarities present in the pig.

Most cases of hypotension or hypoxia during LNF are the result of either prolonged periods of reverse Trendelenberg position or the creation of a capnothorax during dissection of the hiatus. Although Talamini and coworkers imply that a capnothorax is always easily diagnosed during LNF by paradoxical motion of the diaphragm, the literature does not support that fact.[1] In fact, 3% to 5% of patients undergoing LNF have a capnothorax recognized either by an increase in airway resistance, an increase in end-tidal carbon dioxide, a decrease in oxygen saturation or by chest radiograph.[1] although it is important to consider the possibility that surgical disruption of the esophageal hiatus could lead to significant changes in cardiopulmonary physiology, the importance of position and capnothorax should not be forgotten, as they are easily treatable.

J.F. Amaral, M.D.

Reference

1. Joris JL, Chiche JD, Lamy ML: Pneumothorax during laparascopic fundoplication: Diagnosis and treatment with positive end-expiratory pressure. *Anesth Analg* 81:993–1000, 1995.

Long-term Comparison of Antireflux Surgery Versus Conservative Therapy for Reflux Esophagitis

Isolauri J, Luostarinen M, Viljakka M, et al (Univ of Tampere, Finland)
Ann Surg 225:295–299, 1997 10–6

Objective.—Endoscopic examination revealed that approximately 50% of patients with gastroesophageal reflux disease have erosive esophagitis. The course of endoscopically proven esophagitis in these patients who were treated surgically or conservatively, and the possible predictive factors of long-term outcome were examined.

Methods.—Between 1982 and 1983, 120 patients (39 women), aged 36.1 to 82.5 years, with severe reflux symptoms and endoscopically proven erosive esophagitis, were treated with conservative management (n = 81) or antireflux surgery (n = 39) (Nissen fundoplication). Standardized interviews, conducted with 105 patients who were followed for 9.1–13.4 years, assessed symptoms, time of referral, and endoscopic observations.

Results.—Most of the 37 patients who had undergone the Nissen procedure had failed conservative treatment within 6–14 months (n = 31). Six patients had failed conservative treatment within 19–78 months. At follow-up, 84% of surgically treated patients had mild or no heartburn, and 89% had no erosive esophagitis, whereas with conservatively treated patients, 53% were heartburn-free and only 45% no longer had erosive esophagitis. Five percent of surgically treated patients were using H_2 antagonists or omeprazole, whereas 21% of conservatively treated patients used such drugs. The surgically treated group had a significantly greater change in symptom score than did the conservatively treated group (5.7 vs. 1.7). At baseline, Barrett's metaplasia was diagnosed in 5 patients who later had surgery and in no patients treated conservatively. At follow-up, Barrett's metaplasia was diagnosed in 12 surgical patients and in 8 conservatively managed patients. Severity of esophagitis or presence of hiatal hernia at baseline was not a predictor of esophagitis or symptoms at follow-up.

Conclusion.—Surgery, rather than conservative management, for esophagitis yielded improved results for patients with gastroesophageal reflux disease. There were no significant predictors of outcome.

► Which is better therapy for gastroesophageal reflux disease (GERD), medical or surgical treatment? This article by Isolauri and associates evaluates this question by analyzing outcomes of either medical or surgical therapy for patients followed for 10 years. Interestingly, patients in the surgical arm were selected from the failures in the medical treatment group.

Remarkably, those in the surgical group, despite worse disease, did better than those in the medical treatment arm. Treatment with surgery also reduced the calculated nondiscounted 10-year cost of therapy from $11,500 with H_2 antagonists or $23,500 with omeprazole to $4,100 with surgery.

It would seem clear from this study that surgery is superior to medical therapy, at least in the treatment of complicated or nonresponsive GERD. What is not clear is whom in the noncomplicated GERD group of patients should be offered surgery. How can we differentiate the 25% of GERD patients whose condition will worsen from the 20% who will not need long-term therapy?

J.F. Amaral, M.D.

Laparoscopic Paraesophageal Hernia Repair

Perdikis G, Hinder RA, Filipi CJ, et al (Creighton Univ, Omaha, Neb; Mayo Clinic, Jacksonville, Fla)

Arch Surg 132:586–590, 1997 10–7

Introduction.—Patients with paraesophageal hernia, which makes up 5% to 10% of all hiatal hernias, are often seen as surgical emergencies. Because excessive bleeding can lead to compromise of the blood supply, sepsis, and shock, surgical correction is required. Results were reported for 65 patients operated on laparoscopically for paraesophageal hernia.

Methods.—Patients ranged in age from 26 to 90 years (average age, 63.6 years). Sixty-four underwent preoperative endoscopy, 60 had a barium esophagogram, 43 were studied with manometry, and 31 had 24-hour pH monitoring. Fifty-three patients were followed for a mean of 18 months for operative complications, postoperative morbidity, and long-term outcome. Forty-six patients had a routine barium esophagogram at 2 months to 4½ years after surgery.

Results.—Preoperative symptoms included regurgitation (77%), heartburn (60%), dysphagia (60%), chest pain (52%), and pulmonary problems (44%). Preoperative studies showed a type III paraesophageal hernia in 86% of patients and a true type II paraesophageal hernia in 14%. In 21 cases, more than 50% of the stomach was in the chest. An incompetent lower esophageal sphincter was present in 56% of those who underwent manometry; pH monitoring yielded a positive 24-hour pH score in 20 of 31 patients (65%). All patients underwent hernia reduction, crural repair, and fundoplication. Two patients required conversion to an open procedure. Duration of surgery averaged 2 hours, and the average length of hospital stay was 2 days. Three patients required early reoperation. There were no deaths.

Forty-nine of 53 patients followed for at least 2 months reported satisfaction with the procedure. When 3 of the first 22 patients were found to have slippage of the wrap into the chest, the fundoplication was tacked to the diaphragm on both the left and right sides in later procedures. Despite this modification, 4 of 24 patients were subsequently found to have a small type I hiatal hernia.

Conclusion.—The repair of paraesophageal hernias is possible laparoscopically, with excellent patient satisfaction and low mortality. Most of these hernias are type III, and a concomitant antireflux procedure is recommended. Extreme care must be taken not to enter the pleural space or to perforate the gastroesophageal junction.

► Perdikis and coworkers provide us with an important series of patients with paraesophageal hernias treated laparoscopically. In this case series of 65 consecutive patients, most with type III hiatal hernia (combined), 3 major points bear emphasis. First and most importantly, these are very difficult procedures which should not be undertaken by the surgeon inexperienced in laparoscopic esophagogastric surgery. Second, despite the large experience of these authors with routine laparoscopic antireflux procedures, repair of paraesophageal hernias is associated with a much higher complication rate compared with regular laparoscopic antireflux procedures. Finally, repair of paraesophageal hernias is associated with a high incidence of recurrence or creation of a new sliding hiatal hernia, even if the wrap is sutured to the crura.

I would add 3 technical points to the discussion of the repair, which would facilitate these difficult cases. First, I prefer to divide the short gastric vessels first and move into the hiatus, rather than looking for the esophagus at the outset. Second, do not try to reduce the hernia by vigorous traction on the stomach. This leads to tears in the stomach. Reduction is accomplished when all the hernia sac has been cut. Finally, closure of very large hiatal openings is better accomplished from both above and below, rather than from below only. The latter tends to kink the esophagus too much, leading to dysphagia.

J.F. Amaral, M.D.

Complications of Pyloromyotomy for Infantile Hypertrophic Pyloric Stenosis

Hulka F, Harrison MW, Campbell TJ, et al (Oregon Health Sciences Univ, Portland; Emanuel Hosp, Portland, Ore)

Am J Surg 173:450–452, 1997 10–8

Introduction.—It has been suggested that pyloromyotomy (PM) for the treatment of infantile hypertrophic pyloric stenosis (IHPS) should be performed only by pediatric surgeons to minimize complications. The frequency and outcome of complications from PM in patients with IHPS were evaluated.

Methods.—One group of patients were from 2 pediatric surgery centers staffed by board-certified pediatric surgeons only. The other group of patients were infants referred from other institutions in whom complications developed after PM for IHPS. A 25-year retrospective chart review was performed and data were collected regarding demographics, clinical information, age at diagnosis, operative and postoperative complications, and postoperative length of stay.

Results.—There were 901 PMs performed between 1969 and 1994. Eighty-seven patients had 92 complications. Forty patients had intraoperative complications: 39 duodenal perforations and 1 difficult intubation. There were no unrecognized duodenal perforations or incomplete PMs. Fifty-two patients had postoperative complications. Eight patients had wound infections and 31 had prolonged postoperative hospitalization beyond 48 hours. One patient died of sepsis because of delayed diagnosis of Hirschsprung's disease. In the time period, 11 patients were referred from other hospitals for postoperative complications. Five patients with persistent vomiting were treated successfully with expectant management. Six patients underwent reoperation 3 for persistent IHPS, 1 for gastric outlet obstruction, 1 for small bowel obstruction secondary to adhesions, and 1 for wound abscess drainage.

Conclusion.—Pyloromyotomy is a frequently performed procedure that should have a low complication rate. A single standard of care should be required of all surgeons who perform PM for IHPS.

▶ Any pediatric surgeon would love to read a report showing that the treatment of hypertrophic pyloric stenosis is best left to the specialist, by demonstrating that the general surgeon has an unacceptably high rate of complications. Although this may have been the idea behind the present paper, the design of the study did not allow any real comparisons. Fortunately, the authors refrain from such conclusions, commenting only on the relatively low morbidity of pyloromyotomy, regardless of who performs it. (Of the 11 "mishaps" later referred to the pediatric surgeon, half did not need anything more than a reassuring pat on the back.) The authors are correct, of course, in stating that the same standard of care should be expected of all, regardless of whether one possesses a certificate of added qualifications in pediatric surgery.

F.I. Luks, M.D.

Gastric Fluid Volume in Infants for Pyloromyotomy

Cook-Sather SD, Tulloch HV, Liacouras CA, et al (Univ of Pennsylvania, Philadelphia)

Can J Anaesth 44:278–283, 1997 10–9

Introduction.—Infants with hypertrophic pyloric stenosis require abdominal surgery and are thought to be at increased risk for vomiting and aspiration at the time of induction of anesthesia. Because of the potential for large gastric fluid volumes (GFVs) in these infants, many anesthetists consider them to have a full stomach and proceed with awake intubation. A study of 75 infants scheduled for pyloromyotomy was designed to document the large GFVs and to validate the efficacy of a blind aspiration technique for gastric fluid recovery.

Methods.—All infants received atropine 15–30 minutes before induction of anesthesia. Nasogastric tubes were aspirated and removed from those who had undergone preoperative nasogastric suction. The anesthetist blindly passed a 14 F multiorificed orogastric tube and aspirated the gastric contents using wall suction. Catheters were inserted and removed 2 or 3 times until little or no gastric fluid was collected. After tracheal intubation, 15 infants underwent gastroscopy to measure residual gastric fluid.

Results.—The infants averaged 5 weeks of age at diagnosis and surgery; boys outnumbered girls at a ratio of 4.8:1. Large volumes of gastric fluid were obtained with the blind aspiration technique. The average volume removed was 4.8 mL·kg^{-1}, and GFVs exceeded 1.25 mL·kg^{-1} in 83% of infants. Fourteen of the 15 infants who underwent gastroscopy had up to 1.0 mL of residual gastric fluid, but 1 had 1.8 mL·kg^{-1}. Based upon endoscopic data for these 15 patients, the recovery of total GFV by blind aspiration was 96%. Thirteen infants (17%) had nasogastric tubes placed preoperatively to reduce GFV, but the tubes were not effective for this purpose. Gastric fluid volume was independent of fasting interval.

Discussion.—Infants with pyloric stenosis have quite large GFVs, exceeding by 10 times that of a fasted, healthy pediatric surgical population. The blind aspiration technique used in these infants was successful in evacuating the vast majority of fluid. A history of barium administration does not further increase GFV or make it more difficult to remove GFV with the blind aspiration technique.

▶ It is traditionally accepted that infants with hypertrophic pyloric stenosis, like all patients with gastric outlet obstruction, have a full stomach, requiring rapid induction of anesthesia or awake intubation. This article elegantly confirms this belief, and shows the inability of gastric suctioning, immediately prior to anesthesia, to empty the stomach completely. Awake intubation of these infants is therefore still the safest, if not the least stressful, route.

F.I. Luks, M.D.

Hepatobiliary, Pancreas, Adrenal, and Spleen

INTRODUCTION

Currently, about 80% of the cases of acute pancreatitis are etiologically related to gallstones or alcohol abuse. Whether choledochal stones initiate or merely maintain biliary pancreatitis is as yet unproved. Most physiologists and surgeons believe that the majority of gallstones that initiate acute pancreatitis pass spontaneously through the ampulla vater into the duodenum; these stones may be recoverable in a few days within the feces.

Early surgical or endoscopic removal of choledochal stones to abrogate potential acute biliary pancreatitis is well documented. Kelly and Wagner[1] in 1988 randomly assigned 165 patients with acute pancreatitis of gallstone origin to early surgery (within 48 hours of admission), or delayed surgery (more than 48 hours after admission). Early surgery resulted in a much higher mortality rate than was observed with delayed surgery (47.8% vs. 11.8%) in individuals with severe pancreatitis. Stone, Fabian, and Dunlop[2] in 1991 observed no differences in mortality, however, for patients undergoing early surgery and delayed procedures. Similar outcomes[3–6] suggest that endoscopic retrograde cholangiopancreatography (ERCP) is the therapy of choice for severe pancreatitis. Complications, but not mortality, are often lower for those who underwent early ERCP. Moreover, the incidence of biliary sepsis was significantly lower with early ERCP and papillotomy.

Early ERCP for the therapy of cholangitis and stone impaction was reported by Leese et al.[7] A new study by Fölsch and colleagues (Abstract 10–10) noted that patients with acute biliary pancreatitis without evidence of obstructive jaundice did not benefit from early ERCP and papillotomy. This controlled, randomized trial suggests that if biliary obstruction or sepsis are not present, invasive endoscopy should not be performed.

Conventional US is a useful first-line investigation for gallstone disease, but it is limited in the investigation of bile duct stones. Successful visualization of the distal common bile duct is often difficult for small stones in the non-dialated duct and is infrequently visualized by means of US. However, ERCP is generally recognized as the gold standard for preoperative recognition of bile duct stones. Endoscopic US allows clear visualization of the entire extrahepatic biliary tree and may be associated with less procedure-related morbidity than ERCP. A prospective study by Norton and Alderson (Abstract 10–11) compared the accuracy of endoscopic US with ERCP in detecting suspected bile duct stones for preoperative patients awaiting laparoscopic cholecystectomy. Both tests were successful in 46 of 50 patients; both tests failed in 2, and ERCP alone failed in 2 patients. The authors concluded that endoscopic US accurately identifies bile duct stones in all patients with a high risk for stones, especially those with histories of ERCP-induced pancreatitis. Moreover, the endoscopic US approach is indicated when other pathology is suspected, when the ERCP has failed technically, or when abnormalities of the bile duct are suspected during pregnancy and in patients with active acute pancreatitis. The new modality may be more cost-effective, but the advantages of endoscopic US must be examined further.

The roles of intraoperative cholangiography (IOCG) and perioperative ERCP continue to evolve. To avoid a second procedure and to remove retained common bile duct stones, a surgeon must decide between IOCG and preoperative ERCP. The possible morbidity relating to a false-positive finding and the unnecessary common bile duct exploration must be balanced with the potential morbidity evident with a negative and nontherapeutic ERCP. To evaluate these concerns, Fiore and associates (Abstract 10–12) evaluated 1,002 consecutive attempted laparoscopic cholecystectomies over the course of 65 months. The authors performed routine cholangiography in 941 of these patients who were at high- or low-risk for choledocholithiasis, concluding that laparoscopic IOCG is highly successful in detecting common bile duct stones in high-risk patients, and that half of these ducts can be cleared laparoscopically. The authors recommended that the incidence of common duct stones detected in the low-risk patients (1.7%) does not warrant routine cholangiography. We agree that ERCP should be reserved only for patients at risk for common bile duct stones in whom IOCG or laparoscopic duct clearance has not been possible.

Therapeutic approaches for a variety of pediatric pancreatic or biliary disorders continue to evolve. Moreover, multidisciplinary measures of traditional (open) surgery, ERCP, and laparoscopic surgery have revolutionized the care of these children. The study by Tagge and colleagues (Abstract 10–13) focused on collaborative efforts to diagnose and treat patients with pancreatic and/or biliary disorders. The most cost-effective and most event-free protocol for managing pediatric choledocholithiasis has not been determined. Routine intraoperative cholangiography continues to be questioned, even in the adult patient, in the presence of an effective and safe ERCP service. In many respects, this approach may simplify the surgical management of complex problems, although ERCP in small children is rarely necessary. The authors concluded that an aggressive, well-organized multidisciplinary approach can be highly successful for the therapy of even young children with these pancreatobiliary disorders.

The most serious consequence of laparoscopic or open cholecystectomy, aside from death, is injury to the common bile ducts. An important group of papers by Savader and associates (Abstract 10–14), Adamsen and associates (Abstract 10–16), and Mirza et al. (Abstract 10–15) evaluated bile duct injury during laparoscopic cholecystectomy.

As observed by Savader and colleagues, the therapy of cholecystectomy-related duct injuries, particularly those that occur during laparoscopic surgery, is significant for the following reasons: (1) laparoscopic procedures exceed those done by the open technique by approximately 4 to 10:1, (2) with more than 500,000 cholecystectomies performed per year in the United States alone, the complication rates of 0.30% to 0.60% suggest that 1,500–3,000 of these patients have significant duct injuries; (3) common duct injuries are technically difficult to treat and will accentuate costly interventional or surgical procedures, or both; (4) the minimally invasive nature of the laparoscopic approach may broaden the indications for cholecystectomy and further increase the total number of procedures performed; (5) therapy of common bile duct injuries often required postoperative stenting up to 1 year, with resultant long-term morbidity; and (6) the long-term overall morbidity may be accentuated from non-monetary issues such as hospitalization time, travel, and loss in quality of life. These investigators concluded that repair of the laparoscopic cholecystectomy-related bile duct injury costs from 4.5 to 26 times that of the uncomplicated approach, with significant mortality. Moreover, the authors emphasized that intraoperative recognition of such an injury requires immediate conversion to an open procedure for definitive repair, to decrease morbidity, mortality, cost, length of hospitalization, and the number of outpatient care days. After treating 27 patients with difficult bile duct injuries following elective laparoscopic cholecystectomies referred from other units,

Mirza and associates also confirmed that the recognized bile duct injury results in significant postoperative morbidity. Most patients referred after attempted repair required further surgery, and all patients with complex high injuries had the greatest risk for long-term morbidity. Adamsen and associates evaluated this malady in a prospective nationwide series in Denmark. Bile duct injury was evident in 0.74% of patients, including nine injuries occurring after open conversion with a difficult laparoscopic procedure. The annual incidence of bile duct injury did not decrease. Of interest, the frequency of bile duct injury in patients who had intraoperative cholangiography was not significantly different from those who did *not* have the procedure. The authors found the incidence of bile duct injury in laparoscopic cholecystectomy to be higher than anticipated, and it did not decrease from 1991 through 1994. It was not easy to detail the obvious risk factors for these injuries using information from the referral sources. Unequivocally, laparoscopic cholecystectomy will remain a major therapeutic modality for decades. Although complication rates may decrease to an acceptable rate, following a steep learning curve, bile duct injury should be avoided at all costs because the morbidity and mortality and cost of its therapy are substantial. All studies confirm the importance of immediate recognition of a bile duct injury and its subsequent conversion to an open procedure to facilitate definitive repair.

Although the outlook for patients with biliary atresia has dramatically improved with the advent of liver transplantation, patients who maintain their native livers show only modest improvement in survival. To clairfy the controversial efficacy of corticosteroids on biliary flow following the Kasai portoenterostomy for biliary atresia, Muraji and Higashimoto (Abstract 10–17) evaluated 14 consecutive patients with biliary atresia who underwent this procedure. Since 1990, the authors have studied the intensive application of coricosteroids in postoperative management of the Kasai portoenterostomy to improve biliary drainage when inadequate drainage is apparent. The authors reported that aggressive corticosteroid therapy is a most important part of the management of the Kasai procedure. Although the initial response to steroids does not always reflect the final outcome, I agree with the authors that prospective trials should be organized.

The transfer of translational research to the clinical setting has also been seen in radiology, with increased application of percutaneous procedures for the diagnosis and treatment of various hepatobiliary disorders. The use of percutaneous approaches has led to a rise in the frequency of iatrogenic hemobilia—40% to 60% of all cases. The incidence of hemobilia is 0.01% to 0.2% after percutaneous liver biopsy, 4% after percutaneous transhepatic cholangiography (PTC), and 3% to 14% after percutaneous biliary drainage. In 1976, selective arterial embolization was described; this is currently the standard technique for the treatment of hemobilia of intrahepatic origin, replacing most surgical approaches for the majority of these patients. However, surgical therapy is required when selective embolization fails to control the bleeding induced by the aforementioned procedures. To study the role of surgery in patients with iatrogenic hemobilia,

Dousset and associates (Abstract 10–18) evaluated 19 patients treated with the disorder initiated by liver biopsy, PTC, or percutaneous biliary drainage. Selective embolization was used for all patients who bled after biopsy and for the majority with PTC. The authors concluded that surgical considerations for iatrogenic hemobilia are limited but should be considered for those for when all else fails or if there are complications of arterial embolization or hemocholecystitis, or in failed afforts at endoscopic or percutaneous biliary decompression when warranted as treatment for obstructive jaundice. Successful management of these bleeding patients has to be tailored to specific management approaches and is best achieved by combined radiologic, endoscopic, and surgical intervention.

After the introduction in 1987 of laparoscopic cholecystectomy, this procedure became the standard therapy for symptomatic cholelithiasis. Many subsequent studies have confirmed its cost-effectiveness and efficacy. With the surge of interest and the rapid development of techniques and instrumentation for advanced laparoscopic cholecystectomy, laparoscopic splenectomy was introduced, adopted, and successfully implemented in adults as well. Tulman and colleagues[8] were among the first to describe the experience with laparoscopic splenectomies in children, in 1993. Other clinics and universities continue to report results from small series of successful laparoscopic splenectomies in children. One such report is contributed by Schleef and associates (Abstract 10–19), who described a new technique for handling the spleen in children to circumvent major difficulties in purchase and manipulation of the spleen. They proposed the loop umbilical band for retraction of the organ during preparation and placement of the spleen into a sterile bag for its removal. This successful technique should serve as a technical advantage to lasso the spleen; the approach appears to be much safer and more technically adept than grasping the organ directly, reducing operating time and providing enhanced comfort for the surgeon, especially for large spleens. Pediatric surgeons using this laparoscopic procedure should try the loop umbilical band.

Kirby I. Bland, M.D.

References

1. Kelly TR, Wagner DS: Gallstone pancreatitis: A prospective randomized trial of the timing of surgery. *Surgery* 104:600–605, 1988.
2. Stone HH, Fabian TC, Dunlop WE: Gallstone pancreatitis: Biliary tract pathology in relation to time of operation. *Ann Surg* 194:305–312, 1981.
3. Safrany L, Neuhaus B: Intraduodenal manipulations of the common bile duct. *Surg Ann* 12:301–315, 1980.
4. Safrany L, Neuhaus B, Portocarrero G, et al: Endoscopic sphincterotomy in patients with Billroth II gastrectomy. *Endoscopy* 12:16–22, 1980.
5. Neoptolemos JP, Carr-Locke DL, London NJ, et al: Controlled trial of urgent endoscopic retrograde cholangiopancreatography and endoscopic sphincterotomy versus conservative treatment for acute pancreatitis due to gallstones. *Lancet* 2:979–983, 1988. 1988.
6. Fan ST, Lai EC, Mok FP, et al: Early treatment of acute biliary pancreatitis by endoscopic papillotomy. *N Engl J Med* 328:228–232, 1993.

7. Leese T, Neoptolemos JP, Baker AR, et al: Management of acute cholangitis and the impact of endoscopic sphincterotomy. *Br J Surg* 73:988–992, 1986.
8. Tulman S, Holcomb GW III, Karamanoukian HL, et al: Pediatric laparoscopic splenectomy. *J Pediatr Surg* 28:689–692, 1993.

Early ERCP and Papillotomy Compared With Conservative Treatment for Acute Biliary Pancreatitis

Fölsch UR, and the German Study Group on Acute Biliary Pancreatitis (Univ of Kiel, Germany; et al)
N Engl J Med 336:237–242, 1997 10–10

Purpose.—Several studies have examined the use of early surgical and endoscopic removal of gallstones retained in the common bile duct of patients with acute biliary pancreatitis. For patients who have acute biliary pancreatitis without obstructive jaundice, it is unclear whether early endoscopic retrograde cholangiopancreatography (ERCP) and papillotomy is the best treatment. A randomized, controlled trial of early ERCP vs. conservative treatment is reported.

Methods.—The study included 238 patients with acute biliary pancreatitis but without signs of obstructive jaundice. One group of 126 patients underwent ERCP within 72 hours after symptom onset, with endoscopic papillotomy to remove stones from the common bile duct, when indicated. The other 112 patients underwent conservative, noninvasive treatment. Patients in the conservative treatment group underwent ERCP within 3 weeks if signs of biliary obstruction or sepsis appeared. The 2 strategies were compared for overall mortality, mortality related to pancreatitis, and complication rate.

Results.—The success rate of early ERCP was 96%. Forty-six percent of patients in the early ERCP group underwent endoscopic papillotomy to remove bile duct stones, which was successful in 98% of cases. In the conservative treatment group, 20% of patients underwent ERCP. Fifty-nine percent of this group underwent successful papillotomy for stone removal. Within 3 months, mortality from acute biliary pancreatitis was 8% in the early ERCP group and 3.5% in the conservative treatment group. Although there was no significant difference in the complication rate, patients undergoing invasive treatment had more severe complications. Patients in the early ERCP group were more likely to have respiratory failure; those in the conservative treatment group were more likely to have jaundice.

Conclusions.—This randomized trial suggests that early ERCP and papillotomy are not beneficial to patients with acute biliary pancreatitis but without biliary obstruction or sepsis. Early ERCP does not reduce the mortality of acute biliary pancreatitis.

► In this study a prospective, multicenter study was conducted in which 126 patients were randomly assigned to early ERCP and endoscopic papillotomy vs. 112 patients who were randomly assigned to conservative treatment. In the conservative treatment group, ERCP was performed within 3 weeks if signs of biliary obstruction or sepsis developed. The significant findings of this study are that early ERCP was successful in the majority of the patients in removing stones. Fourteen patients in the invasive treatment group and 7 in the conservative treatment group died within 3 months (P = 0.10). Of note, 10 patients in the invasive treatment group and 4 patients in the conservative treatment group died of acute biliary pancreatitis. The overall rate of complications was similar in the two groups, but patients in the invasive treatment group had more severe complications. Respiratory failure was more frequent in the invasive treatment group, and jaundice was more frequent in the conservative treatment group. The authors have concluded that early ERCP and papillotomy were not beneficial in patients with acute biliary pancreatitis but without obstructive jaundice. Our own experience would tend to support the findings of the study. Our protocol is that patients with acute gallstone pancreatitis have ERCP after resolution of their acute pancreatitis but before a laparoscopic cholecystectomy, which is performed during the initial hospitalization. Should signs and symptoms of acute cholangitis develop, an emergency ERCP with decompression of the common bile duct is performed.

H.H. Simms, M.D.

Prospective Comparison of Endoscopic Ultrasonography and Endoscopic Retrograde Cholangiopancreatography in the Detection of Bile Duct Stones

Norton SA, Alderson D (Bristol Royal Infirmary, England)

Br J Surg 84:1366–1369, 1997 10–11

Background.—Although endoscopic retrograde cholangiopancreatography (ERCP) is the gold standard for evaluating bile duct stones, it may cause complications. A less risky procedure is endoscopic US, which can visualize the entire extrahepatic biliary tree. These 2 methods were compared for identifying bile duct stones in patients undergoing laparoscopic cholecystectomy.

Methods.—Fifty patients (34 women and 16 men; median age, 63 years) who were suspected of having bile duct stones were examined by both methods. First, for endoscopic US, the scope was introduced into the duodenum and stones were recognizable by their hyperechoic image and acoustic shadows. Then, within 24 hours, ERCP was performed. Endoscopic sphincterotomy or (in 1 case) open cholecystectomy was performed if either ERCP or endoscopic US suggested that stones were present. The diagnostic accuracies of both tests were calculated and compared.

Findings.—Both tests were successful in confirming or ruling out bile duct stones in 46 patients. In 2 patients both procedures failed, 1 because of intolerance of the procedure and 1 because of choledocholithiasis. Endoscopic retrograde cholangiopancreatography failed in 2 patients because the common bile duct could not be cannulated; in 1 of these, endoscopic US indicated stones and sphincterotomy was successfully performed. Stones were identified in 24 patients; 19 were identified by ERCP (sensitivity 79%) and 21 were identified by endoscopic US (sensitivity 88%). Endoscopic retrograde cholangiopancreatography identified stones in 2 patients who did not have stones (specificity 92%), and endoscopic US did so in 1 patient (specificity 96%). No complications were related to endoscopic US, while pancreatitis developed in 2 patients after ERCP.

Conclusions.—Endoscopic US was slightly more sensitive and specific than ERCP in identifying bile duct stones in these patients. Furthermore, endoscopic US was not associated with any complications. Nonetheless, because endoscopic US cannot be performed coincidentally with surgery, it does represent an extra step for these patients. Thus, endoscopic US seems most useful in evaluating patients with a history of pancreatitis, in those in whom previous ERCP has failed, and when other pathologic conditions or abnormalities are expected, especially in a pregnant woman.

▶ In this manuscript, the authors have prospectively evaluated both ERCP and endoscopic US with regard to their ability to detect common bile duct stones. Fifty patients underwent endoscopic US followed by ERCP and the results between the 2 tests were relatively comparable. The sensitivity for detecting common bile duct stones was 95% both for ERCP and endoscopic US. The specificity was 92% for ERCP and 96% for endoscopic US. The authors have concluded that endoscopic US is capable of identifying common bile duct stones and would be indicated in patients who have ERCP-induced pancreatitis or when ERCP has failed. Our experience at this institution is that endoscopic US is indeed a sensitive and specific way of detecting common bile duct stones; however, there is a fairly steep learning curve associated with this procedure and, therefore until more widespread experience is obtained with this modality in specifically looking for common bile duct stones, ERCP will continue to remain the gold standard in terms of detecting pathologic conditions of the common bile duct. In the future, however, it would not surprise me if endoscopic US to a large extent replaces ERCP for the evaluation of either preoperative or postoperative common bile duct abnormalities.

H.H. Simms, M.D.

An Analysis of Perioperative Cholangiography in One Thousand Laparoscopic Cholecystectomies

Fiore NF, Ledniczky G, Wiebke EA, et al (Indiana Univ, Indianapolis; Wishard Mem Hosp, Indianapolis, Ind; JW Riley Hosp for Children, Indianapolis, Ind; et al)

Surgery 122:817–823, 1997 10–12

Introduction.—The roles of intraoperative cholangiography (IOCG) and perioperative endoscopic retrograde cholangiopancreatography (ERCP) in laparoscopic cholecystectomy are still evolving, and recommendations for the timing and use of IOCG and ERCP have varied. A retrospective study of patients undergoing laparoscopic cholecystectomy for symptomatic cholelithiasis was conducted to determine the proper role of perioperative cholangiography.

Methods.—The study group included 1,002 patients who underwent laparoscopic cholecystectomy between July 1990 and December 1995. Patients were divided into "high-risk" and "low-risk" groups and stratified according to the use or nonuse of IOCG or preoperative or postoperative ERCP. Factors contributing to high risk designation were jaundice, pancreatitis, elevated bilirubin, alkaline phosphatase, serum glutamic-oxaloacetic transaminase, and radiographic evidence of common bile duct stones (CBDSs).

Results.—Laparoscopic IOCG was attempted in 272 patients and successfully completed in 234. Preoperative evaluation placed 62 of these 234 patients (26%) at high risk for choledocholithiasis and 172 (73.5%) at low risk. Only 3 of the low-risk patients (1.7%), but 21 of the high-risk patients (34%) were found to have choledocholithiasis. Sixty-seven patients, including 64 of the high-risk group, underwent preoperative ERCP. In 25 patients (39%), CBDSs were found and removed. The 3 low-risk patients had undergone ERCP before surgical consultation; none had stones.

Conclusion.—In low-risk patients, the incidence of CBDSs was only 1.7%, a risk that does not warrant the use of routine cholangiography. Laparoscopic IOCG is indicated, however, for the detection of CBDSs in high-risk patients, and more than half of these ducts can be cleared laparoscopically. The use of ERCP should be limited to high-risk patients in whom IOCG or laparoscopic duct clearance has failed.

▶ Will the question of routine vs. selective cholangiography during cholecystectomy ever be put to rest? Fiore and colleagues attempt to shed new light on this question by retrospectively analyzing 1,002 patients with symptomatic gallstones undergoing laparoscopic cholecystectomy with selective cholangiography. Criteria the authors considered to put the patient at high risk for CBDSs were jaundice, dilated common duct, elevated liver function tests, and elevated amylase and lipase. Based on these criteria, only 1.7% of patients deemed to be in the low-risk group by the absence of risk factors had CBDSs on cholangiography. In fact, this percentage may be even lower, as only 2 of the 3 patients with positive results on cholangiograms in the low-risk group actually had stones. This incidence of unsuspected stones is certainly equivalent to reported incidences in the literature of false positive cholangiograms and, more importantly, false negative cholangiograms.[1, 2]

My practice is to perform selective rather than routine cholangiograms. In addition to the criteria noted by the authors, I believe the size of the cystic duct is extremely important and should enter into the decision for or against cholangiography. In my opinion, patients with cystic ducts greater than 5 mm should always have a cholangiogram performed.

Proponents of routine cholangiography will argue that the incidence of CBDSs in the patients not undergoing IOGC is unknown and may be large. Although that is certainly true in the long term, short-term follow-up provided in this series suggests it is small, as only 0.5% of patients not undergoing cholangiography presented with CBDSs in the postoperative period. Recent advances and skill in ERCP have made this occurrence of low risk easily treatable.

Finally, advocates of routine cholangiography will argue that cholangiography will avoid common duct injuries. As the authors point out, routine IOCG has never been shown to lessen the incidence. Furthermore, my admonition to the residents remains true: Cholangiography does not replace meticulous blunt dissection without electrosurgery of the cystic duct.

J.F. Amaral, M.D.

References

1. Voyles CR, Sanders DL, Hogan R: Common bile duct evaluation in the era of laparoscopic cholecystectomy: 1050 cases later. *Ann Surg* 219:744–750, 1994.
2. Duensing RA, Williams RA, Collins JC, et al: Managing choledocholithiasis in the laparoscopic era. *Am J Surg* 170:619–623, 1995.

Multidisciplinary Approach to the Treatment of Pediatric Pancreaticobiliary Disorders

Tagge EP, Tarnasky PR, Chandler J, et al (Univ of South Carolina, Charleston)
J Pediatr Surg 32:158–165, 1997 10–13

Introduction.—The advantages of endoscopic retrograde cholangiopancreatography (ERCP) are well documented in the adult literature. Information on the experience with therapeutic ERCP in childhood pancreaticobiliary disorders is scant. A large series of children with pancreaticobiliary disease who underwent a multidisciplinary approach using traditional open surgery, ERCP, and laparoscopic surgery was retrospectively reviewed.

Methods.—The medical records of all children with pancreaticobiliary disorders who underwent ERCP and endoscopic or surgical treatment from 1990–1995 were reviewed for information regarding clinical history, diagnosis, radiologic imaging, laboratory values, ERCP results, surgical technique, postoperative and post-ERCP complications, length of hospital stay, and eventual outcome.

Results.—Of 26 children identified 1 had chronic pancreatitis, 4 had a choledochal cyst, 4 had pancreaticobiliary trauma and 17 had cholelithiasis. The mean patient age was 10.1 years (range, 6 months–19 years). There was successful visualization of the pancreaticobiliary tree in 25 patients (96%). Fifteen patients also underwent attempted therapeutic endoscopic procedures. Of these, 13 (87%) were performed successfully. Stents were placed preoperatively for cholangitis in 3 patients with choledochal cyst; all underwent successful choledochal cyst excision. Two patients who underwent unsuccessful stenting, one for traumatic bile leak and the other for bile duct stricture, required surgical correction. Ten of 17 patients who underwent ERCP to rule out choledocholithiasis had common duct stones. Stones were removed in all patients endoscopically, including those in a 6-month-old infant. Overall survival was 96%. The 1 death was unrelated to pancreaticobiliary disorder.

Conclusion.—Even very young children with pancreaticobiliary disorders can be treated successfully using a multidisciplinary approach with traditional open surgery, ERCP, and laparoscopic surgery.

► In summary, ERCP can now be performed in small children—but it is rarely necessary. The authors are to be commended for making this technique work even in the very young. They rightly point out that, unlike in adults, ERCP is still not routinely performed in the pediatric population. When they tried to use it for specific indications, such as pancreaticobiliary trauma, however, they were forced to concede that it was rarely diagnostic and never therapeutic. As for children with choledocholithiasis, preoperative ERCP successfully demonstrated and retrieved stones in 70%; but as the authors later state, this may have been overkill. Possibly because of a more functional papilla of Vater, choledocholithiasis in children is usually transient, and aggressive treatment (common duct exploration, sphincterotomy) is not warranted. In our own experience with cholelithiasis, ERCP is rarely, if ever, necessary postoperatively, even when intraoperative cholangiography demonstrates the presence of a common duct stone: spontaneous passage of the stone is the rule.

F.I. Luks, M.D.

Laparoscopic Cholecystectomy–related Bile Duct Injuries: A Health and Financial Disaster

Savader SJ, Lillemoe KD, Prescott CA, et al (Johns Hopkins Med Institutions, Baltimore, Md)

Ann Surg 225:268–273, 1997 10–14

Introduction.—The most common cause of bile duct trauma is iatrogenic injury during cholecystectomy, and there are reports that such injuries occur more frequently during laparoscopic cholecystectomy (LC) vs. open cholecystectomy (OC). Because LC procedures now outnumber OC procedures and bile duct injuries (BDIs) can result in significant long-term morbidity, the costs associated with LC-related injuries need to be examined.

Methods.—The study group included 49 patients with LC-related BDI: 39 women (mean age, 38 years) and 10 men (mean age, 55 years). Complete departmental and hospital billing records were obtained in each case so that costs for different injuries and treatment patterns could be analyzed. Also included were all related outpatient visits for chronic biliary tube care. Patients were categorized into 1 of 5 groups on the basis of the nature of their injury and the course of treatment.

Results.—Thirty-two patients had bile duct strictures, 11 had bile duct transections, 2 had bile duct ligations, and 4 had bile duct leaks or lacerations. With the exception of patients who were converted to OC after the intraoperative complication was recognized, percutaneous transhepatic cholangiography followed by percutaneous biliary drainage was performed. Most patients (84%) were then treated by a hepaticojejunostomy with Roux-en-Y loop reconstruction. Two patients, both with a major bile leak, died after extended ICU stays and before reparative surgery could be performed. Patients with LC-related BDIs incurred mean costs of $51,411 for all care related to repair of their BDI. Inpatient hospitalization averaged 32 days and outpatient care 10 days. Long-term chronic biliary intubation averaged 378 days. Both hospitalization and outpatient care days and total costs were considerably less when the BDI was recognized at the initial surgery.

Conclusion.—Although an uneventful LC shortens hospital stay and decreases postoperative pain and duration of at-home recovery time compared with OC, the increased rate of BDIs with LC significantly increases overall costs and mortality. Immediate recognition of the bile duct injury and conversion to OC can reduce complications and costs.

Bile Duct Injury Following Laparoscopic Cholecystectomy: Referral Pattern and Management

Mirza DF, Narsimhan KL, Ferraz Neto BH, et al (Queen Elizabeth Hosp, Birmingham, England)

Br J Surg 84:786–790, 1997 10–15

Introduction.—Although laparoscopic cholecystectomy (LC) offers a number of significant advantages over an open procedure, the risk of bile duct injury (BDI) is greater with the laparoscopic approach. Some patients with BDI will have long-term problems, with recurrent cholangitis and a risk of secondary biliary cirrhosis. The management and outcome of BDIs was reviewed in a series of 27 patients.

Methods.—The patients, 18 women and 9 men, were referred for the treatment of major BDIs sustained during elective LC. Surgery had been described as uneventful in 14 cases and difficult because of adhesions in 13. Only 6 injuries were recognized at operation. All patients were followed regularly with liver biochemistry; further imaging studies were performed when patients had symptoms or cholestatic liver biochemistry.

Results.—Patients were transferred to a tertiary hepatobiliary and liver transplant center at a median of 26 days after LC. Fifteen patients underwent additional surgery before referral, 3 had endoscopic cholangiography and stent insertion, and 5 had external drainage of bile collection; 5 patients were managed conservatively. After referral, surgical reconstruction was performed in 19 patients, percutaneous cholangiography with dilatation and stent placement in 3, percutaneous drainage in 2, endoscopic cholangiography and stent insertion in 2, and laparotomy with drainage in 1; 2 patients were managed conservatively. The duration of inpatient stay after referral ranged from 7 to 78 days (median, 14 days).

With a median follow-up of 30 months, 4 of the 9 patients with complex high injuries continue to have episodes of cholangitis. There was 1 death and 1 case of secondary biliary cirrhosis. Twenty of 27 patients are asymptomatic and well.

Conclusion.—Bile duct injury associated with LC continues to be a major problem, despite greater experience with the laparoscopic technique. Most injuries are the result of inadvertent clipping and division of the common duct when it has been mistaken for the cystic duct. Early recognition of BDI and transfer to a specialized center can help to prevent significant, long-term morbidity. The investigations of choice in cases of suspected injury are abdominal US followed by early endoscopic cholangiography.

Bile Duct Injury During Laparoscopic Cholecystectomy: A Prospective Nationwide Series

Adamsen S, Hansen OH, Funch-Jensen P, et al (Hillerød Hosp, Denmark; Hvidovre Hosp, Denmark; Sundby Hosp, Denmark; et al)

J Am Coll Surg 184:571–578, 1997 10–16

Introduction.—Although the risk of bile duct injury (BDI) in laparoscopic cholecystectomy is well known, there have been no randomized trials to determine whether the risk is greater with the laparoscopic method than with conventional open cholecystectomy (OC). An unselected cholecystectomy population was assessed for the incidence, types, and treatment of laparoscopic BDI.

Methods.—Patients were identified through prospective case registration in a national database which included all laparoscopic cholecystectomy (LC) procedures performed in Denmark, from the first operation in January 1991 through 1994. Case notes were requested if BDI was reported. Laparoscopic BDIs were classified according to extent, from type A (bile leak from a minor duct still in continuity with the common bile duct) to type E (circumferential injury of major bile ducts).

Results.—During the study period, 7,654 patients underwent LC and 57 (0.74%) cases of BDI were reported. Forty-eight injuries (84%) occurred before conversion to OC and 9 occurred after conversion. The incidence of BDI did not decrease over the 4-year period of review. Incisions accounted for 39% of laparoscopic BDIs, transections for 39%, and clip injuries or strictures for 12%. The incidence of BDI was greater in patients who underwent LC for acute cholecystitis (1.3%) than for those with other indications (0.62%). Preoperative endoscopic retrograde cholangiography or IV cholangiography, performed in 26% of patients undergoing LC, did not reduce the risk of BDI. Eleven patients with laparoscopic BDI experienced intraoperative difficulties and 1 patient with BDI died (1.8% of those with BDI).

Conclusion.—The incidence of BDI in patients undergoing LC is higher than previously anticipated, and the rate of injury did not decrease over the

4-year review period. One previous study reported an incidence of 0.6%, vs. 0.2% to 0.3% for OC. Prospective studies are needed to determine risk factors for BDI in LC.

► Common BDI during LC or OC is the most serious injury possible, other than death. Adamsen and colleagues (Abstract 10–16) from Denmark provide us with an excellent analysis of common BDIs since the inception of LC there. Importantly, they found a higher incidence of injuries than previously anticipated, and one that did not change significantly over the 4-year study period. Unlike others, these researchers were not able to document any benefits from intra-operative cholangiography. They did note, however, a greater frequency in acute cholecystitis than in chronic cholecystitis. Interestingly, the incidence of 0.74% in this study is not very different from the 1.07% incidence reported by Madsen in Denmark for OC.[1]

Savader and coworkers (Abstract 10–14) have evaluated the impact of common BDI in the laparoscopic era. Unsurprisingly, injury that was immediately detected accounted for a much lower cost, morbidity, and length of hospital stay compared with that in which diagnosis was delayed. Although these authors provide data to support their contention that common BDI is greater with LC, the results of Adamsen and colleagues dispute that concept.

The results of Savader and colleagues are striking with regard to a mean length of hospital stay of 32 days in the 49 patients treated. In contrast, Mirza and coworkers (Abstract 10–15) reporting on a series of 27 patients treated with similar injuries, report a mean length of hospital stay of only 14 days. In large part, this difference appears to be related to the frequent use of interventional radiologic services by Savader and colleagues, and in large part also accounts for the high cost of therapy in their series. Given the excellent results obtained by Mirza and colleagues, it appears as though interventional radiologic services may not be as important as indicated by Savader et al. However, the best way to reduce cost and limit hospitalization is by avoidance of the injury. In this regard, the importance of blunt dissection without electrosurgery in the triangle of Calot, to identify clearly the junction of the cystic duct with the gallbladder, cannot be overemphasized.

J.F. Amaral, M.D.

Reference

1. Madsen CM, Sorensen HR, Truelsen T: The frequency of operative bile duct injuries, illustrated by a Danish County Survey. *Acta Chir Scand* 119:110–111, 1960.

The Improved Outlook for Biliary Atresia With Corticosteroid Therapy

Muraji T, Higashimoto Y (Kobe Children's Hosp, Japan; Chiba Children's Hosp, Kobe, Japan)

J Pediatr Surg 32:1103–1107, 1997 10–17

Introduction.—Liver transplantation has dramatically improved the outlook for patients with biliary atresia (BA), but survival has improved only moderately in patients with native livers. Outcomes in a series of patients treated with an intensive course of postoperative corticosteroids after Kasai portoenterostomy to enhance bile drainage when it was inadequate were evaluated.

Methods.—Fourteen consecutive infants evaluated for biliary atresia between November 1990 to March 1996 underwent Kasai portojejunostomy. A 50-cm Roux-Y limb of the jejunum without exteriorization was used to perform reconstruction. An intussusception "valve" was made in the Roux-Y limb (shortened to 30 cm) from October 1990 to March 1993. Patients were managed postoperatively with adequate hydration and prophylactic antibiotics. Prednisolone, 20 mg/day (4 mg/kg), was administered when bile drainage was inadequate for 6–8 days after portoenterostomy, then reduced by half. The regimen was repeated when stool was less cholic, even if the previous dose was not completed.

Results.—The age range of 10 girls and 4 boys was 41–113 days (median, 72 days). One patient had excellent postoperative bile drainage and required no steroid support. The remaining 13 patients received corticosteroids for inadequate bile drainage. Three of the 13 patients did not respond to corticosteroids (1 died, 2 survived after liver transplantation). The remaining patients had varying degrees of response. When their serum total bilirubin level reached below 3 mg/dL, patients who responded were discharged 29–75 days after Kasai operation. One child, who was discharged with a total serum bilirubin of 2.5 mg/dL after reoperation, died. At 5-month to 5-year follow-up, the remaining 10 patients were alive and anicteric with their native livers. There was no difference in pathologic analysis between steroid responders and nonresponders.

Discussion.—It is likely that the first month after surgery is when the microscopic communicating ducts are formed into the epithelialized fistula, so it is important that bile flow be adequate during this time. The dose of corticosteroids should be manipulated on a daily basis according to the color of the stool and the bilirubin level. With this approach, bile drainage becomes steady within 1–2 months in most patients, once the microscopic communicating ducts successfully open after transecting the fibrous remnant.

Conclusion.—Aggressive corticosteroid therapy is crucial in the postoperative management of Kasai portoenterostomy. It is recommended that initial therapy be 20 mg/dL of prednisolone (minimum 10 mg for 1 dose). Multiple trials are recommended.

► We have another encouraging report on the benefits of postoperative steroids in biliary atresia. The mechanisms of this effect (if true effect there is) are still unknown, and are not necessarily related to the anti-inflammatory properties of corticosteroids. At least, no infections or other complications were noted, justifying the use of corticosteroids in these patients—every little bit helps. This is a relatively short-term follow-up on a limited number of patients, however, and the results (1 cure, 3 failures, and 10 intermediate results) may not be statistically different from the commonly accepted outcome in this disease.

F.I. Luks, M.D.

Selective Surgical Indications for Iatrogenic Hemobilia

Dousset B, Sauvanet A, Bardou M, et al (Hôpital Cochin, Paris; Hôpital Beaujon, Clichy, France)
Surgery 121:37–41, 1997 10–18

Objective.—Iatrogenic hemobilia is an increasingly common problem, brought on by the increased use of percutaneous procedures. Selective arterial embolization is the standard treatment for hemobilia, but surgery may be needed if embolization fails to control the bleeding. An experience with the treatment of iatrogenic hemobilia was reported, focusing on the use of surgical treatment.

Methods.—The experience included 19 adult patients with hemobilia occurring after a percutaneous procedure. The procedure was liver biopsy in 11 patients, transhepatic cholangiography in 5, and percutaneous biliary drainage in 3. In 13 of 15 cases in which it was attempted, selective embolization was successful. Surgery was performed in 3 patients with active bleeding because selective embolization was technically impossible or because there was no recognizable vascular lesion. Four patients had delayed surgery, 3 because of hemocholecystitis and 1 because of inadvertent gallbladder embolization. Only patients who had undergone transhepatic cholangiography underwent biliary decompression. None of the patients died or had recurrent bleeding.

Conclusions.—Few patients with iatrogenic hemobilia will require surgery. Indications for surgery include failed or complicated arterial embolization, hemocholecystitis, and failed endoscopic or percutaneous biliary decompression in patients with obstructive jaundice. Successful management of bleeding patients with hemobilia relies on a combination of radiologic, endoscopic, and surgical expertise.

► This study was undertaken to assess the place for surgery in patients with iatrogenic hemobilia. It deals with 19 patients who were treated for hemobilia caused by percutaneous liver biopsy, percutaneous transhepatic cholangiography, or percutaneous biliary drainage. Selective embolization was successful in 15, (87%,) of the patients. Technical impossibility of selective embolization and the absence of recognizable vascular lesions were the reasons for surgery in 3 actively bleeding patients. Indications for delayed surgery included hemocholecystitis and inadvertent embolization of the gallbladder. After percutanous biliary drainage, repeat irrigation and tube replacement were used to stop the bleeding and to decompress the biliary tract without embolization or surgery. None of the 19 patients died. The authors conclude that surgical indications for iatrogenic hemobilia are limited and include failure or complication of arterial embolization, hemocholecystitis, and failed attempt at endoscopic or percutaneous biliary decompression in the case of obstructive jaundice. I would agree that most cases of iatrogenic hemobilia can be handled nonoperatively, primarily with selective embolization. However, it is imperative for the surgeon to recognize that if selective embolization is not successful, most of these remaining patients, if they are bleeding, will require surgical intervention to stop the bleeding.

H.H. Simms, M.D.

Technical Aspects of Laparoscopic Splenectomy in Children

Schleef J, Morcate JJ, Steinau G, et al (Univ of Münster, Germany)
J Pediatr Surg 32:615–617, 1997 10–19

Introduction.—Laparoscopic splenectomies have been successfully performed in children. One of the major problems during the procedure is grasping and handling of the spleen. Described is a technique designed to minimize bleeding and damage to the capsule.

> *Surgical Technique.*—With the patient supine, 4 trocars are introduced. With the lower portion of the organ mobilized, an umbilical tape is passed around the lower portion of the spleen and tightened with a grasping forceps. The organ is dissected and placed in the pelvis of the patient. The laparoscope is changed to the left lateral trocar and a sterile bag is used to remove the spleen. After the bag is exteriorized through the umbilicus, the abdominal cavity is inspected and accessory spleens can be removed if detected.

Results.—The age range of 11 patients who underwent laparoscopic splenectomy was 4–16 years. The indications for surgery were hereditary spherocytosis in 9 children and idiopathic thrombocytopenia purpura in 2. Accessory spleens were removed in 3 children. The average operative time was 174 minutes (range, 149–245 minutes). The operative time was an average of 165 minutes (range, 149–175 minutes) in the last 7 patients.

Conclusion.—The loop technique can be useful in laparoscopic splenectomy. It can significantly reduce the operative time required for reinsertion of the forceps and changing position of the forceps.

► The value of reports like this is not in the numbers: 11 patients do not a series make. However, this and other papers help budding laparoscopists develop better techniques, as all of us struggle with the same problems: how do you manipulate the spleen without tearing it (risking splenosis); how do you find accessory spleens; and, most of all, *how do you get that spleen in the bag and out of the abdomen*?! Professor Willital and his group describe a self-made sling, which is not unlike a commercially made splenic grasper available in this country. They found, as we did, that lassoing the spleen is better than grasping it directly. They leave their patient in the supine position; many others seem to favor the right lateral decubitus position, which uses the best retractor of all—gravity. Another point worth mentioning: they perform the operation through 4 ports (not 5, as is usually described in adults). As for accessory spleens, the authors looked for them at the end of the procedure. It is our experience, however, that they're best sought early on, before small mesenteric and omental hematomas, hemorrhages, or cautery scars make the task more difficult.

F.I. Luks, M.D.

Comparison of Laparoscopic and Open Splenectomy in Children With Hematologic Disorders

Farah RA, Rogers ZR, Thompson WR, et al (Univ of Texas, Dallas)
J Pediatr 131:41–46, 1997 10–20

Introduction.—Because of the morbidity related to surgery, the use of laparoscopic techniques is considered for children who require splenectomy for nonmalignant hematologic disorders. Laparoscopic splenectomy may result in less postoperative discomfort and smaller abdominal wall scars, allowing a shorter hospital stay and a faster return to daily activities. A retrospective review of 36 splenectomies was conducted to compare laparoscopic and traditional open splenectomy in children with nonmalignant hematologic disorders.

Methods.—The splenectomies were performed at a single pediatric institution between January 1993 and January 1996. Children were not randomized; the choice of technique was based upon preference or chronologic presentation. Laparoscopic splenectomy was performed with the patient under general anesthesia. Four trocar cannulas were inserted, three 5-mm trocars in the supraumbilical area, the left upper quadrant, and along the midline and one 10-mm trocar in the left lower quadrant. Open and laparoscopic procedures were compared for intraoperative morbidity, postoperative course, postoperative morbidity, and costs.

Results.—Twenty children (mean age, 9.7 years) had an open procedure performed and 16 (mean age, 10.3 years) underwent laparoscopic splenectomy. Five in the open group and 7 in the laparoscopic group had a concomitant cholecystectomy. Although the mean anesthesia and operative times were significantly longer in the laparoscopic group, these patients required an average of 32 fewer hours of postoperative analgesia than those in the open group. Children who had a laparoscopic splenectomy were discharged home 1.4 days earlier than those having an open splenectomy, and 93% resumed a regular diet during the first 2 postoperative days. Mean estimated intraoperative blood loss was similar in the 2 groups (after excluding 1 child in the laparoscopic group who had to be converted to an open procedure after laceration of the splenic artery). Operating room charges were higher for laparoscopy, but total hospitalization costs did not differ significantly in the 2 groups.

Conclusion.—Laparoscopic splenectomy is a safe procedure in children with nonmalignant hematologic disorders, achieving a hematologic response comparable to that of open splenectomy. The laparoscopic procedure is superior with regard to duration of postoperative analgesia, length of hospital stay, and postoperative bowel function.

► There is a notable change of emphasis in recent articles on laparoscopy. Only 1 or 2 years ago, one had to justify the feasibility of the laparoscopic approach, particularly for more advanced procedures such as splenectomy. Now, its cost-effectiveness is being addressed, which can be seen as a coming of age. In this series, laparoscopic splenectomy took 1 to 1.5 hours longer than the open procedure, but patients stayed in the hospital 1 less day. In this study from Dallas, the earlier discharge almost made up for the increased operative costs. Unfortunately, the exact cost of hospitalization, patient charge for laparoscopic instruments, and even the actual cost of the instruments (what with discounts for bulk purchase and exclusivity contracts) are highly institution-dependent, and therefore difficult to extrapolate to other centers. Still, the authors of this series are correct in stating that gradual reduction in laparoscopy time and cost-conscious use of (reusable) instruments will eventually make laparoscopic operations cost-effective. This is particularly true for those indications where either little specialized instrumentation is necessary (fundoplication, for example), or postoperative recovery is much faster.

F.I. Luks, M.D.

Abdomen and Small Bowel

INTRODUCTION

Surgeons of the forthcoming millenium will have access to larger databases than their predecessors. Applications of cellular, biochemical, and molecular medicine have speeded progress in the management of diseases of the abdomen and small bowel. Mucosal injury as a consequence of the ischemia/reperfusion (IR) injury has been studied to reveal its natural history, progression, and therapy. Intestinal ischemia initiates the depletion of cellular energy substrates, with the subsequent accumulation of metabolic toxins and cytokines recognized as early mucosal injury. Further, reperfusion of the ischemic intestine, while necessary to salvage tissues, exacerbates early ischemic injuries by the release of reactive oxidative species, with subsequent accumulation of activated neutrophils. This injury is classically described as an IR injury that occurs in various clinical scenarios: (1) in necrotizing enterocolitis of the newborn; (2) in the harvesting of small and large bowel for transplantation; or (3) more commonly in the mesenteric insufficiency evident in elderly individuals. Although these substrate depletion events are complex and not fully understood, the common denominator of the inciting event is tissue hypoxia (mucosa and submucosa). With proper oxygen delivery the events that initiate IR may be reversed. O'Donnell and associates (Abstract 10–21) examined IR injury to intestinal mucosa in several common clinical situations (e.g., nonocclusive mesenteric insufficiency and necrotizing enterocolitis), evaluating four animal groups to determine whether oxygenated perfluorocarbon (PFC), when administered during ischemia alone, ameliorated IR-induced mucosal injury. It became evident that when oxygenated PFC was delivered during reperfusion alone, the mucosal injury intensified. The authors contended that intraluminal perfusion of oxygenated PFC during ischemia may preserve mucosal function and integrity and greatly improve outcomes and mortality for patients with a variety of mesenteric ischemic disorders.

Smith and associates (Abstract 10–22) reported on the urologic management of cloacal exstrophy. Considerable progress has been made in treating patients with this disorder since the first report of a child surviving correction in 1960. Unequivocally, the foundation of success has rested upon intensive nutritional support and staged reconstructive efforts based upon a greater understanding of this anomaly. Current survival rates approach 90%, and therapy of cloacal exstrophy has now shifted from a focus on improving survival to enhancing quality of life. The authors used modern principles of continent urinary diversion to ameliorate the consequences of cloacal exstrophy to enhance the quality of survival. The use of gastric flaps with preservation of intestinal length has become central to this important urologic reconstructive effort. Suboptimal compliance of these neourinary reservoirs is evident when stomach alone is used. State-of-the-art approaches employ composite ileogastric reconstruction when the gastric flaps are of marginal size. Advanced urologic principles, combined with general surgical methods, are considered safe and effective.

Management of the patient with meconium ileus has progressed significantly. This condition, which occurs in 15% of children with cystic fibrosis, has in various reports suggested a worse prognosis in the individual with cystic fibrosis who also has this malady. Previously, many infants were known to die postoperatively, with survival rates that approximated those of cystic fibrosis without meconium ileus. Coutts and associates (Abstract 10–23) evaluated 49 children with meconium ileus who were confirmed to have cystic fibrosis either by a positive sweat test or histologic study. The authors confirmed that children with cystic fibrosis born with meconium ileus had higher early mortality rates than did other children with the disease; however, when deaths attributable to postoperative complications were discounted, the authors noted a similar prognosis to the general cystic fibrosis population. The authors further emphasized that *early* clinical presentation of meconium ileus may improve long-term survival for this group of infants and may enhance the quality of life over and above that for individuals who are first seen with late symptoms.

The remarkable progress in the evolving field of fetal surgery continues to demonstrate that intrauterine repairs of specific congenital malformations may provide alternative management options. Saiki and associates (Abstract 10–24) assessed the fetal physiologic responses to CO_2 pneumometrium during fetoscopy using a chronically instrumented fetal lamb model to examine whether hyperventilation of the mother can offset fetal hypercarbic acidosis. While there is concern for the outcomes of this work, many authors advocate endoscopic fetal surgery using amnioinfusion and a more natural amniotic environment.

Rescorla and associates (Abstract 10–25) reported on the role of laparoscopy in the management of the contralateral groin of neonates, infants, and children who are seen with unilateral inguinal hernia. This pediatric surgical group evaluated the role of diagnostic laparoscopy performed synchronously with repair of the clinically apparent hernial sac to identify a contralateral exploration only to infants having CPPV-positive findings. Sixty-four percent of patients under 6 months old had a CPPV, compared with 30% older than 6 months ($P = 0.001$). Girls more frequently had a CPPV than did boys (67% vs. 44%; $P = 0.087$). This approach seems a safe and effective measure to identify the presence of a CPPV, leading to improved diagnosis and the need for a bilateral approach. It is also cost-effective.

Atresia of an intestinal segment as a consequence of an in utero vascular accident was first confirmed by Leuw and Bernard in 1955. Dilated bowel is one factor inducing disturbed intestinal transit in duodenal atresia-stenosis patients. Takahashi and associates (Abstract 10–26) determined whether dilated bowel proximal to the obstruction associated with duodenal atresia and stenosis is related to feeding problems after surgical correction of the obstruction. This relationship between disturbed transit and function of the dilated duodenum is unclear. The authors concluded that dilated bowel is related to disturbed transit during the postoperative period and that the low contraction amplitude of the dilated bowel was the main pathophysiologic feature. Tapering or plication may be indicated for a markedly dilated bowel after surgical correction of the obstruction. Intestinal tapering during the initial operation may avoid this postoperative complication.

An additional paper in this YEAR BOOK OF SURGERY also evaluates altered gastrointestinal function after repair of gastroschisis, especially those associated with atretic intestinal segments. Cheng and associates (Abstract 10–27) evaluated this abdominal wall defect, studying gastric and small-bowel myoelectric activity in a child with prolonged inability to tolerate oral intake after stage repair of the gastroschisis and an associated ileal atresia. The authors concluded that myoelectric recordings via implanted electrodes are safe for children and may provide important information regarding underlying alterations of intestinal motility. Roles for myoelectric activity in clinical medicine are not fully established; however, the knowledge that motility disorders exist in the presence of abdominal wall defects is important and may guide subsequent interventions.

NO POSTAGE
NECESSARY
IF MAILED
IN THE
UNITED STATES

BUSINESS REPLY MAIL

FIRST-CLASS MAIL PERMIT NO 135 ST LOUIS MO

POSTAGE WILL BE PAID BY ADDRESSEE

SUBSCRIPTION SERVICES
MOSBY–YEAR BOOK, INC.
11830 WESTLINE INDUSTRIAL DRIVE
ST. LOUIS MO 63146-9988

NO POSTAGE
NECESSARY
IF MAILED
IN THE
UNITED STATES

BUSINESS REPLY MAIL

FIRST-CLASS MAIL PERMIT NO 135 ST LOUIS MO

POSTAGE WILL BE PAID BY ADDRESSEE

Mosby

PAT NEWMAN
11830 WESTLINE INDUSTRIAL DRIVE
PO BOX 46908
ST. LOUIS MO 63146-9934

Want to speed up the process?

To order the *Year Book*,
you also may call 1-800-426-4545

To subscribe to the journal today,
call toll-free in the U.S.:
1-800-453-4351
or fax 314-432-1158
Outside the U.S., call: 314-453-4351

Visit us at:
www.mosby.com/Mosby/Periodicals

Mosby–Year Book, Inc.
Subscription Services
11830 Westline Industrial Drive
St. Louis, MO 63146 U.S.A.

Mosby

McKernan and Laws[1] and Felix et al.[2] recently described laparoscopic techniques for the repair of inguinal hernias. In several small trials, these techniques have proved superior to open repair with regard to postoperative pain and recovery. However, these studies are too small to determine differences in recurrence rates. Liem and associates (Abstract 10–28) compared conventional anterior surgery to laparoscopic surgery for repair of inguinal hernias in a randomized multicenter trial. No standardized interior hernia repair approach was used. The authors concluded that as recurrence rates were lowest at 2 years with the laparoscopic method, laparoscopic hernia repair on a large scale seems warranted, when supervised by experienced surgeons. A companion paper by Cunningham and associates (Abstract 10–29) assessed postoperative pain in this prospective trial as a portion of a larger study evaluating recurrence rates and other morbidity of the Bassini-McVey and Shouldice repairs. Pain or numbness were late sequelae of the traditional external surgical repairs. Two years postoperatively, more than half of the patients had pain, with 10.6% reporting moderate to severe pain. The authors of this paper advocated using various strategies to reduce complications and morbidity.

The presence of adynamic ileus after major abdominal surgery, characterized by an absence of abdominal sounds and evidence of loss of neuromuscular motility, is caused by neuronal inhibition following sympathetic overreactivity. Simple bowel trauma, intestinal evisceration, infection, and so on, are common etiologic mechanisms that initiate adynamic ileus. Routine application of postoperative nasogastric decompression after major surgery continues to be challenged. Studies exist that repudiate the routine measures for decompression in elective abdominal surgery without detriment to patient recovery and outcome. The recent application of early oral feedings after abdominal surgery suggests that this is a safe and generally well-tolerated measure. Moreover, it is cost-effective if early feedings are tolerated and the hospital stay is shortened. To evaluate the role of early postoperative feeding after elective colorectal surgery, Hartsell and associates (Abstract 10–30) performed a prospective, randomized trial to determine whether early postoperative feeding would shorten hospital stays. No significant differences were seen in nausea and vomiting or length of hospital stay between the early-fed group and the patients treated with postoperative decompression and traditional progression of feeding. Thus, while early feedings may be safe, they seem to be of little advantage in clinical surgery.

Inflammatory bowel disease (IBD) remains a cause of major morbidity in children and adults. Crohn's disease is a chronic, transmural, panintestinal inflammatory disorder of small and large bowel that typically progresses despite surgical or medical management and has no known etiology or cure. Approximately half of patients managed medically will eventually require surgical intervention. The surgical treatment of IBD is designed to alleviate symptoms uncontrolled by medical therapy or to correct complications such as perforation, abscess, fistula, or obstruction. Resection remains the choice for long-term cure; the 10-year reoperative rates for recurrent disease have been static at one third to one half of the patients so managed. Delays in surgery with prolonged use of corticosteroids may prolong unnecessarily the disease state and risk complications secondary to both the medication and fistulization, obstruction, or bleeding of diseased segments. Kim and colleagues (Abstract 10–31) studied long-term clinical outcomes of patients undergoing ileocecal resection for Crohn's IBD. The results suggest that ileocecal resection of Crohn's IBD has a high rate of disease control with low morbidity and few multiple bowel resections. The authors admonished that resection of ileocecal Crohn's should *not* be unduly delayed for fear of risking short bowel syndromes, as the overall patient satisfaction and outcomes are excellent.

With increase in size of an adrenal mass, the likelihood of a malignancy increases. Kloos and associates (Abstract 10–32) noted that large incidentally discovered adrenal masses (more than 3 cm diameter) are easy to characterize with MRI or CT. Functional characterization with adrenocortical scintigraphy, positron emission tomography (PET), or tissue characterization by CT-guided adrenal biopsy, are all useful. As smaller masses (up to 3-cm diameter) may easily be misdiagnosed, Kloos and associates evaluated the utility of NP59 scintigraphy for evaluation of small adrenal lesions. Diagnostic accuracy was excellent (90%); specificity was 100%. The authors emphasized the importance of analyzing small incidentally discovered adrenal masses.

Kirby I. Bland, M.D.

References

1. McKernan JB, Laws HL: Laparoscopic repair of inguinal hernias using a totally extraperitoneal prosthetic approach. *Surg Endosc* 7:26–28, 1993.
2. Felix EL, Michas CA, McKnight RL: Laparoscopic herniorrhaphy: Transabdominal preperitoneal floor repair. *Surg Endosc* 8:100–103, 1994.

Oxygenated Intraluminal Perfluorocarbon Protects Intestinal Muscosa From Ischemia/Reperfusion Injury

O'Donnell KA, Caty MG, Zheng S, et al (Children's Hosp of Buffalo, NY)
J Pediatr Surg 32:361–365, 1997 10–21

Background.—Patients with necrotizing enterocolitis or nonocclusive mesenteric insufficiency may have ischemia/reperfusion (I/R) injury to the intestinal mucosa. It might be possible to avoid I/R injury by delivering oxygen to the newly ischemic intestine. Perfluorocarbon (PFC) has a unique mechanism of oxygen delivery and is already approved for use as a gastrointestinal imaging agent. Continuous intraluminal flow of oxygenated PFC was tested for its ability to prevent I/R injury in the intestinal mucosa of rats.

Methods and Results.—Four groups of rats were studied. One group underwent laparotomy only, and 3 groups underwent experimental I/R.

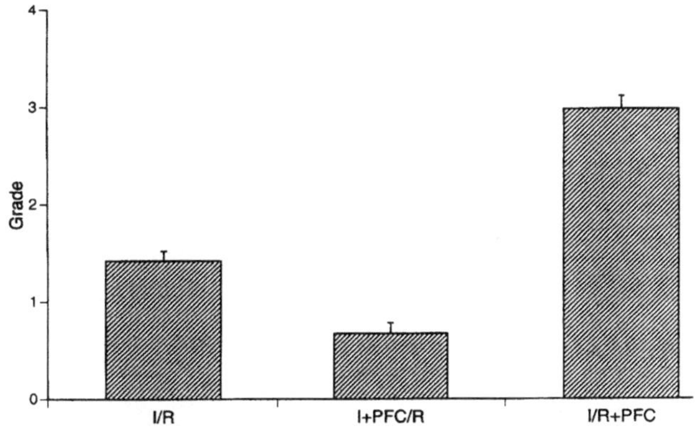

FIGURE 2.—Comparison of the mean histological scores between the I/R−, I + PFC/R−, and I/R + PCF-treated groups. The distribution of grading frequencies is significantly different between the groups. (Courtesy of O'Donnell KA, Caty MG, Zheng S, et al: Oxygenated intraluminal perfluorocarbon protects intestinal mucosa from ischemia/reperfusion injury. *J Pediatr Surg* 32:361–365, 1997.)

One group had I/R alone, another group received oxygenated PFC during the ischemic interval only, and another group received PFC only during reperfusion. Mucosal I/R injury was reduced in animals that received PFC during ischemia only. In contrast, those receiving PFC during reperfusion only had worse mucosal injury (Fig 2).

Conclusions.—In this rat model, giving oxygenated PFC by intraluminal perfusion during periods of ischemia can reduce I/R-induced mucosal injury. This may offer a new approach to the treatment of patients with mesenteric ischemic disorders.

► This study deals with the effect of intestinal I/R injury on mucosal integrity in a rat model. Animals were divided into four groups—sham, IR, ischemia with oxygenated intraluminal perfluorocarbon during ischemia, and IR, with oxygenated intraluminal perfluorocarbon administered only during reperfusion. Oxygenated perfluorocarbon when administered during ischemia alone ameliorated IR-induced mucosal injury; however, when it was delivered during reperfusion alone, mucosal injury was worsened. These data are representative of the findings shown in Figure 2, which demonstrates significant histological preservation when intraluminal perfluorocarbon is given during periods of ischemia. This appears to be a novel use for the use of the oxygenated intraluminal perfluorocarbon, and a mechanism behind the fact that mucosal injury was worsened when perfluorocarbon was given during reperfusion probably relates to the increased number of oxidants produced with restoration of molecular oxygen at the mucosal level. This technique clearly needs to be investigated in larger animal models but might have significant applicability in preventing not only mucosal injury but possibly bacterial translocation after periods of significant intestinal IR.

H.H. Simms, M.D.

Current Urologic Management of Cloacal Exstrophy: Experience With 11 Patients

Smith EA, Woodard JR, Broecker BH, et al (Emory Univ, Atlanta, Ga)
J Pediatr Surg 32:256–262, 1997 10–22

Introduction.—The once-fatal diagnosis of cloacal exstrophy now has a survival rate approaching 90%. The focus of treatment has shifted from improving survival to improving quality of life. The quality of life of 12 patients who underwent lower urinary tract reconstruction for cloacal exstrophy was evaluated.

Methods.—Of the 12 patients, 1 patient died as a neonate from severe pulmonary hypoplasia before reconstruction. Seven of 11 patients underwent either bladder augmentation or construction of a continent urinary reservoir. Four patients were able to void volitionally. Five patients had a purely gastric reservoir constructed (of these, 2 subsequently had ileal augmentations producing composite reservoirs) and 2 had closure of the bladder neck and an augmentation gastrocystoplasty. Patient records were reviewed for stability of the upper urinary tract and for quality of life, using a continence score with a range of 0 (worst) to 6 (best).

Results.—The mean age at reconstruction was 6 years, and the mean postreconstruction follow-up was 3.5 years. Reconstruction was successful without reflux in patients who underwent ureteral reimplantation into the gastric reservoir. Six of the 9 patients with continence had upper tract stability. Creatinine was normal in all patients. Two patients with gastric reservoirs and 1 with an augmentation gastrocystoplasty required hospitalization for dehydration with hyponatremia, hypochloremia, and hypokalemia. Of 7 patients with urinary reconstruction with gastric or bowel segments, 4 had continence scores of 3 and 2 who had an abdominoperineal pull-through procedure had a score of 4. Continent reconstruction failed in 1 patient who had a score of 2 with stomas. Two patients with variant features had a continence score of 5.

Conclusion.—Quality of life can be improved in patients with cloacal exstrophy using gastric flaps. If the gastric flap is of marginal size, composite ileogastric construction should be considered.

► Less than 40 years ago, cloacal exstrophy was uniformly fatal. In light of this, a survival rate of more than 90% is remarkable. This, unfortunately, is when things become complicated. Infants born with cloacal exstrophy have grossly abnormal or nonexistent urinary and stool continence mechanisms, foreshortened bowel, and a small bladder, to name only a few problems. As survival increased, urologists and general surgeons began a tug-of-war, each side claiming hollow viscera as their own. If one uses a portion of the small bowel to construct a urinary reservoir, short-bowel syndrome may ensue; if the bladder is to be used as a neovagina, what then of a urinary reservoir?

In the end, it is difficult to optimize 1 function without jeopardizing the other. This is essentially 1 of the authors' conclusions: a perfect "6" (both urinary and intestinal continence) can never be achieved, and even a single continent system occurs only if the patient has a milder variant of the disease. The authors are certainly to be commended for their excellent results. However, as infant mortality has been all but eradicated in this disease, one should keep in mind a not infrequent cause of delayed mortality: teen suicide, caused by deep-rooted feelings of inadequacy.

F.I. Luks, M.D.

Clinical Course of Patients With Cystic Fibrosis Presenting With Meconium Ileus

Coutts JAP, Docherty JG, Carachi R, et al (Royal Hosp for Sick Children, Yorkhill, Glasgow, Scotland)

Br J Surg 84:555, 1997 10–23

Introduction.—The prognosis for infants with meconium ileus has improved because of better management before and after surgery. The surgical outcome in children with cystic fibrosis with and without meconium ileus was evaluated.

Methods.—Survival and severity of subsequent disease were compared in a group of 47 children with cystic fibrosis and meconium ileus and 88 children with cystic fibrosis without meconium ileus.

Results.—Ten of 47 children with cystic fibrosis and meconium ileus died within the first 30 days of life. Mean group survival was significantly different: 10.1 years in children with meconium ileus and 13.8 in children without meconium ileus (Fig 1). When perioperative deaths were excluded, mean survival in children with meconium ileus was similar to children without meconium ileus (12.8 years).

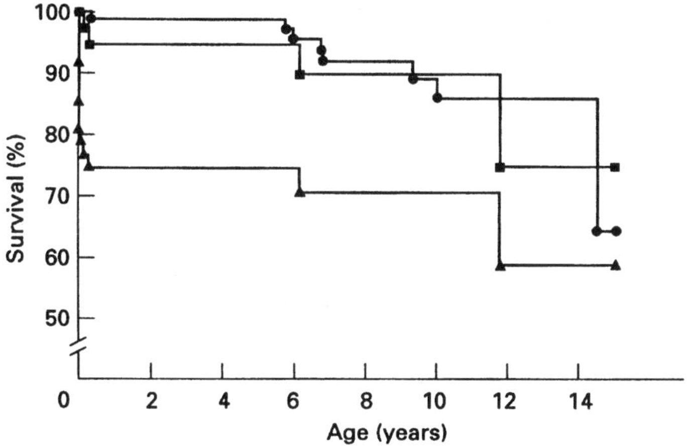

FIGURE 1.—Kaplan-Meier survival curves for children born with meconium ileus (*solid triangle*; n = 47); children born with meconium ileus who survived the first 30 days (*solid square*; n = 37), and children with cystic fibrosis without meconium ileus (*solid circle*; n = 88) (Courtesy of Coutts JAP, Docherty JG, Carachi R, et al: Clinical course of patients with cystic fibrosis presenting with meconium ileus. *Br J Surg* 84:555, 1997, Blackwell Science Ltd.)

Conclusion.—Children with cystic fibrosis and meconium ileus had a significantly higher early mortality rate than children with cystic fibrosis and no meconium ileus. The subsequent clinical course did not differ between groups of survivors after the first month of life. With continued improvements in medical and surgical treatment, the rate of deaths attributable to postoperative complications should diminish.

► A very short but elegant report that answers an often-asked question: Does the presence of meconium ileus indicate a worse form of cystic fibrosis? Yes and no. A number of infants (20%!) with meconium ileus went on to die postoperatively (not necessarily, one assumes, due to the underlying cystic fibrosis). The survivors, however, had a survival rate similar to those children with cystic fibrosis without meconium ileus. The authors further speculate that, if it is true that early detection and treatment of cystic fibrosis are beneficial, meconium ileus may be regarded as the earliest possible screening test—and that, in the long run, these children should fare better.

F.I. Luks, M.D.

Reducing the Deleterious Effects of Intrauterine CO_2 During Fetoscopic Surgery

Saiki Y, Litwin DEM, Bigras J-L, et al (Hosp For Sick Children, Toronto; Univ of Toronto)

J Surg Res 69:51–54, 1997 10–24

Objective.—Videoscopic or fetoscopic techniques are less-invasive approaches to fetal intervention. Videoscopic techniques require distention of the amniotic cavity, usually with CO_2, for adequate visualization of the fetus. But CO_2 pneumometrium causes fetal hypercarbia and acidosis. Results of a study in which the fetal physiological response to CO_2 pneumometrium during fetoscopy was assessed by using a chronically instrumented fetal lamb model and examining whether maternal hyperventilation can offset the fetal hypercarbic acidosis are presented herein.

Methods.—The right carotid arteries of 7 fetal lambs, 98- to 115-days-old, were cannulated in utero with a polyvinyl catheter (i.d. 0.030 inch). At gestational ages from 107 to 119 days, a Veress needle was inserted into the uterus through a small maternal laparotomy and CO_2 was insufflated slowly at 10 mmHg of intraamniotic pressure, with continuous monitoring of maternal end-tidal CO_2 ($ETCO_2$). After 30 minutes, ewes were hyperventilated at 22–24 breaths/min. The uterus was deflated, and the procedure was repeated 1 hour later. Fetal and maternal arterial blood was sampled every 15 minutes during the procedure.

Results.—Fetal $PaCO_2$ increased significantly during both insufflation periods (from 51 to 72 mmHg), but reverted to baseline values after maternal hyperventilation (from 72 to 52 mmHg). During the insufflation period, fetal blood pH decreased significantly from 7.350 to 7.236. Fetal and maternal systolic blood pressure remained stable throughout the procedure. The increase in fetal heart rate during the procedure was not significant.

Conclusion.—Significant changes in fetal and maternal pH and $PaCO_2$ result from CO_2 insufflation into the uterus. The fact that fetal acidosis can be reversed by maternal hyperventilation suggests that the $PaCO_2$ gradient between maternal and fetal circulation helps to preserve fetal $PaCO_2$ within normal values.

► After having been confined to a semi-experimental status for more than a decade, fetal surgery is enjoying a renaissance with the application of minimally invasive techniques. This is one of many papers detailing the steps needed to make endoscopic fetal surgery clinically applicable. The authors confirm the nefarious effects of carbon dioxide pneumoamnios: the fetus has to rely on his mother, through placental exchange, to eliminate the excess carbon dioxide, which so readily diffuses through the amniotic membrane and the fetal epidermis. Contrary to the present study, however, our own experiments did not show a significant improvement of the fetus' hypercapnia with maternal hyperventilation.[1] Whether it succeeds in correcting fetal hypercarbia, maternal hypercapnia could be detrimental to the fetus, as it causes a decrease in uterine artery blood flow (and therefore fetal oxygen delivery). Working in a gas medium might have other side effects for the fetus, such as dehydration or gas embolization. Most authors are therefore advocating endoscopic fetal surgery via amnioinfusion and a *more natural* fluid environment.

F.I. Luks, M.D.

Reference

1. Luks FI, Deprest JA, Marcus M, et al: Carbon dioxide pneumoamnios causes acidosis in the fetal lamb. *Fetal Diagn Ther* 9:105–109, 1994.

The "Other Side" of Pediatric Hernias: The Role of Laparoscopy

Rescorla FJ, West KW, Engum SA, et al (Indiana Univ, Indianapolis; James Whitcomb Riley Hosp for Children, Indianapolis, Ind)

Am Surg 63:690–693, 1997 10–25

Introduction.—Contralateral inguinal exploration is performed to prevent the occurrence of a future hernia on that side. Arguments for and against this approach abound. One of the issues influencing choice of contralateral inguinal exploration is the presence of a contralateral patent processus vaginalis (CPPV). The role of nonpuncture laparoscopy performed through the symptomatic hernia sac for identification of a CPPV was evaluated in neonates, infants, and children undergoing unilateral inguinal hernia repair.

Methods.—Laparoscopic evaluation for a CPPV through the ipsilateral hernia sac was performed in 100 children who would have undergone routine exploration of the contralateral side. Age range of 79 boys and 21 girls was 4 weeks to 11 years. If a CPPV was identified, the other side was explored.

Results.—Of 100 children, 48 had a CPPV identified. These children underwent contralateral repair with operative findings of a sac larger than 2 cm in length. Fifty-two children without CPPV did not undergo exploration. There were no significant differences in the rate of CPPV based on the side of the initial hernia. Girls had a higher rate of CPPV than boys (67% vs. 44%). Infants age 6 months and younger had a significantly higher rate of CPPV than older children (64% vs. 30%). At an average follow-up of 7 months postoperatively, there were no episodes of contralateral hernias or hydroceles in patients who did not have a CPPV detected at laparoscopy and subsequently did not undergo contralateral exploration.

Conclusion.—Laparoscopic evaluation through the symptomatic hernia sac is safe and accurate and may be used to avoid contralateral exploration in infants and children who would otherwise need to undergo routine contralateral exploration. Because it is not possible to predict which patients with CPPV will have a hernia, all must undergo repair. Infants 6 months and younger are more likely than other children to have CPPV.

► In the days when general anesthesia was less safe for small children, a routine bilateral inguinal exploration was recommended in all boys younger than 2 years and in all girls, regardless of the age (because there is no vas deferens to be injured here). At present, a more selective approach may be warranted. This is one of several articles in the last few years that have attempted to identify, by laparoscopy, which infants and children with a unilateral inguinal hernia are at risk of developing a contralateral hernia. The use of a 70-degree telescope is difficult, but elegantly exposes the internal inguinal ring on the other side through the ipsilateral hernia sac, thereby avoiding an additional (umbilical) incision. The findings are similar to those of other recent studies, in that roughly 50% of patients have a contralateral patent processus vaginalis. In the end, however, the authors are forced to admit that a patent processus is not synonymous with a hernia; a true contralateral hernia may not develop in more than 5% to 15% of the children, and nobody knows which ones. In light of this, the recommendations of this study (laparoscopy in all, and contralateral exploration in those with a patent processus) seem excessive.

F.I. Luks, M.D.

The Relationship Between Disturbed Transit and Dilated Bowel, and Manometric Findings of Dilated Bowel in Patients With Duodenal Atresia and Stenosis

Takahashi A, Tomomasa T, Suzuki N, et al (Gunma Children's Med Ctr, Japan; Gunma Univ, Japan)

J Pediatr Surg 32:1157–1160, 1997 10–26

Introduction.—Disturbed gastrointestinal transit occurs in some patients after surgical correction of duodenal atresia and stenosis (DA-S). It has been suggested that the disturbed transit in patients with DA-S is associated with impaired function of dilated duodenum proximal to the obstruction. The contractile profile of duodenum proximal to the anastomosis and risk factors for disturbed transit in patients with DA-S were evaluated.

Methods.—Records of 18 patients with duodenal atresia and 12 patients with duodenal stenosis were reviewed retrospectively for information concerning gestational age, birth weight, gender, presence or absence of heart anomaly, Down's syndrome, postoperative complications, and degree of descending dilatation before and 2 weeks after surgery (dependent variables). A multivariate analysis was performed using the degree of disturbed features as independent variables. Physiologic function of the dilated bowel was evaluated by manometry of dilated bowel in 8 patients. The duration and frequency of phase 1, 2, and 3 contraction, the migration velocity of phase 3, and the mean amplitude of contraction were compared with data from normal infants.

Results.—The presence of postoperative complications and existence of bowel dilatation 2 weeks after surgery were determined to be risk factors for disturbed transit. Six of 8 patients who were measured had 1 or 2 episodes of phase 3 during the recorded period. Low contraction amplitude of phase 2 and 3 was the most distinctive manometric finding.

Conclusion.—There was a relationship between dilated bowel and disturbed transit during the postoperative period. Low contraction amplitude of the dilated bowel was the most remarkable finding. Patients with markedly dilated bowel may benefit from tapering or plication of dilated bowel.

► Infants with duodenal atresia often experience prolonged postoperative feeding difficulties, sometimes lasting months to years. The high overall incidence of intestinal dysmotility has often been blamed on the frequent association of this condition with Down's syndrome (present in one third of the patients, according to this and most other series). The authors of the present article did not find the association with trisomy 21 to be an independent risk factor for disturbed duodenal transit. Rather, they believe that (chronic, antenatal) dilation of the duodenum is at fault. This is a hopeful conclusion, because intestinal tapering during the initial operation may treat the problem.

F.I. Luks, M.D.

Gastrointestinal Myoelectric Activity in a Child With Gastroschisis and Ileal Atresia

Cheng G, Langham MR Jr, Sninsky CA, et al (Univ of Florida, Gainesville; VA Med Ctr, Gainesville, Fla)

J Pediatr Surg 32:923–927, 1997 10–27

Background.—Impaired intestinal transit and atresia are commonly associated with repair of gastroschisis, but little is known about how this occurs. Electrodes were placed in the stomach and proximal small bowel of a child who didn't respond to gastroschisis repair, and myoelectric activity was correlated with the clinical course after repair.

Case Report.—Boy, 37 weeks' gestation, had gastroschisis diagnosed prenatally. He underwent repair immediately after birth, and a Ladd's procedure with abdominal wall closure at 4 days. The child underwent enterolysis at 2 months of age, but subsequently had such severe reflux that he was unable to tolerate feedings. Reoperation at 5 months of age involved a wedge resection of bowel with an end-to-end ileoileostomy and a Stamm gastrostomy. At this time, 2 electrodes were sutured to the jejunum at the ligament of Treitz and 20 cm distally, and 2 electrodes were sutured to the anterior gastric wall near the greater curvature. Electrodes exited through stab incisions in the left abdominal wall. Bipolar myoelectric activity (a total of 1,877 minutes [31.3 hours]) was recorded regularly during the next 13 days.

Findings.—Gastric dysrhythmias were common, including tachygastria, retrograde migrating myoelectric complex propagation, and retrograde propagated jejunal activity fronts. The electrodes provided important information about the clinical response to gastrostomy tube feedings. On day 8, Pedialyte delivered via a gastrostomy tube caused jejunal myoelectric activity to mimic that of the fed state, although tachygastria persisted. On day 10, quarter-strength Progestimil was begun and the fedlike pattern remained. The gastrostomy tube feedings were stopped on day 10 and the electrodes were removed on day 13 because of abdominal distension and persistent fever, respectively.

After the abdominal distension resolved, the gastrostomy tube feeding resumed, and by 4 weeks the child was tolerating Progestimil at 25 mL/hr. As the child responded positively or negatively, the Progestimil dose was changed until at discharge 4 months later, he was receiving 40 mL/hr. The gastrostomy tube feedings were weaned until he was taking all food by mouth at 20 months of age.

Conclusions.—Gastric and small bowel electrodes gave useful information on myoelectric activity in this young child. This information helped shape clinical decision making, with no adverse effects noted. Although more research is needed, the placement of monitoring electrodes seems a feasible way in which to examine altered gastrointestinal motility in children.

▶ This case report proves that a detailed and meaningful study can be obtained from a single case. The authors have elegantly described the intestinal dysmotility at the myoelectric level in this complicated case of gastroschisis, and have documented the reversal to a more normal peristaltic pattern. Let's hope that a future paper will report on the systematic use of this direct, yet minimally invasive technique, so that it's predictive value and therapeutic relevance can be evaluated.

F.I. Luks, M.D.

Comparison of Conventional Anterior Surgery and Laparoscopic Surgery for Inguinal-hernia Repair

Liem MSL, van der Graaf Y, van Steensel CJ, et al (Univ Hosp Utrecht, The Netherlands; Ikazia Hosp, Rotterdam, The Netherlands; St Clara Hosp, Rotterdam, The Netherlands; et al)

N Engl J Med 336:1541–1547, 1997 10–28

Introduction.—Postoperative recovery for inguinal hernias may be slow, but results of surgical repair often are satisfactory. In terms of postoperative pain and recovery, laparoscopic techniques for the repair of inguinal hernia have proved to be superior to open repair in small studies. This multicenter, randomized study compares conventional anterior repair with extraperitoneal laparoscopic repair in terms of recovery, complications, and recurrence rates in patients with primary or first recurrent unilateral hernias.

Methods.—Extraperitoneal laparoscopic repair was done in 487 patients and conventional anterior repair in 507 patients. At 1 week, 6 weeks, 6 months, and 1–2 years after surgery, follow-up was conducted to record information about postoperative recovery, complications, and recurrences.

Results.—Wound abscesses were found in 6 patients in the open-surgery group, but in none in the laparoscopic group. A more rapid recovery was seen in the laparoscopic group. Resumption of normal daily activity occurred in a median of 6 days in the laparoscopic group compared with 10 days in the open-surgery group. The laparoscopic group returned to work at a median of 14 days and the open-surgery group returned to work at a median of 21 days. Athletic activities were resumed at 24 days for the laparoscopic group and at 36 days for the open-surgery group. The laparoscopic group reported less pain after surgery than the open-surgery group. On the day of surgery, 33% of the open-surgery group did not require analgesic drugs for postoperative pain, whereas in the laparoscopic group, 59% did not require drugs. In the open-surgery group, 31 patients (6%) had recurrences with a median follow-up of 607 days, whereas 17 patients (3%) in the laparoscopic group had recurrences. In the laparoscopic group, all but 3 of the recurrences occurred within 1 year after surgery and were related to surgeon errors. During the first year, 15 patients in the open-surgery group had recurrences and 16 had them in the second year.

Conclusion.—Patients who have open-surgical repair with inguinal hernias recover more slowly and have more recurrences than those who have laparoscopic repair.

Cooperative Hernia Study: Pain in the Postrepair Patient

Cunningham J, Temple WJ, Mitchell P, et al (Dalhousie Univ, Halifax, NS; Univ of Calgary, Alta)

Ann Surg 224:598–602, 1996 10–29

Introduction.—Inguinofemoral hernia repairs are very common surgical procedures, but the long-term outcome of this treatment has not been evaluated in prospective, randomized trials. Such a design was used in The Cooperative Hernia Study, which assessed postoperative pain and numbness in 3 standard hernia repairs.

Methods.—From a group of 818 patients scheduled for elective hernia repair, 276 (315 hernia repairs) met entry criteria and were seen at follow-up. Patients were randomized during the operative procedure to 1 of 3 standard hernia repairs: Bassini, McVay, or Shouldice. Follow-up information was obtained at 6 months, then annually for 5 years. Pain was classified as mild, moderate, or severe. Patients were examined at 1 and 2 years for recurrence, new hernia, testicular atrophy, and distribution of pain and paresthesia.

Results.—Moderate or severe pain was reported by 55.5% of patients in the immediate postoperative period, by 11.9% at 1 year, and by 10.6% at 2 years. The incidence of any groin or inguinal pain was 62.9% at 1 year and 53.6% at 2 years. Variables associated with long-term pain were the absence of a palpable, visible bulge preoperatively, the presence of moderate or severe immediate postoperative discomfort, and the need for a medical leave of absence for 4 weeks or more after surgery. At both 1 and 2 years, numbness alone was more common than pain or pain with numbness. There was no relationship between type of repair and the presence of numbness. Three types of chronic pain were identified: somatic ligamentous (the most common and severe); neuropathic; and visceral, ejaculatory pain (described by a single patient).

Conclusion.—Long-term pain and numbness are common sequelae of standard hernia surgical repair. Many patients remain debilitated, even 2 years postoperatively. Numbness, although reported frequently, was not a cause of morbidity. Somatic pain might be prevented by avoiding periosteal sutures at the insertion of the inguinal ligament at the pubic tubercle.

▶ The role of laparoscopic surgery in repair of inguinal hernia remains unsettled. This multicenter, randomized trial (Abstract 10–28) of laparoscopic vs. conventional anterior surgery attempts to settle the debate. Unfortunately, despite success in enrolling patients in this randomized trial, no standardized anterior approach was used for repair. Reconstruction of the inguinal floor was accomplished with nonabsorbable sutures, and only if necessary was a mesh prosthesis implanted. Not surprisingly, recurrence rates were lower at 2 years for the laparoscopic approach, given the use of a tension-free repair.

One of the most important findings of the study, however, may be the decrease in chronic pain after repair by the laparoscopic technique compared with the open technique. This is especially important considering the report of Cunningham and coworkers (Abstract 10–29) from the Cooperative Hernia Study, in which 53.6% of patients had pain at 2 years after repair, with 10.6% of patients reporting moderate-to-severe pain. Reduction of chronic pain syndromes after hernia repair, in combination with early return to work, certainly may make up for the added expense of laparoscopic repair.

W.G. Cioffi, M.D.

Early Postoperative Feeding After Elective Colorectal Surgery

Hartsell PA, Frazee RC, Harrison JK, et al (Texas A&M Univ, Temple)

Arch Surg 132:518–521, 1997 10–30

Background.—Research has shown that routine nasogastric decompression after abdominal surgery is not necessary and can be eliminated safely. One study has demonstrated the safety of early oral feedings. The hypothesis that successful early feeding would shorten the duration of hospitalization and reduce costs after elective colorectal surgery was tested.

Methods.—Fifty-eight patients undergoing elective colorectal surgery were randomly assigned to early feeding (group 1) or traditional feeding (group 2). All patients in group 1 began a liquid diet the day after surgery and progressed to a regular diet after consuming 1,000 mL in 24 hours. All group 2 patients began a liquid diet after the postoperative ileus was resolved and progressed to a regular diet after consuming 1,000 mL in 24 hours. These treatments were ended after two thirds of the regular diet could be tolerated. Both groups had intraoperative orogastric tubes removed at the end of surgery. Persistent postoperative vomiting was treated by means of nasogastric tube insertion.

Findings.—Rates of nausea or vomiting in the 2 groups were comparable (occurring in about half the patients in each group). Aspiration pneumonia developed in 1 patient in group 1. One patient in group 2 had an anastomotic leak resulting in sepsis and death. Length of hospitalization did not differ between the groups.

Conclusions.—Most patients tolerate early oral feeding after elective colorectal surgery. Although this such feeding is safe, it does not significantly reduce length of hospital stay.

▶ This prospective, randomized study of the 58 patients undergoing elective colorectal operations concludes that early oral postoperative feeding is safe; however, it does not significantly affect the length of hospital stay. Several interesting points for discussion have been raised by recent studies analyzing hospital length of stay after major gastrointestinal operations, in particular, colorectal surgical procedures. The technical feasibility of laparoscopy-assisted colorectal surgery led many surgeons to anticipate significantly shorter lengths of stay. Although laparoscopy-assisted colorectal surgery is commonly performed, a significantly shorter length of stay has generally not been observed. An abdominal incision is still generally required to extract an often-voluminous intestinal specimen, and the duration of postoperative ileus has generally not been found to be any shorter. The relative merit of laparoscopic surgery has been to feed patients in the postoperative period without waiting for return of bowel function, as evidenced by bowel evacuations. If the same rules are applied to patients who have undergone traditional open surgical techniques, no differences in the length of stay are generally observed. Other technical points, such as use of oral gastric decompression limited to the intraoperative phase, as well as use of epidural catheters for postoperative analgesia, may play a role in the shortening of postoperative hospital stay after major operations on the colon and rectum. In summary, it appears that the only effective method to significantly shorten hospital length of stay after elective colorectal surgery is to discharge patients home while they are still receiving a liquid diet and before objective return of bowel function. The safety and feasibility of this method may be related to the need for closer home care by a visiting nurse.

V.E. Pricolo, M.D.

Long-term Outcome After Ileocecal Resection for Crohn's Disease

Kim NK, Senagore AJ, Luchtefeld MA, et al (Ferguson-Blodgett Digestive Disease Inst, Grand Rapids, Mich; Michigan State Univ, East Lansing)

Am Surg 63:627–633, 1997 10–31

Background.—Concerns about early recurrence and the potential for multiple small bowel resections resulting in gastroenteric crippling usually affect the decision to operate on patients with ileocecal Crohn's disease. However, delaying surgical treatment may unnecessarily prolong a patient's disease state and increase the risk of complications from medication or unchecked disease. The long-term clinical outcomes of patients undergoing ileocecal resection for Crohn's disease between 1970 and 1993 are reported.

Methods and Findings.—One hundred eighty-one patients undergoing ileocecal resection for Crohn's disease were reviewed. Median follow-up was 14.3 years. Mean age at first resection was 32.7 years. Initial resection was indicated by intractability in 68.4%, obstruction in 25.9%, enteric fistula in 15.5%, perforation in 9.2%, intra-abdominal abscess in 4%, and hemorrhage in 2.9%. Postoperative complications included prolonged ileus in 7.5%, pneumonia/atelectasis in 8.6%, wound infection in 6.3%, urinary tract infection in 5.7%, intra-abdominal abscess in 4%, and wound dehiscence in 0.6%. No operative deaths occurred. Recurrence necessitating additional surgery occurred in 30.9% of the patients, at a mean interval of 72.3 months. A second recurrence developed in 10.5% of the patients, at a mean interval of 52.3 months. The sites of first recurrences were the preanastomotic ileum in 87.5% of the patients, postanastomotic colon in 17.9%, other colonic sites in 28.6%, other small bowel sites in 3.6%, and other sites in 7.1%. Types of resection for first recurrences were ileal in 50%, right hemicolectomy in 30.4%, segmental colectomy in 10.7%, total proctocolectomy in 5.4%, and proximal small bowel resection in 3.6%. By the end of follow-up, 69.1% of the patients had only 1 resection, 20.4% had 2, 8.3% had 3, and 2.2% had 4.

Conclusions.—Ileocecal resection of Crohn's disease is associated with a high rate of disease control, low morbidity, and a low frequency of 3 or more bowel resections. Thus surgical resection of ileocecal Crohn's disease should not be delayed unduly because of concerns about the possibility of short bowel syndrome. Such an approach should minimize overall disease-related patient morbidity by avoiding long periods of chronic disease.

► In this review of a large cohort of Crohn's disease patients undergoing ileocecal resection (the most common operation for this condition), several interesting observations are made. The recurrence rate requiring further surgery (30.9%) and a second recurrence (10.5%) found the preanastomotic ileum to be by far the most common site (87.5%), more so than the postanastomotic colon (17.9%). In addition, even patients who required multiple resection for re-recurrences had an excellent rate of disease control obtained with low morbidity and a very low frequency of 3 or more bowel resections (2.2%)*. These findings should encourage our gastroenterology colleagues not to unduly delay referral of patients for resectional surgery for fear of inevitable recurrence or short-gut syndrome, once "end-stage" Crohn's disease or its complications are detected.

* These data are generally more encouraging than the usually quoted 50–50 risk of reoperative surgery, after small bowel resection, for recurrent Crohn's disease.

V.E. Pricolo, M.D.

Diagnostic Dilemma of Small Incidentally Discovered Adrenal Masses: Role for ^{131}I-6β-Iodomethyl-Norcholesterol Scintigraphy

Kloos RT, Gross MD, Shapiro B, et al (Univ of Michigan, Ann Arbor)
World J Surg 21:36–40, 1997 10–32

Introduction.—Up to 5% of patients who undergo CT have incidentally discovered adrenal masses. In the absence of known extra-adrenal primary malignancy, most of these masses are benign. Small masses 3 cm in diameter or smaller, however, can be difficult to characterize with various imaging methods. The patients in this study underwent ^{131}I-6β-Iodomethyl-norcholesterol (NP59) scintigraphy in at attempt to determine the nature of their small adrenal masses.

Methods.—The study group included 166 patients with unilateral adrenal masses discovered incidentally at CT. Most patients underwent CT because of abdominal pain or for staging of known or suspected malignancy. None had clinically suspected adrenal disease. All received NP59 (1 mCi) injected IV, followed by abdominal scans performed 1 or more times between 5 and 10 days after injection. Various combinations of blood and urine biochemical measurements were also obtained.

Results.—There were 82 men and 84 women with a mean age of 59.0 years. Masses were right-sided in 76 cases and left-sided in 90. In 28 patients, a final diagnosis of adenoma was made by adrenalectomy or CT-guided adrenal biopsy. Adenoma was confirmed in 104 patients who had no change in adrenal appearance on repeat CT scans or at clinical follow-up of 6 months or more. Adrenalectomy or specimens from CT-guided adrenal biopsy detected and confirmed the presence of 14 intra-adrenal space-occupying or destructive lesions other than adenomas. Seven of these masses were caused by metastatic lung carcinoma; other conditions responsible were adrenal cysts, leukemia, metastatic colon adenocarcinoma, metastatic renal carcinoma, pheochromocytoma, and an adrenal hematoma.

Conclusion.—Small, incidentally discovered adrenal masses need to be examined to determine their origin. Although most of these masses are simple nonhypersecretory adenomas, a proportion prove to be a primary adrenal malignancy or metastatic disease in the adrenals. Findings in this series of patients confirm the value of NP59 scintigraphy in the evaluation of adrenal masses.

► With the increased use of CT and MRI for the evaluation of various disease states, an increased number of adrenal masses are now being incidentally discovered. Although size of the mass serves as a discriminator between malignant and nonmalignant lesions, adrenal malignancies of less than 3 cm have been well described. The role of NP59 imaging in patients with incidentally discovered small adrenal lesions appears to be superior to that of conventional imaging techniques.

The enthusiasm of the authors, however, must be tempered, as the sensitivity of this technique in lesions of less than 3 cm was only 39%.

Although the diagnostic accuracy was respectable (90%), and the specificity was 100%, the true utility of NP59 scintigraphy as a cost-effective means of investigating small adrenal masses remains unproven. The results of this study would suggest that NP59 scintigraphy may certainly be valuable in the decision-making process for patients with incidentally discovered small adrenal masses and a nonadrenal primary neoplasm.

W.G. Cioffi, M.D.

Improved Long-term Outcome for Patients With Jejunoileal Apple Peel Atresia

Waldhausen JHT, Sawin RS (Univ of Washington, Seattle)

J Pediatr Surg 32:1307–1309, 1997 10–33

Introduction.—The rarest type of intestinal atresia is apple peel deformity (type IIIb), in which the distal ileum receives its blood supply from the ileocolic or right colic artery in a retrograde manner. This congenital anomaly has been associated with a high rate of mortality, and is caused by significant loss of small intestine and feeding intolerance. At the study institution, however, surgical management has achieved excellent long-term outcome.

Methods.—In a retrospective review of 12 patients treated over an 11-year period, investigators examined short- and long-term complications and outcome, evolution in care, and current recommendations for therapy. Children were assessed for weight gain and growth, dietary needs, bowel function, and overall development.

Results.—The 10 girls and 2 boys were born at a mean gestational age of 35.9 weeks. Associated anomalies were present in 6 infants. Surgery revealed evidence of utero bowel perforation in 5 cases, malrotation in 3, and additional bowel atresias in 4. The mean intestinal length from the ligament of Treitz to the proximal atresia was only 29.3 cm; the segment of bowel distal to the atresia ending at the ileocecal valve had a mean length of 32.1 cm. Seven infants underwent a primary anastomosis, 3 had end enterostomies, and 2 had a Bishop-Koop anastomosis. Enterostomy closure occurred at an average of 2 months after operation. The mean period of hospitalization was 67 days; an average of 39 days of hyperalimentation was required. Nine infants were discharged on oral feeds alone. With a mean follow-up of 5.1 years, 8 of 11 children available for review are gaining weight and growing along a stable curve between the 5th and 50th percentile. Three children, including 2 with chromosomal abnormalities, require gastrostomy supplementation to maintain adequate growth. All have acceptable bowel function and none have short bowel physiology.

Conclusion.—Improvements in surgical and feeding techniques have led to an improved outlook for children with apple peel atresia. Initial operative management should include the use of hyperalimentation, a gastrostomy tube, and primary anastomosis with enteroplasty or resection of the dilated proximal segment.

▶ This optimistic article reflects the many improvements in surgical technique (tapering enteroplasty, more liberal use of primary anastomosis) and parenteral nutrition that have changed the outlook for infants with extensive intestinal atresia. Still, these patients may have been exceptionally lucky: Apple-peel atresia and multiple intestinal atresias, which likely result from catastrophic in utero vascular accidents, are sometimes associated with severe malfunction and malabsorption of the remaining intestine. In these cases, even the optimal management reported here may not allow these children to be weaned off parenteral nutrition, exposing them to all the complications of short bowel syndrome.

F.I. Luks, M.D.

Necrotizing Enterocolitis: Diagnosis With CT Examination of Urine After Enteral Administration of Iodinated Water-soluble Contrast Material

Rencken IO, Sola A, Al-Ali F, et al (Univ of Carolina, San Francisco)
Radiology 205:87–90, 1997 10–34

Introduction.—The diagnosis of necrotizing enterocolitis in neonates has depended upon demonstration of intramural air in the bowel, portal venous air, or pneumoperitoneum on abdominal radiographs. These findings, however, are not always present or certain, and clinical signs may not be specific or sensitive. To develop a safe and objective diagnostic test, researchers measured in vitro the CT attenuation coefficient of imaged excreted urine after administration of water-soluble contrast material.

Methods.—Thirty-five neonates were studied. Group 1 included 13 premature infants who were imaged without contrast material. The 10 neonates in group 2 underwent upper gastrointestinal studies for diagnostic purposes. Infants in groups 1 and 2 had no clinical evidence of necrotizing enterocolitis. The 5 neonates in group 3 had suspected (stage I) necrotizing enterocolitis, and the 7 neonates in group 4 had definite (stage II) necrotizing enterocolitis. Mean gestational ages in the 4 groups ranged from 34.2 to 36.2 weeks. Neonates in groups 2, 3, and 4 received an oral solution of iohexol diluted with sterile water. The solution was administered via an indwelling orogastric tube over 30 minutes. To allow passage of the solution into the bowel, gastric suction was discontinued for 2 hours. The attenuation coefficient of each urine specimen was determined with CT.

Results.—There was a slight increase in CT attenuation coefficients with increasing specific gravity of urine. Neonates who did not receive iohexol had a mean CT attenuation coefficient of urine of 5.6 Hounsfield units (HU). In neonates without necrotizing enterocolitis who underwent upper gastrointestinal study, the mean value was 6.7 HU. In patients with suspected or definite necrotizing enterocolitis, mean CT attenuation coefficients of urine were 26.0 HU and 71.0 HU, respectively. The difference between neonates with and without the disease was significant. No infants had side effects from enteral administration of contrast material. In some cases, CT examination of urine samples enabled positive prediction of necrotizing enterocolitis at least 24 hours before surgery.

Conclusion.—Prompt diagnosis of necrotizing enterocolitis is essential, but early radiographic signs are often absent. Examination of urine with CT after enteral administration of iohexol may allow very early detection of the disease.

► This is a truly creative method to obtain a very early diagnosis of necrotizing enterocolitis. The use of a CT scanner to measure the urinary concentration of iodine seems rather peculiar (that's a very big gantry for such a small specimen cup). The test's principle, however, is similar to the measurement of urinary lactulose or other macromolecules to evaluate bowel wall integrity in inflammatory bowel disease or after small bowel transplantation.

F.I. Luks, M.D.

Colon, Rectum, and Anus

INTRODUCTION

Differentiating various abdominal pathologic disorders from appendicitis continues to challenge the general surgeon. The use of high-frequency compression sonography in children and adults with acute abdominal pain has improved diagnostic accuracy and outcomes. Rarely is the appendix visualized on routine abdominal sonography. Further, acute appendicitis cannot be conclusively identified sonographically without high-frequency linear transducers and carefully graded compression. The diagnosis of acute appendicitis is based typically on clinical findings only; diagnosis of atypical presentations may be assisted by the use of plain abdominal films, barium enemas, and abdominal sonography. Computed tomography (CT) has been widely used in adults to diagnose appendicitis, with accuracy equal to or higher than that of US. In children, however, CT has been littled used, with no large series addressing its findings. Jabra and associates (Abstract 10–35) attempted to clarify the role of CT for evaluating appendicitis in children. The authors found that CT helped in their diagnosing of appendicitis in children, especially if US findings were negative or equivocal. The major role of CT may be for cases with complicated appendicitis, to define the extent of the pathologic process. The authors further emphasized the importance of CT scanning with thin sections, intravenous contrast material, and well-opacified bowel loops. Cost-effectiveness and possible overuse of CT were not discussed.

In 1886, Reginald H. Fitz of the Boston City Hospital consolidated opinion and treatment philosophies regarding the pathophysiology of appendicitis. As emphasized in the review of Hale and associates (Abstract 10–36), current approaches for diagnosis and early treatment remain a paradox. Perforation rates of 20% to 30% have remained constant for 70 years despite many technological improvements since the 1930s. Most cases of appendiceal perforation had not received preoperative surgical evaluation, suggesting that early evaluation and access to care are important criteria. As emphasized, however, by Berry and Malt,[1] modern surgical therapy reduced mortality of appendicitis from 26% to less than 1%. Hale and associates report an overall mortality rate of 0.08%, but rates of perforation and negative appendectomies remain unchanged, as they are influenced primarily by factors outside the realm of technology and physician intervention. Perforation disproportionately affects the very young and the very old, perhaps related to delays in presentation and diagnosis due to confounding medical conditions, decreased suspicion, and lack of communication. The authors conclude that reduction in the rate of perforation will not occur until patients seek earlier evaluation and intervention.

Brasel and associates (Abstract 10–37) performed a decision- and cost-utility analysis for contaminated appendectomy wounds, recommending primary closure over delayed primary closure for management of contaminated right lower quadrant incisions. The potential negative impact of forced cost-effectiveness in this era of managed care and cost-restructing is paramount to a large number of ongoing prospective studies that are attempting to clarify the literature relative to morbidity, mortality, and quality-of-life issues.

Since the original description by Swenson and Bill[2] in 1948 of the reconstructive procedure to treat Hirschsprung's disease, neonates have been treated soon after diagnosis with a defunctioning colostomy. The three-stage procedure designed for older patients was a more definitive pull-through procedure followed by colostomy closure. The latter procedure was advocated because it was thought unsafe to perform a definitive operation in neonates. Wilcox and associates (Abstract 10–38) report on a 10-year experience for the treatment of Hirschsprung's disease during the neonatal period with a one-stage pull-through procedure. Short- and long-term results were equivalent to those with the three-stage procedure; benefits are that there are fewer procedures, no stoma is required, and the hospital stay is shorter. This one-stage approach promises a reduction in morbidity and should be performed by pediatric surgical teams experienced in this procedure. Evaluation of the long-term outcomes of this series is advisable.

Rintala and associates (Abstract 10–39) compared bowel function in normal healthy children to bowel function in children after repair of a low anorectal malformation. The need for careful follow-up and documentation cannot be overemphasized. Only half of the children with low anorectal malformations had age-appropriate normal bowel function after attempted repairs. The authors further suggested that long-term follow-up is essential to manage the major functional problem, constipation, which is also the etiology of soiling. Late diagnosis of low anorectal malformations may predispose patients to functional abnormalities. Awareness and recognition of mild anorectal anomalies are essential for pediatricians and other primary care physicians.

In this YEAR BOOK, at least four papers deal with inflammatory bowel disease (IBD), pouch ileoanal construction, and their outcomes. The management of patients with mucosal ulcerative colitis and familial adenomatous polyposis frequently includes a restorative proctocolectomy after ileal pouch–anal anastomosis. The procedure has also been utilized, with limited success, in the management of megarectum and megacolon. Despite the complexity of the pouch reconstructions that are apparently utilized internationally, complications are low (3.5% to 12%). Typical etiologies for pouch failure are anastomotic leaks/dehiscence, pelvic abscess and sepsis, strictures and pouch fistulas, as well as diminished pouch function as a consequence of the aforementioned events. Ogunbiyi and colleagues (Abstract 10–40) reported on their attempts to salvage ileal pouch function, concluding that salvage surgery for major complications following ileoanal pouch construction is warranted in the absence of major pelvic sepsis. Success was achieved in half of the patients, of whom the majority had acceptable results. Although significant perianal disease is a relative contraindication to the pelvic pouch procedure for concern of misdiagnosis of Crohn's disease, the procedure has been infrequently offered to selected patients. Despite this adopted policy, in some clinics throughout the world, the effect of preexisting perianal pathology on the outcome and function of pelvic pouches is not well understood. To delineate these issues, Richard and associates (Abstract 10–41) compared 52 patients who had previous pelvic pouch reconstruction and were known prospectively to have perianal disease with a large group of pouch patients *without* prior perianal disease. Pouch failure was not significantly different between the two groups, nor was the subsequent diagnosis of Crohn's disease different. There was no significant difference in outcome according to the type of perianal lesion or the history of perianal surgery, suggesting that the pelvic pouch may be acceptable for select individuals with colitis and prior perianal disease. The continuing concern with neoplastic transformation in the neorectal ileal mucosa for patients with ulcerative colitis who had previously required an ileal-pelvic pouch with ileoanal anastomosis (IPAA) was addressed by Gullberg and colleagues (Abstract 10–42), who evaluated whether persistent severe villous atrophy in the IPAA mucosa was a risk for subsequent neoplastic development. The authors determined that patients with ulcerative colitis and a long-standing IPAA who developed this pathologic mucosal atrophy are at risk for neoplastic transformation of mucosa within the pouch. Additional approaches include evaluation with flow cytometry and oncogene protein expression to determine the early molecular events that indicate neoplastic alterations. Intensive follow-up with biopsy is warranted when this pathologic transformation is evident. A similar evaluation was conducted by Marcello and associates, who studied patients with idiopathic IBD to determine the implications of pathologic diagnosis on the subsequent complications and outcomes. Marcello and colleagues (Abstract 10–43) attempted to define the evolving natural history of patients with indeterminate colitis and Crohn's disease who have undergone reconstruction with an IPAA. This is one of the largest prospective analyses (n = 543 patients) with idiopathic IBD that evaluates changes in the pathologic diagnosis with time and its ultimate effect on outcome. This paper emphasized the importance of accurate diagnostic differentiation and caution by the surgeon in advising the IPAA procedure for individuals with indeterminate colitis, and the complications that are inevitable with misdiagnosis.

Fecal incontinence confers physiologic, monetary, and social consequences on its sufferers. While many patients' conditions can be managed with medical measures alone, variations in activity and demanding work and social schedules are often unsatisfactory. Moreover, those with severe incontinence cannot have a normal lifestyle in the absence of surgical correction. Two new surgical procedures increase the probability for restoration of continence for those for whom conventional management has failed. The gracilis muscle transposition, which can be electrically stimulated, shows promise. Christiansen and Lorentzen[3] recently reported on a successful artificial anal sphincter. Wong and associates (Abstract 10–44) used a fully implantable artificial anal sphincter in 12 patients who had previously had conventional management of fecal incontinence that failed. Continence can be restored with acceptable morbidity. Long-term studies are not yet available but are essential. Lehur and associates (Abstract 10–45) evaluated the identical artificial sphincter reported by Wong and associates, and also recommended it for treatment of severe anal incontinence where local therapies are not applicable or have failed.

Lord (Abstract 10–46) found the frequency of anorectal disease in homosexual males infected with HIV to be 6% to 34%. It is the most common reason for surgical intervention in these patients. The incidence of anorectal disease is much higher in this population than in the general community, as are human papilloma virus–related diseases and AIDS-related cancers. Studies have examined anorectal disease in HIV-infected patients, but the natural history and etiology remain unclear, with no definitive treatment yet established. Lord noted that when CD4+ T-lymphocyte counts were less than 50 cells µL, healing was significantly impaired. Wound repair remains a significant problem in these patients infected with HIV, when this lymphoctye population is depleted. Little or no benefit was found from invasive operations in cases with CD4+ counts less than 50/µL, but Lord recommended thorough examination with adequate biopsies, performed with the patient under general anesthesia. This important paper suggested that severe immunosuppression indicated by a low CD4+ count (less than 50 cells/µL) predicts impaired wound healing and is expected in those with chronic, usually posterior midline fissures or ulcers, such as HIV patients with suppressed lymphocyte populations.

Kirby I. Bland, M.D.

References

1. Berry JJ, Malt RA: Appendicitis near its centenary. *Ann Surg* 200:567–575, 1984.
2. Swenson O, Bill AH Jr: Resection of rectum and rectosigmoid with preservation of the sphincter for benign spastic lesions producing megacolons: An experimental study. *Surgery* 24:212–220, 1948.

3. Christiansen J, Lorentzen M: Implantation of artificial sphincter for anal incontinence. *Lancet* 1:244–245, 1987.

CT of Appendicitis in Children

Jabra AA, Shalaby-Rana EI, Fishman EK (Johns Hopkins Med Institutions, Baltimore, Md; Children's Natl Med Ctr, Washington, DC)

J Comput Assist Tomogr 21:661–666, 1997 10–35

Background.—Although CT is often used to help diagnose appendicitis in adults, there are few reports of its usefulness for this purpose in children. The CT findings of appendicitis were reviewed in a large series of children.

Methods.—Computed tomography was performed in 22 of 732 children with acute appendicitis to confirm clinical findings of pain, fever, vomiting, diarrhea, and a palpable abdominal mass. A positive CT finding was based on appendiceal wall thickening of more than 1 mm or the presence of an abscess, phlegmon, or pericecal inflammation in association with an appendicolith. In 14 children, ultrasound was also performed within 48 hours of CT, and ultrasound findings were correlated with those of CT.

Findings.—Computed tomography allowed visualization of the appendix in 4 of 22 children (18%), abscesses in 13 (59%), appendicoliths in 10 (45%), bowel wall thickening in 7 (32%), phlegmon in 5 (23%), and pericecal inflammation in 2 (9%). Based on defined diagnostic criteria, CT findings indicated the presence of appendicitis in 11 of 22 children (50%). Compared with ultrasound, CT was slightly better in diagnosing appendicitis, visualizing the abnormal appendix, and defining the presence and extent of abscess and inflammation.

Conclusions.—Computed tomography aided in the diagnosis of appendicitis in half of the children. Its performance was slightly better than that of ultrasound, and its advantages are particularly evident in complicated cases involving fistulas, abnormal air collections, or abdominal wall inflammation. Thus CT should be considered a useful adjunct in diagnosing appendicitis in children.

► The appendix was visualized in only 4 of 22 cases, hardly a stellar performance. Between the availability and growing accuracy of ultrasonography and the ease of surgical exploration (particularly with the advent of laparoscopy), the statement that "CT has a definite role in the diagnosis of appendicitis" seems disingenuous. Computed tomography is most helpful, of course, when an abscess or other complication is suspected.

F.I. Luks, M.D.

Appendectomy: A Contemporary Appraisal

Hale DA, Molloy M, Pearl RH, et al (Quality Assurance Office, Assistant Secretary of Defense [Health Affairs], Washington, DC)

Ann Surg 225:252–261, 1997 10–36

Introduction.—Despite advances in technology over the past 50 years, appendicitis presents a diagnostic challenge, and rates of perforation and negative appendectomy remain unchanged. A 12-month review of appendectomies performed in the 147 Department of Defense hospitals was undertaken to present a comprehensive overview of the practice of appendectomy in the 1990s and to identify factors responsible for inaccurate diagnoses.

Methods.—Medical records of all patients undergoing nonincidental appendectomy over a 12-month period (February 1992 through January 1993) were collected for analysis. The hospitals, located throughout the world, varied considerably in size and surgeons' level of experience. Appendectomies were performed on 4,950 patients during the study period.

Results.—The patients ranged in age from 6 months to 82 years at the time of appendectomy (mean age, 25.5 years). Males outnumbered females (64.4% vs. 35.6%), and whites made up 80.4% of the sample. An operative diagnosis of acute appendicitis was confirmed pathologically in 66.0% of cases; 20.8% had pathologic confirmation of perforated appendicitis. The remaining patients (13.2%) were found to have a normal appendix. Patients younger than 8 years of age and older than 45 had the highest risk of perforation; the negative appendectomy rate was highest in patients younger than 5 years. Males were somewhat more prone to perforation, and females had a significantly higher rate of normal appendices. Race appeared to have little influence on the rates of perforation and normal appendices. Although 90% of patients with appendicitis had an elevated leukocyte count preoperatively, this finding was present in 60% of those with a normal appendix. Relatively few patients in all 3 diagnostic groups had an elevated temperature. Neither type nor size of hospital had any influence on perforation and normal appendix rates. Only 4 deaths (0.08%) occurred in this series; the complication rate was 5.2% (about half were wound infections). Twenty-seven patients, all with acute appendicitis or perforated appendix, required reoperation within 45 days.

Conclusion.—The rates of perforated appendix have remained consistent (20% to 30%) over the last 70 years, but surgical advances have lowered the mortality rate from 26% overall to less that 1% over the same period. Perforation occurs most often in the youngest and oldest age groups, the result of delays in diagnosis. Negative appendectomy rates have remained stable because of the lack of a test or objective physical finding to accurately rule out appendicitis.

13.2 %

▶ As much as things change, things remain the same. The authors have shown that although mortality rates from appendicitis have decreased significantly over 50 years, perforation and negative appendectomy rates remain unchanged. Not surprisingly, the same factors associated with an increased risk of perforation have been noted in earlier studies. Given that technological advances, including advanced imaging techniques, have not altered the rates of these complications, reliance on education and clinical acumen should take precedence over the use of expensive testing modalities in this era of cost consciousness.

W.G. Cioffi, M.D.

Cost-Utility Analysis of Contaminated Appendectomy Wounds

Brasel KJ, Borgstrom DC, Weigelt JA (Univ of Minnesota, St Paul)

J Am Coll Surg 184:23–30, 1997 10–37

Introduction.—Contaminated and dirty surgical wounds are typically left open to reduce the incidence of wound infection and its sequelae. Open wounds are more labor intensive, and expensive to care for, and they limit patient activities. Infected appendectomy incisions have been treated successfully with primary closure (PC). A decision and cost-utility analysis was conducted to determine the effect of right lower quadrant surgical wound infection on quality of life and total cost of wound management in patients treated with PC or delayed primary closure (DPC).

Methods.—A MEDLINE search was conducted of postappendectomy wound infection literature. Institution-specific cost data were collected and utility assignments were made. Studies used included information regarding perforated appendix or gangrenous appendicitis; use of perioperative antibiotics active against aerobic and anaerobic bacteria; and data stratified by wound management, operative findings, and infection rate.

Results.—Compared with DPC and secondary closure (Table 5), the least expensive wound management option and the 1 with greatest utility was PC (Table 4) for all contaminated appendectomy wounds. Decision favored PC over DPC.

TABLE 5.—Cost-Utility Analysis

Wound management	*Incremental cost savings, $**	*Incremental effectiveness†*	*Cost-utility‡ $/QALY*
SC	—	—	—
DPC	DPC cost–SC cost=936	DPC utility–SC utility=0.04	22,340§
PC	PC cost–DPC cost=197	PC utility–DPC utility=0.01	22,635‖

*Costs from Table 4.

†Utility from Table 4.

‡Cost-utility equals incremental cost savings divided by incremental effectiveness.

§Cost savings per population (24 points) treated to gain 1 quality-adjusted life year.

‖Cost savings per population (115 patients) treated to gain 1 quality-adjusted life year.

Abbreviations: QALY, quality-adjusted life year; *SC*, secondary closure; *DPC*, delayed primary closure; *PC*, primary closure.

(By permission of the *Journal of the American College of Surgeons*, courtesy of Brasel KJ, Borgstrom DC, Weigelt JA: Cost-utility analysis of contaminated appendectomy wounds. *J Am Coll Surg* 184:23–30, 1997.)

TABLE 4.—Ultimate Utility and Cost of Wound Management Per Patient

Wound management	*Utility**	*Cost, $*
PC	A+B+C 0.99	2,680
DPC	D+E+F+G+H 0.98	2,877
SC	I+J 0.94	3,813

*Capital letters are weighted utilities from Figure 1 of the original article.
Abbreviations: PC, primary closure; *DPC*, delayed primary closure; *SC*, secondary closure.
(By permission of the *Journal of the American College of Surgeons*, courtesy of Brasel KJ, Borgstrom DC, Weigelt JA: Cost-utility analysis of contaminated appendectomy wounds. *J Am Coll Surg* 184:23–30, 1997.)

Conclusion.—In a challenge to traditional surgical dogma, PC was the preferred method of managing contaminated right lower quadrant incisions in a cost-utility analysis. Findings are specific to right lower quadrant incisions.

▶ The conclusions of this paper have already been adopted by many, if not most, pediatric surgeons. Save for a few exceptions, all appendectomy wounds (even after perforation) can be closed primarily without increasing the risk of wound infection and its sequelae. This study tries to take an unbiased, scientific look at the benefits, in terms of cost and patient comfort (utility). Although assigning utility weight to the various options (PC, DPC, or secondary closure) ends up being somewhat arbitrary, 2-way sensitivity analysis shows that the conclusions remain valid over a wide range of utility values.

Of course, this analysis is only relevant because of its basic tenet: nowadays, secondary infection of a right lower quadrant wound does not lead to necrotizing fasciitis, sepsis, or an incisional hernia; it only converts a closed wound to an open one. If, as the authors suggest, the risk of wound infection after appendectomy is at worst 27%, the vast majority of patients can avoid the nuisance of prolonged open wound care without an increased risk of dreadful complications. And treating patients this way is cheaper.

F.I. Luks, M.D.

One-Stage Neonatal Pull-Through to Treat Hirschsprung's Disease

Wilcox DT, Bruce J, Bowen J, et al (Royal Manchester Children's Hosp, England)

J Pediatr Surg 32:243–247, 1997 10–38

Introduction.—Hirschsprung's disease has historically been treated by a 3-stage procedure because of concerns about performing definitive procedures in the neonatal period. The 3-stage procedure is associated with stoma problems, 3 episodes of hospitalization, and the disadvantage of delayed passage of feces via the rectum. The results of a 1-stage neonatal pull-through were evaluated in 51 patients treated over a 10-year period.

Methods.—Records were reviewed retrospectively to determine results of neonatal pull-through in the treatment of Hirschsprung's disease. The Swenson and the Soave (endorectal pull-through) procedures were used in this patient cohort.

Results.—Eight of 51 children had associated anomalies; 6 had Down's syndrome. Thirteen and 38 patients, respectively, underwent a Soave or a Swenson procedure. Disease was rectosigmoid in 39 patients and the remaining patients had sigmoid, descending colon, or total colonic involvement. Thirteen patients required a mean volume of 55 mL of transfused blood. The mean surgical time was 181 minutes. Complications included wound infection in 3 patients and an anastomotic leak in 2 patients with Down's syndrome who required a second laparotomy and colostomy. There were 2 delayed deaths related to other congenital anomalies. Overall, 2 of 3 patients who required reoperation had a stoma (1 needed a repeat pull-through and 1 had an ileostomy for enterocolitis). The total average length of hospital stay was 20.4 days. The mean follow-up was 3.73 years. Of the 21 patients with follow-up greater than 4 years, 4 patients soiled themselves at least once a week and 17 had normal bowel function.

Conclusion.—Hirschsprung's disease may be successfully treated in the neonatal period using either the Soave or the Swenson 1-stage pull-through procedure. Short- and long-term results of this approach are similar to those of children who undergo the 3-stage procedure with its accompanying need for a stoma and 2 extra hospital stays.

▶ This homogeneous series of infants who underwent a primary pull-through operation for Hirschsprung's disease reflects the general trend in the surgery of this and other congenital conditions. As stated by the authors, the tradition of performing lesser, temporizing operations (such as a colostomy) at birth stems from the days when perioperative care of the newborn was primitive. Now that it has been established that operating at birth is safe, many surgeons have discovered that it can also be advantageous. It is often technically easier (the authors pointedly comment on the shallow pelvis, which greatly facilitates low rectal dissection) and may be beneficial for the neurocortical development of stooling patterns as well.

Although most surgeons agree on this general philosophy, the actual treatment may still vary between, and even within, centers. In this series, some infants were operated on at birth, whereas others had their "neonatal" pull-through at 1 month of age. In the interim, some children will need daily rectal irrigations; a (small?) group will still require a colostomy.

F.I. Luks, M.D.

Do Children With Repaired Low Anorectal Malformations Have Normal Bowel Function?

Rintala RJ, Lindahl HG, Rasanen M (Univ of Helsinki; Alder Hey Children's Hosp, Liverpool, England)

J Pediatr Surg 32:823–826, 1997 10–39

Background.—Recent reports have suggested that bowel problems occur in patients who underwent low anorectal malformation repair as children. Other reports claim that functional defects in this population are rare. Current bowel function was examined in patients who had undergone bowel surgery between 1983 and 1992.

Methods.—Questionnaires regarding bowel function were completed by or on behalf of 40 patients (median age 7 years, range 3–13 years) who had undergone low anorectal repair surgery in the newborn period (in 7 children, diagnosis had been delayed up to 2 years). The control group consisted of 54 age-matched children (median age 6 years, range 3–12 years) who also completed the questionnaire. The maximal bowel function score was 20. Two clinicians also evaluated clinical status as excellent, good, or poor. All participants were toilet trained.

Findings.—The maximal bowel function score was achieved by 54% of the controls (median score 20, mean 19.1 ± 1.3), and a tenth percentile score of the maximal (i.e., 18 points) was set as the lower limit of normality for the patient group. With this criterion, 52% of patients (median score 19, mean 19.3 ± 0.7) also had normal bowel function. Clinical outcomes were excellent in 21 (52%) patients, good in 15 (38%) patients (median bowel function score 17, mean 16.3 ± 2.4; significantly worse than in controls), and fair in 4 patients (10%) (median bowel function score 10, mean 10.5 ± 2.9; significantly worse than in controls). Clinical outcome at the last patient visit correlated strongly with the bowel function score.

Constipation was the most problematic concern; 17 of 40 patients (42%) reported constipation, compared with only 4 of 54 controls (7%). Nine patients (23%) reported social problems because of bowel function, and in 4 of these (10% of the total patient group) fecal soiling substantially curtailed the child's social life. The mean age at toilet training did not differ significantly between the 2 groups, nor did the occurrence of occasional urinary incontinence.

Conclusions.—When compared with healthy controls, only half of patients who had undergone earlier surgical repair of low anorectal malformations had normal bowel function. Constipation was a significant problem and required dietary or medical treatment in 42% of patients. Thus, physicians caring for pediatric patients should examine for bowel dysfunction in patients who have undergone surgical repair. Better results were more likely in patients in who were diagnosed and treated at an early age. Pediatricians should be alert for anorectal anomalies in newborns, and should ensure that any anomalies detected receive prompt treatment.

► Another example of how careful follow-up tempers the initial enthusiasm about a treatment that was previously felt to be "curative." The patient's expectations, as well as ours, should not be too high in these conditions and, to paraphrase Dr. Jan Molenaar (Rotterdam, Netherlands), if we can't render these children continent, let's at least make them content. The only critique of this study has to do with its patient population, which is a somewhat mixed bag of "lesser" anal conditions with a strong male preponderance, which contrasts with the commonly accepted female preponderance of low imperforate anus.

F.I. Luks, M.D.

Pouch Salvage: Long-term Outcome

Ogunbiyi OA, Korsgen S, Keighley MRB, et al (Univ of Birmingham, Edgbaston, England)

Dis Colon Rectum 40:548–552, 1997 10–40

Background.—An increasing number of surgeons are performing restorative proctocolectomy with ileal pouch-anal anastomosis as the procedure of choice in the elective treatment of ulcerative colitis and familial adenomatous polyposis. The complication rate is low, ranging from 3.5% to 12%. The outcome of pouch salvage surgery and the factors that may influence it were investigated.

Methods and Findings.—One hundred ninety-eight patients who had had restorative proctolectomy at 1 center during an 11-year period were reviewed retrospectively. Twenty-seven patients (13.6%) had pouch-specific complications requiring pouch salvage. Another 5 patients needing pouch salvage were referred from other centers. Outcomes of salvage surgery were successful in half of the 32 patients undergoing the procedure. Of the remaining patients, 37.5% had pouch excision, and 9% continue to be defunctionalized. One patient died, for a mortality of 3%. Pelvic sepsis was a major cause of pouch failure, occurring in half the failed procedures and accounting for 58% of pouch excisions.

Conclusions.—In the absence of major pelvic sepsis, salvage surgery for major complications after ileoanal pouch construction is beneficial. The overall success rate is 50%, which may be acceptable to highly motivated patients.

► This retrospective review of approximately 200 patients during an 11-year period deals with the difficult problem of salvaging an ileoanal pouch after severe complications such as fistulas, outlet problems, anastomotic leaks, ischemia, and incontinence. A salvage rate of 50% is described by the authors as not significantly different from figures reported by other major institutions, such as the Mayo Clinic or Cleveland Clinic (50% to 67.5% salvage rate, when all reoperations related to pouch problems are included). The important point that is stressed by the authors is that major pelvic sepsis remains the worst postoperative complication and 1 that is least likely to be associated with a satisfactory attempt to salvage the anatomical and physiologic integrity of the pouch. Performing a temporary ileostomy in the majority of patients at a time of ileoanal pouch reconstruction procedures still remains a very safe option to minimize these potentially disastrous complications. Even after pouch salvage procedures, the functional results may be less than ideal but still preferable to some patients than a conventional ileostomy.

V.E. Pricolo, M.D.

Outcome of the Pelvic Pouch Procedure in Patients With Prior Perianal Disease

Richard CS, Cohen Z, Stern HS, et al (Univ of Toronto)

Dis Colon Rectum 40:647–652, 1997 10–41

Background.—For most patients with ulcerative colitis requiring surgery, the preferred treatment is the pelvic pouch procedure. However, patients with presumed ulcerative colitis and significant perianal disease may in fact have Crohn's disease, which is a contraindication to a pelvic pouch procedure. The effect of prior perianal disease on pelvic pouch outcome was determined.

Methods.—Of 753 patients undergoing a pelvic pouch procedure between 1982 and 1994, 52 (6.9%) were identified as having perianal disease. Outcomes of pelvic pouch surgery in these 52 patients (group 1) were compared with those of the 701 patients with no previous perianal disease (group 2). The perianal diseases in group 1 patients were fissure-in-ano in 17, perianal abscesses in 13, fistula-in-ano in 7, rectovaginal fistula in 3, and significant hemorrhoids and skin tags in 25. Twenty-one percent of these patients had more than 1 type of perianal disease. A total of 33 perianal operations were performed in 27 patients (52%).

Findings.—The 2 groups were comparable in age, pathology, pouch design, and type of ileoanal anastomosis. An ileoanal anastomosis leak developed in 21% of group 1 patients and in 11.4% of group 2 patients. Perianal complications occurred in 11.5% and 1.7%, respectively, after surgery. The 2 groups did not differ significantly in total pouch failure rate (11.5% and 7.6%, respectively). Crohn's disease was diagnosed subsequently in 1.9% of group 1 patients and in 2.7% of group 2 patients. A subgroup analysis of patients in group 1 indicated no significant difference in outcomes according to type of perianal lesion or history of perianal surgery.

Conclusions.—Although prior perianal disease significantly increases the risk of developing an ileoanal anastomotic leak and postoperative perianal complications, a pelvic pouch procedure may be an acceptable surgical alternative for selected patients with ulcerative colitis with prior perianal disease. The overall pouch failure rate is not increased significantly in such patients.

► This interesting report deals with the doubt that arises when considering a patient who may be a candidate for restorative proctolectomy, carries a diagnosis of ulcerative colitis, but presents with perianal disease. This latter finding alone certainly raises one's suspicions of Crohn's disease, which would greatly increase the risk of long-term pouch failure, and represents a general contraindication to the performance of this procedure. In this large review of the University of Toronto experience on 753 patients, the individuals (*n* = 52) presenting with perianal problems had a significantly higher incidence of anastomotic leak and perianal postoperative complications. Nonetheless, the total pouch failure rate was not found to be significantly different, and the later diagnosis of Crohn's disease was not identified in a significantly higher number of patients with prior perianal disease. This paper should not therefore discourage colorectal surgeons from performing restorative proctocolectomy in patients with perianal disease, provided that the integrity of the anal sphincteric complex can be maintained, and that the diagnosis of ulcerative colitis is reasonably certain. Nonetheless, a word of caution should be remembered. These patients appear to have higher incidences of complications, therefore, a longer period of temporary ileostomy diversion may be warranted, along with routine use of pouchogram and pouchoscopy prior to ileostomy closure.

V.E. Pricolo, M.D.

Neoplastic Transformation of the Pelvic Pouch Mucosa in Patients With Ulcerative Colitis

Gullberg K, Ståhlberg D, Liljeqvist L, et al (Huddinge Univ, Sweden; Karolinska Inst, Stockholm; Univ Hosp Malmö Allmänna Sjukhus, Sweden)
Gastroenterology 112:1487–1492, 1997 10–42

Background.—Persistent, severe villous atrophy develops in the pouch mucosa of some patients receiving an ileal pelvic pouch with ileoanal anastomosis (IPAA) for ulcerative colitis (UC). The present study examines whether mucosal atrophy is a risk factor for subsequent neoplastic transformation of the ileal pouch mucosa.

Methods.—Seven patients with UC, an IPAA, and persistent severe atrophy (type C) and 14 control subjects with no or only slight atrophy (type A) were studied prospectively. Flexible videoendoscopy was performed with multiple biopsies to assess possible neoplastic changes.

Findings.—In both groups, the median time of the pouch in function was 9 years. Dysplasia occurred in 5 of 7 patients (71%) in the type C group and in none of the type A group. Four patients had low-grade dysplasia. One patient had sequential multifocal development of high-grade dysplasia. Two patients had multifocal aneuploidy—low grade in 1 and high grade in 1.

Conclusions.—The development of persistent severe mucosal atrophy in patients with UC and a long-standing IPAA indicates a risk of neoplastic transformation of the pouch mucosa. Thorough follow-up with long-term endoscopic surveillance would be prudent, including multiple biopsy samples for the assessment of possible dysplastic development. Flow-cytometric analysis may also be useful for detecting DNA aneuploidy.

▶ This communication from Swedish colleagues raises concerns about the long-term potential for malignant transformation of the ileal mucosa in the pelvic pouch. Although no case of cancer has ever been reported in the pelvic pouch mucosa in patients who, in some cases, have a more than 20-year follow-up, this study used histologic findings of dysplasia as well as flow cytometry to assess the presence of aneuploidy. In a small subset of patients, multifocal aneuploidy was detected, which leads the authors to conclude that a neoplastic transformation was under way. Although one may argue with these findings, on the basis of the observation that aneuploidy and genetic mutations have been found in several nonmalignant states, one has to agree that in the majority of cases, genetic mutations as well as aneuploidy and dysplasia are associated with premalignant states. The reasonable conclusion would be to follow-up very closely with patients after restorative proctocolectomy with routine endoscopic biopsies of the pouch mucosa over time.

V.E. Pricolo, M.D.

Evolutionary Changes in the Pathologic Diagnosis After the Ileoanal Pouch Procedure

Marcello PW, Schoetz DJ, Roberts PL, et al (Lahey Hitchcock Med Ctr, Burlington, Mass)

Dis Colon Rectum 40:263–269, 1997 10–43

Background.—Failure to initially differentiate between ulcerative colitis and Crohn's disease can result in a diagnosis of indeterminate colitis. In those patients who have Crohn's disease, ileoanal pouch construction may result in significant morbidity and pouch failure. The current study documented these changes in pathologic diagnosis and examined the implication of pathologic diagnosis on the development of pouch-related complications and eventual pouch failure.

Methods and Findings.—Five hundred forty-three patients with idiopathic inflammatory bowel disease were included in the prospective study. The preoperative diagnosis was ulcerative colitis in 499 patients, indeterminate colitis in 42, and Crohn's disease in 2. Fifty-eight percent of those with ulcerative colitis and all those with indeterminate colitis and Crohn's disease had had colectomy previously. After surgery, the diagnosis was changed in 20 patients with ulcerative colitis: 13 were changed to indeterminate colitis and 7 to Crohn's disease. Evidence of Crohn's disease was also found in the resected rectal specimens of another 2 patients with indeterminate colitis. During follow-up, another 13 patients proved to have Crohn's disease. Considering the current diagnosis, perineal complications occurred in 23% and pouch failure in 2% of patients with ulcerative colitis, in 44% and 12% of those with indeterminate colitis, respectively, and in 63% and 37% of those with Crohn's disease. Overall, the pathologic diagnosis in 6% of the patients was changed, resulting in a 12-fold increase in the diagnosis of Crohn's disease. Diagnoses were changed to Crohn's disease in 3% of those with ulcerative colitis, compared with 13% with indeterminate colitis.

Conclusions.—A significant number of patients initially diagnosed as having indeterminate colitis had pouch-related complications, eventual pouch failure, and a subsequent change in diagnosis to Crohn's disease. Thus surgeons should be cautious in recommending the ileoanal pouch procedure to patients with indeterminate colitis.

► This review from the Lahey Hitchcock Medical Center also draws the surgeon's attention to the likelihood of Crohn's disease eventually manifesting itself after a diagnosis of so-called "indeterminate colitis." This finding of indeterminate colitis may occur in approximately 10% of patients with inflammatory bowel disease limited to the large intestine, and may make the decision of performing a restorative proctocolectomy more difficult. Generally, most authors have still recommended performance of the ileoanal pouch procedure in this subcategory of patients, with a caveat that the complication rate as well as eventual emergence of clear-cut Crohn's disease in the pouch may be greater. In this review, 42 of 543 patients were believed to have indeterminate colitis. In this subgroup of patients, the diagnosis was eventually changed to Crohn's disease in 7, and they experienced a significantly higher number of pouch-related complications and eventual pouch failure. The option of preserving the rectum and performing an ileorectal anastomosis in a subgroup of patients with indeterminate colitis is certainly limited by the degree of involvement of the rectum, as well as by its compliance and ability to maintain a decent reservoir function. The choice of restorative proctocolectomy in patients with indeterminate colitis should be carefully discussed with patients and made with the awareness of a higher failure risk.

V.E. Pricolo, M.D.

Artificial Anal Sphincter

Wong WD, Jensen LL, Bartolo DCC, et al (Univ of Minnesota, Minneapolis; Royal Infirmary, Edinburgh, Scotland)

Dis Colon Rectum 39:1345–1351, 1996 10–44

Background.—Patients with fecal incontinence unresponsive to medical or conventional surgical treatments face the distressing prospect of living with their condition or undergoing a diverting stoma. However, 2 new recently reported surgical procedures may provide hope for such patients. The current study determined the efficacy of a fully implanted artificial anal sphincter in patients with severe fecal incontinence.

Methods.—Twelve patients failing conventional management for severe fecal incontinence underwent implantation of an artificial anal sphincter. Mean follow-up was 58 months. Manometric assessment was done before and after surgery, and function and patient satisfaction were assessed by questionnaire.

Findings.—Four patients (33%) had a total of 3 infections and 3 mechanical complications. Nine patients (75%) had a successful outcome. Postoperative manometric studies showed increased high-pressure zone compared with preoperative resting pressures. All 7 patients returning the questionnaire (at a mean 40 months after sphincter activation) reported continence to solid stool. Two patients reported some problems controlling liquid stool. Three had occasional incontinence to flatus. Six of the 7 survey respondents rated their bowel control as good to excellent. All 7 respondents reported satisfaction with the improvement in function.

Conclusions.—This preliminary experience shows that continence can be restored in patients with severe fecal incontinence with an artificial anal sphincter. Associated morbidity was considered acceptable.

▶ Patients with incapacitating fecal incontinence who have failed medial and surgical options face distressing prospects with their incontinence and often have to resort to a diverting stoma. The important contributions to the literature by Wong et al. (Abstract 10–44) and Lehur et al. (Abstract 10–45) provide an early experience that is short-term, which suggests that this artificial sphincter can restore continence with acceptable morbidity in patients with this distressing disorder. As with the introduction of any new medical device, proper testing in a prospective analysis should be followed with careful review by the FDA and various clinics before its recommendation to the general surgical community for implantation. We await the long-term results of these ongoing studies. As with any new medical device, unequivocally there will be improvement in its design, function, and outcomes. Proper evaluation of these reports is essential to determine the role of this novel device in the surgical management of incontinence.

K.I. Bland, M.D.

Results of Artificial Sphincter in Severe Anal Incontinence: Report of 14 Consecutive Inplantations

Lehur P-A, Michot F, Denis P, et al (Hôpital Laënnec, Nantes, France; Hôpital Charles Nicolle, Rouen, France)

Dis Colon Rectum 39:1352–1355, 1996 10–45

Introduction.—Severe anal incontinence, constituting a serious digestive infirmity, is a physical and psychological disability. Restoration of sphincteric capacity can be compatible with a normal social life. To provide an adequate therapeutic response with functional results that are reliable and stable, new techniques for treating severe anal incontinence need to be developed. A new alternative is a totally implanted prosthesis that recreates an active and controlled sphincteric mechanism. Results from perianal implants of artificial sphincters for severe anal incontinence are reported.

Methods.—There were 13 patients with total incontinence for stool who had urinary artificial sphincters implanted. The causes for incontinence were traumatic or postoperative, congenital, neurologic, or idiopathic. One patient had a proximal stoma already present before implantation.

Results.—Two patients developed sepsis. Three patients needed removal of sphincter and colostomy; sepsis had developed in 1 of these patients. Another patient had severe pain in a radiation-injured anorectum, and the other had perineal ulceration before activation of the sphincter in a severely scarred perineum. Sphincter-related failure occurred once, in a constipated woman, by rupture of the cuff after 2 years of satisfactory function. This patient had normal continence with reimplantation of a new cuff. Nine of 10 patients with a functioning sphincter were continent for stool after a median follow-up of 20 months; 5 also were continent for gas. Failure occurred in 1 patient, because the cuff was too large to occlude the anal canal and this patient is awaiting reimplantation. Easily controlled difficulties with evacuation of feces occurred with 4 patients. With inflated cuff, anal pressure varied from 43 to 94 cm H_2O.

Conclusion.—When local therapies are not applicable or have failed, an artificial sphincter has a role in the treatment of severe anal incontinence. Predictable postoperative functional results occurred with this technique, more than with others. The artificial sphincter is the primary therapeutic choice for anal incontinence with a poor prognosis, such as a sphincter rupture affecting more than 50% of the anal circumference, multifocal ruptures of the internal sphincter with very low anal pressures, or internal and external sphincter ruptures.

► This interesting new technique appears to be most promising in achieving satisfactory control over a very disabling problem. The experience is now limited to selected centers that performed the operation as an investigational method. The early results appear superior to reconstruction performed with autologous tissue and to the electrically stimulated autologous muscle transfers.

V.E. Pricolo, M.D.

Anorectal Surgery in Patients Infected With Human Immunodeficiency Virus: Factors Associated With Delayed Wound Healing

Lord RVN (St Vincent's Hosp, Sydney, Australia)

Ann Surg 226:92–99, 1997 10–46

Introduction.—Up to 34% of homosexual men infected with HIV have anorectal disease, which is the most common reason for surgical intervention. There is no consensus on how anorectal disease in patients infected with HIV should be treated. There is considerable variance in the results of wound healing in these patients. In these patients, the predictive value of

TABLE 1.—Wound Healing

Operation or Diagnosis	Total Number of Operations	Number of Operations, Wound Healing Known	% of Wounds Healed at 3 Months
All operations	161	106	40
First operations	101	74	43
Repeat operations	60	32	31
Abscess†	48	30*	40
Chronic fissure	36	19*	16
Fistula†	34	16*	31
Cancer	12	9*	33
Condylomata	17	10*	90

*First operations only.
†Includes operations at which both abscess and fistula are present.
(Courtesy of Lord RVN: Anorectal surgery in patients infected with human immunodeficiency virus: Factors associated with delayed wound healing. *Ann Surg* 226:92–99, 1997.)

$CD4^+$-T-lymphocyte count is uncertain. The incidence, variety, and clinical course of anorectal disease in patients infected with HIV was assessed. Several factors that influence wound healing were identified, including $CD4^+$ T-lymphocyte cell counts.

Methods.—A retrospective evaluation was conducted of 101 patients infected with HIV who had 161 anorectal operations during a 7-year period. There were 98 patients who were homosexuals and 3 who were bisexuals, and 5 also had IV drug use as an additional risk factor. More than 1 operation was performed on 37% of patients. At operation, 72% of patients had Centers for Disease Control category group 4 disease, 27% were group 2, 1% was group 3, and none were group 1.

Results.—For 74% of first operations, accurate information about wound healing was available. Healing was significantly retarded when the $CD4^+$ T-lymphocyte count was below 50 cells/μL. Significant predictors of wound healing were not patient age, serum albumin, or the Centers for Disease Control group. Impaired wound healing was not associated with the interval between HIV diagnosis and operation. Significantly better wound healing was associated with recognition of AIDS more than 1 year before operation when compared with those in whom AIDS developed within the year before operation. Only 40% of patients had healing of wounds by 3 months after operation in the patients for whom accurate wound healing information was available (Table 1). Patients with chronic fissures had the worst wound healing rate (16% at 3 months). Repeat operations had a worse wound healing rate than first operations. Anorectal malignancies were found in 10% of patients, none of which were diagnosed clinically before or during operation.

Conclusion.—In patients infected with HIV, especially when the CD4 count is below 50 μL, wound healing is a significant problem after anorectal operations. Thorough examination with adequate biopsies is required in all cases, although there seems to be little or no benefit from more invasive operations in some patients. The best management of anorectal disease in patients infected with HIV is still unclear.

► The issue of wound healing after anorectal operations in patients infected with HIV has generally been underestimated. In this very informative review of this unfortunately common problem from an Australian institution, the author accurately defines several factors that have been associated with delayed wound healing, in particular a $CD4^+$ count below 50 μL. The implications for ideal management are difficult to articulate; nonetheless, these data warrant consideration and would induce surgeons to be rather conservative in the treatment of anorectal problems in this high-risk subset of patients.

V.E. Pricolo, M.D.

11 Oncology

Introduction

This past year has seen advances in the incorporation of molecular markers in the management of patients with malignant disease. New techniques and clinical trials attempting to define parameters for these new management strategies are presented in this section of the YEAR BOOK.

Molecular markers such as *bcl*-2, which is a proto-oncogene, can be incorporated into the prognostic scheme for patients with pancreatic adenocarcinomas. This information can be obtained on core biopsy and may well form the basis of selection of patients for neoadjuvant therapy. Similarly, immunohistochemistry can be utilized for evaluation of lymph node micrometastases. Once again, this will more accurately stage disease as well as form the basis for adjuvant therapy studies. As these molecular and genetic studies are more commonly introduced into clinical practice, it will be important for the practicing surgeon to understand the limitations and interpretation of these tests. Alliance with genetic counselors and utilization of informed consent will be the foundation for incorporating these new techniques into everyday practice.

We have entered the age of obtaining more information from less tumor sample; stereotactic core needle biopsy for malignancy of the breast is becoming routine. Controversy may arise over whether this is the venue of the radiologist or the treating surgeon, but the fact remains that utilizing stereotactic core needle biopsy can be safer, simpler, and certainly less invasive than past practices. It will also, however, necessitate a change of surgical practice for the treating surgeon. For example, subsequent definitive surgical excision may require localization with multiple wires, whereas previous surgical excision would be reliant upon scar tissue surrounding the incisional biopsy. As mentioned previously, core biopsy is now being utilized in the management of other malignancies, such as soft tissue sarcoma. As pathologic interpretation improves the management of soft tissue sarcoma, it will also be made simpler by the use of these new techniques.

Another major area of advancement over the past year has been in defining the parameters for more tissue conservation, but with adequate treatment of the primary malignant disease. Here, defining the parameters of mesorectal excision and margin assessment, and establishing new techniques such as ultra low anterior resection and coloanal pouch reconstruction are increasing our ability to preserve function without increasing the risk of recurrence. Similarly, in the management of breast cancer, we are defining the role of breast conservation in young women as well as the management of patients with specific histologic findings, such as lobular carcinoma in situ.

Innovations are also playing an important role in the management of patients with malignancy. For example, sentinel lymph node biopsy is becoming the standard of practice for patients with malignant melanoma. While a multi-institutional randomized prospective trial is pending, controversy still surrounds the use of gamma irradiation or blue dye techniques. This technology has also found its way into the management of malignancy of the breast. Here, lymphatic mapping is less definitive, but with meticulous attention to the detail of sentinel node mapping this technology will find its role in the management of breast cancers. The past year has also seen a resurrection of old techniques attempting to find new applications. For example, cryosurgery is being utilized in the management of patients with metastatic disease in the liver.

Surgeons are always interested in improving the technical aspects of their craft, and this year has seen advances in intestinal anastomoses, coloanal anastomosis, and laparoscopic resection of colon tumors.

Finally, surgeons are in the forefront of developing new therapeutic interventions. These advances may be in defining the parameters of neoadjuvant therapy, in the development of new vaccines, or in understanding the basic pathobiology or immune response to malignancy. All of these advances will predict for future success in the management of patients with malignant disease.

This year's selections will undoubtedly help the practicing surgeon to contemporize his or her practice by incorporating new techniques and new technology. Emphasis has been placed on improving functional and cosmetic outcomes and utilizing newer molecular and biologic parameters to predict for recurrence, as well as the need for additional adjuvant therapies. As would be expected, surgeons will continue to be at the center of development of new strategies for the treatment of malignant disease.

Timothy J. Eberlein, M.D.

Breast

Large-Core Needle Biopsy of Nonpalpable Breast Cancers: The Impact on Subsequent Surgical Excisions

Smith DN, Christian R, Meyer JE (Brigham and Women's Hosp, Boston)
Arch Surg 132:256–259, 1997 11–1

Purpose.—Large-core needle biopsy (LCNB) under image guidance has become an increasingly popular technique for the evaluation of nonpalpable breast abnormalities. It is about as accurate as surgical excision at as little as one third the cost. For patients found to have occult breast cancer after preoperative wire localization followed by surgical excision, at least

1 surgical re-excision is usually required to ensure that the surgical margins are free of cancer. For lesions discovered by LCNB, it may be possible to perform a total excision of the lesion in 1 procedure. The number of subsequent surgical excisions required after LCNB or surgical excision was compared in women with nonpalpable breast cancers.

Methods.—The retrospective study included 677 women with nonpalpable breast cancers initially detected on mammography. The lesion was diagnosed as breast cancer by LCNB in 67 women and by surgical excision after wire localization in 610. The 2 groups were compared for the number of surgical excisions required after tumor diagnosis.

Results.—Seventy-three percent of patients in the LCNB group underwent just 1 surgical procedure, whereas 81% of patients in the surgical biopsy group had 2 procedures. The average number of procedures per patient was 1.25 in the LCNB group and 2.01 in the surgical excision group.

Conclusion.—In women with nonpalpable breast cancers, LCNB can reduce the need for subsequent surgical procedures, compared with surgical biopsy after wire localization. The increased use of LCNB would lead to significant cost reductions. At the authors' hospital, charges for LCNB are about one third as high as for outpatient surgical excisional biopsy.

► This is a retrospective analysis of a large group of patients undergoing LCNB. The authors found that subsequent surgical procedures are decreased after LCNB. This is partially because the previous habits of surgeons who performed needle-directed excisional biopsies were to perform a standard second operation or re-excision. There is now a trend among surgeons to perform wide excision at the time of needle-directed excisional biopsy, obtain frozen section, obtain margin assessment, and then perform the axillary dissection. In theory, this can be done in 1 step.

Large core needle biopsy obviously is the most attractive procedure for benign lesions as no further intervention is necessary. This would occur approximately 75% of the time. One cautionary note is that interductal hyperplasia with atypia is difficult to fully assess by LCNB, and this is probably 1 of the few indications for needle-directed excisional biopsy after LCNB. The other caveat is that patients who have lesions very close to the chest wall are oftentimes not amenable to LCNB.

Our institution has switched almost exclusively to use of LCNB. Although this clearly reduces costs, it also requires retraining of surgeons who then will require wider excision and careful margin assessment at the time of definitive surgical excision.

T.J. Eberlein, M.D.

Risk of Recurrence After Treatment of Early Breast Cancer With Skin-sparing Mastectomy

Kroll SS, Schusterman MA, Tadjalli HE, et al (Univ of Texas, Houston)

Ann Surg Oncol 43:193–197, 1997 11–2

Background.—No published long-term data support the oncologic safety of the increasingly popular skin-sparing mastectomy combined with immediate breast reconstruction. The long-term oncologic risk of skin-sparing mastectomy was evaluated.

Patients and Methods.—Records were reviewed for all patients who underwent treatment of T1 or T2 breast cancer by mastectomy and immediate breast reconstruction and who were observed for at least 5 years to compare the risk of local and systemic recurrence with that in patients treated with conventional non–skin-sparing mastectomy. Patients were also grouped by T stage and nuclear grade to determine whether these parameters were associated with different recurrence risks.

Results.—Of 104 patients treated with skin-sparing mastectomies, 6.7% had local recurrences develop (mean interval to recurrence was 32.5 months), 12.5% had distant metastases develop, 88.5% remained free of disease, and 7.7% died of their disease (Table 1). Of the 27 patients who did not have skin-sparing mastectomies, 7.4% had local recurrences, 25.9% had distant metastases, 74.1% remained free of disease, and 15.5% died of their disease. Average T stage in the skin-sparing mastectomy group was 1.41, whereas in the conventional mastectomy group it was 1.37. The average nuclear grade in the skin-sparing mastectomy group was 1.71, whereas in the conventional mastectomy group it was 1.72. The recurrence rates are similar to those reported elsewhere after treatment with conventional mastectomy and without reconstruction.

Conclusion.—Neither immediate reconstruction nor skin-sparing mastectomy confers any increased risk of tumor recurrence, either local or systemic.

TABLE 1.—Local Recurrence, Distant Metastases, and Disease Status of Patients With Early Breast Cancer After Skin-sparing Mastectomy and Immediate Reconstruction

Group	n	Percentage of patients: Local recurrences	Distant metastases	Free of disease	Died of disease
All undergoing SSM patients	104	6.7	12.5	88.5	7.7
T1 tumors	61	3.3	14.8	88.5	8.2
T2 tumors	43	11.6	9.3	88.4	7.0
Black's grade I*	31	12.9	19.4	80.6	19.4
Black's grade II	48	6.3	10.4	91.7	0.0
Black's grade III	6	0.0	0.0	100.0	0.0

*Black's nuclear grade, which was not known for all patients. The lower the grade, the more anaplastic the tumor.
Abbreviation: SSM, skin-sparing mastectomy.

(Courtesy of Kroll SS, Schusterman MA, Tadjalli HE, et al: Risk of recurrence after treatment of early breast cancer with skin-sparing mastectomy. *Ann Surg Oncol* 43:193–197, 1997. Copyright © the Society of Surgical Oncology, Inc.)

► This is an *Annals of Surgical Oncology* article. Immediate breast reconstruction has now become more commonly performed in the management of patients with breast cancer requiring mastectomy. This has led to the obvious extension of utilizing a skin-sparing technique, that is, preserving as much of the skin of the breast as is possible. Obviously one of the concerns when using a skin-sparing technique is the risk of local and/or distant recurrence. This study, from the M.D. Anderson Cancer Center, included 131 patients. Of those, 104 underwent a skin-sparing mastectomy and 27 patients did not. Obviously, these were selected patients because it appears that for all stages of tumor, there was a higher rate of disease-free status in the patients with skin-sparing mastectomies. Nonetheless, as seen in Table 1, patients with skin-sparing mastectomy had a numerically lower rate of local recurrence and distant metastases than patients with non–skin-sparing mastectomies. Although not published, our own institutional series of skin-sparing mastectomies verifies this data.

Although patients with T3 and T4 tumors were excluded from this study, other contraindications such as a superficial tumor or dermal skin involvement or both were not mentioned as contraindications to a skin-sparing mastectomy. Another possible relative contraindication may be the patient with a relatively large tumor, yet extensive lymphatic vessel invasion associated with the tumor.

It certainly seems from this report, utilizing a minimum follow-up of 5 years, that the rate of local recurrence is not increased if skin-sparing mastectomy is appropriately utilized. We will still need to better define the other relative contraindications to this technique.

T.J. Eberlein, M.D.

Management of Microcalcifications That Develop at the Lumpectomy Site After Breast-conserving Therapy

Vora SA, Wazer DE, Homer MJ (Tufts Univ, Boston)

Radiology 203:667–671, 1997 11–3

Introduction.—In women undergoing breast-conserving therapy (BCT) for breast cancer, early detection of breast recurrence may improve survival. The mammographic appearance of recurrences may be affected by surgery and breast irradiation, causing calcifications among other abnormal findings. It would be helpful to have some way of selecting those patients at high risk of recurrent tumors for biopsy. Guidelines for the diagnostic management of microcalcifications appearing after BCT were developed.

Methods.—The study included 504 women with early breast carcinoma treated with BCT. Patients who had microcalcifications with probably benign morphological features within 3 years after BCT were followed up closely with mammography. Those with less than 4 probably benign microcalcifications developing more than 3 years after BCT received either mammographic follow-up or biopsy. Biopsy was done in all patients who

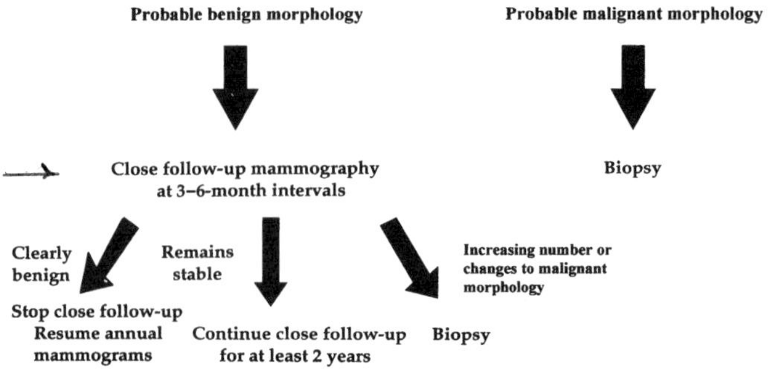

FIGURE 1.—Algorithm for the management of microcalcifications that develop at the lumpectomy site within 3 years of breast-conserving therapy. (Courtesy of Vora SA, Wazer DE, Homer MJ: Management of microcalcifications that develop at the lumpectomy site after breast-conserving therapy. *Radiology* 203:667–671, 1997. Reprinted by permission of the Radiological Society of America.)

had malignant-appearing microcalcifications or microcalcifications developing after 3 years (Figs 1 and 2).

Results.—Microcalcifications confined to the lumpectomy site developed in 29 breasts of 28 patients. In 15 breasts of 15 patients, the microcalcifications developed within 3 years of treatment; follow-up was by mammography. In 14 breasts of 13 patients, the microcalcifications developed after more than 2 years. Of 4 breasts with late microcalcifications that appeared malignant, 3 proved on biopsy to be recurrences. Mammographic follow-up was used in the other 10 breasts. There was no evidence of local treatment failure among the breasts that were followed up mammographically.

Conclusions.—In women undergoing BCT, the management of microcalcifications developing at the lumpectomy site depends on the time since treatment, site, morphological appearance, and number of microcalcifications. Patients with benign-appearing microcalcifications developing within 3 years after BCT should be followed up by mammography. This can avoid unnecessary biopsy for many patients. Biopsy is needed for

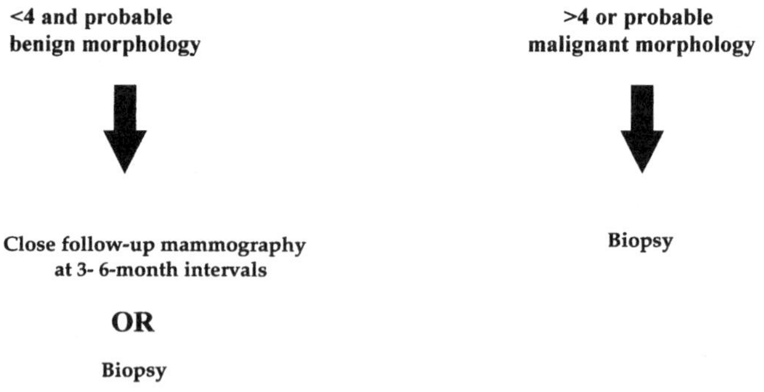

FIGURE 2.—Algorithm for the management of microcalcifications that develop at the lumpectomy site more than 3 years after breast-conserving therapy. (Courtesy of Vora SA, Wazer DE, Homer MJ: Management of microcalcifications that develop at the lumpectomy site after breast-conserving therapy. *Radiology* 203:667–671, 1997. Reprinted by permission of the Radiological Society of America.)

patients with malignant-appearing microcalcifications and/or a larger number of microcalcifications.

▶ This is one of the most difficult management problems in patients who have had BCT or radiation therapy. It requires an experienced breast radiologist. The characteristics and number of calcifications are extremely important. Figures 1 and 2 show a very reasonable algorithm. If the calcifications are few and appear benign, close mammographic follow-up is a reasonable approach, especially if they appear relatively soon after surgery. If the calcifications have indeterminate and/or potentially malignant morphological characteristics, biopsy is the prudent approach. In our institution, we have frequently utilized core needle biopsy because it is much less invasive, does not cause increased scarring, and allows documentation of the presence of the calcifications in the core samples. Obviously, in patients who have mammographic follow-up, biopsy should be recommended if the calcifications are increasing, even if they have relatively benign morphological features.

T.J. Eberlein, M.D.

Sentinel Lymphadenectomy in Breast Cancer

Giuliano AE, Jones RC, Brennan M, et al (Saint John's Health Ctr, Santa Monica, Calif)

J Clin Oncol 15:2345–2350, 1997 11–4

Background.—There is ongoing debate over the value of routine axillary lymphadenectomy (ALND) for patients with potentially curable breast cancer. Intraoperative lymphatic mapping and sentinel lymphadenectomy (SLND) have been performed in patients with breast cancer at the study institution for about 5 years. That experience suggests that SLND plus immunohistochemical examination can increase detection of axillary metastases. The results of this "mature" SLND technique were evaluated.

Methods.—The experience included 107 consecutive patients undergoing surgery for potentially curable breast carcinoma. The patients' mean age was 57 years. The typical patient was a postmenopausal woman with a palpable primary tumor undergoing a breast-conserving operation. After SLND, a standard ALND was performed through the same incision. The sentinel nodes underwent intraoperative examination by frozen section. After surgery, the specimens were studied by hematoxylin and eosin staining, as well as by immunohistochemical staining with antibody to cytokeratin. Histologic but not immunohistochemical examination was performed in the nonsentinel nodes.

Results.—One hundred of the 107 patients had an identified sentinel node. The sentinel node showed metastatic involvement in 42 patients, 28 of whom had no other involved axillary nodes (Table 2). The average number of nodes examined per patient was 1.8 sentinel nodes and 20.2 nonsentinel nodes. Six of the 7 patients with no identified sentinel nodes

TABLE 2.—Detection of Sentinel Node Metastases

Variable	No.
SLND procedures	107
Detecting sentinel node(s)	100 (93.5%)
Tumor-involved axillae	42
Containing tumor-positive sentinel node(s)	42
With macrometastases	23
With micrometastases	19
Detected by H&E staining	10
Detected by IHC staining	9

Abbreviations: SLND, sentinel lymphadenectomy; *H&E*, hematoxylin and eosin; *IHC*, immunohistochemical.

(Courtesy of Giuliano AE, Jones RC, Brennan M, et al: Sentinel lymphadenectomy in breast cancer. *J Clin Oncol* 15:2345–2350, 1997.)

had no axillary tumor involvement. In this subgroup, axillary status was 100% predicted by SLND. Primary tumor size was related to sentinel lymph node status.

Conclusions.—Sentinel lymphadenectomy, with examination by frozen section and immunohistochemistry, is a minimally invasive, accurate predictor of axillary status in patients with operable breast cancer. Studies are being conducted to see if it is possible to avoid routine ALND for patients with negative sentinel nodes. Most women with primary breast cancer probably do not need routine ALND.

▶ This is a follow-up report by one of the leaders of sentinel lymph node biopsy techniques. Dr. Giuliano utilizes an isosulfan blue dye technique. As can be seen from Table 2, 93% of the sentinel nodes were detected. No sentinel lymph node specimen was tumor-negative if the corresponding axillary lymph node dissection specimen from the same patient was tumor-positive. However, 31 sentinel lymph node specimens (35 nodes) were tumor-positive when the remaining axillary lymph nodes were negative. Thus, in this series with probably the most experienced surgeon, sentinel lymph node biopsy produced no false negative results and was 100% predictive of axillary metastases.

Other groups have recommended radiolymphoscintigraphy because it may be more technically reproducible. Obviously, it is hard to imagine improving on the results of Dr. Giuliano's group.

Another important point from this paper that helps to improve accuracy is the fact that these investigators utilized immunohistochemistry with antibodies for specific breast epithelial antigens such as cytokeratin, mucin, and milk fat globulin. In this series, most of the patients with small tumors had metastases detected by immunohistochemistry alone. Detection of occult micrometastases using these techniques is usually considered an indication of adjuvant systemic therapy. This may particularly alter the therapy of patients with T1 breast cancers.

T.J. Eberlein, M.D.

The Role of Contralateral Prophylactic Mastectomy in Invasive Lobular Carcinoma

Babiera GV, Lowy AM, Davidson BS, et al (Univ of Texas MD Anderson Cancer Ctr, Houston)

Breast J 3:2–6, 1997 11–5

Introduction.—Contralateral prophylactic mastectomy (CPM) in patients with unilateral breast cancer is controversial and data are conflicting, particularly in patients with primary invasive lobular carcinoma (ILC). The value of CPM was retrospectively analyzed in 133 patients with unilateral ILC.

Methods.—Of 133 patients, 18 were treated with CPM and 115 were treated with observation of the contralateral breast. Data for the CPM and contralateral observation (CO) groups were compared regarding development of distant disease, follow-up time, vital status, and survival times.

Results.—Patients in the CPM group underwent modified radical mastectomy of the involved breast and total mastectomy of the contralateral breast. About one third of patients in both groups had a positive family history of breast cancer. Three patients in the CPM group had occult noninvasive cancer, and no patients had occult invasive lesions in the contralateral breast. Three patients in the CO group had metachronous breast cancer at 11, 34, and 101 months. Distant disease was detected in 3 and 25 patients, respectively, in the CPM and CO group. Five-year disease-free survival was 80% and 90%, for the CPM and CO groups, respectively (Fig 1). There was no significant between-group difference in disease-specific survival.

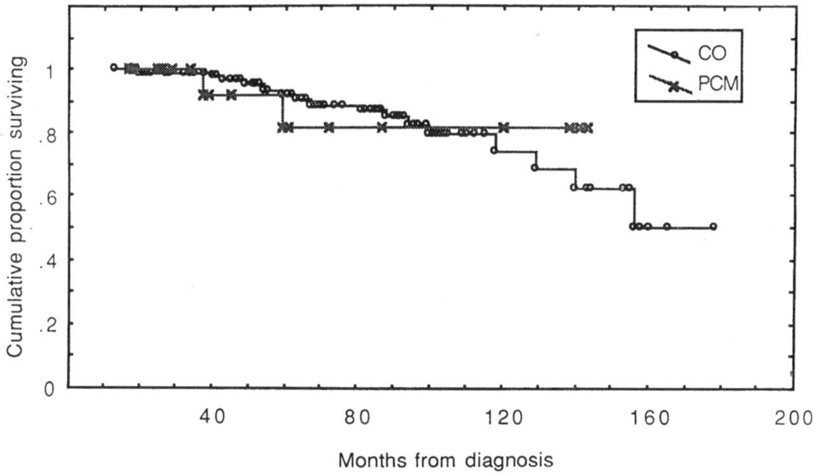

FIGURE 1.—Disease-specific survival curves for patients who underwent contralateral prophylactic mastectomy (*PCM*) and those who had observation of the contralateral breast (*CO*). (Courtesy of Babiera GV, Lowy AM, Davidson BS, et al: The role of contralateral prophylactic mastectomy in invasive lobular carcinoma. *Breast J* 3:2–6, 1997.)

Conclusions.—Careful observation with a yearly mammogram and physical examination may be considered appropriate management for patients with ILC.

▶ The role of CPM is controversial in ILC. In fact, some surgeons still prefer to treat patients with bilateral modified radical mastectomies. This study, from M.D. Anderson Cancer Center, retrospectively reviewed 133 patients treated for ILC. The goal of the study was to evaluate CPM vs. observation. As seen in Figure 1, there was no survival advantage. It is interesting that in this study, only 2.6% of the patients undergoing observation had metachronous invasive breast cancer, and none of the patients in the prophylactic mastectomy group had occult invasive breast cancer. Lobular carcinoma in situ, however, was found in the prophylactic mastectomy group; however, most of us would consider this a benign marker of risk for disease. This study supports the recommendation for conservative clinical observation consisting of a yearly physical examination and mammogram. Obviously, if symptoms develop or some abnormality is identified, a lower threshold for core needle biopsy is prudent.

T.J. Eberlein, M.D.

Lymphatic Mapping and Sentinel Node Biopsy in the Patient With Breast Cancer

Albertini JJ, Lyman GH, Cox C, et al (Univ of South Florida, Tampa)
JAMA 276:1818–1822, 1996 11–6

Introduction.—The most powerful and predictive prognostic factor for most solid tumors is the status of the regional lymph nodes; however, there is controversy over removing the axillary lymph nodes. The first node in the lymphatic basin that receives primary lymphatic flow is the sentinel lymph node, and the histologic characteristics of the sentinel lymph node may predict the histologic characteristics of the remaining lymph nodes in the axilla. Lymphatic mapping and sentinel lymph node biopsy is described in women with invasive breast cancer.

Methods.—A combination of vital blue dye and filtered technetium-labeled sulfur colloid was used for intraoperative lymphatic mapping in 62 women with newly diagnosed invasive breast cancers. A definitive cancer operation, including a complete axillary node dissection, was performed after the sentinel lymph node was identified and removed. In women with occult nodal disease, the metastatic distribution in the axilla was determined.

Results.—The sentinel lymph node was identified in 57 (92%) of 62 women with the 2 lymphatic mapping procedures. Eighteen women (32%) were found to have metastatic disease after localization. In all 18 women, the sentinel lymph node test result was positive. There was no occurrence of a sentinel lymph node with negative test results with higher nodes that had tested positive. The sentinel lymph node was the only site of disease in

12 (67%) of 18 women. Sentinal lymph node involvement was significantly favored by the metastatic distribution. The probability of observing the distribution of sentinel lymph node involvement by chance is very small among women with discordant nodal involvement.

Conclusion.—In women with breast cancer, the histologic characteristics of the sentinel lymph node probably reflect the histologic characteristics of the rest of the axillary lymph nodes, confirming that lymphatic mapping is technically possible. The histologic examination can be focused on 1 or 2 nodes by the pathologist, which can potentially increase the accuracy of staging and the yield of positive dissections.

► Sentinel lymph node biopsy was first described for patients with melanoma. In extremity melanoma where the lymphatic drainage is predictable, sentinel lymph node biopsy has rapidly become an accepted practice. There are current randomized prospective trials comparing this technique with elective lymph node dissection. My suspicion is that sentinel lymph node biopsy will eventually become the standard of practice in the treatment of extremity melanoma.

In breast cancer, however, the lymphatic drainage is much more variable. There are several points of emphasis to be made about this study. The first is that a combination of techniques for lymphatic mapping was used in this study—vital blue dye and technetium-labeled sulfur colloid. Addition of these two techniques resulted in a 92% ability to identify the sentinel lymph node. The sentinel lymph node was positive in all the patients with positive lymph nodes. No patients had a skipped metastasis. There were some patients with upper outer quadrant tumors that had sentinel lymph nodes in the level 2 distribution.

In breast cancer, a combination of techniques in the same patient results in the highest success in identifying a sentinel lymph node. There is clearly a learning curve associated with this technique, but once mastered, it may potentially save the necessity of performing full axillary dissections. Techniques are now being perfected using immunohistochemistry and genetic markers on the sentinel lymph node to obtain maximal pathologic information for utilization of further medical management.

T.J. Eberlein, M.D.

The Conservative Management of Paget's Disease of the Breast With Radiotherapy

Pierce LJ, Haffty BG, Solin LJ, et al (Univ of Michigan, Ann Arbor; Yale Univ, New Haven, Conn; Univ of Pennsylvania, Pa; et al)

Cancer 80:1065–1072, 1997 11–7

Background.—Paget's disease is characterized by eczematous changes of the nipple, almost inevitably followed by tumor development in the affected breast. Mastectomy has long been the treatment of choice for Paget's disease. There is current interest in establishing the usefulness of conservative surgery and radiotherapy as a breast-conserving alternative to mastectomy when a palpable breast mass is not present at the time of treatment. However, few data exist regarding the success of treating Paget's disease conservatively. The outcome of patients who received breast-conserving therapy for Paget's disease in the absence of clinical evidence of breast masses is reviewed in this report.

Methods.—Thirty women with Paget's disease of the nipple without palpable breast masses or mammographic densities who had been treated with definitive radiotherapy in 7 institutions between 1980 and 1994 were included in the study. Twenty-nine women had clinical Tis N0 M0, stage 0 Paget's disease, and the remaining woman had clinical T1 N0 M0, stage I disease. The patients had been treated with partial or complete nipple excision, with or without excision of the areola and retroareolar tissue. Each patient was subsequently treated with external-beam radiotherapy. Irradiation was tangential and at a median dose of 50 Gy to the entire breast.

Results.—Three (10%) patients suffered a recurrence in the breast as the sole site of initial failure after a median follow-up of 62 months, and an additional 2 (7%) patients experienced a recurrence in the breast concurrently with regional or distant failure. The 5- and 8-year actuarial estimate of treatment failure were 9% and 16%, respectively, for local failure, and 9% and 23%, respectively, for local failure as a component of first failure. Of the 5 patients experiencing local recurrence, 4 were subsequently salvaged by mastectomy. Cause-specific survival was 100% at 8 years.

Conclusions.—Resection of the nipple–areola complex with subsequent definitive radiotherapy is an effective alternative to mastectomy in the treatment of Paget's disease. Rates of local control, disease-free survival, and cause-specific survival are high with this treatment option, justifying consideration of the conservative, breast-conserving option.

► This study is a collaborative review, which is retrospective. Patients were excluded who had either a palpable mass or a mammographic density. In spite of the fact that it is a multi-institutional study, there is a relatively small number of patients, and therefore they are highly selected. However, the 5-year overall survival is 95% and is 88% at 8 years. In fact, the cause-specific survival rate at both 5 and 8 years was 100%. The actuarial breast recurrence rate was 9% and 15% at 5 and 8 years, respectively. These are very consistent with what is seen and has been reported for ductal carcinoma in situ treated definitively but with radiotherapy.

There are several caveats in this highly selected group of patients: (1) the authors believe that treatment of Paget's disease should include complete excision of the entire nipple as well as areolar complex; (2) the margins should be microscopically negative; and (3) all suspicious microcalcifications should be confirmed as associated with negative pathology or be included in the excision specimen with negative. Another potential drawback to this study is the fact that there was no central pathologic review as well as mammographic review. It does appear, however, that in selected patients without mammographic abnormalities and/or a palpable mass, that breast conservation may be offered with the expectation of producing a high rate of disease-free and overall survival in addition to adequate local control.

T.J. Eberlein, M.D.

Association of Breast Cancer With the Finding of Atypical Ductal Hyperplasia at Core Breast Biopsy

Moore MM, Hargett CW III, Hanks JB, et al (Univ of Virginia, Charlottesville)
Ann Surg 225:726–733, 1997 11–8

Introduction.—Among women in the United States, breast cancer is the most common cancer not involving the skin. To investigate mammographically detected nonpalpable breast lesions, core needle biopsy has become the procedure of choice. Atypical ductal hyperplasia of the breast is a premalignant lesion and may frequently coexist with ductal carcinoma in situ in the same lesion. Involvement of at least 2 ducts is the usual criterion for ductal carcinoma in situ; otherwise, it is identified as atypical ductal hyperplasia. Atypical ductal hyperplasia that is found in a core needle breast biopsy may be identified as ductal carcinoma in situ at surgical excision. The prevalence of occult breast carcinomas found using surgical breast biopsies was evaluated. The biopsies were performed on nonpalpable breast lesions that were diagnosed originally by core needle biopsy as atypical ductal hyperplasia.

Methods.—Using a 14-gauge automated device with an average of 7.5 cores obtained per lesion, physicians performed image-guided core biopsies of 510 mammographically identified lesions in a 2-year period. In 23 of 510 lesions (4.5%), atypical ductal hyperplasia was found, and in 21 of these patients, surgical excisions were subsequently performed. Histopathologic results from core needle and surgical biopsies were reviewed and correlated in these 21 patients.

Results.—Seven of the 21 (33.3%) surgically excised lesions having atypical ductal hyperplasia in their core needle specimens had ductal carcinoma in situ; 5 had atypical ductal hyperplasia (23.8%) (Table 1).

TABLE 1.—Correlation of Mammographic and Surgical Histopathologic Appearance in 21 Cases of ADH at Core Needle Biopsy

	Surgical			
Mammographic	Benign	ADH	Carcinoma	Total
Calcifications	4	5	6	15
Mass	3	0	1	4
Mass with calcifications	1	0	0	1
Architectural distortion	1*	0	0	1
Total	9	5	7	21

*Case containing focal LCIS.

Abbreviations: ADH, atypical ductal hyperplasia; *LCIS*, lobular carcinoma in situ.

(Courtesy of Moore MM, Hargett CW III, Hanks JB, et al: Association of breast cancer with the finding of atypical ductal hyperplasia at core breast biopsy. *Ann Surg* 225:726–733, 1997.)

Other findings showed specific benign entities in 273 (52.6%) and invasive malignant lesions in 112 (21.9%).

Conclusion.—An occult carcinoma was found in one third of patients with atypical ductal hyperplasia at core biopsy. A recommendation for excisional biopsy is warranted by a core needle breast biopsy finding of atypical ductal hyperplasia for nonpalpable lesions.

▶ This is a study of core needle biopsies of which approximately 4.5% (23) showed atypical ductal hyperplasia (ADH). The policy of this group was to perform excisions on all patients with ADH. Subsequent review of the pathologic features of the excision specimens showed 7 with ductal carcinoma in situ (DCIS).

Several points from this manuscript need emphasis. Atypical ductal hyperplasia is associated with a high incidence of DCIS and therefore warrants open biopsy. Unfortunately, there is no pathognomonic lesion that is associated with ADH that can be detected mammographically.

In our own institution, core needle biopsy is performed preferentially unless the lesion is very close to the chest wall or there is some other technical reason that core needle biopsy cannot be performed.

Depending on the skill and experience of the individual performing a core needle biopsy, the false-negative rate can range between 0% and 18% for the first 100 procedures. However, an individual's technique continues to improve, and, for example, in our institution, the false-negative rate approaches 0%.

Using this technique has a major impact, however, on surgical education because far fewer needle-directed excisional biopsies are then performed. The most successful approach has been to use a combination of radiologists and surgeons involved in recommending the performance of these procedures; afterward, these patients are followed up.

T.J. Eberlein, M.D.

---

c-*erb*B-2 Oncoprotein Detected by Automated Quantitative Immunocytochemistry in Breast Carcinomas Correlates With Patients' Overall and Disease-free Survival

Charpin C, Garcia S, Bouvier C, et al (Faculté de Médecine, Marseilles, France; Hôpital Nord Marseilles, France; Hôpital de la Conception, Marseilles, France)

Br J Cancer 75:1667–1673, 1997 11–9

Introduction.—Patients with operable breast cancers have extremely variable prognoses. One of the most important prognostic factors is axillary nodal status; however, 30% of those with negative nodes relapse and die within 10 years. New and more accurate prognostic indicators are needed for patients with breast carcinomas. Some oncogenes in breast cancers have been amplified and overexpressed through molecular biological studies. Several studies have found that the c-*erb*B-2 oncogene has

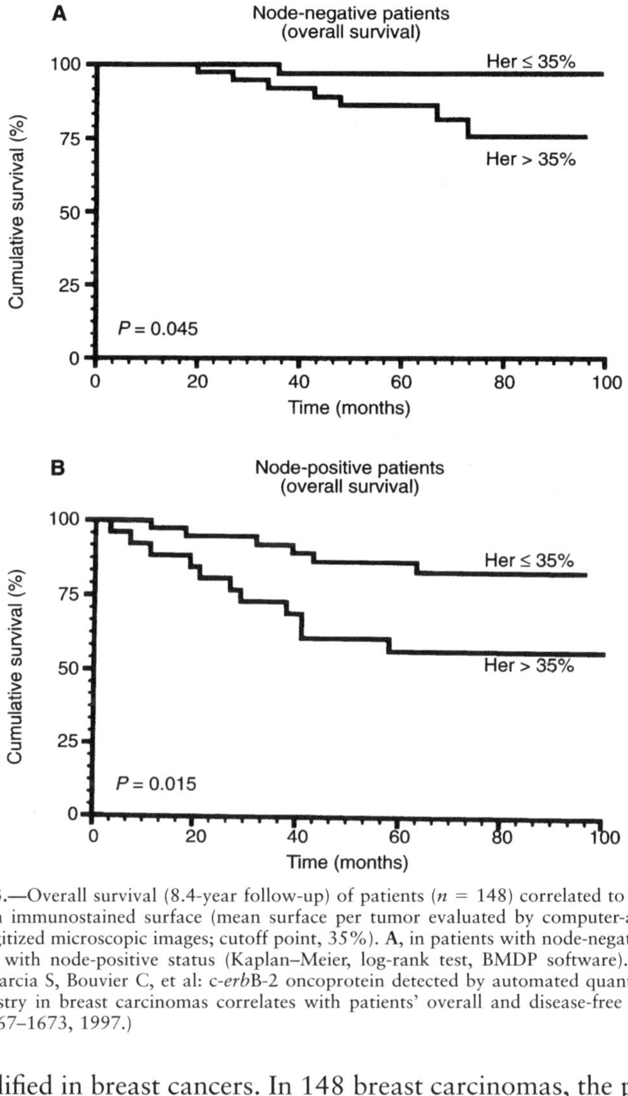

FIGURE 3.—Overall survival (8.4-year follow-up) of patients (n = 148) correlated to c-*erb*B2 (Her-2/neu) protein immunostained surface (mean surface per tumor evaluated by computer-assisted image analysis of digitized microscopic images; cutoff point, 35%). **A**, in patients with node-negative status and **B** in patients with node-positive status (Kaplan–Meier, log-rank test, BMDP software). (Courtesy of Charpin C, Garcia S, Bouvier C, et al: c-*erb*B-2 oncoprotein detected by automated quantitative immunocyctochemistry in breast carcinomas correlates with patients' overall and disease-free survival/ *Br J Cancer* 75:1667–1673, 1997.)

been amplified in breast cancers. In 148 breast carcinomas, the prognostic significance of c-*erb*B-2 oncoprotein overexpression detected in tumors by immunocytochemical assays was investigated.

Methods.—Using frozen-tissue section, immunocytochemical assays were performed under optimal technical conditions. The analysis included an automated immunoperoxidase technique and densitometry of digitized colored microscopic images. The patients' follow-up examinations in axillary lymph node-positive and node-negative subgroups were correlated with the results of quantitative immunocytochemical assays (expressed in percentages of c-*erb*B-2–positive surfaces and mean optical densities).

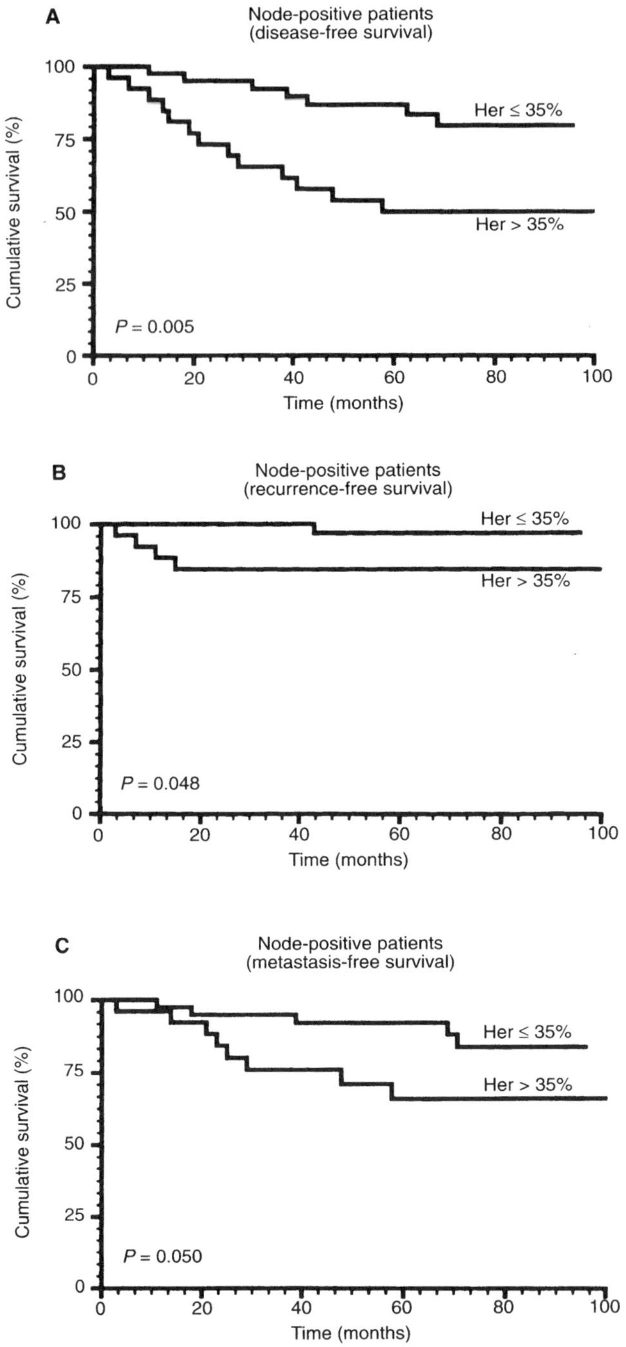

FIGURE 4.—A, disease-free survival and **B** recurrence-free survival and metastasis-free survival (8.4-year follow-up) of patients (n = 148) correlated to c-*erb*B2 (Her-2/neu) protein immunostained surface (mean surface per tumor) evaluated by computer-assisted analysis (SAMBA) of digitized colored microscopic images, cutoff point 35% in patients with node-positive status. (Ordinate, percent of patients; abscissa, percent of immunostained surface vs. counterstained surface.) (Courtesy of Charpin C, Garcia S, Bouvier C, et al: c-*erb*B-2 oncoprotein detected by automated quantitative immunocytochemistry in breast carcinomas correlates with patients' overall and disease-free survival/ *Br J Cancer* 75:1667–1673, 1997.)

There was a mean overall follow-up of 62.5 months, and it ranged from 9 months for the first death to 101 months for the 121 living patients.

Results.—Significantly correlated with the patients' poor overall survival seen in axillary lymph node-positive and node-negative subgroups was marked c-*erb*B-2 immunocytochemical expression in tumors with a cutoff point of 35% (Fig 3). In patients with node-positive status, there was a correlation between marked c-*erb*B-2 immunohistochemical expression and short disease-free, recurrence-free, and metastasis-free survival, but this was not seen in the subgroups with node-negative findings (Fig 4).

Conclusion.—In terms of overall and disease-free survival, c-*erb*B immunohistochemical expression under optimal conditions is a significant prognostic indicator.

► c-*erb*B-2 oncoprotein overexpression is seen in many epithelial-based malignancies, specifically breast, ovarian, non–small-cell lung, gastric, and pancreatic malignancies. This manuscript used immunocytochemical assays under optimal conditions with frozen-tissue sections. Quantitative overexpression of c-*erb*B-2 is significantly correlated with poor survival in patients with either node-negative or node-positive status (Fig 3). It is also interesting that there is a shorter disease-free survival, recurrence-free survival, and metastasis-free survival in patients with node-positive status who have marked c-*erb*B-2 overexpression. This is not seen, however, in patients with node-negative status (Fig 4). There may be biological significance to this finding, or it may simply be the result of there being fewer deaths in the node-negative subset of patients when compared with the node-positive subset of patients in this study.

A major technical issue in this paper is the use of frozen sections, which enabled the elimination of technical bias as a result of tissue fixation and paraffin embedding. The authors strongly believe that immunocytochemical assays should be performed on frozen-tissue samples to standardize the methodologies.

T.J. Eberlein, M.D.

Effect of Preoperative Chemotherapy on Local-Regional Disease in Women With Operable Breast Cancer: Findings From National Surgical Adjuvant Breast and Bowel Project B-18

Fisher B, Brown A, Mamounas E, et al (Univ of Pittsburgh, Pa; Mt Sinai Ctr for Breast Health, Cleveland, Ohio; St Luc Hosp, Montreal; et al)

J Clin Oncol 15:2483–2493, 1997 11–10

Introduction.—The treatment of breast cancer has been evolving over the past 3 decades, and there is interest now in the use of preoperative chemotherapy. A study of women with primary breast cancer who were participants in the National Surgical Adjuvant Breast and Bowel Project (NSABP) B-18 sought to determine whether preoperative doxoru-

TABLE 6.—Comparison Between Postoperative and Preoperative Therapy Groups Relative to Clinical Nodal Status, Clinical Tumor Size, and Pathologic Nodal Status

	Regardless of Clinical Nodal Status or Tumor Size (%)		Clinical Nodal Status* (%)				Clinical Tumor Size,* cm (%)			
			Negative		Positive		≤ 2		≥ 2.1	
Pathologic Nodal Status†	Postop (n = 743)	Preop (n = 735)	Postop (n = 554)	Preop (n = 543)	Postop (n = 189)	Preop (n = 192)	Postop (n = 200)	Preop (n = 211)	Postop (n = 540)	Preop (n = 524)
Negative	43	59	52	67	14	36	54	73	39	54
Positive	57	41	48	33	86	64	46	27	61	46
1–3	30	24	29	21	34	33	30	18	30	27
4–9	17	12	14	9	28	21	12	7	19	14
≥ 10	10	4	5	2	23	9	4	1	12	5
P value, pathologic nodal status (negative/positive)	< .001		< .001		< .001		.001		< .001	

*Before randomization (excludes 3 patients with unknown tumor size in the postoperative group).
†Excludes 16 patients in the postoperative group and 12 patients in the preoperative group with unknown status.
Abbreviations: postop, postoperative; *preop*, preoperative.
(Courtesy of Fisher B, Brown A, Mamounas E, et al: Effect of preoperative chemotherapy on local-regional disease in women with operable breast cancer: Findings from National Surgical Adjuvant Breast and Bowel Project B-18. *J Clin Oncol* 15:2483–2493, 1997.)

TABLE 7.—Comparison Between Postoperative and Preoperative Therapy Groups Relative to Frequency of Lumpectomy Proposed and Performed According to Nodal Status and Tumor Size

Clinical Nodal Status and Tumor Size (cm)*	Lumpectomy Proposed* (%)		Lumpectomy Performed (%)	
	Postop	Preop	Postop	Preop
All patients	66	65	60	67
≤ 2.0	83	89	79	81
2.1–5.0	71	68	63	71
≥ 5.1	3	3	8	22
Negative	70	71	64	70
≤ 2.0	85	90	80	83
2.1–5.0	73	73	65	73
≥ 5.1	4	4	8	14
Positive	53	49	48	59
≤ 2.0	74	82	76	68
2.1–5.0	67	57	56	66
≥ 5.1	2	2	9	33

*At time of patient entry and before randomization.

(Courtesy of Fisher B, Brown A, Mamounas E, et al: Effect of preoperative chemotherapy on local-regional disease in women with operable breast cancer: Findings from National Surgical Adjuvant Breast and Bowel Project B-18. *J Clin Oncol* 15:2483–2493, 1997.)

bicin and cyclophosphamide (AC) permits more lumpectomies to be performed and decreases the incidence of positive nodes.

Methods.—Eligible women had primary palpable, operable breast cancer (T1, T2, T3, N0, N1, M0). Tumors were confined to the breast and axilla. Patients were stratified by age (49 years or younger or 50 years or older), clinical tumor size, and positive or negative nodal status. Preoperative AC was administered to 747 patients, and postoperative AC was administered to 759. All patients received AC therapy every 21 days for 4 courses. Tumor response to preoperative therapy was classified as *clinically complete* (cCR), *partial* (cPR), *stable* (cSD), or *progressive disease* (cPD). In patients with cCR, tissue was examined for pathologic complete response (pCR).

Results.—In the group randomized to preoperative AC, breast tumor size was reduced in 80% of patients, and 36% had cCR. Younger women with clinically positive nodes and smaller tumor size (up to 2.0 cm) were most likely to have cCR. A pCR was obtained in 26% of women with cCR. Clinical nodal response occurred in 89% of node-positive patients, and there was a 37% increase in the incidence of pathologically negative nodes (Table 6). Compared with the postoperative AC group, patients who received preoperative AC had 12% more lumpectomies than had been proposed before randomization (Table 7). In the subgroup with larger (at least 5.1 cm) tumors, there was a 175% increase in lumpectomies.

Conclusion.—Preoperative therapy has been reported on since the early 1980s, but few patients were included in these studies. Findings in the large number of patients in the NSABP B-18 support the consideration of preoperative therapy for the initial management of breast tumors too large for lumpectomy. Preoperative therapy reduced the size of most tumors and decreased the incidence of positive nodes.

► Relatively little information is available from randomized, prospective trials of preoperative chemotherapy in breast cancer. The NSABP B-18 trial is the largest trial. In fact, it is larger than a summation of all previously performed trials. Approximately 80% of the patients demonstrated decrease in size of their breast tumor. This confirms the findings from studies conducted by other investigators. In this study, 36% of the patients had a clinical complete response, although on pathologic review, many of these patients had a microscopic tumor. It is particularly interesting that the most significant effect of preoperative chemotherapy was, as one might expect, in patients with the largest tumors. As seen in Table 7, of patients who had tumors 5.1 cm. or larger, only 2% of these had proposed lumpectomy, and 9% actually underwent lumpectomy and then subsequently received postoperative chemotherapy. On the other hand, of the preoperative tumor group, 33% of patients who started out with tumors 5.1 cm. or larger had lumpectomies.

Another important finding is that patients who had preoperative chemotherapy seem to have a higher incidence of pathologically negative axillary nodes (Table 6).

We are still awaiting results from this trial and other trials that demonstrate preoperative therapy having equivalent or superior results with respect to distant disease-free survival or survival, compared with postoperative therapies. Certainly at this time, it seems that at the very least, preoperative therapy may be used to reduce the size of a breast cancer in order to make a patient eligible for breast conservation therapy.

T.J. Eberlein, M.D.

Does Breast Conservation Therapy in Young Women With Breast Cancer Adversely Affect Local Disease Control and Survival Rate? The MD Anderson Cancer Center Experience

Bouvet M, Babiera GV, Tucker SL, et al (Univ of Texas, Houston)

Breast J 3:169–175, 1997 11–11

Purpose.—In general, young women with breast cancer do not do as well as older patients. Some previous retrospective studies suggested that the results of breast-conserving surgery are worse in young women, including a high local recurrence rate. One cancer center's experience with breast-conserving therapy (BCT) in young women was reviewed.

Methods.—The study included 219 patients with breast cancer aged 35 years or younger treated at a major cancer center between 1978 and 1993. All women included in the analysis were free of distant metastases at diagnosis, had received no previous treatment, and had no concurrent cancers. Breast conserving therapy was used in 79 patients and modified radical mastectomy in 140. The 2 groups were compared for demographic

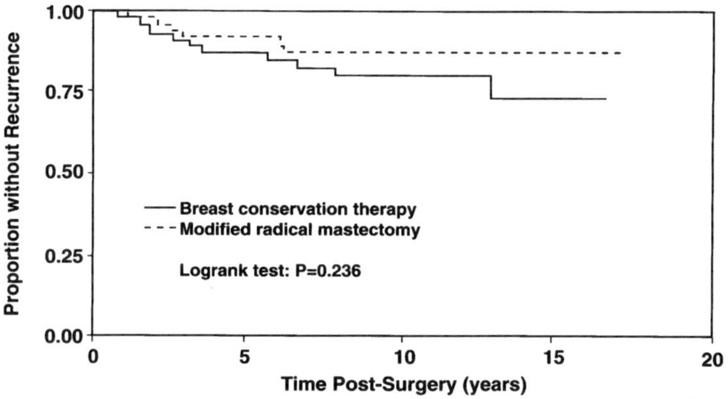

FIGURE 1.—Time to locoregional disease recurrence according to type of surgery in the matched cohort study. (Courtesy of Bouvet M, Babiera GV, Tucker SL, et al: Does breast conservation therapy in young women with breast cancer adversely affect local disease control and survival rate? The MD Anderson Cancer Center Experience. *Breast J* 3:169–175, 1997.)

characteristics, TNM stage, use of adjuvant therapy, locoregional recurrences, distant metastases, and vital status. The survivors were followed up for a median of 8 years. Univariate and multivariate analyses were performed.

Results.—There were 27 locoregional recurrences, 12 in the BCT group and 15 in the modified radical mastectomy group. After matching for stage was carried out, the type of surgery performed did not influence either the locoregional recurrence rate or disease-specific survival (Fig 1). Overall disease-specific survival rate at 5 years was 84%. The only factor related to both locoregional recurrence rate and disease-specific survival on multivariate analysis was TNM stage.

Conclusions.—In young patients with breast cancer, type of surgery—BCT vs. modified radical mastectomy—is not significantly correlated with either locoregional recurrence risk or disease-specific survival rate. Young age should not be considered a contraindication to BCT. This form of local treatment should be considered for women aged 35 years or younger who have breast cancer.

► This is a retrospective study covering some 15 years. It is interesting that during the period of this study more patients were treated with mastectomy than breast conservation. I would venture to say that these numbers would be reversed if a later period of time were utilized. Nonetheless, as seen in Figure 1, as might be expected, modified radical mastectomy provided numerically better, but statistically no different local control rates when compared with breast conservation. Similarly, the disease-specific survival was virtually identical.

What is most significant about this study is that it was confined to women younger than 35 years. it is also interesting that in univariate analysis, positive tumor margin on final pathologic examination was associated with local recurrence. However, only disease stage correlated with either locoregional relapse, or distant specific survival rate.

There are still regions of the United States where breast conservation is recommended infrequently. However, this study further verifies that breast conservation can be expected to have equivalent results to mastectomy, even in the young patient population who might be expected to have a higher degree of interest in breast conservation.

T.J. Eberlein, M.D.

Segmental Mastectomy and Tamoxifen Alone Provide Adequate Locoregional Control of Breast Cancer in Elderly Women

Yeh S, Tan LR, O'Connell TX (Kaiser Permanente Med Ctr, Los Angeles)

Am Surg 63:854–857, 1997 11–12

Background.—Breast cancer incidence increases with patient age, with women aged 70 years or older accounting for 10% to 30% of all cases. Older patients also are at a relatively high risk for having complications during or after surgery, because of comorbid conditions or physical disability. In addition, breast cancer is often less aggressive in older women than in perimenopausal or premenopausal women, and is responsive to tamoxifen. Therefore, cause exists to seek less aggressive surgical interventions concurrent with hormone therapy for older women with breast cancer. The ability of segmental mastectomy with tamoxifen therapy to achieve locoregional control of breast cancer was evaluated.

Methods.—Medical records were reviewed for 36 women aged 70 years or older (mean age, 80.6 years) who, between 1985 and 1995, had been treated for breast cancer with segmental mastectomy and tamoxifen, 10 mg administered twice daily for a minimum of 3 years. Patients were contacted for continued follow-up until July 1996 or until death.

Results.—Recurrent cancer was not detected in 28 (78%) patients, 5 of whom had positive margins at the time of surgery. The average duration of disease-free survival was 39.3 months. Distant metastasis occurred in 7 (19%) patients and was the cause of death in 2. The average time of onset and the average survival time for recurrence were 30.6 months and 45.6 months, respectively. Local recurrence occurred in 1 patient, requiring reexcision of the biopsy site and additional tamoxifen therapy 18 months after the initial procedure. Regional recurrence occurred in 1 patient, requiring modified radical mastectomy and chemotherapy. This patient died as a result of metastatic lesions after 17 months. Tumor size, histologic grade, hormone receptor status, and margin status were not predictive of distant metastasis or locoregional recurrence.

Conclusions.—Local excision of breast tumors with subsequent tamoxifen therapy provided locoregional control comparable to that achieved with more aggressive therapy in this select group of patients studied. Ongoing clinical trials will determine whether this therapeutic regimen is suitable for routine use in a larger population of elderly women with breast cancer.

▶ This is a relatively small study, confined to patients older than 70 years. The patients were treated with breast conservation and tamoxifen treatment. Several points about this study require emphasis. It is a highly selected patient population. Adequate surgical margin of the initial procedure is necessary. In this study, the patients with locoregional recurrence were able to be treated with further surgical intervention. The mean follow-up in this study was only 44 months; thus if the patients were followed up longer, a higher rate of locoregional recurrence might have been seen. As it was, the patients were elderly, and almost 17% died of unrelated causes, without evidence of breast cancer.

In selected patients, treatment with excision and tamoxifen offers an alternative and may even be desirable, especially in the very elderly patient with multiple co-morbid problems.

T.J. Eberlein, M.D.

Colorectal

Ultra-low Anterior Resection and Coloanal Pouch Reconstruction for Carcinoma of the Distal Rectum

Guillem JG (Mem Sloan-Kettering Cancer Ctr, New York)
World J Surg 21:721–727, 1997 11–13

Introduction.—Low anterior resection has been compared with an abdominoperineal resection in several studies; no significant differences in rates of pelvic recurrence were found. Local recurrence rates vary between 6% and 28% for restorative resection of upper and midrectal cancers. There is considerable variation in long-term functional results after a low anterior resection and coloanal anastomosis; there is poor function with regard to stool frequency, soiling, and urgency.

Pouch.—To increase reservoir capacity, investigators in various studies have shown that creation of a colonic reservoir with a coloanal anastomosis may be beneficial. An inverse relation between the frequency of defecation and the maximum tolerated volume of the neorectum was found in this study, which proved that improved function was partly a result of increased maximum tolerated volume. A significant reduction in the number of stools per day was found in patients with a pouch vs. a straight coloanal anastomosis.

Reconstruction.—The most common type of anastomosis after a low anterior resection is the straight double-stapled technique, but caution must be exercised to avoid anastomotic leaks. Some patients may require a diverting colostomy to avoid pelvic sepsis, anastomotic disruption, and poor function secondary to pouch fibrosis, rigidity, and noncompliance. Clear contraindications to a coloanal anastomosis are a bulky tumor that cannot be lifted off the pelvic floor and a lesion located near the uppermost part of the anorectal ring. One study found female sex as a contraindication.

Conclusion.—For coloanal reconstruction, proper patient selection is essential. Limited bowel function after a coloanal anastomosis can be related to limited preoperative sphincter function. A colonic pouch should be used selectively, even if it is easy to perform. A colonic pouch may not be indicated for patients with a capacious descending colon and a narrowing pelvis. A patient with a wide pelvis and a narrow caliber colon would benefit from a colonic pouch.

Local Excision of Rectal Cancer

Bleday R (Harvard Med School, Boston)

World J Surg 21:706–714, 1997 11–14

Introduction.—Patients with rectal cancer often fear radical resection and a permanent colostomy, which is often performed for cancers of the low or middle rectum. Significant morbidity and mortality is also associated with radical resection, particularly the abdominoperineal type. Less radical alternatives would seem appealing; thus, the use of local excision for treating small rectal cancers is being examined.

Local excision.—To remove a small rectal cancer completely, a surgeon can use any of 3 local excision techniques, and selection criteria are critical when matching the technique with the patient. Tumors must take up less than 40% of the rectal wall circumference and must be less than 4 cm in diameter. Tumors must have no evidence of any invasion into the mesorectum or perirectal nodes, and they need to be relatively close to the dentate line. Appropriate patients can be selected with preoperative staging with endorectal US, CT, and digital examination. The 3 types of excisions are the transanal excision, the transcoccygeal excision, and the transsphincteric excision.

Results.—Significant success using local excision techniques has been found in retrospective series with local recurrence rates ranging from 0% to 11% for early-stage lesions. Similar recurrence rates have also been found with prospective studies. Other studies have shown that adjuvant radiation therapy or adjuvant chemo-irradiation can increase survival because radiation therapy may sterilize any potential microscopically positive circumferential margins and positive lymph nodes.

Conclusion.—Preservation of the anal sphincters is the goal of local excision, and reports have shown good or satisfactory sphincter function in 80% to 100% of patients who had local excision performed. Any future reports on local excision techniques and other rectal cancer treatment studies should focus on postoperative function with or without adjuvant therapy, as well as quality-of-life issues. In well-selected patients, local excision seems to provide adequate treatment and is a alternative causing less morbidity than radical resection.

► These 2 manuscripts are very nice reviews of alternative surgery for abdominoperineal resection. In the paper by Dr. Bleday (Abstract 11–14), the following important selection criteria are emphasized: tumors should be less than 4 cm in diameter and should take up less than 40% of the rectal wall circumference. I usually try to limit the size of the tumor to no more than one third of the rectal wall circumference. This paper also has some very nice technical suggestions as well as an excellent review of the literature.

In the paper by Dr. Guillem, (Abstract 11–13) the importance of total mesorectal excision is emphasized, and the historical and functional outcomes of various pouch reconstructions are nicely reviewed. Dr. Guillem also discusses several contraindications to coloanal anastomosis, these being preoperative diminished sphincter tone, a bulky tumor, and lesions located near the uppermost part of the anorectal ring.

As surgeons familiarize themselves with these alternative techniques, abdominoperineal resection will become less frequently used. The key, however, will be the careful selection of patients, meticulous attention to technical detail, and a willingness to convert to a more radical resection with a permanent colostomy if an adequate resection is not possible using these alternative techniques.

T.J. Eberlein, M.D.

Early Postoperative Results of a Prospective Series of Laparoscopic vs. Open Anterior Resections for Rectosigmoid Cancers

Goh YC, Eu KW, Seow-Choen F (Singapore Gen Hosp)

Dis Colon Rectum 40:776–780, 1997 11–15

Introduction.—Laparoscopic colorectal surgery is widely used in the treatment of benign colorectal conditions, but its use in colorectal cancer is controversial. Early postoperative data were compared in patients who underwent laparoscopic anterior resection (LAR) and open anterior resection (OAR) for rectosigmoid cancer.

Methods.—Forty patients were randomized to undergo either LAR (20 patients) or OAR (20 patients). Patients with nonpalpable tumors were more likely to undergo LAR and patients with palpable tumors were more likely to undergo OAR. Use of parenteral analgesia, start of fluids, resumption of a solid diet, first bowel movement, and time to discharge were recorded.

Results.—The median age for the LAR group was 62 years, and the median age for the OAR group was 61 years. The median length of the distal margin of clearance was 4.0 for the LAR group and 4.5 cm for the OAR group. The lateral margins in all resection specimens were histologically clear of tumors in both groups. The median number of lymph nodes harvested for the LAR group was 20, and the median number for the OAR group was 19. The median length of surgery was 90 minutes for the LAR group and 73 minutes for the OAR group. The median blood loss for both

TABLE 1.—Postoperative Recovery After Surgery for Rectal Cancer

Postoperative Event (Postoperative Days)	Laparoscopic (n = 20)		Open (n = 20)		P
Parenteral analgesia	2	(1–4)	3	(1–4)	0.45
Start fluids	2	(1–3)	2	(2–5)	0.40
Resume solid diet	3.5	(2–5)	3.5	(1–5)	0.70
First bowel movement	3	(1–5)	3	(1–5)	0.90
Discharge from hospital	5	(3–10)	5.5	(4–29)	0.13

Note: Postoperative days are expressed in median (range).
(Courtesy of Goh YC, Eu KW, Seow-Choen F: Early postoperative results of a prospective series of laparoscopic vs. open anterior resections for rectosigmoid cancers. *Dis Colon Rectum* 40[7]:776–780, 1997.)

LAR and OAR was 50 mL. There were no intraoperative complications in either patient group. No patients who underwent LAR needed conversion to an open procedure. The median length of the surgical incision was 5.5 cm for LAR and 18 cm for OAR. There were no significant between-group differences in duration of parenteral analgesia, start of fluid and solid diet after surgery, time to first bowel movement after surgery, or time to discharge from hospital (Table 1). Postoperative complications were: 1 wound infection in the OAR group and 1 wound infection, 1 case of atelectasis, and 2 cases of prolonged ileus (both recovered 6th postoperative day) in the LAR group.

Conclusion.—Laparoscopic surgery for rectosigmoid cancer is feasible and safe. The same standards of tumor excision and clearance can be expected for LAR as for conventional OAR. Significant improvement in postoperative function after LAR compared with OAR was not demonstrated in this preliminary report.

► This is a very provocative paper by an experienced group of laparoscopic surgeons. Somewhat surprisingly (Table 1), there was no significant difference between laparoscopic and open resection, with respect to resumption of a solid diet, the first bowel movement, or time of discharge from the hospital. Of note, however, the experience of these surgeons is documented by the median operating time: 90 minutes for the laparoscopic group and 73 minutes for the open resection group. Blood loss was approximately 50 mL in each group.

In this series, the adequacy of the oncologic resection was not addressed; however, it will be addressed in the multi-institutional, randomized trial, now ongoing. Perhaps the most significant difference between these 2 groups will be in the return to functional activity levels, which may be sooner in the laparoscopic group.

T.J. Eberlein, M.D.

The DCC Protein and Prognosis in Colorectal Cancer

Shibata D, Reale MA, Lavin P, et al (Harvard Med School, Boston; Yale Univ, New Haven, Conn; Boston Biostatistics Research Found, Farmingham, Mass; et al)

N Engl J Med 335:1727–1732, 1996 11–16

Objective.—Allelic loss of chromosome 18q is linked to a poor outcome in individuals with stage II of Dukes' stage B2 colorectal cancer. The *DCC* (deleted in colorectal cancer) gene is suspected of being the gene inactivated by this loss. The expression of the *DCC* protein in stage II and III colorectal cancers was studied histochemically to determine its importance as a prognostic marker of colon cancer.

Methods.—Antibody studies were performed on 132 formalin-fixed, paraffin-embedded samples from patients (66 female) with stage II or III colorectal cancers. Status of the *DCC* gene was determined by immunohistochemical analysis. The Cox proportional hazards model was used to determine the contributions of age, sex, tumor site, degree of differentiation of the tumor, presence of radiation or chemotherapy, TNM stage, and *DCC* status.

Results.—*DCC* positivity was found in 59% of sections from female patients and 41% from male patients. Tumors were well or moderately well differentiated in 86% of patients. TNM stage and *DCC* status were not related. Patients were followed for an average of 95.7 months for *DCC*-positive tumors and 85.1 months for *DCC*-negative tumors. Overall survival depended on disease stage and *DCC* positivity or negativity (Fig

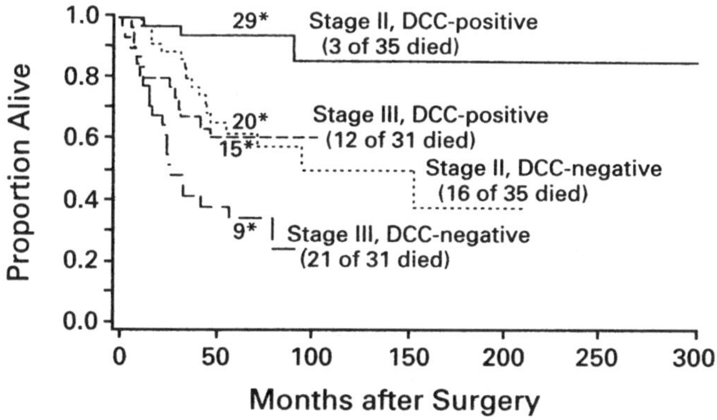

FIGURE 3.—Kaplan-Meier Life-Table Analysis of the Overall Survival of Patients with Colorectal Cancer. According to TNM Stage and the Expression of *DCC*. Patients with stage II disease whose tumors were *DCC*-positive had a significantly better prognosis than patients with stage II disease whose tumors were *DCC*-negative ($P < 0.001$). Similarly, in stage III disease, patients with *DCC*-positive tumors had a significantly better overall survival rate than patients with *DCC*-negative tumors ($P = 0.03$). The number of patients who died of colorectal cancer during the entire study is shown in parentheses. The asterisks indicate the number of patients at risk at 60 months. (Reprinted by permission of The New England Journal of Medicine, from Shibata D, Reale MA, Lavin P, et al: The DCC protein and prognosis in rectal cancer. *N Engl J Med* 335:1727–1726. Copyright 1996, Massachusetts Medical Society. All rights reserved.)

TABLE 2.—Multivariate Analysis of Maximum-Likelihood Estimates of Selected Clinical Variables in 132 Patients Evaluated for DCC

Variable	Risk Ratio for Mortality (95% CI)*	P Value
Age (≤65 vs. ≥65)	0.906 (0.503–1.632)	0.74
DCC status (negative vs. positive)	3.155 (1.700–5.852)	<0.001
TNM stage (III vs. II)	3.112 (1.696–5.710)	<0.001
Degree of differentiation of the tumor (poor vs. good or moderately good)	2.218 (1.119–4.397)	0.02
Sex (male vs. female)	1.280 (0.720–2.275)	0.40
Tumor site (colon vs. rectum)	0.868 (0.476–1.583)	0.64
Adjuvant therapy (yes vs. no)	1.209 (0.633–2.309)	0.56

*CI denotes confidence interval.

3). Tumor stage and *DCC* status were independent predictors of death (Table 2).

Conclusion.—In patients with colorectal cancer, the absence of *DCC* is a marker for poor outcome. Patients with stage II colorectal cancer and no *DCC* expression have tumors that behave like stage III cancers. Determination of *DCC* status may help clinicians select patients with stage II tumors who would benefit from adjuvant therapy.

▶ The *DCC* gene is on chromosome 18q21.2. In this article the authors attempt to show association of this gene with prognosis in stage II and stage III colorectal cancer. As seen in Figure 3, stage II patients who were *DCC* negative had a survival that was very similar to a stage III patient. In contrast, *DCC*-positive stage II patients had a significantly prolonged survival. One of the limitations of this study is that immunohistochemical analysis of a protein by an antibody (as used in this study) does not fully establish the function of the gene producing the protein. Currently, it is not known whether *DCC* has a regulatory control of the cell. It is also not known whether a particular threshold level of production of protein is necessary to associate with prognosis. Again, in this study, the staining was present or absent. Therefore, quantification of the level of *DCC* protein was not performed. As can be seen from Table 2, *DCC* status and TNM stage were predictive of mortality in multivariate analysis. Thus, assessment of *DCC* in colorectal tumors may identify patients who may benefit from adjuvant therapy.

T.J. Eberlein, M.D.

Transanal Surgery With a New Anal Retractor and a Stapler for Tumours in the Proximal Rectum

Maeda K, Hashimoto M, Nakajima K, et al (Fujita Health Univ, Toyoake, Japan; Social Insurance Saitama Chuo Hosp, Urawa, Japan)

Eur J Surg 163:219–221, 1997 11–17

Introduction.—Nineteen patients with rectal tumors underwent transanal surgery during which a new E-type anal retractor (Fig 1) was used. This retractor was connected to an Octopus retractor holder (22-inch long type) to provide a better field of operation than that provided with the usual anal retractor.

Technique.—The 3-bladed E-type anal retractor has a cylinder that allows smoother insertion into the anus and exposes the field

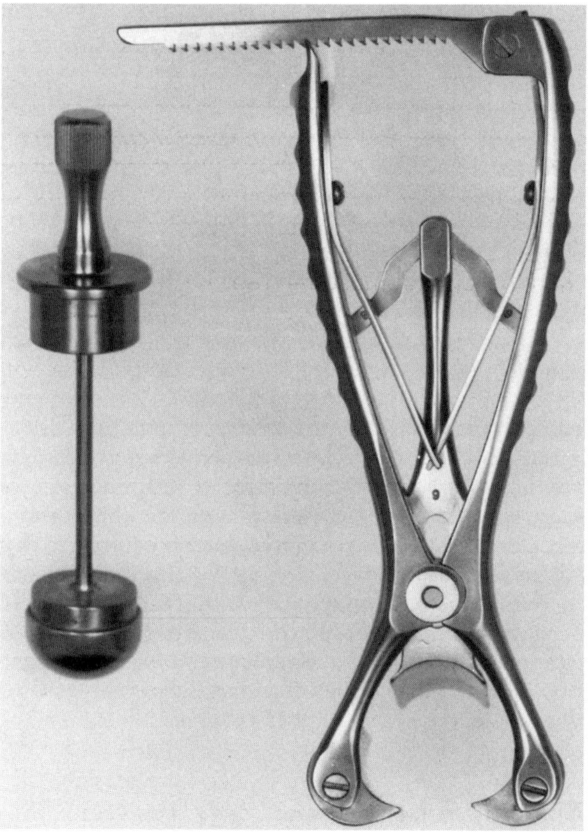

FIGURE 1.—E-type anal retractor is a triblade device with a cylinder that permits smooth insertion through the anus and allows for a wider field of vision to an approximate inner diameter of 37 mm. (Courtesy of Maeda K, Hashimoto M, Nakajima K, et al: Transanal surgery with a new anal retractor and a stapler for tumors in the proximal rectum. *Eur J Surg* 163:219–221, 1997.)

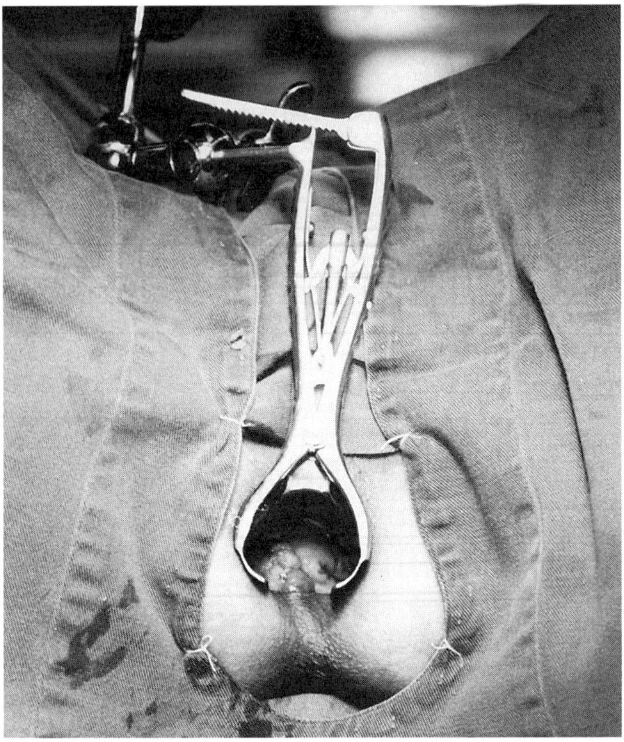

FIGURE 2.—A villous tumor 6 cm from the anal verge can be seen with an E-type anal retractor connected to an Octopus retractor holder under the main theater light. (Courtesy of Maeda K, Hashimoto M, Nakajima K, et al: Transanal surgery with a new anal retractor and a stapler for tumors in the proximal rectum. *Eur J Surg* 163:219–221, 1997.)

of surgery to a diameter of approximately 37 mm. A ratchet keeps the surgical field exposed, and a bar connected to the Octopus holder fixes the retractor. The operation is performed after whole gut lavage, with the patient under epidural anesthesia and in the lithotomy or prone jackknife position. After the lubricated head of the retractor is inserted into the anus and rolled to pull the rectum in, the mandrin is removed. Optimal exposure of the tumor (Fig 2) is obtained with the retractor fully dilated and fixed in place. A stay suture is applied to the distal side of the tumor for extracting it. The automatic suture clamp (ENDO TA or ENDO GIA) is applied under the retraction stitches and fired while the rectum is being extracted (Fig 3).

Results.—Thirteen of the patients had early rectal carcinoma and 6 had sessile adenoma with moderate or severe dysplasia. Eleven lesions were located above the peritoneal reflection. The mean tumor diameter was 26 mm; mean operating time and blood loss were 26 minutes and 27 g, respectively. A single case of transient bleeding was the only complication.

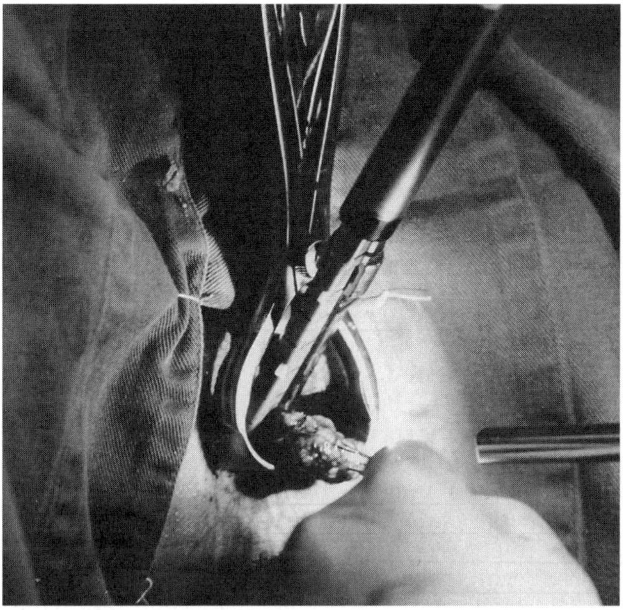

FIGURE 3.—The tumor is excised and anastomosed with an ENDO TA 60 instrument. (Courtesy of Maeda K, Hashimoto M, Nakajima K, et al: Transanal surgery with a new anal retractor and a stapler for tumors in the proximal rectum. *Eur J Surg* 163:219–221, 1997.)

In all cases but 1, an adenoma, free surgical margins were confirmed histologically. This patient underwent a further curative resection 12 months later. Three patients with high risk T1 cancer had additional anterior resection immediately after local resection. During a mean follow-up of 18 months, no recurrences were observed.

Conclusion.—This method of transanal excision with a mechanical device allows simultaneous excision and anastomosis to be performed under excellent vision. Patients are selected for this minimally invasive surgical procedure after colonoscopic examination and double-contrast barium enema studies.

► It is not often that I select a manuscript on surgical technique. However, as more and more conservative operations are performed on the rectum transanally, difficulty with exposure is often quite limiting. This new retractor has a triblade device and allows for almost a 3.5 cm inner diameter that would be quite adequate for most tumor excisions. Obviously, these excisions are restricted to in situ cancers or very superficial T1 lesions. Another unique feature of this retractor is its connection to an octopus retractor, thereby eliminating the need for an assistant to maintain the retractor exposure. For surgeons interested in local tumor excision of rectal cancers, this retractor seems like an excellent alternative to existing retractors.

T.J. Eberlein, M.D.

Sphincter Preservation Therapy for Distal Rectal Carcinoma

Ng AK, Recht A, Busse PM (Harvard Med School, Boston)

Cancer 79:671–683, 1997 11–18

Introduction.—For patients with low-lying rectal carcinoma, sphincter-preserving therapy may be performed in the interests of improving quality of life while preserving local control and survival. This may be done through local therapy alone, local excision plus adjuvant therapy, or preoperative radiation with or without chemotherapy. For patients with early-stage rectal carcinoma, the results of sphincter-preserving therapy are comparable to those of abdominoperineal resection (APR). The techniques and outcomes of sphincter-preserving therapy for distal invasive rectal carcinoma are reviewed.

Methods and Findings.—The study looked at retrospective and prospective clinical series of patients treated with various sphincter-preserving approaches to determine the rates of local control, salvage, and treatment complications. The data suggest that local excision alone is a suitable treatment for patients with well or moderately differentiated small T1 tumors, provided there is no lymphatic or vascular invasion and if resection can achieve negative margins. Chemoradiation therapy is needed for patients with T2 lesions or "unfavorable" T1 lesions. For patients with T3 lesions, local recurrence may occur in 20% of cases even with adjuvant chemotherapy and radiation after local excision. The decision to provide sphincter-preserving therapy in this situation must be carefully considered. There have not been and are unlikely to be any randomized studies comparing sphincter-preserving therapy and APR in this situation.

The best techniques of delivering radiation and chemotherapy after local excision of rectal cancers have not yet been determined. Good local control and survival, good anorectal function, and low complication rates have been achieved with high-dose radiotherapy followed by sphincter-sparing circumferential resection. The patient selection criteria are unclear, although pretreatment staging with endorectal ultrasound provides helpful information. The evaluation of sphincter function as an endpoint needs to be standardized. The addition of preoperative chemotherapy to radiation therapy needs to be further studied, but again, randomized comparison with APR is unlikely. Two current randomized trials will compare preoperative chemoradiation with postoperative combined-modality treatment. The findings should help to clarify the ability of preoperative therapy to downstage tumors, and the ability to perform sphincter-preserving surgery rather than APR.

Discussion.—The available data on sphincter-preserving treatment for distal rectal carcinoma are reviewed. At the authors' clinic, patients who are candidates for this type of treatment receive preoperative chemotherapy and radiotherapy by the same techniques and in the same doses as used postoperatively. The decision to perform sphincter-preserving therapy vs. APR is made 4 to 8 weeks later, at the time of surgery—posttreatment, preoperative imaging studies are not accurate enough to make this decision.

► This very clearly written review is from the Joint Center for Radiation Therapy in Boston. It offers a very clear discussion of local excision alone, local excision with adjuvant radiation, with and without chemotherapy, as well as the role of preoperative radiation therapy followed by either local excision or circumferential resection. Survival, complication rates, and functional results are discussed. Certainly for surgeons who treat a significant number of colorectal tumors, this review will prove beneficial.

T.J. Eberlein, M.D.

Analysis of Prognostic Risk Factors in Hepatic Resection for Metastatic Colorectal Carcinoma With Special Reference to the Surgical Margin

Shirabe K, Takenaka K, Gion T, et al (Kyushu Univ, Fukuoka, Japan)

Br J Surg 84:1077–1080, 1997 11–19

Introduction.—For metastatic colorectal cancer, the effectiveness of liver resection is well established. There is still some debate about whether the surgical margin from the tumor edge to the cut surface of the liver is a significant prognostic factor in hepatic resection for colorectal metastatic liver cancer. Some studies have indicated that a surgical margin of 10 mm would be beneficial. In resection of colorectal metastasis to the liver, an attempt was made to identify the prognostic factors with special attention being paid to microscopic intrahepatic invasion and the surgical margin.

Methods.—There were 31 patients who underwent curative hepatic resection for metastatic colorectal cancer in a 10-year period. A retrospective examination was conducted to determine the clinical and pathologic factors. Univariate and multivariate analyses were performed to clarify the prognostic risk factors in hepatic resection for colorectal metastasis.

Results.—One-year survival rates were 92%, 3-year survival rates were 42%, and 5-year survival rates were 39%. In 2 of 15 patients, hepatic vein invasion by cancer cells was found among the 16 resected specimens that had a solitary liver tumor. Three patients had portal vein invasion, 2 patients had microsatellite lesions, and 6 had biliary tract invasion. One of these factors was observed in only 2 of 9 patients who had resected specimens with a solitary tumor measuring less than 4 cm in diameter. These factors were observed in 6 of 7 patients who had specimens with a solitary tumor measuring more than 4 cm in diameter. Less than 10 mm was the distance from the tumor edge to the intrahepatic invasion. Significant factors that indicated a poor prognosis were tumor size of 4 cm or more in diameter, 4 or more gross tumors, an interval of 6 months or less between colorectal and hepatic resection, and bilobar involvement and a resection margin from the tumor of less than 10 mm.

Conclusion.—Because occult intrahepatic invasion was always found to be located within 10 mm from the edge of the tumor, the surgical margin should be more than 10 mm when treating metastatic colorectal cancer to the liver. In previous reports, adjuvant therapy has also been found to be effective in preventing recurrence.

▶ This paper emphasizes the importance of adequate surgical resection margins when performing liver resections for metastatic colorectal cancer. As is seen in previous studies, the disease-free interval is a major predictor of survival. Also in this report, multiple metastases and large tumor size are also correlated with poor survival rates, which confirms findings from previous studies. This study is unique in that it measured the distance from the tumor to the area of occult invasion, which was detected microscopically. That distance, from occult invasion to the tumor edge, was within 10 mm. Careful attention to the technical details of resections will maximize the ability to ensure local control.

T.J. Eberlein, M.D.

Sphincter-saving Resection, or Not, for Cancer of the Midrectum

Huguier M, Chastang C, Houry S, et al (Université Paris VI; Université Paris V)

Am J Surg 174:11–15, 1997 11–20

Objective.—There is disagreement regarding whether sphincter-saving resection (SSR) or abdominoperineal resection (APR) is more appropriate for cancer of the midrectum. Results of a study comparing time to pelvic recurrence and survival in patients with midrectal cancer who underwent SSR or APR were presented.

Methods.—Between 1970 and 1993, 119 patients (58 males), aged 15–88 years, were operated on for cancer of the midrectum. The surgery involved an APR in 76 cases and an SSR in 43 cases. Patients were followed for as long as 5 years. Baseline prognostic covariates were adjusted to eliminate bias in the nonrandomized retrospective comparison.

Results.—Four SSR patients and 1 APR patient died in the hospital. Overall, the postoperative mortality rate was 26% (14 patients) in the SSR group and 18% (11 patients) in the APR group. There were 4 complications after SSR and 1 after APR. There were 10 recurrences in the SSR group and 16 in the APR group. Time to recurrence was similar in the 2 groups (Fig 1). There were 18 deaths in the SSR group and 23 deaths in the APR group. Overall survival was similar in the 2 groups (Fig 2).

Conclusion.—Results of SSR and APR for midrectal cancer are similar.

▶ This is a study of 119 patients with cancer of the midrectum. The authors have attempted to eliminate the bias that is inherent in a nonrandomized retrospective comparison by adjusting for baseline prognostic covariants. However, 20% of the patients who underwent APR had poorly differentiated tumors whereas only 7% with poorly differentiated tumors underwent SSR. Nonetheless, there was no difference between pelvic recurrence or overall

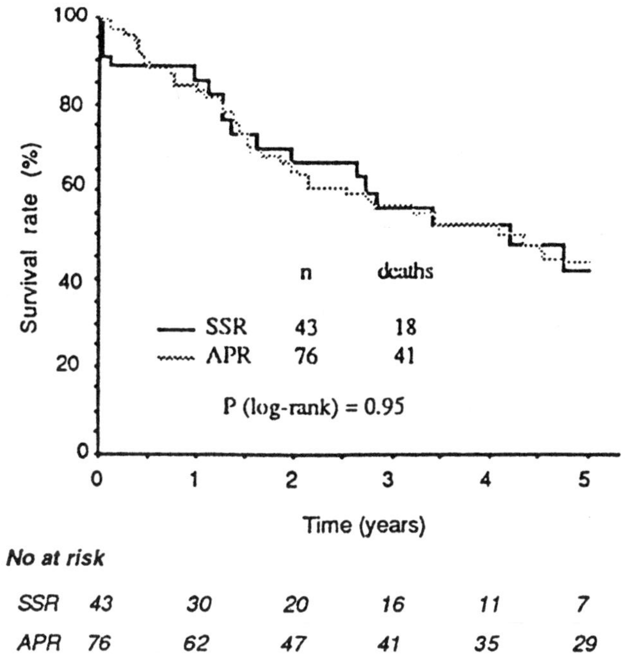

FIGURE 1.—Pelvic recurrence rates related to the type of resection, sphincter-saving resection (*SSR*) or abdominoperineal resection (*APR*). (Reprinted by permission of the publisher, courtesy of Huguier M, Chastang C, Houry S, et al: Sphincter-saving resection, or not, for cancer of the midrectum. *Am J Surg* 174:11–15, copyright 1997 by Excerpta Medica Inc.)

survival (Figs 1 and 2). It is interesting that selection of patients for SSR paralleled the practice of most active rectal surgeons; that is, they increased with the advent and improvement of stapling instruments and reappraisal of the distal resection margin. As surgeons become more familiar with the technical details of midrectal resection, nerve preservation, and evaluation of distal margins, APR may well become a minimally used therapeutic approach.

T.J. Eberlein, M.D.

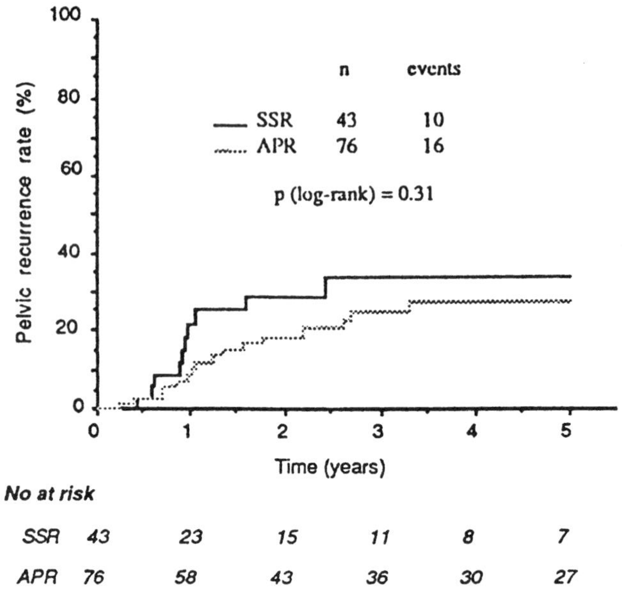

FIGURE 2.—Survival rates related to the type of resection, sphincter-saving resection (*SSR*) or abdominoperineal resection (*APR*). Reprinted by permission of the publisher, courtesy of Huguier M, Chastang C, Houry S, et al: Sphincter-saving resection, or not, for cancer of the midrectum. *Am J Surg* 174:11–15, copyright 1997 by Excerpta Medica Inc.)

The National Cancer Data Base Report on Carcinoma of the Anus

Myerson RJ, Karnell LH, Menck HR (Washington Univ, St Louis; Univ of Iowa, Iowa City; American College of Surgeons, Chicago)
Cancer 80:805–815, 1997 11–21

Objective.—Anal carcinoma is rare and carries a low mortality rate. Management of the disease centers around preserving anorectal function. Data or disease characteristics, care, and outcome from the National Cancer Data Base (NCDB) were reviewed.

Methods.—Patterns of care, longterm outcome, and trend data on patients with anal carcinoma from 1988 (n = 1,050) to 1993 (n = 1,289) were analyzed statistically.

Results.—The average age at diagnosis declined from 62.8 in 1988 to 61.8 in 1993. About half the patients were female in both years; 87.2% of patients were non-Hispanic whites in 1993. The use of the "cloacogenic zone" category increased from 0.3% in 1988 to 8.9% in 1993 and the "overlapping lesion" category decreased from 29.2 to 18.8%. The proportion of epidermoid carcinomas increased from 74.3% to 79.1%, whereas the percentage of adenocarcinomas declined from 21.9% to 16.5%. The proportion of early-stage carcinomas increased from 66.6% to 73.4%, and the number of cases not staged decreased from 43.9% to

17.8%. Patients with epidermoid carcinoma were 67.1% female, whereas patients with adenocarcinoma were 42.0% female.

The use of resection decreased during this period; the use of radiation therapy increased from 67.4% to 72.6% and chemotherapy increased from 57.4% to 64.8%. The overall use of surgery declined from 53.8% in 1988 to 49.1% in 1993, but increased for adenocarcinoma. The overall 5-year survival rate was 53.9% in 1988. Other statistics for that year were 57.6% for epidermoid carcinoma and 41.3% for adenocarcinoma, 56.2% for females and 49.6% for males, 71/3% for Stage I disease and 23.1% for Stage IV, and 64.0% for nonsurgical treatment of Stage I–II epidermoid carcinoma and 65.4% for surgical treatment.

Conclusion.—Radiochemotherapeutic treatment of epidermoid carcinoma of the anus is increasing. Surgery plus radiotherapy and/or chemotherapy is becoming more common. Studies confirm the efficacy of conservative radiation plus chemotherapy for treatment of epidermoid carcinoma. Early stage epidermoid carcinoma and female sex favor increased 5-year survival.

▶ This large study compares over 1,000 patients from 1988 with over 1,000 patients from 1993 according to data from the National Cancer Data Base Commission on Cancer of the American College of Surgeons. It shows that for early-stage epidermoid carcinomas, the 5-year survival rate for patients treated with radiation and chemotherapy was equivalent to that of patients who received surgery. Analysis of this data base confirms the treatment algorithm that radiation/chemotherapy is the treatment of choice for epidermoid carcinomas, and surgery would be used for patients with residual tumor after neo-adjuvant therapy. Also seen in this study is an increasing trend of multimodality therapy for adenocarcinoma of the rectum. This trend, coupled with the experience of rectum-saving surgery, will result in a potentially higher survival rate, without the stigma of a permanent colostomy.

T.J. Eberlein, M.D.

Treatment of Liver Metastases

Cryosurgical Ablation of Hepatic Metastases From Colorectal Carcinomas

Yeh KA, Fortunato L, Hoffman JP, et al (Fox Chase Cancer Ctr, Philadelphia)
Am Surg 63:63–68, 1997 11–22

Objective.—Almost half of the individuals with colon or rectal cancer die of their disease. Because curative resection is contraindicated in patients with hepatic metastases or close surgical margins, cryoablation has been used. A review of outcomes in these patients is presented.

Methods.—Between February 1992 and May 1995, 24 patients (10 women), aged 34–84, with metastatic colon and rectal carcinoma underwent cryoablation of metastatic tumors ($n = 12$) or cryoablation for close resection margins ($n = 12$). Surgery was palliative in 3 patients and curative in 21. Disease-free and overall survival rates were calculated.

Results.—The average hospital stay was 8.4 days. Pleural effusions developed in 7 patients in each group, 1 cardiac dysrhythmia in each group, stroke in 1 patient, and line sepsis in 1 patient who underwent cryoablation of central lesions, atelectasis in 1 patient, and myocardial infarction in 1 patient who underwent cryoablation for close or positive surgical margins. Overall survival was 31 months, and disease-free survival was 19.5 months for patients receiving cryoablation for close surgical margins. The overall survival for patients with central lesions was 31 months and the mean disease-free survival period was 23 months. At last follow-up (37 months) there were 20 survivors; 2 patients died of complications and 2 of their disease. Nine survivors were disease free and 11 were alive with their disease, including the 3 patients who received palliative treatment. Recurrent disease that developed in 10 patients included extrahepatic metastases in 6, hepatic in 2, and combined in 2. The median time to recurrence in these patients was 9.5 months and median survival was 14 months. Overall survival and disease-free survival for all patients were 32.7 and 23.5 months, respectively.

Conclusion.—In patients with metastatic colon and rectal cancer, cryoablation of hepatic metastases or close resection margins is a safe alternative that increases survival and has an acceptable complication rate.

► This article is selected mainly to present a possible alternative to patients with unresectable hepatic metastases from colon and rectal carcinoma. Twelve of the ablations were for unresectable central hepatic metastases and 12 were for gross or microscopically positive resection margins. The overall survival was 32.7 months with a mean disease-free survival of 23.5 months. This study had a median follow-up of 19 months. Therefore, a longer follow-up period and a direct comparison to patients undergoing resection would be helpful. Complications were quite acceptable.

Another caveat in this study was that the majority of the lesions were 3 cm or smaller, which represents another possible limitation for cryosurgery. Although not done in this present study, some surgeons are performing this technique laparoscopically.

Until further studies with longer follow-up are performed, directly comparing this technique with resection, I believe cryosurgery is still to be used in a palliative setting. However, with further study, this may change.

T.J. Eberlein, M.D.

Hepatic Cryosurgery for Liver Metastases: Long-term Follow-up

Korpan NN (Internatl Inst of Cryosurgery, Vienna; State Med Univ of Kiev, Ukraine; Evangelisches Krankenhaus Wein-Währing, Vienna)

Ann Surg 225:193–201, 1997 11–23

Introduction.—Cryosurgery has been used for the treatment of many benign and malignant tumors, but this is the first report of long-term clinical outcome for hepatic cryosurgery in patients with liver metastases

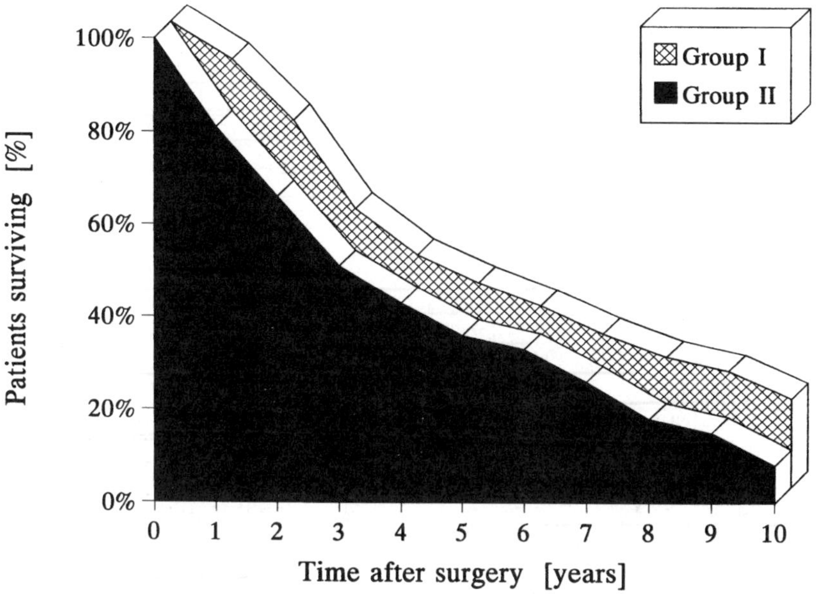

FIGURE 5.—Survival curves after cryogenic and conventional hepatic surgery. (Courtesy of Korpan NN: Hepatic cryosurgery for liver metastases. *Ann Surg* 225:193–201, 1997.)

(LM). Study subjects were participants in a prospective, randomized trial comparing tumor reduction and survival after cryogenic and conventional surgery.

Methods.—The study group included 123 patients, 87 men and 36 women with a mean age of 41.3 years. Sixty-three were treated with cryogenic surgery and 60 with conventional surgical techniques. All had solitary metastases in the liver or multiple nodules in one or both lobes. Most were free of symptoms at the time of evaluation. The cryogenic and conventional surgery groups did not differ significantly in age, gender distribution, presence of symptoms, LM distribution, or disease-free interval. Patients in both groups received systemic chemotherapy and were monitored at regular intervals postoperatively with liver function tests, ultrasonography of the liver, chest x-ray films, and computed tomography.

Results.—Approximately two thirds of patients in each treatment group had colorectal cancers metastatic to the liver. The extent of resection was determined by the size and site of the lesion. In the cryosurgery group, 29 had cryoextirpation, 20 had cryoresection, and 14 had cryodestruction. Cryoextirpation was used for smaller lesions (mean, 2.1 cm), cryoresection for larger lesions (mean, 3.1 cm), and cryodestruction for nonresectable LM. The most commonly used conventional surgery techniques were wedge resection (40%), anatomic lobectomy (28%), and exploratory laparotomy (20%). There was no operative mortality in either group. Cryosurgery was associated with reduced postoperative pain and significantly greater improvement in laboratory and clinical parameters. Three- and

5-year survival rates after cryosurgery vs. conventional surgery were, respectively, 60% vs. 51% and 44% vs. 36% (Fig 5). Disease-free survival was 30% with cryosurgery and 18% with conventional surgery. More patients in the cryosurgery group survived 10 years (19% versus 8%).

Conclusion.—Hepatic cryosurgery was found to be effective in the treatment of resectable and nonresectable LM. Compared with conventional surgical procedures, hepatic cryosurgery offers improved survival and disease-free survival.

► Cryosurgery has been used as a treatment for both benign and malignant neoplasms of the liver. What is unique about this report is that it represents a large series of patients (123) with long follow-up. As can be seen from the survival curves of Figure 5, the patients treated with cryosurgery did as well as patients with conventional hepatic surgery. In this study, patients in both treatment groups received systemic chemotherapy with 5-fluorouracil. It is interesting that patients with cryosurgery seemed to have a more precipitous decrease in carcinoembryonic antigen titers when compared with conventional surgery groups. This implies that at least in the hands of these experienced surgeons, cryosurgery may more effectively remove all of the tumor burden with an adequate margin. However, it remains to be proved whether chemotherapy after cryosurgery improves survival. Further studies may better define the role of cryosurgery in the treatment of liver metastases, but this article emphasizes the fact that at least in experienced hands cryosurgery may be an alternative modality.

T.J. Eberlein, M.D.

Liver Resection for Colorectal Metastases

Fong Y, Cohen AM, Fortner JG, et al (Mem Sloan Kettering Cancer Ctr, New York)

J Clin Oncol 15:938–946, 1997 11–24

Introduction.—Because the liver is often the only site of metastases from colon cancer, early and aggressive surgical excision of hepatic colorectal metastases may benefit a large number of patients. To determine the safety and efficacy of liver resection for colorectal metastases, investigators analyzed data for 456 consecutive resections performed during a 6-year period at a single institution. Previously published studies have often represented heterogenous clinical approaches and may not reflect current surgical practice (Table 1).

Methods.—Patients underwent liver surgery at Memorial Sloan-Kettering Cancer Center between July 1985 and December 1991. All had tumors that were anatomically confined within the liver and had no imaging evidence of disseminated disease. Patient data were extracted from the Department of Surgery Liver Resection database, hospital and office charts, and interviews. Specific items of interest included demographics,

TABLE 1.—Results of Hepatic Resection for Metastatic Colorectal Cancer

First Author/Year	No. of Patients	Years	No. of Institutions	Lobectomy or More No.	Lobectomy or More %	Operative Mortality (%)	5-Year Survival (%)
Foster,[12] 1978	168	—	99	45	27	5	20
Adson,[13] 1984	141	35	1	46	33	2	25
Fortner,[14] 1984	75	11	1	51	68	7	35
Butler,[15] 1986	62	31	1	22	35	10	34
Iwatsuki,[16] 1986	60	10	2	49	82	0	45
Hughes,[17] 1986	607	38	24	—		—	33
Nordlinger,[18] 1987	80	16	2	43	54	5	25
Schlag,[19] 1990	122	9	1	49	40	4	30
Doci,[20] 1991	100	9	1	50	50	5	30
Scheele,[9] 1991	219	28	1	87	33	6	39
Rosen,[21] 1992	280	28	1	69	25	4	25
Gayowski,[22] 1994	204	11	1	170	83	0	32
Current series	456	6	1	259	57	3	38

(Courtesy of Fong Y, Cohen AM, Fortner JG, et al: Liver resection for colorectal metastases. *J Clin Oncol* 15:938–946, 1997.)

pathologic condition of the primary colorectal lesion, pathologic findings of the liver lesion, operative details, hospital course, and outcome.

Results.—The median age of the 456 patients was 62 years. At the last follow-up examination, 212 patients had died at a median of 22 months from the time of liver resection. Median follow-up of survivors was 37 months. The perioperative mortality rate was 2.8%; for resections that involved a lobectomy or more (57% of cases), the mortality rate was 4.6%. Median hospital stay was 12 days (Table 3), but patients undergoing a lobectomy or more had a significantly longer hospital stay in addition to higher 30-day mortality rates and more complications. The 5-year survival rate in this patient series is 38%; median survival duration is 46 months. In univariate analysis, predictors of poorer outcome were nodal status of the primary lesion, a short disease-free interval before detection

TABLE 3.—Overall Perioperative Results

Variable	All Resections (n = 456)	Lobectomy or More (n = 259)	Less Than Lobectomy (n = 197)
Hospital stay (days)			
Median	12	13	11
Range	1-70	1-70	6-32
30-day mortality			
No.	13	12	1
%	2.8	4.6	0.5
Complications (%)	24	31	16
1-year survival (%)	88	87	89
3-year survival (%)	59	55	60
5-year survival (%)	38	37	42
Median survival, months	46	42	54

(Courtesy of Fong Y, Cohen AM, Fortner JG, et al: Liver resection for colorectal metastases. *J Clin Oncol* 15:938–946, 1997.)

TABLE 6.—Multivariate Predictors of Recurrence

Variable	Hazard	Coefficient	P
Positive margin	2.3	0.8	.00006
Size > 10 cm	1.8	0.59	.001
Disease-free interval < 12 months	1.5	0.41	.004
> 1 tumor	1.5	0.4	.005
Extrahepatic disease	1.6	0.45	.05
Node-positive primary	1.2	0.16	.4
CEA > 200 ng/mL	1.2	0.15	.5
Bilateral tumor	1.1	0.1	.5

Abbreviation: CEA, carcinoembryonic antigen.
(Courtesy of Fong Y, Cohen AM, Fortner JG, et al: Liver resection for colorectal metastases. *J Clin Oncol* 15:938–946, 1997.)

of liver metastases, carcinoembryonic antigen (CEA) level greater than 200 ng/mL, multiple liver tumors, extrahepatic disease, large tumors, and a positive resection margin. Independent predictors of poorer outcome in multivariate analysis were positive margin, size larger than 10 cm, disease-free interval less than 12 months, multiple tumors, and extrahepatic disease (Table 6).

Conclusion.—Liver resection for colorectal metastases, now the only potentially curative therapy for metastatic colorectal cancer, is safe and effective. Extrahepatic disease is the only absolute contraindication to resection. Despite an association between short disease-free interval or multiple tumors and poorer outcome, patients with these findings had a mean 5-year survival rate higher than 24%.

► Metastatic disease to the liver from colorectal cancer is a common problem. This is one of the largest series of patients who have been prospectively evaluated with hepatic resection (Table 1). As previously published in other series, a significant portion of patients will have a 5-year survival. This series had a 38% 5-year survival rate. Multivariate analysis of predictors of recurrence show that by far the margin of resection is extremely important as is the size of the tumor, the disease-free interval, and the number of tumor nodules (Table 6). An aggressive surgical strategy for the management of colorectal metastases to the liver, however, comes at a price. Even in the hands of this very experienced group, lobectomies were associated with a complication rate of approximately 30% (Table 3).

The majority of patients, with disease recurrence have liver metastases. This brings up several issues: (1) adequacy of imaging study to ensure that no small lesion is left unresected; (2) emphasis on the importance of adequate surgical margins; and (3) the issue of use of either regional or systemic chemotherapy. Unfortunately, no prospective study has adequately addressed the utility of adjuvant systemic chemotherapy after resection. Regional chemotherapy is clearly feasible. An ongoing, randomized, prospective trial will hopefully better define the role of adjuvant treatment after resection.

T.J. Eberlein, M.D.

Repeat Hepatectomy for Colorectal Liver Metastases

Adam R, Bismuth H, Castaing D, et al (Université Paris Sud)

Ann Surg 225:51–62, 1997 11–25

Objective.—After surgical resection for isolated liver metastases, approximately 60% of patients have a recurrence requiring repeat resections. Whether repeat resection actually increases survival and long-term benefit has not been thoroughly studied. Results of a retrospective analysis of a 12-year experience in hepatic resection of colorectal metastases to define longterm patients outcome and survival are presented.

Methods.—Between January 1984 and June 1995, of 243 patients who had liver resection, 64 (20 women), aged 31–73, underwent 83 repeat hepatectomies (64 second, 15 third, and 4 fourth) after primary colon cancer (n = 45) or primary rectal cancer (n = 19). Extrahepatic disease was present in 3 patients at first resection and 17 at repeat resection. All patients had chemotherapy after first resection. Survival and the variables associated with it were analyzed statistically.

Results.—Curative resection was not possible in 16 repeat surgeries. Extrahepatic surgery was required in 6 second resections and 2 third resections. Intraoperative bleeding did not increase significantly with repeat resection. No patients died during or within 2 months after surgery. There were 13 complications after second resections and 3 complications after the third and fourth resections (Table 4). Patient survival was determined at 1, 3, and 5 years (Figs 2, 3, and 4). Univariate analysis showed that 5-year survival was significantly better when the length of time between first and second resection was longer than 1 year, when the resection was curative, fewer than 3 nodules were found at second resection, and serum carcinoembryonic antigen levels were less than 30 IU/L. The presence of synchronous resectable extrahepatic disease significantly decreased survival. Multivariate analysis showed that more than 1 year between first

TABLE 4.—Operative Mortality and Postoperative Morbidity Following Repeat Hepatic Resection

	Hepatectomy			
	First	Second	Third-Fourth	p Value
Operative mortality (<2 mo)	0/64	0/64	0/19	—
Operative blood transfusion (units) [mean (range)]	1.2 ± 1.8 (0–6)	2.0 ± 2.7 (0–12)	2.1 ± 2.8 (0–10)	NS
Complications (no.)				
Postoperative bleeding	1	3	—	NS
Biliary fistula	1	2	2	
Abdominal infection	3	2	1	
Fluid collection	2	2	—	
Pleuropneumopathy	3	4	—	
Total	10 (16%)	13 (20%)	3 (16%)	
Hospital stay (days)	13.9 ± 8.1	13.3 ± 4.2	13.1 ± 5.7	NS
Mean Range	7–63	7–25	7–30	

(Courtesy of Adam R, Bismuth H, Castaing D, et al: Repeat hepatectomy for colorectal liver metastases. *Ann Surg* 225:51–62, 1997.)

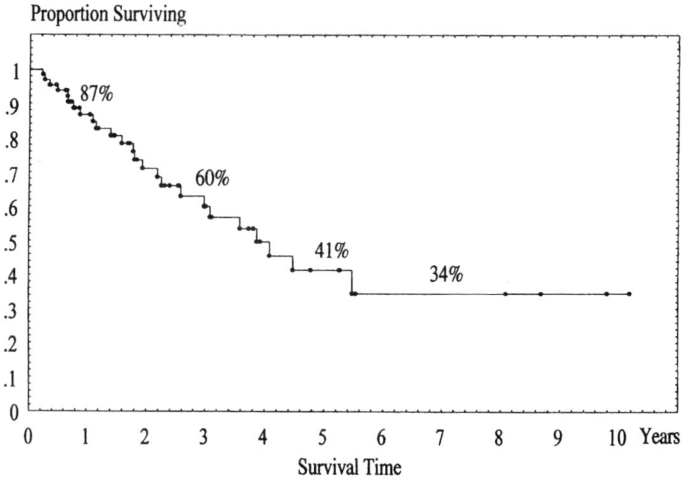

FIGURE 2.—Cumulative survival of 64 patients with recurrent metastases of colorectal cancer after a second hepatectomy. (Courtesy of Adam R, Bismuth H, Castaing D, et al: Repeat hepatectomy for colorectal liver metastases. *Ann Surg* 225:51–62, 1997.)

and second resections and a curative second resection were independently and significantly related to survival.

Conclusion.—Repeat, curative resection for colorectal metastases can increase survival provided no extrahepatic disease is present.

► As experience with resection for recurrent metastatic colorectal cancer is obtained, the question of whether repeat resection for re-recurrent disease is often undertaken. This article, by Adam and colleagues from Université

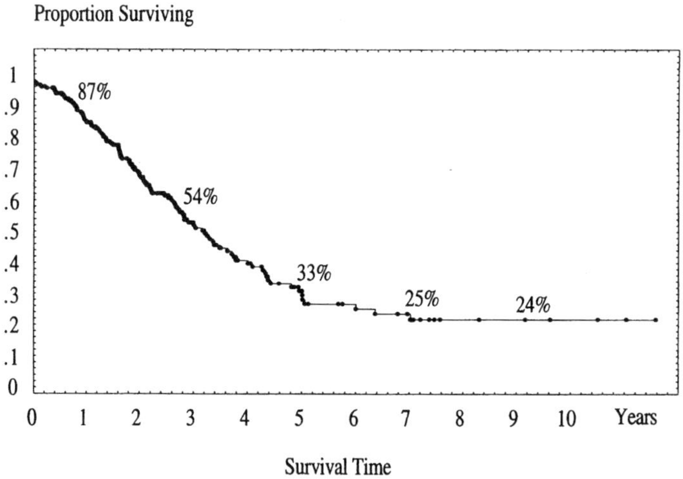

FIGURE 3.—Cumulative survival of 243 patients with metastases of colorectal cancer after a first hepatectomy. (Courtesy of Adam R, Bismuth H, Castaing D, et al: Repeat hepatectomy for colorectal liver metastases. *Ann Surg* 225:51–62, 1997.)

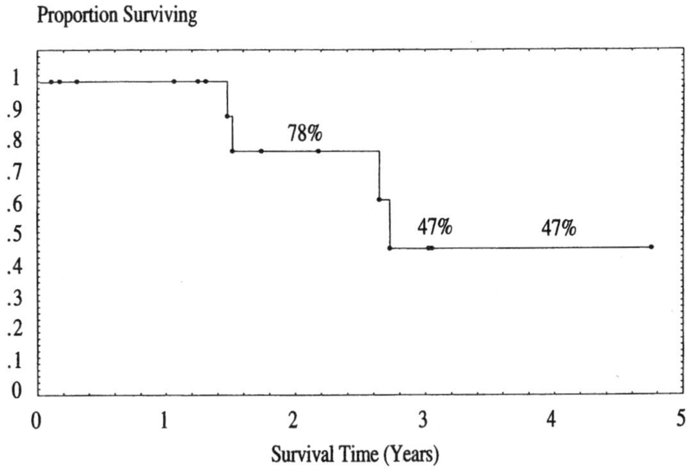

FIGURE 4.—Cumulative survival of 15 patients with recurrent metastases of colorectal cancer after a third hepatectomy. (Courtesy of Adam R, Bismuth H, Castaing D, et al: Repeat hepatectomy for colorectal liver metastases. *Ann Surg* 225:51–62, 1997.)

Paris Sud at Villejuif, showed that in fact second and even third resections are possible. In the hands of these very experienced surgeons, the morbidity for repeat resection is not significantly different than for initial hepatic resection (Table 4); the morbidity is very acceptable. As seen in Figure 3, the cumulative long-term survival after initial hepatectomy is approximately 25%. However, in selecting patients for repeat resection, multivariate analysis shows that the length of time between first and second resection, as well as the curative intent of the re-resection, is associated with an excellent long-term survival advantage (Figure 2). Once again, in highly selected patients, even after a third hepatectomy, nearly 47% of the patients are alive at 5 years (Figure 4).

To duplicate these results would require careful patient selection and careful operative technique, both related to the experience of the operating surgeon.

T.J. Eberlein, M.D.

Pancreas

Adenocarcinoma of the Ampulla of Vater: A 28-Year Experience
Talamini MA, Moesinger RC, Pitt HA, et al (Johns Hopkins Med Insts, Baltimore, Md)
Ann Surg 225:590–600, 1997 11–26

Introduction.—Adenocarcinoma of the ampulla of Vater is considered to be the most curable of all carcinomas of the upper gastrointestinal tract. Reported series are small and treatment of periampullary cancer has changed significantly in recent years. The experience with adenocarcinoma

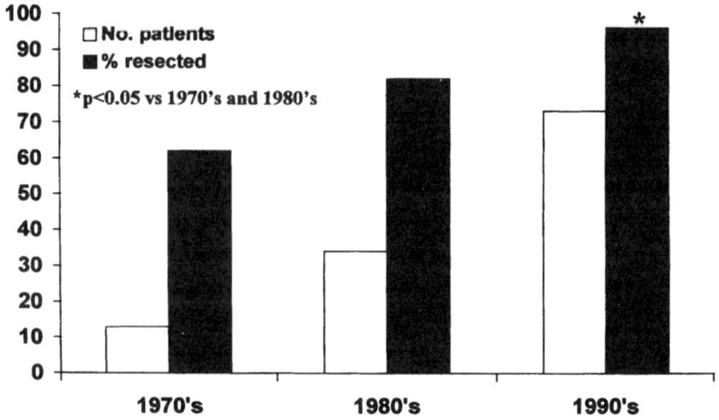

FIGURE 3.—Number of patients resected and resection rate by decade. (Courtesy of Talamini MA, Moesinger RC, Pitt HA, et al: Adenocarcinoma of the ampulla of Vater: A 28-year experience. *Ann Surg* 225:590–600, 1997.)

of the ampulla of Vater was evaluated during a 28-year period to determine which factors influence patient outcome.

Methods.—Medical records from 1969 to 1996 of 120 patients with adenocarcinoma of the ampulla of Vater were reviewed for demographics,

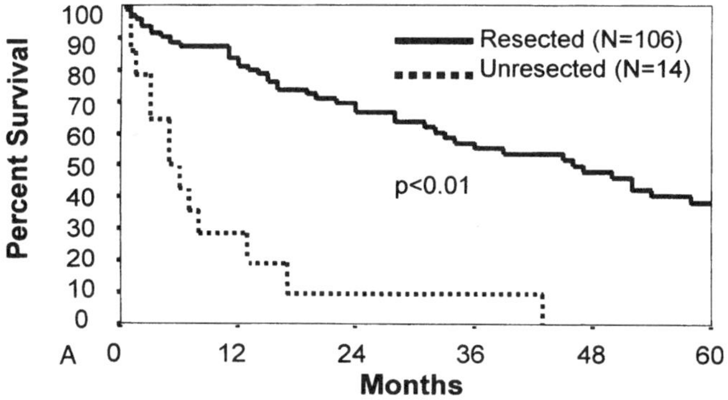

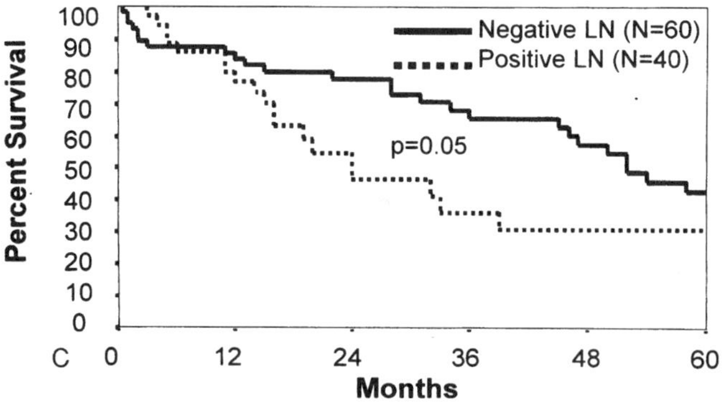

(Continued)

FIGURE 5 (cont.)

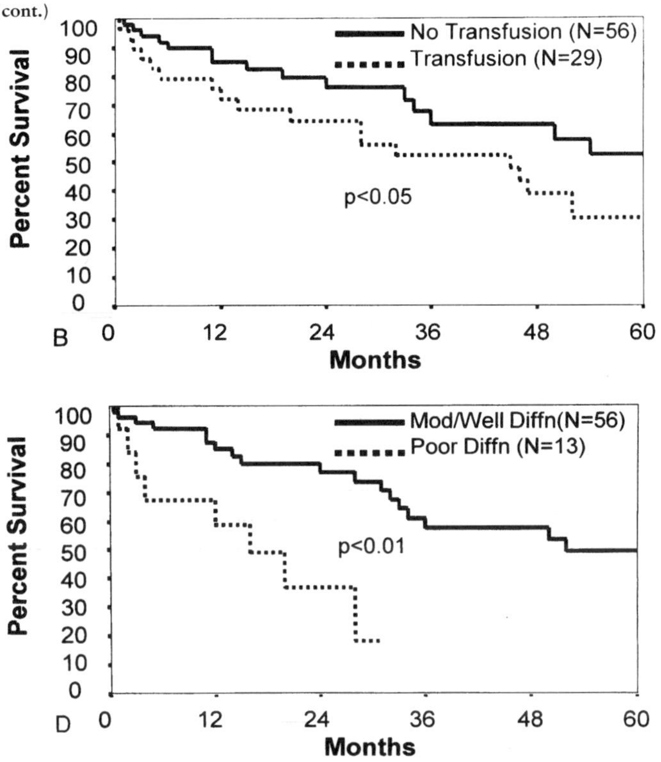

FIGURE 5.—A, influence of resection on outcome for ampullary carcinoma. B, influence of blood transfusion on outcome for ampullary carcinoma. C, influence of lymph node status on outcome for ampullary carcinoma. D, influence of tumor differentiation for ampullary carcinoma. (Courtesy of Talamini MA, Moesinger RC, Pitt HA, et al: Adenocarcinoma of the ampulla of Vater: A 28-year experience. *Ann Surg* 225:590–600, 1997.)

history and physical findings, laboratory data, radiologic evaluation, procedures, pathologic evaluation, complications, and treatment. Morbidity and long-term survival were calculated. Factors influencing patient outcome were evaluated.

Results.—One-hundred six (88%) of 120 patients underwent resection. Of these, 105 (99%) underwent pancreaticoduodenal resection (103) or total pancreatectomy (2). The number of patients who underwent resection increased from 62% in the 1970s to 82% in the 1980s, to 96% in the 1990s (Fig 3). The 5-year survival rate for patients who were unable to undergo resection was 5 months, and the mean survival rate was 0%. For patients who underwent resection, these numbers were 46 months for the 5-year survival rate and 38% for the mean survival rate (Fig 5). The number of transfusions significantly decreased from 1.5 in the 1980s to 0.82 in the 1990s (Table 4). The 5-year survival rate of patients with blood transfusions was 30% and the survival rate of patients without transfusions was 53%, which indicated a significant adverse effect of transfusions

TABLE 4.—Operative Time, Blood Loss, and Transfusions

	1980s (N = 28)	1990s (N = 70)
Operative time (min)	448	421
Blood loss (mL)	686	653
Transfusions (units)	1.5	0.62*

**P* < 0.05 vs. 1980s.
(Courtesy of Talamini MA, Moesinger RC, Pitt HA, et al: Adenocarcinoma of the ampulla of Vater: A 28-year experience. *Ann Surg* 225:590–600, 1997.)

on survival. There was a significant decrease in morbidity from 70% before to 38% after December 1992. Factors influencing long-term outcome were resection, no perioperative blood transfusions, negative lymph node status, and moderately or well-differentiated tumors. The best predictor of prolonged survival was the absence of perioperative blood transfusions.

Conclusion.—This is the first time that the use of perioperative transfusions has been shown to be a significant factor affecting the long-term survival in patients with adenocarcinomas of the ampulla of Vater. Survival rates were also better in patients with resectable tumors, negative lymph nodes, and moderately or well-differentiated histologic features.

► This is a superb single-institution experience describing 120 patients with adenocarcinomas of the ampulla of Vater. Although this is not a randomized experience, this group has had an interest in these types of tumors as well as pancreatic tumors. Figure 3 documents that, as the experience of the group increased over 3 decades, the number of patients undergoing resection and the percentage of patients undergoing resection increased significantly. Once again, the experience of this operative team had an impact on survival. Although blood loss was not significantly less in the 1990s compared with the 1980s, transfusions were (Table 4), but this had a significant impact on survival (Fig 5B).

The overall survival rate of this group of patients is among the best in the series reported. This is no doubt a result of the technical expertise developed by this group. Clearly, the take-home message is that these results are obtainable only with experienced surgeons who frequently do these operations, which thereby improves the resectability rates, even in marginal cases. The other issue, of course, is the question of what happens to the other 60% of patients who undergo successful resections but who have recurrences. Thus, these patients will probably form the basis of a randomized trial of adjuvant therapies. Unfortunately, no single institution is large enough to adequately answer the question about adjuvant therapy in a reasonable period of time; therefore, the study of this issue will probably benefit from a collaborative effort.

T.J. Eberlein, M.D.

Pancreaticoduodenectomy for Pancreatic Adenocarcinoma: Postoperative Adjuvant Chemoradiation Improves Survival. A Prospective, Single-Institution Experience

Yeo CJ, Abrams RA, Grochow LB, et al (Johns Hopkins Med Insts, Baltimore, Md)

Ann Surg 225:621–636, 1997 11–27

Introduction.—Chemoradiation after pancreatic resection for adenocarcinoma of the pancreas significantly improves median and long-term survival rates, according to limited data from the Gastrointestinal Tumor Study Group (1985 and 1987). Many patients still do not receive adjuvant therapy after this procedure. Survival after pancreaticoduodenectomy for pancreatic adenocarcinoma was prospectively compared in patients receiving 1 of 2 different combined-modality adjuvant protocols or no adjuvant therapy.

Methods.—During a 4-year period, all patients with resected, pathologically confirmed adenocarcinoma of the head, neck, or uncinate process of the pancreas were evaluated by a multidisciplinary team. Patients were offered 3 treatment options: standard therapy: external beam radiation to the pancreatic bed (4,000–4,500 cGy) during two 3-day fluorouracil (5-FU) courses, then a weekly 5-FU bolus for 4 months; intensive therapy: external beam radiation to the pancreatic head (5,040–5,760 cGy) with prophylactic hepatic irradiation (2,340–2,700 cGy) with 5-FU plus leucovorin for 5 of 7 days for 4 months; or no therapy: no radiation or chemotherapy.

Results.—Of 174 patients, 99 elected standard, 21 elected intensive, and 53 elected no therapy. A tumor diameter less than 3 cm, intraoperative blood loss of less than 700 mL, an absence of intraoperative blood transfusions, and use of adjuvant chemoradiation therapy were associated with significantly longer survival. The most powerful predictors of outcome were tumor diameter, intraoperative blood loss, status of resected margins, and use of postoperative adjuvant therapy (Table 7). Compared with no therapy, patients who underwent postoperative adjuvant radiation therapy survived significantly longer (mean, 13.5 vs. 19.5 months) (Fig 2). The

TABLE 7.—Multivariate Analysis

Factor	p Value	Hazard Ratio	95% Confidence Intervals
Tumor diameter ≥3 cm	<0.001	2.278	1.433–3.623
Intraoperative blood loss ≥700 mL	0.014	1.754	1.119–2.749
Positive resection margins	0.055	1.586	0.990–2.542
Intensive therapy	0.04	0.495	0.253–0.967
Standard therapy	<0.001	0.347	0.211–0.572

(Courtesy of Yeo CJ, Abrams RA, Grochow LB, et al: Pancreaticoduodenectomy for pancreatic adenocarcinoma: Postoperative adjuvant chemoradiation improves survival: A prospective, single-institution experience. *Ann Surgery* 225:621–636, 1997.)

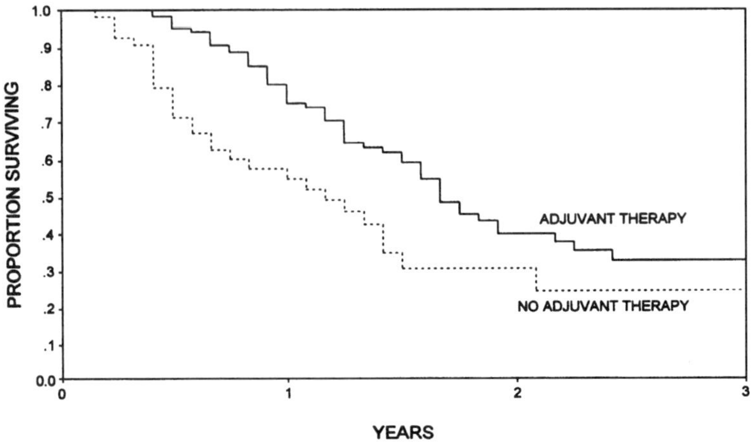

FIGURE 2.—The actuarial survival curves for patients undergoing pancreaticoduodenectomy comparing patients receiving adjuvant therapy (n = 120) to those declining adjuvant therapy (n = 53; P = 0.003). (Courtesy of Yeo CJ, Abrams RA, Grochow LB, et al: Pancreaticoduodenectomy for pancreatic adenocarcinoma: Postoperative adjuvant chemoradiation improves survival: A prospective, single-institution experience. *Ann Sur* 225:621–636, 1997.)

intensive therapy group did not have any survival advantages over the standard therapy group (mean, 21 vs. 17.5 months).

Conclusion.—Compared with no therapy, the survival rate was significantly improved in patients who received adjuvant chemoradiation after pancreaticoduodenectomies for pancreatic adenocarcinomas. There was no significant treatment advantage of intensive over standard therapy.

► This is a single-institution experience. Although it is prospective, it is not randomized. As seen in Figure 2, patients receiving adjuvant therapy had an improved survival rate compared with patients that received no adjuvant therapy. However, the patients receiving intensive treatment (higher pancreatic bed radiation and prophylactic hepatic radiation with combination chemotherapy) initially had an improved survival rate, but long term this improved survival rate did not hold up. Whether this is because of longer term toxicities is not addressed in this report, but it also seems to support the observation that more treatment is not necessarily better.

A tumor diameter of more than 3 cm was a strong independent predictor for decreased survival (Table 7). Intraoperative blood loss also negatively influenced survival as did positive resection margins. Although both intensive and standard adjuvant therapies improved survival, standard therapy appeared to be a more powerful predictor of survival than did intensive therapy.

Giving the patients the option of treatment potentially allowed bias into the results because younger, healthier patients with the easiest recovery would have the opportunity to pick participation in the adjuvant therapy arms. Another issue involves the question of whether, with longer follow-up, the 2 curves will begin to merge together.

As follow-up of this study increases, it will also be interesting to address the specific question of why the intensive adjuvant arm had no better, and possibly a worse, survival rate than did the standard adjuvant arm. This would seem to be related to the effects of the intensive adjuvant treatments.

T.J. Eberlein, M.D.

Stomach

Immunohistochemical Evaluation of Lymph Node Micrometastases From Gastric Carcinomas

Ishida K, Katsuyama T, Sugiyama A, et al (Shinshu Univ, Matsumoto, Japan)
Cancer 79:1069–1076, 1997 11–28

Objective.—Whereas discrete carcinoma cells or occult metastases of primary gastric carcinoma are difficult to detect in ordinary preparations stained with hematoxylin and eosin (H&E), the immunoperoxidase method—which stains for cytokeratin and carcinoembryonic antigen (CEA)—is able to detect micrometastases.

Methods.—A total of 2,446 lymph nodes were removed from 109 patients with primary gastric carcinoma stages I, II, and III. Tissues were fixed in 20% phosphate-buffered formalin and stained with H&E; Alcian blue pH 2.5 with periodic acid-Schiff stain (AB-PAS); CAM5.2, an antibody against cytokeratin; and an antibody against CEA. The ability of the staining methods to detect micrometastases were compared statistically. Surviving patients were followed for an average of 1,833 days.

Results.—Staining methods H&E, AB-PAS, CAM5.2, and CEA detected metastases in 230, 258, 427, and 287 lymph nodes, respectively. Eleven patients had lymph node micrometastases only. Micrometastases were found in the marginal sinus, the medullary sinus, or both. The number of micrometastases increased with the depth of invasion of the primary carcinoma. Patients with pathologic stage II disease and no micrometastases survived significantly longer than did patients with micrometastases (Fig 6).

Conclusion.—Identification of micrometastases in patients with stage I or II gastric carcinoma is predictive of decreased survival.

▶ This paper raises a very important issue: if more careful evaluation of lymph nodes is performed, more biologically accurate staging of patients is performed, as seen in Figure 6. For both stage II and stage III carcinoma, identification of micrometastases can identify patients who will have a much worse prognosis. Utilization of this type of technique will be important not only in gastric cancer, but in other gastrointestinal malignancies. In reviewing future articles, surgeons will need to pay particular attention to the detailed methodology for identification of micrometastatic disease in lymph nodes

Whereas this technology will increase the accuracy for biologically present micrometastatic disease, it would also suggest a patient population that may

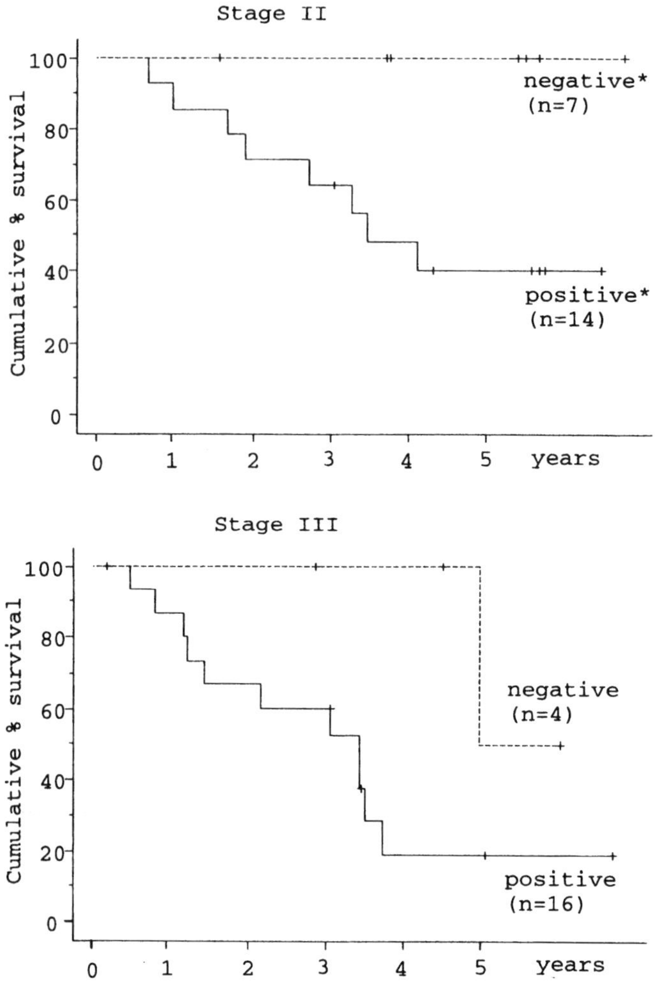

FIGURE 6.—Survival curves are shown for patients who tested positive or negative for micrometastases at stages II and III. Patients with micrometastases had a significantly worse prognosis at stage II. (*Asterisk* indicates $P < 0.05$, log rank test). (Courtesy of Ishida K, Katsuyama T, Sugiyama A, et al: Immunohistochemical evaluation of lymph node micrometastases from gastric carcinomas. *Cancer* 79:1069–1076, copyright 1997, American Cancer Society. Reprinted by permission of Wiley Liss, Inc., a subsidiary of John Wiley & Sons, Inc.)

benefit from more intensive adjuvant therapy. Whereas these authors used immunostaining for cytokeratin (or CEA), other authors have used polymerase chain reaction to amplify the presence of microscopic tumor.

As these improved techniques become more widespread, the opportunity to study larger numbers of patients for longer periods will help to define the importance of microscopic metastatic disease in lymph nodes. In the meantime, it will behoove the practicing surgeon to carefully evaluate the methodology for detection of pathologic spread of tumor in lymph nodes.

T.J. Eberlein, M.D.

Factors Predicting Hospitalization After Operative Treatment for Gastric Carcinoma in Patients Older Than 70 Years

Schwarz RE, Karpeh MS, Brennan MF (City of Hope Natl Med Ctr, Duarte, Calif; Mem Sloan Kettering Cancer Ctr, New York)

J Am Coll Surg 184:9–15, 1997 11–29

Objective.—More than half the diagnoses of gastric carcinoma are made in patients older than age 70. There is little information about the length of hospitalization and cost of care for these patients. Results of a study assessing morbidity, patient characteristics, perioperative mortality rates, and factors influencing length of hospitalization and survival are presented.

Methods.—A prospective review of information in the Memorial Sloan-Kettering Cancer Center Department of Surgery identified 385 patients (151 women), age 71–92, with gastric carcinoma diagnosed between July 1985 and July 1995. Length of stay, long-term survival, and disease specific survival were determined. Univariate and multivariate analyses were performed to compare groups.

Results.—Resection was performed in 310 patients; procedures included 138 distal gastrectomies, 111 proximal gastrectomies, and 61 total gastrectomies. Lymphadenectomies were performed in 281 patients. There were 22 deaths (7.1%) and 146 (47.1%) complications including 78 infections. The median hospital stay was 13 days with complications, particularly infectious complications, increasing hospital stays significantly. Univariate analysis showed that complications, resection type, primary cancer site, and infection were significantly related to longer hospitalization. Complications increased the hospital stay by an average of 11.5 days. Patients older than age 70 had significantly longer hospital stays than did patients age 70 or younger. According to multivariate analysis the presence of complications did not have an independent influence on survival.

Conclusion.—Resection for gastric carcinoma in the elderly increases survival, although the surgery carries a higher morbidity and mortality. Careful patient selection is important. Complications significantly increase the length of hospitalization.

► In the United States, gastric cancer is frequently associated with elderly patients. This article is therefore timely in its analysis of factors predicting for hospitalization in the treatment of patients older than 70 years who have gastric carcinoma. Hospitalization in the present study was approximately 17.8 days. Almost half the patients (47.1) had some complication. The occurrence of any complication was the most important factor leading to increased length of hospitalization.

This study underscores the necessity for carefully selecting and preoperative preparation of patients before attempted resection for gastric carcinoma.

T.J. Eberlein, M.D.

Quality of Life After Gastrectomy for Gastric Carcinoma: Controlled Study of Reconstructive Procedures

Svedlund J, Sullivan M, Liedman B, et al (Sahlgrenska Univ, Gothenburg, Sweden; Univ Hosp, Linköping, Sweden)

World J Surg 21:422–433, 1997 11–30

Introduction.—For patients with gastric cancer, radical resection is the only treatment that offers a chance of cure. Total gastrectomy may be preferred to ensure total tumor elimination, but this operation is often followed by postprandial symptoms leading to impaired dietary intake. Some authors have recommended subtotal gastrectomy in an attempt to prevent some of these adverse sequelae. The use of an enteric reservoir has been proposed as well. These 3 surgical alternatives for the treatment of gastric cancer were compared in a randomized clinical trial.

Methods.—The study included 64 patients eligible for curative surgery for gastric cancer. They were randomized to undergo total gastrectomy (31 patients), subtotal gastrectomy (13 patients), or gastric reconstruction with a jejunal S-shaped pouch (20 patients). Quality of life was assessed using a wide range of instruments selected to evaluate the subjective physical, mental, and social consequences of stomach cancer and its treatment. The patients completed this battery of tests the week before surgery and 3 and 12 months afterward.

Results.—There were few serious complications in any of the 3 groups. The patients lost 10% of their preoperative body weight within the first 3 months after surgery; after that, body weight stabilized. There was no evidence of tumor recurrence or progression during the 12-month study. Patients in all 3 groups reported alimentary symptoms and functional limitations in daily life, including eating dysfunction, indigestion symptoms, and diarrhea. After surgery, mental well-being was significantly improved. Patients undergoing total gastrectomy, with or without a gastric substitute, had significantly more overall gastrointestinal symptoms than those undergoing subtotal gastrectomy. Patients in the subtotal gastrectomy group also had significantly less diarrhea.

Conclusion.—Patients undergoing gastrectomy for gastric cancer experience significant unfavorable effects, including alimentary symptoms and functional limitations. Mental well being is improved after surgery. Patients undergoing total gastrectomy have more gastrointestinal sequelae than those undergoing subtotal gastrectomy. Pouch reconstruction does not appear to offer improvement in quality of life after total gastrectomy. The option of subtotal gastrectomy must be considered for patients with gastric cancer, whenever feasible.

▶ This is a very interesting study of 64 consecutive patients who were randomized to have either a total gastrectomy, subtotal gastrectomy, or jejunal S-shaped pouch implanted as a gastric substitute. As has been previously published, total gastrectomy is associated with an increase in morbidity that is best prevented by subtotal gastric resection, even if only a small cuff of stomach is preserved. However, these authors found no significant benefit, nutritionally, among the 3 groups.

One potential issue with this study is the fact that the patients were assessed at 3 and 12 months after surgery. Some believe that quality of life will continue to improve and probably will not stabilize until approximately 3 years after surgery. Obviously, in patients who present with advanced-stage disease, 3-year assessment would be impossible.

T.J. Eberlein. M.D.

Melanoma

Mortality, Major Amputation Rates, and Leukopenia After Isolated Limb Perfusion With Phenylalanine Mustard for the Treatment of Melanoma
Taber SW, Polk HC Jr (Univ of Louisville, Ky)
Ann Surg Oncol 4:440–445, 1997 11–31

Background.—This review examined the risks of isolated limb perfusion (ILP) chemotherapy for advanced primary, regionally recurrent, or metastatic melanoma of the extremity.

Study Design.—A MEDLINE search of the English language medical literature from 1980 to 1995 was conducted to obtain all reports of patients treated with phenylalanine mustard ILP for cutaneous melanoma of the extremities. This search identified 13 articles, 11 retrospective case studies, and 2 prospective trials, which were analyzed for mortality rates, major amputations, and leukopenia incidence. There were 1,315 women and 667 men included in this study.

Findings.—The overall 30-day mortality rate was 0.6%. The incidence of major amputation was 0.8%. Leukopenia occurred in 0.7% of the patients in this study group.

Conclusions.—A review of 35 years of reported experience with phenylalanine mustard ILP therapy for patients with cutaneous malignant melanoma of the extremity indicated that the risk of mortality, limb amputation, and leukopenia following this therapy was low.

▶ This is a well-written educational review. Although it does not address the issue of efficacy of isolated limb perfusion in extremity melanoma, it does document that there is a less than 1% risk of mortality, severe leukopenia, or major amputation following isolated limb perfusion.

Some studies suggest improvement in local and regional disease control. The World Health Organization may help define isolated limb perfusion's use for thick or high-risk primary lesions in this patient population. Meanwhile, it is probably beneficial for use in regionally confined, recurrent melanoma.

T.J. Eberlein, M.D.

Recent Advances in the Care of the Patient With Malignant Melanoma

Reintgen D, Balch CM, Kirkwood J, et al (Univ of South Florida, Tampa; Univ of Pittsburgh, City of Hope Natl Med Ctr, Duarte, Calif)

Ann Surg 225:1–14, 1997 11–32

Background.—Important advances in the treatment of melanoma have occurred in the past 3 years. The advances in surgical care, staging, and adjuvant treatment of melanoma were reviewed.

Methods and Findings.—Recently reported surgical techniques, elective node dissection, and sentinel lymph node (SLN) biopsy, were reviewed. Findings from the Eastern Cooperative Oncology Group 1684 trial, the basis for the FDA approval of adjuvant interferon alfa-2b (IFN-α-2b), also were reviewed. In the Intergroup Melanoma Trial, a survival benefit was associated with elective node dissection in patients with melanoma and tumor thickness of 1–2 mm or in patients younger than 60 years of age. Six reports show an order to melanoma nodal metastases and that the SLN histology reflects the histology of the rest of the nodal basin. Thus, the more conservative SLN biopsy can be done for adequate nodal staging of patients with melanoma. Adjuvant IFN-α-2b is most beneficial in patients with nodal metastases who are disease free after surgical resection. When only lymph node–positive patients are considered, the survival benefit associated with adjuvant IFN is significant.

Conclusions.—Adjuvant IFN-α-2b therapy is associated with a survival benefit in patients at high risk for melanoma recurrence. It may be argued that all patients with melanoma larger than 1 mm should have a nodal staging procedure. The least morbid procedure for obtaining this information is selective lymphadenectomy with SLN biopsy.

► I would recommend this paper for any practicing general surgeon who treats patients with melanoma. It is a very clearly written manuscript and in a few pages reviews the Intergroup Melanoma Trial looking at lymph node dissection. It also reviews the most recent data on SLN biopsy and discusses adjuvant therapy consisting of IFN-α-2b. There is also an excellent introduction consisting of a discussion of prognostic factors and biology in malignant melanoma.

T.J. Eberlein, M.D.

Localizing the Sentinel Node in Cutaneous Melanoma: Gamma Probe Detection Versus Blue Dye

Kapteijn BAE, Nieweg OE, Liem IH, et al (The Netherlands Cancer Inst, Amsterdam)

Ann Surg Oncol 4:156–160, 1997 11–33

Objective.—There is debate over the use of elective lymph node dissection in patients with primary melanoma of the skin without palpable metastases. One proposed technique of avoiding unnecessary lymph node dissection is biopsy of the sentinel node (SN), the first node into which the melanoma drains. Two methods of finding the SN have been proposed—intradermal injection of a radioactive tracer around the melanoma and injection of patent blue dye (PBD). These 2 techniques for the localization of SNs were compared.

Methods.—The study included 110 patients with a clinically localized melanoma with a Breslow thickness of 1 mm or greater. All patients had undergone excision less than 3 months previously. The day before surgery, each patient underwent lymphoscintigraphy using the radiopharmaceutical ^{99m}Tc-nanocolloid to determine the position of the SN. On the day of surgery, PBD was injected at the same site. During surgery, blue-stained nodes were sought. When they were found, the radioactivity level of the node was measured with the gamma probe. If no blue nodes were found, the SN was traced with the probe.

Results.—A total of 219 SNs in 141 basins were identified by preoperative lymphoscintigraphy. Of these SNs, 8 were not explored and 1 could not be found. The remaining 210 SNS were excised, as were 27 additional nodes detected during surgery. Eighty-four percent of the excised nodes were detected using PBD alone, and the remaining nodes were localized using the gamma probe. Thus, the combination of PBD and the gamma probe identified 99.5% of all SNs. Melanoma was found in the SN in 23 patients. Three patients had SNs that were false negative for metastasis.

Conclusion.—In patients with cutaneous melanoma, intraoperative use of the gamma probe combined with PBD injection identifies more SNs than lymphatic mapping with PBD alone. The PBD provides information useful in distinguishing between SN and second-echelon nodes. It is almost always possible to identify the SN, and the operation to excise it is usually simple. A randomized trial to determine the impact of SN excision on regional tumor control and survival is underway.

► This is a study of 110 patients who underwent lymphoscintigraphy, then PBD injection, followed by gamma probe detection of the SN. The results are interesting and confirm other studies, that is, it appears that there are more SN identified by gamma probe than by PBD methodology. However, the combination of these techniques rendered a 99.5% localization of SNs.

Clearly, a high proportion of patients can have SN identification using PBD methodology. However, gamma probe technology seems to be easier to apply with a quicker learning curve. An advantage of PBD is that it is able to distinguish afferent from efferent lymphatics. Gamma probe might be utilized alone in the patient in whom dynamic lymphoscintigraphy clearly distinguishes first echelon nodes from second echelon nodes. As with radiopharmaceutical development, gamma probe technology will undoubtedly become easier. By means of polymerase chain reaction and molecular markers, false negative lymph nodes will be minimized. The prospective, randomized multicenter trial initiated by Morton and colleagues will more thoroughly evaluate this new technology in patients with melanoma.

T.J. Eberlein, M.D.

Sarcoma

Core Needle Biopsy for Diagnosis of Extremity Soft Tissue Sarcoma

Heslin MJ, Lewis JJ, Woodruff JM, et al (Mem Sloan-Kettering Cancer Ctr, New York)

Ann Surg Oncol 4:425–431, 1997 11–34

Background.—Open biopsy is traditionally used for diagnosis of extremity masses suspicious for soft-tissue sarcoma. The disadvantages of this technique are cost, time, and morbidity. The advantages of core needle biopsy are minimal morbidity, cost, and time. However, the diagnostic accuracy of core needle biopsy has not been reliably established under these circumstances. The diagnostic accuracy of core needle biopsy was compared with open biopsy for the diagnosis of primary extremity masses suspicious for soft-tissue sarcoma.

Study Design.—From 1990 through 1995, 164 patients with extremity masses suspicious for soft-tissue sarcoma underwent biopsy at a single institution. Two patients in this group underwent both types of biopsies. Of these 164 patients, 111 were derived from a prospective soft-tissue sarcoma database and 55 with a benign diagnosis were derived from a clinical information center. Pathology reports were reviewed. Statistical analyses were performed only for adequate biopsy specimens.

Findings.—For this group of 164 patients, the initial diagnostic approach was 60 core needle, 44 incisional, 36 frozen section, and 26 excisional biopsies. Two patients underwent 2 biopsy procedures. Of the core needle biopsy specimens, 93% were adequate for diagnosis. Of these adequate specimens, 95% correlated with the final resection diagnosis for malignancy, 88% for grade and 75% for histologic subtype (Table 3). Of the frozen-section biopsy specimens, 94% were adequate for diagnosis. Of these adequate specimens, 88% correlated with the final resection diagnosis for malignancy, 62% for grade, and 47% for histologic subtype. The false-negative rate for core needle biopsy was 5% and the false-positive

TABLE 3.—Comparison of Biopsy Type for Malignancy of Adequate Biopsy Specimens

Biopsy	Resection	Core (n = 56)	Incisional (n = 45)	Frozen section (n = 34)
Malignant	Malignant	42	38	15
Malignant	Benign	0	0	2
Benign	Malignant	3	0	2
Benign	Benign	11	7	15
Sensitivity (%)		93	100	88
Specificity (%)		100	100	88
Accuracy (%)		95	100	88
Positive predictive value (%)		100	100	88
Negative predictive value (%)		79	100	88

(Courtesy of Heslin MJ, Lewis JJ, Woodruff JM, et al: Core needle biopsy for diagnosis of extremity soft tissue sarcoma *Ann Surg Oncol* 4:425–431, 1997. Copyright © the Society of Surgical Oncology, Inc.)

rate was 0%. Two core needle biopsy specimens that were graded low were actually high, and 1 graded high was actually low.

Conclusions.—When read by an experienced pathologist, core needle biopsy is accurate for the preoperative diagnosis and grading of extremity masses suspicious for soft-tissue sarcoma. If adequate tissue sampling cannot be achieved, open biopsy is required.

▶ This manuscript from the Memorial Sloan-Kettering Group documents the adequacy of core needle biopsy for diagnosis of soft tissue sarcoma. As can be seen from Table 3, incisional biopsy showed no false-positive and no false-negative biopsy results. However, there were several core needle biopsies that were falsely negative. All of these turned out to be well-differentiated liposarcoma, a difficult pathologic distinction even after incisional biopsy. Core needle biopsy showed no false-positive biopsy results.

There are obvious disadvantages to open biopsy techniques such as morbidity, inadequacy of the specimen, inappropriately placed incisions, as well as the need for an operating room environment.

Another issue with core needle biopsy for soft-tissue sarcoma is whether the grade is accurately predicted. Even in these experienced pathologists' hands, grade was underestimated, in which case patients would receive additional radiation therapy, but their treatment would be otherwise unaltered. However, the possibility where biopsy results in high grade when the tumor on resection is actually low grade may result in increased morbidity and cost, especially if preoperative chemotherapy is advised. Thus, for this technique to be widely adapted, the importance of an experienced pathologist is emphasized.

T.J. Eberlein, M.D.

Other and New Technology

The Use and Interpretation of Commercial *APC* Gene Testing for Familial Adenomatous Polyposis

Giardiello FM, Brensinger JD, Petersen GM, et al (Johns Hopkins Univ, Baltimore, Md; LabCorp, Research Triangle Park, NC)

N Engl J Med 336:823–827, 1997 11–35

Background.—Commercial tests are available to test for the adenomatous polyposis coli (*APC*) gene, which causes familial adenomatous polyposis. But how effective is such testing. These authors examined the use of clinical *APC* testing in one commercial laboratory in 1995.

Methods.—Data are based on 177 members of 125 families who underwent *APC* testing. The *APC* gene was analyzed by in vitro synthesized-protein assay. The test has two valid indications: (1) to confirm familial adenomatous polyposis in patients with typical colorectal adenomatous polyposis or multiple adenomas and (2) to test their first-degree relatives. The laboratory collected patient data prospectively by telephone and returned a standardized written report that briefly summarized the results.

TABLE 3.—Features of the Gene-testing Process

Feature	Percent	No. of Patients/Total
Valid indication for testing*	83.0	147/177
Appropriate strategy for pre-symptomatic testing among patients at risk†	79.4	50/63
Genetic counseling provided before testing	18.6	33/177
Written informed consent obtained‡	16.9	28/166
Test results interpreted correctly	68.4	121/177

*Fifty-four patients had familial adenomatous polyposis, 30 had multiple colorectal adenomas, and 63 were at risk for familial adenomatous polyposis.

†The appropriate strategy was one in which a family member with familial adenomatous polyposis, if available, was tested before a family member who was at risk for the disease.

‡There was no response to our request for documentation of written informed consent for 11 patients.

(Courtesy of Giardiello FM, Brensinger JD, Petersen GM, et al: The use of interpretation of commercial *APC* gene testing for familial adenomatous polyposis. *N Engl J Med* 336:823–827, 1997.

Findings.—Eighty-three percent of the tests were performed for valid indications; 9.6% of tests were ordered because of colorectal cancer (family or personal history). Table 3 revealed that in only about one fifth of cases was genetic counseling provided before testing or was informed consent for the procedure obtained. In almost one third of cases, the physician incorrectly interpreted the results of the test (mainly, that failure to detect a mutation could be a false-negative result). *APC* gene mutations were identified in about two thirds (68.5%) of 54 patients with clinically identified familial adenomatous polyposis, and in one fourth of patients with at least 20 colorectal adenomas but no family history of polyposis. Of 44 patients who were tested for other indications, a mutation was identified in only 1 patient.

Conclusions.—Almost 20% of tests were ordered for invalid indications, and in only about 20% of cases was genetic counseling provided and informed consent obtained. Importantly, because colorectal cancer develops in almost all patients with familial adenomatous polyposis, a failure to find an *APC* gene mutation in about 20% of this patient population could lead to false-negative results, with disastrous consequences.

► This study evaluates 177 patients that underwent a commercial laboratory test for the *APC* gene during the calendar year 1995. An overwhelming majority of the patients (83%) had valid indications for being tested. As seen in Table 3, however, only 18% of the patients received genetic counseling before testing, and only approximately 17% gave written informed consent. Additionally, 20% of clinically unaffected patients considered at risk underwent pre-symptomatic testing before the *APC* mutation was identified in affected family members. This would be expected to be eliminated if genetic counseling were performed before the testing.

Because APC gene mutations are not detected in 20% of patients with familial adenomatosis polyposis, false-negative results occur. Most disturbing in this study is that some patients at risk for familial adenomatous polyposis would have been given false-negative results.

As genetic testing increases, physicians who order these tests should include genetic counseling and obtain written informed consent for all of their patients.

T.J. Eberlein, M.D.

Efficacy and Safety of Enoxaparin *Versus* Unfractionated Heparin for Prevention of Deep Vein Thrombosis in Elective Cancer Surgery: A Double-Blind Randomized Multicentre Trial With Venographic Assessment

Bergqvist D, for the ENOXACAN Study Group (Univ Hosp, Uppsala, Sweden)
Br J Surg 84:1099–1103, 1997 11–36

Introduction.—Patients undergoing elective abdominal surgery for malignant disease are at high risk for venous thromboembolic complications and require perioperative antithrombotic prophylaxis. A randomized, double-blind trial was designed to evaluate the efficacy of enoxaparin, a low-molecular-weight heparin, with that of unfractionated low-dose heparin (UFH) when administered for the prevention of deep vein thrombosis in abdominal or pelvic surgery for cancer.

Methods.—Patients eligible for the multicenter trial were 40 years of age or older, scheduled for surgery expected to exceed 45 minutes in duration and to require at least 6 days of postoperative hospitalization, and had an expected survival of at least 6 months. Randomization was to UFH (5,000 units administered subcutaneously with the first injection 2 hours before surgery, then 3 times daily until venography) or to enoxaparin (40 mg administered subcutaneously with the first injection 2 hours before surgery, then once daily until venography). Venography was performed at a mean of 10 days after operation. The primary end point was the development of documented venous thromboembolism; hemorrhage was a secondary end point.

Results.—The evaluable study population included 631 patients, 319 who received UFH and 312 who were treated with enoxaparin. Demographic variables, types of surgery, and mean duration of operation were similar in the 2 groups. Thromboembolic complications developed in 104 patients (16.5%), 58 (18.2%) in the UFH group and 46 (14.7%) in the enoxaparin group. The incidence of hemorrhage was also similar in the UFH and enoxaparin groups (17.1% and 18.7%, respectively), and there were no differences between the groups in 30-day or 3-month mortality.

Discussion.—The low-molecular-weight heparin enoxaparin, administered once daily, was equivalent to 3-times-daily UFH for thromboprophylaxis in patients undergoing surgery for abdominal or pelvic cancer. The 2 regimens were also equivalent in safety.

▶ Patients with malignancy have a higher risk of venous thromboembolic complication. Low–molecular weight heparin has been used for thromboprophylaxis. Recently, enoxaparin has been used as an effective prophylaxis in hip surgery. This double-blind, randomized, multicenter trial studied enoxaparin in patients with abdominal malignancies undergoing curative surgery. Enoxaparin was shown to be equivalent to UFH given three times daily for thromboprophylaxis. Not only was the frequency of deep venous thrombosis similar in the 2 groups (deep venous thrombosis was documented by a filling defect seen in 2 projections on venographic studies), but there also was no change in the rate of bleeding complications in either group. Thus, it appears that enoxaparin can be safely used in patients with abdominal malignancy as well as orthopedic surgery.

T.J. Eberlein, M.D.

A Multivariate Analysis of Factors Contributing to Leakage of Intestinal Anastomoses

Golub R, Golub RW, Cantu R Jr, et al (Flushing Hosp, NY; State Univ of New York, Brooklyn)

J Am Coll Surg 184:364–372, 1997 11–37

Introduction.—Morbidity and mortality increase dramatically in patients with anastomotic leaks. Previous investigators have used univariate analysis to identify perioperative risk factors for anastomotic breakdown. Factors contributing to leakage of small and large bowel anastomoses were evaluated in a retrospective, multivariate analysis.

Methods.—A wide range of possible determinants of anastomotic leaks were analyzed retrospectively in 764 patients who underwent 813 intestinal anastomoses. End points were clinically significant anastomotic leaks and mortality. All variables underwent univariate and multivariate analysis.

Results.—Of 764 patients, 27 had 28 anastomotic dehiscences (overall rate, 3.4%). Leaks were clinically evident at an average of 12.2 days. There were no differences in the rate of leakage among different types of anastomoses or among anastomotic levels. Hand sewn and stapled anastomoses did not differ in leakage rates. The rate of anastomotic leakage in patients undergoing a protecting ostomy was nonsignificantly greater, compared with that in patients without ostomies (5.6% vs. 3.4%). Six significant predictive variables were identified by multivariate analysis: serum albumin level of less than 3.0 g/L, use of corticosteroids, peritonitis, bowel obstruction, chronic obstructive pulmonary disease, and perioperative transfusions of more than 2 units of packed red blood cells (Table 5). The mortality rate of hospitalized patients was 37% for patients with

TABLE 5.—Multivariate Analysis*

Variable	*Odds ratio*	*95% Confidence intervals*			*p Value*
Chronic obstructive pulmonary disease	3.22	1.14	to	9.09	.03
Bowel obstruction	2.79	1.17	to	6.62	.02
Peritonitis	8.46	2.46	to	29.13	.0007
Corticosteroids	6.46	1.87	to	22.28	.003
Transfusion >2 U	7.25	2.35	to	22.33	.0006
Albumin <3.0 g/L	2.73	1.29	to	5.81	.009

*Hosmer-Lemeshow goodness of fit chi-square equals 2.128, degrees of freedom equals 8, P = 0.9768.

(Courtesy of Golub R, Golub RW, Cantu R Jr, et al: A multivariate analysis of factors contributing to leakage of intestinal anastomoses. *J Am Coll Surg* 184:364–372, 1997. By permission of the *Journal of the American College of Surgeons*.)

leakage and 6.8% for patients without leakage. The presence of an anastomotic leak was a strong independent predictor of in-hospital mortality.

Conclusions.—Multivariate analysis revealed 6 factors predictive of anastomotic leaks: malnutrition, use of corticosteroids, peritonitis, bowel obstruction, chronic obstructive pulmonary disease, and use of more than 2 units of packed red blood cells. Anastomotic leak was a strong independent predictor of in-hospital mortality.

► Intestinal anastomotic leak is a major source of morbidity and mortality for patients. This is a retrospective, multivariate analysis of more than 750 patients who underwent various types of intestinal anastomoses. It was interesting that technique and location of the anastomosis did not seem to make a difference. However, as seen in Table 5, the presence of infection (peritonitis), poor nutrition, the use of corticosteroids, multiple blood transfusions, as well as bowel obstruction and/or presence of chronic obstructive pulmonary disease all significantly contributed to anastomotic breakdown and leak. Interestingly, proximal diversion did not decrease the frequency of leak.

While no new striking information is obtained from this review, there are certainly elements that are either preventable or treatable which will mitigate the impact on intestinal anastomosis. Issues of bowel preparation have been somewhat controversial. These authors showed a substantially reduced risk of anastomotic leak of colocolic anastomoses when there was proper bowel cleansing. Of note also, these authors found no increased risk of anastomotic leak when more than 1 anastomosis was performed in a particular patient.

As has been previously identified, anastomotic leak in this study was associated with a four-fold increase in hospital stay which, in this era of cost-effective medical care, would be best avoided.

T.J. Eberlein, M.D.

Dendritic Cells Pulsed With RNA Are Potent Antigen-presenting Cells In Vitro and In Vivo

Boczkowski D, Nair SK, Snyder D, et al (Duke Univ, Durham, NC)

J Exp Med 184:465–472, 1996 11–38

Background.—Because the dendritic cell (DC) network is specialized to present antigen to T cells, immunization with DCs that have been loaded with tumor antigens is potentially an effective method for inducing immunity to tumors. Although such immunization has been limited to those cancers with defined tumor rejection antigens, an approach that uses unfractionated tumor peptides could work with any type of tumor. This approach is limited by the amount of tumor material available and the possibility of reaction against "self" antigens. To overcome these problems, messener RNA (mRNA) from tumor cells represents a potential source of tumor antigen for immunization. This RNA can be amplified from a small amount of source material and can be enriched in tumor-specific material by subtractive hybridization with mRNA from normal tissue. This study was performed to determine whether dendritic cells pulsed with RNA are effective in inducing CTL responses and tumor immunity in a mouse model.

Methods.—Mouse splenocytes were harvested and used as source material for the purification of DC and B cells. The cationic lipid, DOTAP, was used to deliver RNA into the dendritic cells. Mice were then immunized with these irradiated, RNA-pulsed cells. After 10–14 days, these mice were challenged with live tumor cells. All mice were killed when tumor size reached greater than 3.5 cm or after 40 days. A separate group of mice were injected in the foot pad with poorly immunogenic F10.9 melanoma cells. When the local tumor was 7–8 mm in diameter, their legs were amputated. Two days after amputation, mice were immunized intraperitoneally with pulsed DC and then received 2 booster vaccinations a week apart. Metastatic loads were assessed by lung weight.

Results.—Splenic DCs pulsed with RNA were assessed for their ability to induce a primary CTL response in vitro in the E.G7–OVA (ovalbumin) tumor system. DCs pulsed with OVA RNA synthesized in vitro were more effective in stimulating primary OVA-specific CTL responses in vitro than were DCs pulsed with OVA peptide. DCs pulsed with unfractionated RNA from OVA-expressing tumor cells were as effective as DCs pulsed with OVA peptide. Induction of the OVA-specific CTL response was eliminated when polyA$^+$ RNA from OVA-expressing tumor cells was treated with antisense OVA oligodeoxynucleotide and RNAse H, which digests the resulting hybrid nucleotide complexes. These results suggest that the RNA taken up by the pulsed DC cells was translated and the protein processed and presented via the class I antigen presentation pathway to stimulate cytotoxic T cells. Mice vaccinated with DCs pulsed with RNA from OVA-expressing tumor cells were protected against a challenge with OVA-expressing tumor cells. In the poorly immunogenic, highly metastatic B16/F10.9 tumor model, mice vaccinated with DCs pulsed with tumor-derived RNA had a significant reduction in tumor lung metastases. The same results were obtained with DCs pulsed with total tumor RNA, polyA$^+$ RNA, but not with polyA$^-$ RNA.

Conclusions.—The results of this study have demonstrated that murine dendritic cells pulsed with RNA are an efficient method to introduce antigens into the major histocompatibility complex (MHC) class I presentation pathway. DCs pulsed with RNA were capable of stimulating a primary CTL response in vitro, and animals immunized with pulsed DCs mounted an effective antitumor and antimetastatic response. Total tumor RNA, polyA$^+$ tumor RNA or RNA transcribed in vitro from complementary (cDNA) cloned into a bacterial plasmid were effective for immunization. Because RNA transcribed in vitro from cDNA cloned into a bacterial plasmid was effective in sensitizing DCs, amplification of antigenic content from a small source of material is possible, expanding the potential usefulness of RNA-pulsed DC vaccines for patients with small tumors.

▶ There has been great effort during the last several years to identify tumor-associated antigens (TAA). However, it has become equally obvious that once these antigens are identified, they are not very helpful in immunization protocols unless there are proper co-stimulatory molecules. In this study, the authors show that DCs pulsed with RNA are highly potent antigen-presenting cells and that they are unable to induce a primary CTL response in vitro that is at least as efficient as the response elicited by peptide-pulsed DCs. Treatment of mice with DCs pulsed with tumor-derived RNA also led to a dramatic reduction in the extent of lung metastases.

I have selected this article because DCs may well play an important role in immunization schema in various malignancies. It also offers the potential that once antigens are identified from a particular tumor, the tumor itself is not necessary for immunizations, but as in the case RNA, naked DNA, or even protein may form a more specific antigen for sensitization of the immune system.

In the very near future, my prediction is that DCs with some form of specific TAA will become a potential adjuvant therapy for many solid tumors such as breast, ovary, melanoma, and pancreas.

T.J. Eberlein, M.D.

12 Plastic, Reconstructive, and Head and Neck Surgery

Introduction

The mixture this year is two thirds head and neck and about one third other topics (breast, truncal-extremity reconstruction, complex wounds). The selections reflect some significant trends in head and neck surgery: the increased use of combined therapy (concurrent chemoradiotherapy) in the treatment of advanced head and neck cancer—with which, unfortunately, a large proportion of patients are initially seen—and the increased incidence of problems seen with this more-aggressive approach to a difficult problem.

I have placed the "other" category in front of the head and neck selections and begin with two relatively controversial topics: the explantation of breast implants and the use of bilateral reconstruction for "prophylactic" (How *do* we define *prophylactic,* anyway?) mastectomy. The incidence and complications with explantation are not trivial. Then follows a subsection on truncal and extremity reconstructive problems, including two papers on reconstruction of the anterior abdominal wall—one with microvascular techniques and the other with an innovative approach to the use of local tissues, two contrasting concepts. A paper discusses an effort to decrease the duration of immobilization in the postoperative care of decubiti patients, and another paper details the peerless experience of Emory with infected median sternotomy wounds.

All surgeons (worth their salt) are interested in wounds. No wounds are more difficult than those inflicted by war, and the authors of one article included here described an aggressive approach to casualties of the Balkan conflict. Another wound paper assessed occlusive dressings, a currently popular choice for difficult wounds. The last of the trio in this wound section tried to quantify infections in bone (When is bone "osteo myelitic?").

Next, we enter the head and neck selection booth and scroll up our choices. The papers this year, as in years past, naturally fall into one (usually) of several subcategories: diagnosis, treatment, secondary problems, reconstruction, and miscellaneous. The diagnosis group is the largest with abstracts and comments on six papers. In a number of other anatomical sites (rectum, prostate, esophagus), US has been employed to evaluate tumor extent. The authors of the first paper discussed in this section did so to determine tumor thickness in carcinoma of the tongue, an important prognostic indication (we think). The next paper highlights that fact by the use of tumor thickness in the prediction of regional lymph node metastases. The authors of the third paper in this group used routine CT of the chest in head and neck cancer patients, with a surprising set of results. The next paper reflects the interest in the use of radiotherapy as a primary modality, and not adjuvant therapy, in an attempt to find biomarkers in those patients that will not respond. Another investigation of parameters to further assess the perioperative management is evaluation of the nutritional status of the patient, an instinctual conclusion on the part of most surgeons but one lacking in hard data. The last paper in this group is a negative diagnostic paper, namely, the lack of efficacy (according to the authors) of sestamibi scanning for parathyroidectomy.

The treatment section addresses the topic mentioned above, concurrent chemotherapy and radiotherapy, with the preliminary results of a phase III trial, and the dark side of the force, morbidity of combining such therapy in supraglottic laryngectomy.

Treatment failure in head and neck cancer foretells a dismal outcome for the patient and misery for the surgeon. One paper addresses the extent of neck disease after regional failure when one obseves an N0 neck, and another advises us on the endovascular management of catastrophic hemorrhage. As a reconstructive surgeon, I am particularly pleased to include abstracts and commentary, on a small group of papers on head and neck reconstruction. These include a discussion of the current role of radial forearm flap in mandibular reconstruction (a controversial choice), the use of the fibula for mandibular placement, and the management of extensive mandibular osteoradionecrosis by immediate reconstruction. The last paper in this group is particularly interesting. It concerns the repair of a complete glottic stenosis with a fibula free flap, a salvage situation that would otherwise culminate in laryngectomy.

The miscellaneous group includes three papers that deal with an aggressive variant of head and neck cancer. The first of these is Merkel cell carcinoma; the second is neurotropic skin cancers; and the third, adenoid cystic carcinoma. A fourth paper is not particularly aggressive, but this can be a difficult management problem. The authors give us some perioperative strategies for the management of carotid body tumors. The final paper in the miscellaneous group is an interesting discussion of paracutaneous vs. surgical tracheostomy.

Last, but not least, is on quality assurance in plastic surgery. If you're interested in the current initiative in quality assurance in medicine, the paper is well worth reading. The very fact that we have included only one paper on plastic surgery as such is reflective of the incredible restraint on the part of your reviewer.

Edward A. Luce, M.D.

Breast Reconstruction

Simultaneous Bilateral Breast Reconstruction With the Transverse Rectus Abdominus Musculocutaneous Free Flap

Khouri RK, Ahn CY, Salzhauer MA, et al (Washington Univ, St Louis; Univ of California, Los Angeles; Mount Sinai Med Ctr, Miami Beach, Fla; et al)

Ann Surg 226:25–34, 1997 12–1

Background.—The use of autogenous tissue in a technically feasible, safe procedure for breast reconstruction may make bilateral prophylactic total mastectomy more acceptable for patients at the highest risk for breast cancer. The outcomes and morbidity associated with simultaneous bilateral transverse rectus abdominis myocutaneous (TRAM) free flap breast reconstruction were reported.

Methods and Findings.—One hundred twenty consecutive patients undergoing 240 simultaneous bilateral TRAM free flap breast reconstructions at several centers were reviewed retrospectively. The mean operating time was 8.6 hours, including the time needed for the breast ablative part of the procedure. The mean length of stay was 7.6 days. However, these figures declined to 7.1 hours and 6.1 days, respectively, for the most recent group of 40 patients. Overall, 28% of the patients needed nonautologous blood transfusions. However, only 1 was needed among the last 40 patients. Thromboses developed in 2.5% of the flaps, including 4 arterial and 2 venous. Re-exploration permitted circulation restoration in 5 flaps, whereas 1 flap had to be replaced. One patient with a history of recurrent deep vein thromboses had an uncomplicated deep vein thrombosis, which did not adversely affect her outcome. Fifteen percent of the patients had minor complications, such as hematoma, partial wound necrosis, wound infection, and prolonged postoperative ileus. These complications did not adversely affect long-term outcome. Abdominal wall weakness or hernias developed in 11.6%. Mean follow-up was 37.2 months. At this time, satisfaction with the procedure was reported to be excellent by 56% of the patients; good by 40%; and fair by 4%.

Conclusions.—Simultaneous bilateral free flap reconstruction is a technically feasible procedure associated with a high success rate and acceptable morbidity. Bilateral prophylactic total mastectomy combined with simultaneous bilateral TRAM flap reconstruction performed by experienced surgeons may be an acceptable option for patients at high risk for breast cancer.

► The most cogent point of this paper from my perspective is that high-quality reconstruction for the "prophylactic" bilateral mastectomy will make this procedure considerably more palatable to both the patient and the general surgeon. The keys to the success in this series of patients was the use of loupes rather than the microscope for the microsurgical anastomosis, and the team approach. One must recall that the extirpative procedure is bilateral and affords the opportunity for bilateral tissue expansion and subsequent implants. The decision for autogenous tissue and the sacrifice of some abdominal wall integrity must be balanced against the probable better aesthetic result with the TRAM flap. Yet where this advantage is clear-cut and distinct is in **unilateral** reconstruction (at least in my opinion), bilateral reconstruction blurs that advantage substantially. Selection is the key. This is a well-illustrated and well-written article.

E.A. Luce, M.D.

Explantation of Silicone Breast Implants

Thomas WO III, Harper LL, Wong SW, et al (Univ of South Alabama, Mobile)

Am Surg 63:421–429, 1997 12–2

Background.—Silicone gel–filled breast implants have been employed successfully for decades. More recently, these implants have been associated with chronic morbidity in some implant recipients. In 1992, the United States Food and Drug Administration placed a moratorium on the use of silicone gel–filled breast implants. A retrospective analysis is reported of 25 patients with silicone gel–filled breast implants who were referred for evaluation and underwent removal of these implants.

Study Design.—Between 1992 and 1994, 25 consecutive female patients underwent bilateral silicone gel–filled breast implant removal at the University of South Alabama Medical Center. Information was obtained from referring physicians, medical records, patient interviews and medical examinations.

Findings.—Patient-reported symptoms included mastodynia, arthralgia, fibromyalgia, xerophthalmia, xerostomia, hypesthesia and amblyopia. Clinical examination and mammography were accurate in diagnosing 44% of ruptured implants. Only re-exploration was accurate in the detection of implant leakage. Histopathologic analysis of tissue samples demonstrated chronic inflammation (Fig 4). Postoperatively, patient-reported symptoms diminished over a course of months. There was no mortality associated with explanation, but the overall morbidity was 20%.

Conclusions.—A small group of silicone gel–filled breast implant recipients will manifest chronic morbidity. There is, as yet, no way to prospectively identify these patients. Symptomatic patients should be considered for removal, although this is associated with some morbidity. Patients

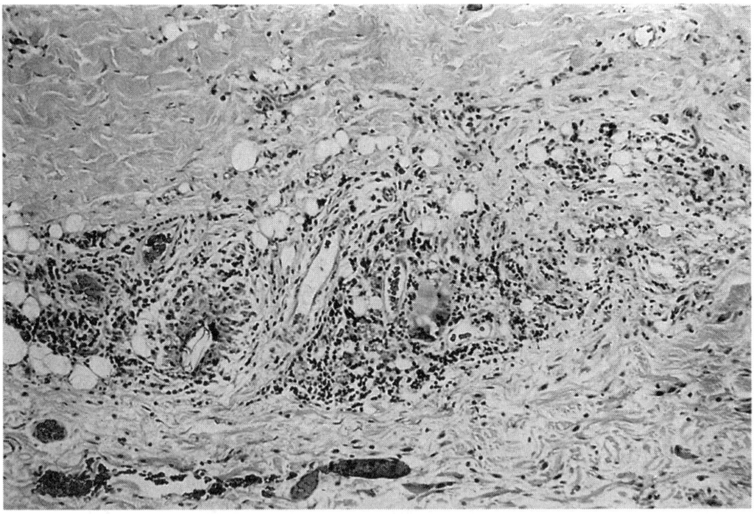

FIGURE 4.—Light microscopic histopathologic analyses of capsulectomy specimens revealed fibrosis and chronic mono- and multinucleated inflammatory cells (× 240). (Courtesy of Thomas WO III, Harper LL, Wong SW, et al: Explantation of silicone breast implants *Am Surg* 63:421–429, 1997.)

currently requiring prosthetics may be better served by saline-filled implants. Patients consenting to these procedures must be made aware of the associated risks.

► Another silicone breast implant paper for the reader's consumption. What was perhaps a little different in the slant of this paper were 2 aspects. First, the morbidity of explantation and replacement was considerably higher than in other studies and quite frankly and candidly presented. These results do demonstrate that the procedure of explantation is not innocuous and should not be offered to the patient in a cavalier fashion. Second, the authors have a reasonably good discussion of the silicone implant controversy up through 1995, although somewhat slanted. They did not cite *The New England Journal of Medicine* editorials by Marcia Angell, M.D., who is quite critical of the lack of science in the efforts to establish relationships between implants and systemic disease.

E.A. Luce, M.D.

Truncal-Extremity Reconstruction

The Tensor Fascia Lata Free Flap in Abdominal-Wall Reconstruction

Williams JK, Carlson GW, Howell RL, et al (Emory Univ, Atlanta, Ga; Indiana Univ, Indianapolis)

J Reconstr Microsurg 13:83–90, 1997 12–3

Background.—When possible, the pedicled tensor fascial lata (TFL) flap is preferred for use in reconstruction of the abdominal wall. However, the size and location of the abdominal defect sometimes preclude use of the

TABLE 1.—Characteristics of the Abdominal Wall Defects

Patient (Age)	*Infection/ Contamination*	*Size (cm^2)*	*Location (per umbillicus)*	*Underlying disorder (Initial Operation)*
1 (59yrs)	No	15 × 15	Infra	Leiomyosarcoma of the jejunum
2 (47yrs)	No	20 × 22	Infra/Supra	Adenocarcinoma Of the Colon
3 (49yrs)	No	13 × 16	Supra	CABG/Sternal Dehiscence
4 (27yrs)	Yes	24 × 12	Infra/Supra	Crohn's Disease
5 (44yrs)	Yes	20 × 12	Supra	Gastroesophageal Reflux/ Nissen Fund
6 (53yrs)	Yes	?	Infra/Supra	Perforated Ulcer of Duodenum
7 (35yrs)	Yes	15 × 25	Infra/Supra	Multiple Abdominal Stab Wounds

Abbreviation: CABG, coronary artery bypass grafting.

(Reprinted with permission from *Journal of Reconstructive Microsurgery* from Williams JK, Carlson GW, Howell RL, et al: The tensor fascia lata free flap in abdominal wall reconstruction. *J Reconstr Microsurg* 13:83–90, 1997. Copyright 1997, Thieme Medical Publishers, Inc.)

TFL flap. In this situation, microsurgical tissue transfer may provide greater reconstructive freedom. Use of the TFL flap as a free flap for reconstruction of full-thickness defects of the abdominal wall is reported.

Methods.—The retrospective study included 7 patients who had full-thickness abdominal wall defects reconstructed with TFL free flaps (Table 1). The wounds ranged in size from 208 to 375 cm^2; most were infected or contaminated. Eighty-six percent of the wounds involved the epigastrum. The TFL free flap had several key advantages, starting with elimination of the arc of rotation. This allowed the flap to be horizontally situated with the fascia placed in the position of greatest tensile strength. There was also less need for undermining than with a pedicled flap. The ability to use a single flap precluded the need for multiple donor sites. There was a 30% rate of donor site complications, including dehiscence of the native skin after skin grafting. No cases of total flap loss occurred.

Conclusions.—For patients with full-thickness defects of the abdominal wall, the TFL free flap is an attractive reconstructive option. Its use is not hindered by a limited arc of rotation, and it results in increased vascularity of the distal part of the flap. Microsurgical transfer of the TFL free flap is a particularly useful option for large defects or those located over the umbilicus.

► As the authors describe, no one has published this size series of the use of free flaps for abdominal wall reconstruction. In terms of reconstructing "like with like," tensor fascia lata flap fills the criterion quite nicely. The problem in this reviewer's experience is the unreliability of the distal portion of the flap, even when not extended further onto the lateral thigh. In fact, 3 of the 7 flaps did develop "tip necrosis," a potentially devastating complication if the integrity of the abdominal wall is lost because of the partial flap necrosis. Sometimes the reliability of the tensor fascia lata flap can be enhanced in length by prior delay. What we know now about delay is that the principle could be applied to the transfer of the tissue as a free flap, particularly on an elective basis.

E.A. Luce, M.D.

Massive Abdominal-Wall Hernia Reconstruction With Expanded External/Internal Oblique and Transversalis Musculofascia

Jacobsen WM, Petty PM, Bite U, et al (Mayo Clinic, Rochester, Minn)

Plast Reconstr Surg 100:326–335, 1997 12–4

Background.—This report describes a technique for expansion and primary closure of chronic, massive middle and lower abdominal-wall hernias. Massive hernias are defined as those at least 20 cm along any dimension, without the possibility of reduction, and repair without prosthetics.

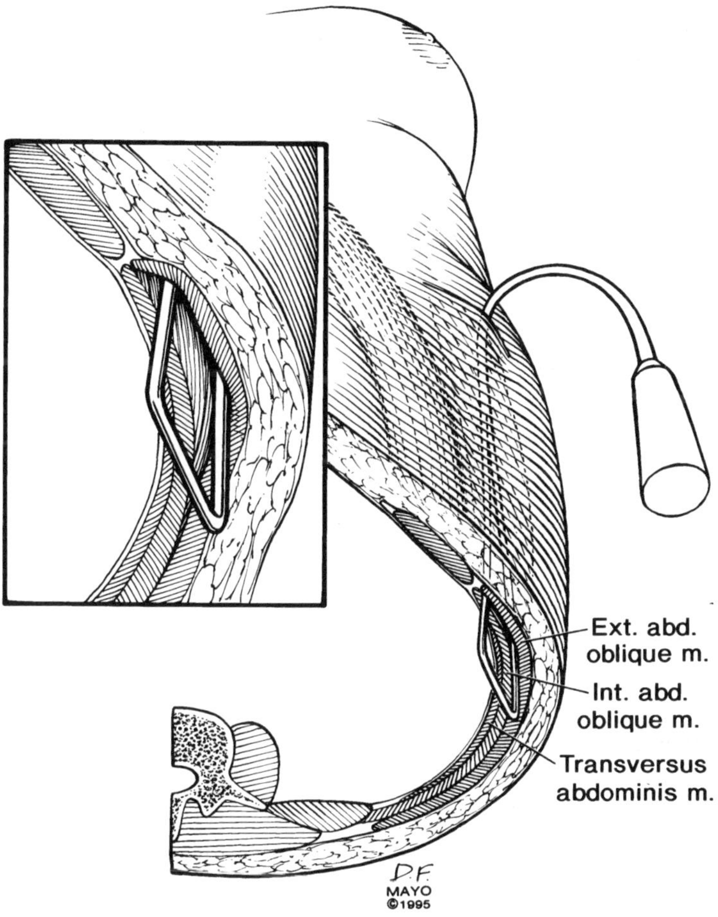

FIGURE 2.—Dissection of the space for tissue expander placement between the external oblique fascia and the complex of the internal oblique-transversalis fasciae. (Reprinted by permission of Mayo Foundation courtesy of Jacobsen WM, Petty PM, Bite U, et al: Massive Abdominal-wall Hernia Reconstruction With Expanded External/Internal Oblique and Transversalis Musculofascia *Plast Reconstr Surg* 100:326–335, 1997.)

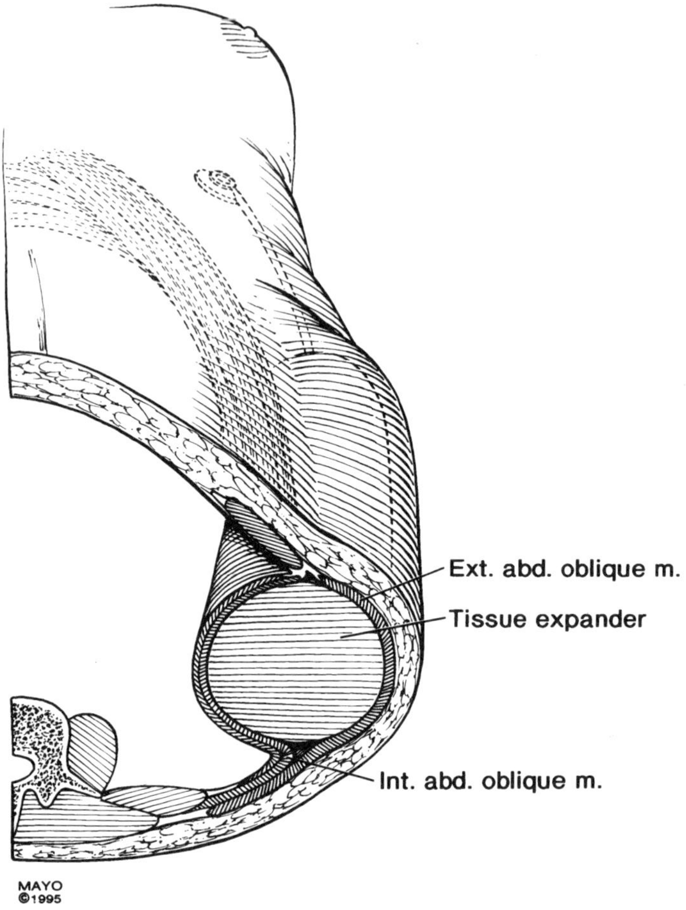

FIGURE 3.—Tissue expanders partially expanded in lateral abdominal wall. (Reprinted by permission of Mayo Foundation, courtesy of Jacobsen WM, Petty PM, Bite U, et al: Massive Abdominal-wall Hernia Reconstruction With Expanded External/Internal Oblique and Transversalis Musculofascia *Plast Reconstr Surg* 100:326–335, 1997.)

Anatomy.—The lateral abdominal-wall fascia and musculature and the rectus abdominis muscle are innervated along the same pathway. A transverse incision at the costal margin through the external oblique fascia will not injure significant nerves or blood vessels of the abdominal wall. The plane between the external and internal oblique fascia is an easily dissected, bloodless space that is convenient for expander placement. Expanders are placed in this area bordered by the inguinal ligament, the lateral margin of the rectus sheath, the midaxillary line, and the costal margin.

Technique.—Patients were examined by means of CT. Skin grafts were applied to the abdominal viscera and allowed to mature for 6 to 12 months. Abdominal wall incisions of 5 cm were made transversely and slightly downward on the costal margin. A 5 cm incision was made in the external oblique fascia (Fig 2). Expanders were placed in the region discussed in the anatomy section beneath the external oblique fascia (Fig 3). Wounds were allowed to heal for 3 weeks before the first expansion. Expansion was performed as tolerated. The fascial hernia borders were identified by intraperitoneal and extraperitoneal exposure. The expanders remained in place until adequate fascia was available for primary closure. The anesthesiologist monitored peak airway pressure throughout closure. The overlying abdominal-wall skin was closed over the fascial repair.

Conclusions.—The technique for repair of chronic, massive abdominal-wall hernias described in this report has several advantages: repair is achieved without destruction of musculature or neurovascular structures; the lateral abdominal wall is uninjured and can be used for expansion; the insertion of expanders is reliable; the operative field can be isolated from open wounds or ostomies in the abdominal wall; the external oblique musculofascial layer is strong enough for expansion; and the expanders are isolated from the operative field and can be left in place until final hernia closure can be achieved. Complications associated with this technique include rupture, early recurrence, and enterotomy. No pulmonary problems were associated with this technique. This technique has been successful in 4 patients.

► I don't know if this technique works consistently or not. The authors admitted to complications in 3 of the 4 patients, and my experience with efforts to expand the abdominal wall has been similar, namely, a significant complication rate. Other plastic surgeons have related a similar experience in informal discussions. Perhaps the error is in not selecting the appropriate plane. The authors emphasized the importance of utilization of the plane between the external and internal oblique that will preserve innervation to the rectus and avoid major blood vessels. Is the internal oblique and transversalis sufficiently strong to resist and direct expansion outward rather than inward into the peritoneal cavity?

E.A. Luce, M.D.

The Gracilis Myofasciocutaneous Flap: Vascular Anatomy and Clinical Application

Whetzel TP, Lechtman AN (Univ of Calif, Davis)

Plast Reconstr Surg 99:1642–1652, 1997 12–5

Background.—Skin perfusion may be unreliable with the gracilis myocutaneous flap. This problem can lead to moderately high partial flap

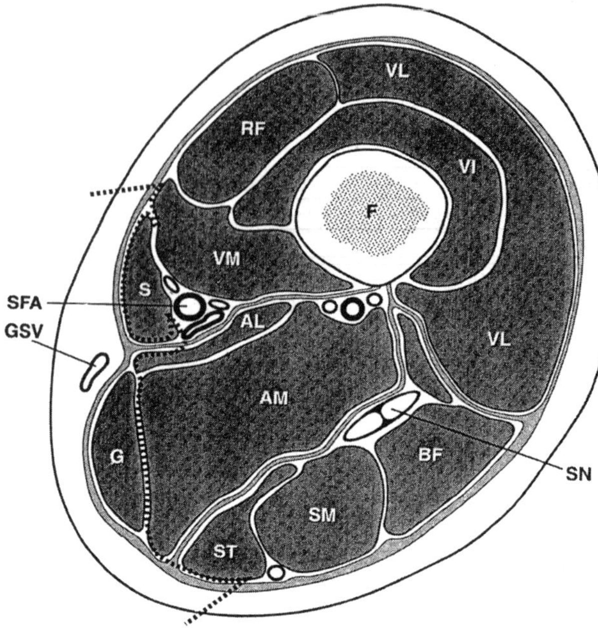

FIGURE 1.—Dissection plane of the gracilis myofasciocutaneous flap in an axial view at midthigh. *Dotted line* shows dissection plane. Skin incisions are beveled to include maximal deep investing fascia of medial thigh muscles. Dissection plane is onto the sartorius muscle fibers and down into the septum between the sartorius and adductor longus, ligating superficial femoral artery perforators close to their origins. Posterior fascia of the gracilis is entirely preserved without direct visualization of gracilis muscle fibers. *Abbreviations: AL,* adductor longus muscle; *AM,* adductor magnus muscle; *F,* femur; *G,* gracilis muscle; *GSV,* great saphenous vein; *RF,* rectus femoris muscle; *SFA,* superficial femoral artery; *ST,* semitendinosus muscle; *VM,* vastus medialis muscle. (Courtesy of Whetzel TP, Lechtman AN: The gracilis myofasciocutaneous flap: Vascular anatomy and clinical application. *Plast Reconstr Surg* 99:1642–1652, 1997.)

necrosis. In an attempt to prevent this problem, the authors have designed a gracilis myofasciocutaneous flap, to include all available regional fascia surrounding and deep to the gracilis muscle.

Methods.—Initial cadaver studies showed arterial connections between the pedicle vessel and fasciocutaneous perforating vessels from the superficial femoral artery (Fig 1). An axially oriented fascial network, supplying the overlaying skin, was partially supplied by perforating vessels (Fig 4). Each perforator had its own primary cutaneous vascular territory, as demonstrated by selective ink injection. The arterial connections between the pedicle and superficial femoral artery perforators were confirmed by specimen radiographs.

This information was used to design gracilis myofasciocutaneous flaps for use in 12 patients with previous pelvic irradiation. A total of 18 longitudinally oriented flaps were harvested; the flaps measured 8 cm in width and up to 30 cm in length. They included all fascia beneath the skin paddle in continuity with the deep fascia around the gracilis muscle. This

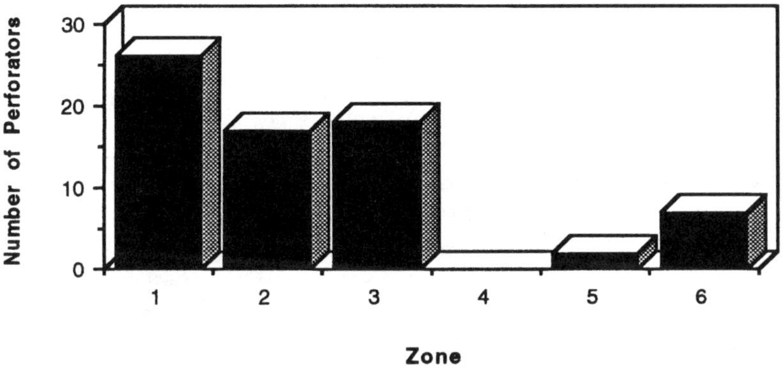

FIGURE 4.—Graph showing number of perforators in each zone. No significant perforating vessels were demonstrated in zone 4. (Courtesy of Whetzel TP, Lechtman AN: The gracilis myofasciocutaneous flap: Vascular anatomy and clinical application. *Plast Reconstr Surg* 99:1642–1652, 1997.)

was done to avoid disturbing the connecting vasculature within the fascia. The average follow-up was 12 months.

Outcomes.—Six of the 12 patients had minor flap-related complications such as seromas, mild infections, and partial dehiscence. However, there were no cases of flap necrosis. All flaps had excellent vascularity with good healing.

Conclusion.—The gracilis myofasciocutaneous flap avoids the skin perfusion problems encountered with the gracilis myocutaneous flap. The former incorporates the fascia around the gracilis muscle en bloc during flap elevation, thus preserving some of the fasciocutaneous blood supply to the skin. The flap should include the fascia deep to the gracilis, as well as the circumferential fascia from the sartorius and adductor muscle, along the entire length of the muscle. Occlusive disease of the profunda artery is a contraindication to the use of this flap, but previous pelvic radiation and surgery are not contraindications.

► Many reconstructive surgeons have become disillusioned with the use of a "standard" gracilis flap for pelvic and perineal reconstruction and may have communicated that discontent with the flap to their general surgical and surgical oncology colleagues. At first blush, the gracilis flap offers a number of advantages: the flap is in the immediate vicinity; can be harvested in a bilateral fashion; and, at least in a thinner patient, is a thin and pliable flap because of the small muscle bulk. Finally, the abdominal wall does not have to be entered to harvest the flap as is necessary in a transverse rectus abdominis myocutaneous reconstruction.

The authors offer hope, based on sound scientific experimentation and analysis, that the vascularity of the gracilis flap can be substantially enhanced by modification to include its adjacent vascularized fascia. The 12 patients in whom they utilized the flap represented difficult reconstructive problems, and all had been previously irradiated. The 25% incidence of problems could be related entirely to the past radiation and difficulty in healing in this area. One caveat, though: the flap depends on the intactness of the superficial femoral artery. Any amount of vascular disease in the femoral system would preclude successful harvest.

E.A. Luce, M.D.

Reducing the Period of Immobilization Following Pressure Sore Surgery: A Prospective, Randomized Trial

Isik FF, Engrav LH, Rand RP, et al (Univ of Washington, Seattle)

Plast Reconstr Surg 100:350–354, 1997 12–6

Background.—Treating pressure sores can be very expensive, partly because of prolonged postoperative immobilization. Because there have been no studies of the superiority of longer vs. shorter periods of immobilization, a prospective trial was done comparing 2 and 3 weeks of postoperative immobilization.

Methods.—Forty-two patients with paraplegia, tetraplegia, or multiple sclerosis and a solitary pressure sore were enrolled in the study during 5 years. By random assignment, each patient received 2 or 3 weeks of postoperative immobilization.

Findings.—The complication rates in the 2-week and 3-week groups were 39% and 47%, a nonsignificant difference. However, time to mobilization and time to sitting were significantly decreased in the 2-week group.

Conclusions.—Two weeks of immobilization after surgery is sufficient for the treatment of uncomplicated solitary pressure sores. In the absence of complications, this shortened period of immobilization may reduce length of stay and total hospital charges.

► This study is sorely needed so that we can reduce the cost of management of these patients. The authors, though, compared 2 vs. 3 weeks of immobilization, and probably missed the point. In this era of managed care, the comparison that needs to be made is against 3 or 4 days of hospitalization and discharge to a skilled nursing home.

E.A. Luce, M.D.

Management of the Infected Median Sternotomy Wound With Muscle Flaps: The Emory 20-Year Experience

Jones G, Jurkiewicz MJ, Bostwick J, et al (Emory Univ, Atlanta, Ga)

Ann Surg 225:766–778, 1997 12–7

Background.—Significant mortality is associated with median sternotomy wound infection after open heart surgery. Patient variables contributing to morbidity and mortality after such infection and the efficacy of treatment by débridement and closure with muscle flaps were investigated.

TABLE 18.—Classification of Sternal Wound Infection

Type	Depth	Description
1a	Superficial	Skin and subcutaneous tissue dehiscence
1b	Superficial	Exposure of sutured deep fascia
2a	Deep	Exposed bone, stable wired sternotomy
2b	Deep	Exposed bone, unstable wired sternotomy
3a	Deep	Exposed necrotic or fractured bone, unstable, heart exposed
3b	Deep	Types 2 or 3 with septicemia

(Courtesy of Jones G, Jurkiewicz MJ, Bostwick J, et al: Management of the infected median sternotomy wound with muscle flaps: The Emory 20-year experience. *Ann Surg* 225:766–778, 1997.)

Methods.—Four hundred nine patients treated during 20 years were reviewed. One hundred eighty-six treated since 1988 were included in the analysis of variables affecting rates of flap closure complications, recurrent sternal wound infection, and mortality.

Findings.—Overall mortality was 8.1%. Five percent of the patients needed additional procedures for recurrent sternal wound infection. Treatment for hematoma was required in 7.6% of the patients and hernia repair in 2.7%. Factors that were strongly associated with death were septicemia, perioperative myocardial infarction, and intra-aortic balloon pump. Intra-aortic balloon pump, hypertension, and a history of smoking were associated with wound closure complications. Recurrent infection was associated with history of sternotomy and treatment for sternal wound infection between 1988 and 1992. The average length of stay after sternal wound reconstruction decreased from 18.6 days between 1988 to 1992 to 12.4 days between 1993 and 1996 (Table 18).

Conclusions.—A significant decrease in mortality associated with sternal wound infection can be achieved by using the principles of sternal wound débridement and early flap coverage. Further improvements will rely on earlier detection of mediastinitis (before the onset of septicemia) and the increased efficacy of critical care of patients with multisystem organ failure.

► These authors tend to treat a more severe group of median sternotomy dehiscences, inasmuch as the cardiothoracic group at Emory probably operates on a fair number of referred difficult problems such as second sternotomies, obese and diabetic patients, etc. These authors attempt to provide us with a longitudinal perspective on the largest series of patients with this problem published. The sheer weight of numbers adds a great deal of quality to this paper. The discussion includes an excellent description of patient management that is clearly experience based. Points are made about postoperative antibiotics (Do we need them for 6 weeks if the sternum is completely débrided?), the deleterious effect of obesity in women on primary healing (Should large, obese, and pendulous breasts be strapped in the poststernotomy period?), and the location of skin necrosis with the use of the pectoralis major muscle (Are there fewer problems if the muscle is turned over than if the perforators are all sacrificed?).

E.A. Luce, M.D.

Complex Wounds

One-Stage Reconstruction of War Wounds With Free Osteocutaneous Flaps

Džepina I, Stanec Z, Škrbić S, et al (Univ of Zagreb, Croatia)
Br J Plast Surg 50:81–87, 1997 12–8

Objective.—High-energy war wounds are devastating. The usual treatment is excision followed by delayed primary closure and stabilization of fractures after wound débridement and external fixation. Secondary autogenous bone grafts and free tissue transfer are performed after wound healing. Management of segmental bone defects, particularly with loss of soft tissue cover can be challenging. Results of long-term follow-up of 31 patients with osteocutaneous defects of upper and lower extremities are discussed.

Methods.—Between July 1991 and May 1993, 369 patients were treated for war wounds of the extremities; 31 of these patients had a segmental bone defect greater than 4 cm. Group 1 patients (n = 8) underwent reconstruction within 3 to 6 days of injury. Group 2 patients (n = 23), referred from other hospitals, had reconstruction after 2 weeks to 12 months. Wounds were reassessed after 48 hours, and débridement was performed as necessary. Injuries were scored according to the Mangled Extremity Syndrome Index (MESI).

Results.—There were 20 wounds caused by explosions and 11 by gunshots. Bone defects ranged from 4 to 12 cm and usually involved the tibia (Fig 1). Types of flaps used for reconstruction included scapular, fibular, radial, deep circumflex iliac artery, and serratus anterior. Grafts were fixed with external fixators, plates, and screws in 10 patients and with K-wires in 9. One group 1 patient had a partial loss of the skin island. Seven patients needed 1 to 2 operations. One group 1 patient required more than 2 operations.

Discussion.—High-energy war wounds require removal of all devitalized tissue. Reexamination of the wound 24 to 48 hours later is necessary to make sure all nonviable tissue has been removed. Soft tissue must be well-healed to facilitate bone grafting. Revascularization is a slow process that may take years and may leave large dead areas in the interior of the graft. Vascular grafts, on the other hand, provide their own blood supply, result in early initiation of remodeling, and produce stronger unions early in the healing process. Osteocutaneous flaps allow immediate reconstruction of large bone defects.

Conclusion.—High-energy war wounds must be treated aggressively and reexamined within 24 to 48 hours to judge the success of débridement. One stage reconstruction using a free vascular flap facilitates the remodeling process and avoids the delay required by a 2-stage procedure.

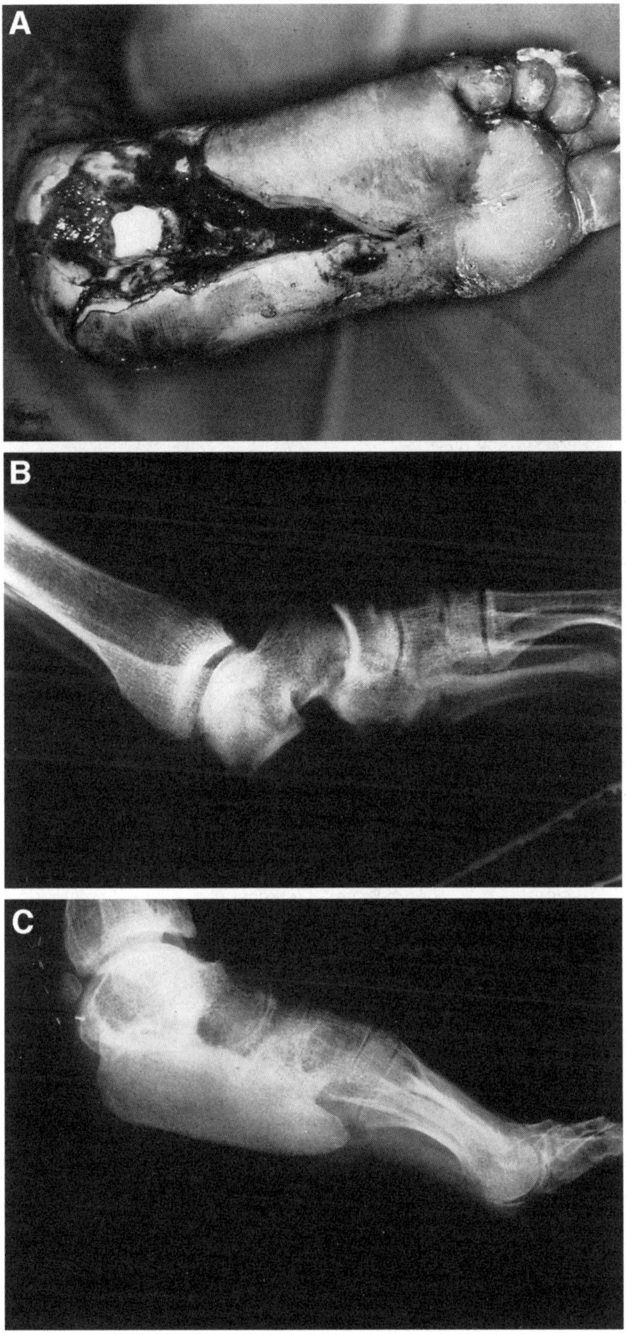

(Continued)

FIGURE 1 (cont.)

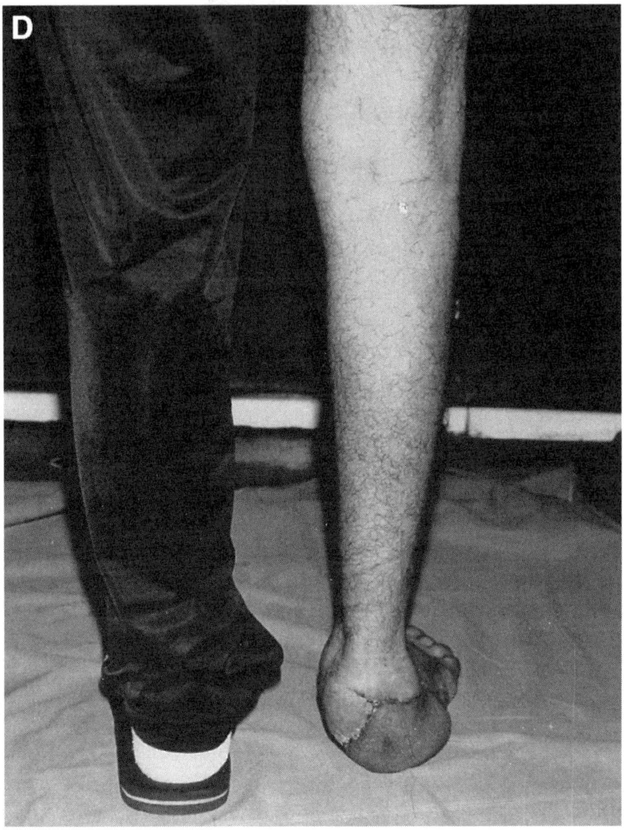

FIGURE 1.—Patient (ZS). **A**, explosive wound of the right foot 3 days after injury. Note the exposed talus. **B**, x-ray of the foot, showing complete destruction of the calcaneum. **C**, x-ray of the foot 6 months after reconstruction with composite groin flap. **D**, posterior view with full weight bearing. (Courtesy of Džepina I, Stanec Z, Škrbić S, et al: One-stage reconstruction of war wounds with free osteocutaneous flaps. *Br J Plast Surg* 50:81–87, 1997).

▶ This paper was not selected because of the superb methodological design and excellent epidemiological analysis, because neither characterize the study. Rather, the selection was done because of the unique (fortunately) patient material, traumatic war wounds. Plastic surgeons have never been particularly pleased with the overall results of a staged approach to combined soft and hard tissue traumatic injuries of the extremities. The use of free tissue transfer (osteocutaneous flap) affords the opportunity for early, aggressive, definitive débridement and early composite wound closure including the bony defect. A number of years ago Godina, before his tragic premature death, published a series of lower extremity injuries managed with such an aggressive approach. Since that series of years ago, techniques in available donor sites have matured, and a fresh look at the problem would be worthwhile.

The paper is a potpourri of different patient groups, and eventually boils down to 8 patients treated acutely with free flaps, 2 of which were lower extremities.

E.A. Luce, M.D.

The Use of Quantitative Bacteriologic Assessment of Bone
Heller WA, Gottlieb LJ, Zachary LS, et al (Univ of Chicago)
Plast Reconstr Surg 100:397–401, 1997 12–9

Background.—The treatment of draining wounds involving bone usually entails multiple surgical débridements followed by coverage with well-vascularized soft tissue. Quantitative bacteriologic assessment of soft tissue in open fractures can be useful in predicting wound infection. A retrospective study was performed to determine whether quantitative bacteriologic assessment of bone is useful in assessing the adequacy of débridement in patients with draining wounds with suspected osteomyelitis.

Methods.—A retrospective review was conducted of 19 patients treated at the University of Chicago Hospitals from 1988 through 1992 for draining wounds involving bone. These wounds were treated with débridement, with the extent of débridement based on vascularity and intraoperative rapid slide quantitative bacteriologic assessment of bone. A negative assessment meant that the bacterial population was no more than 10^5 organisms/g of tissue. If the bacteriologic assessment was negative, the wound was closed with a well-vascularized tissue flap. If bacteriologic balance could not be ensured in the operating room, the wound was treated with topical antimicrobial agents and closed secondarily.

Results.—Of the 19 patients in this series, 5 had gram-negative infections and 3 had multiple organisms isolated from bone cultures. The initial rapid slide quantitative bacteriologic assessment was positive in 8 patients. At follow-up, none of these patients had recurrent wound drainage. Two patients required a secondary procedure to drain recurrent soft-tissue infections.

Conclusions.—The results of this study suggest that rapid slide quantitative bacteriologic assessment of bone can be used to determine the extent of débridement necessary before closure of draining wounds involving bone.

► The authors have given us a method to accomplish 1 stage of reconstruction of wounds that are combined soft and hard tissue. Characteristically, because of the unpredictability of adequate débridement of the hard tissue component, bone, a multi-stage approach has been adopted by most reconstructive surgeons. The authors offer a semi-quantitative method of assessment adopted and modified from similar procedures in the soft-tissue world to definitively débride and close such wounds. This paper should be regarded as a preliminary report, in my opinion. Sixty percent of the patients actually were not osteomyelitic if 10^5 bacterial colony count is used as the standard, and perhaps 2 of the 8 who were osteomyelitic were complicated by secondary infections (my extrapolation—I couldn't tell from the paper). But the authors were not attempting to duplicate results elsewhere, but rather to describe the technique.

E.A. Luce, M.D.

A Comparative Study of Three Occlusive Dressings in the Treatment of Full-Thickness Wounds in Pigs

Ågren MS, Mertz PM, Franzén L (Univ of Miami, Florida; Faculty of Health Sciences, Linköping, Sweden)

J Am Acad Dermatol 36:53–58, 1997 12–10

Objective.—Whereas occlusion encourages healing of surgically excised partial-thickness wounds, not much information is available on the healing effect of occlusive dressings on full-thickness wounds. Results of a study of tissue response to and effects of hydrocolloid dressing A, hydrocolloid dressing B, and film dressing on the quality and rate of closure of full-thickness wounds in domestic pigs was examined.

Methods.—Punch wounds (20 mm) were made in the muscular layer of 3 white, female domestic pigs and dressed with 8 × 8 cm hydrocolloid dressing A, hydrocolloid dressing B, and film dressing. After 4 days, the wounds were cleaned and redressed, and after 10 days, wound contracture was determined using the equation $(A_{Day\ 0} - A_{Day\ X})/A_{Day\ 0} \times 100$ where X = 4 or 10 in day X. Wound sections were evaluated by light spectroscopy and planimetry.

Results.—Wound exudate leaked from the 2 hydrocolloid dressings. Hydrocolloid dressing A and film dressing were easy to remove but hydrocolloid dressing B stuck to the skin and the wound. Significantly more foam cells were found in wounds covered with the hydrocolloid dressings than in film dressing. Significantly more extracellular vacuoles, often surrounded by granulomas, were present in wounds covered by hydrocolloid dressing B but not by the other 2 dressings. Wounds covered by hydrocolloid dressing had a stronger inflammatory reaction than wounds covered by the other dressings, although the inflammatory response was less severe with hydrocolloid dressing A than the other 2 dressings. Percent wound contracture and epithelialization were similar for all dressings. The average wound surface covered, (57%), was similar for all dressings.

Conclusion.—There was no difference in wound contracture or epithelialization of full-thickness wounds in pigs treated with 3 different occlusive dressings.

► The proliferation of wound dressings is a multi-billion dollar industry. Do we actually know what we are using when we order a particular type of dressing on patients? This study defines some of the different properties of occlusive wound dressings, both the absorbent and non-absorbent types. One particular and popular wound dressing (Brand B) provokes an inflammatory wound response that the authors interpreted as beneficial but an entirely different conclusion could be reached.

These wounds had 57% re-epithelialization at ten days! **Please** let me see some controls (dry dressings closed with non-adherent gauze).

E.A. Luce, M.D.

Head and Neck Surgery

DIAGNOSIS

Intraoral Ultrasonography Is Useful to Evaluate Tumor Thickness in Tongue Carcinoma

Shintani S, Nakayama B, Matsuura H, et al (Aichi Cancer Ctr, Nagoya, Japan)
Am J Surg 173:345–347, 1997 12–11

Background.—In patients with oral cancers, tumor thickness is an important prognostic factor, particularly as an indicator of lymph node metastasis. However, previous studies have assessed tumor thickness postoperatively, in histologic specimens. There has been no available technique of measuring the thickness of oral tumors preoperatively. Intraoral ultrasonography was evaluated for its ability to measure the thickness of tongue cancers.

Methods.—The study included 24 patients with tongue cancers, ranging from T1, N0, M0 to T4, N0, M0. Measurements of tumor thickness were performed by intraoral ultrasound—from the surface to the maximal thickness of the tumor—and on histologic sections. The relationship between the 2 measurements was then assessed.

Results.—Intraoral ultrasound clearly depicted the tongue carcinomas, even lesions as thin as 1 mm. The thickness measurements ranged from 1.0 to 37.4 mm on ultrasound and from 1.0 to 33.0 mm on histologic section. The correlation between the 2 measurement techniques was significant. The measurements were concordant for tumors thinner than 10 mm, but discordant for most tumors thicker than 20 mm, because of tissue shrinkage in formalin.

Conclusion.—Intraoral ultrasound is useful in depicting and measuring the thickness of tongue carcinomas. It is a noninvasive, quick, and repeatable technique that can measure tumor thickness within 0.1 mm. Intraoral ultrasound will be useful in monitoring the response of tongue carcinomas to radiotherapy or chemotherapy.

► Who of the patients with an N0 neck should have a neck dissection and who should not? Tumor thickness has been advocated by some authors, including these, as a predictive variable. Ultrasound is a noninvasive technique and in the 9 patients with less than a 10-mm thick lesion, it correlated highly with later absolute measurements by histologic investigation. What is provocative about this paper is its speculation regarding other uses of ultrasonic technique to assess response to neoadjuvant therapy such as radiotherapy or chemotherapy. A great deal more experience, though, will be necessary and that perhaps, underlines the point that ultrasound here, as elsewhere, is interpreter dependent.

E.A. Luce, M.D.

Depth of Invasion as a Predictive Factor for Cervical Lymph Node Metastasis in Tongue Carcinoma

Fukano H, Matsuura H, Hasegawa Y, et al (Aichi Cancer Ctr, Nagoya, Japan)
Head Neck 19:205–210, 1997 12–12

Objective.—Although predictions for neck node metastasis in patients with oral cancer have been based on histopathologic variables and imaging studies, imaging results lack specificity. Depth of invasion is one of the most important predictors of cervical metastasis. Clinical and pathologic data on surgically-treated tongue carcinomas was reviewed retrospectively to determine the incidence of neck disease based on tumor thickness.

Methods.—Records of 34 patients (17 women), age 22–79, who had surgery, postoperative chemotherapy, irradiation, or all of these between 1980 and 1991 were reviewed. Patients were followed for an average of 4 years. Thirty patients were clinically N0 and 4 were N1. Histologic sections were examined by 1 pathologist to confirm the initial diagnosis of squamous-cell carcinoma and to determine tumor thickness. Clinical histologic variables or both were correlated with metastasis.

Results.—Tumors were located on the lateral border in 26 patients, on the inferior surface in 7, and on the dorsum in 1. There were 7 local and 5 regional recurrences. Tumor depth ranged from 0 to 18.2 mm. No

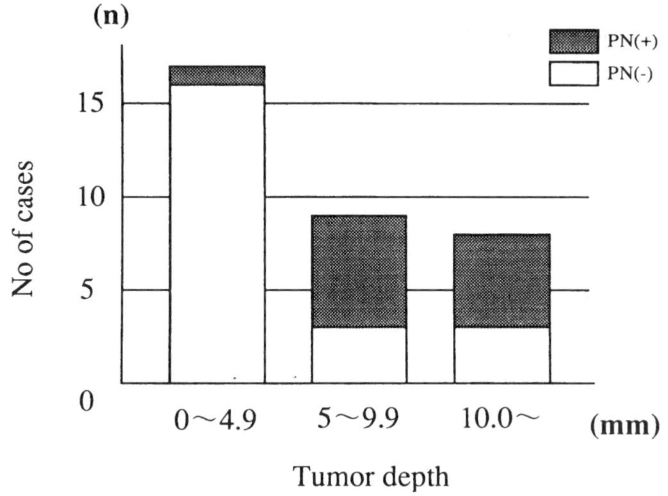

FIGURE 1.—Relation of depth of invasion and cervical lymph node metastasis. (Reprinted by permission of John Wiley & Sons, Inc. from Fukano H, Matsuura H, Hasegawa Y, et al: Depth of invasion as a predictive factor for cervical lymph node metastasis in tongue carcinoma. *Head Neck* 19:205–210, 1997. Copyright 1997, John Wiley & Sons, Inc.)

cervical metastasis was found for tumor depths less than 3 mm (Fig 1). In the 30 clinically N0 patients, 17 tumors were less than 5 mm and 13 were greater than 5 mm in depth. Nine (30%) clinically N0 necks were pathologically positive. One (5.9%) of 17 patients with a tumor depth less than 5 mm had metastatic disease, whereas 8 (61.5%) of 13 patients with a tumor depth greater than 5 mm had metastatic disease. Although 18 (82%) of 22 patients with pathology-negative (PN−) nodes and 6 (50%) of 12 patients with PN+ nodes had T1/T2 tumors, the difference of histologic differentiation between PN− and PN+ was not significant.

Conclusion.—As reported in other studies, there was a significant relationship between depth and lymph node metastasis between tumors less than 5 mm and greater than 5 mm. In this study, the subclinical metastasis rate was 30%. Elective dissection should be an option for tongue tumors greater than 5 mm. Measurement of tumor depth at excision may provide useful information regarding the necessity for neck dissection in clinically N0 patients.

► The really worthwhile information in this paper is the correlation between the depth and the incidence of lymph node metastasis. Yet I see no effort to do a multivariate analysis to consider effect, for example, of T-stage (one third of the group had T-3, T-4 primaries). I also doubt the practicality of the authors' recommendation about excision of the primary and frozen section for a decision about lymph node dissection. Because the difference between a yes or no decision about radical neck dissection was essentially 2 millimeters, more than likely the pathologist will equivocate (perhaps more than usual). What is needed is a larger series, because this was but 34 cases over eleven years, to more clearly confirm and delineate this relationship between the thickness of the primary and the incidence of regional node metastases.

E.A. Luce, M.D.

The Impact of Routine CT of the Chest on the Diagnosis and Management of Newly Diagnosed Squamous Cell Carcinoma of the Head and Neck

Reiner B, Siegel E, Sawyer R, et al (Univ of Maryland, Baltimore; Baltimore Veterans Affairs Med Ctr, Md)

AJR 169:667–671, 1997 12–13

Background.—About one fourth of deaths in patients with squamous cell carcinomas of the head and neck are caused by second primary tumors. Early detection of these second primary neoplasms therefore has a major influence on prognosis; however, chest radiographs do not show the tumors while they are still resectable. The value of chest CT in detecting second primary tumors in patients with newly diagnosed squamous cell carcinoma of the head and neck was studied.

Methods.—The study included 189 consecutive patients at initial diagnosis of squamous cell carcinoma of the head and neck. Within 1 week, all patients were studied by both conventional radiography and CT of the chest. Before CT was performed, the chest radiographs were prospectively read by board-certified radiologists. The CT scans were subsequently read by certified radiologists with specialized training in cross-sectional imaging. Sixty-six patients had a significant abnormality on chest CT; a tissue diagnosis was obtained in 42 of these cases.

Results.—Thirty-five percent of patients had abnormal findings on chest CT scan. Fifty-five percent of patients with CT abnormalities were found to have additional primary or metastatic lesions; only 29% of these malignancies appeared on chest radiographs. Of intrathoracic malignancies, 35% of those detected on chest CT scans were also seen on radiographs. Seven of 10 patients discovered to have synchronous pulmonary lesions had stage IV disease in the neck. Eight of 10 primary lung tumors were squamous cell carcinomas. In all 10 patients, the recognition of a synchronous lung tumor significantly altered clinical management. Twenty patients were found to have distant metastases; 11 of them had a primary tumor located within the oral cavity. Just 45% of cases of metastatic disease were detected on chest radiographs, compared with 70% of synchronous primary lung neoplasms.

Conclusion.—Additional malignancies are common in patients with newly diagnosed squamous cell cancer of the head and neck but are frequently missed by conventional chest radiographs. Thus, chest CT should be a routine part of the evaluation of such patients. The additional malignancies detected by chest CT almost always lead to alterations of surgical or medical management. Early detection of such tumors will help to avoid the high mortality rate associated with distant metastases or second primary tumors.

▶ This is an important study because the detection of a second primary tumor or metastatic disease made a significant difference in the management of most patients, yet chest x-ray studies were unable to accomplish that objective when compared with routine CT of the chest. Although one half the index tumors were laryngeal-hypopharyngeal, conclusions about this relationship are difficult to establish in the absence of information about the distribution and the patient universe study. Another piece of information that would have been of interest: three fourths of the patients who had metastases determined on CT had stage IV disease (and the remainder stage III), and 70% of the synchronous primaries had stage IV disease. More information about the distribution of advanced disease in the universe of 190 patients would have been helpful.

E.A. Luce, M.D.

Markers of Radioresistance in Squamous Cell Carcinomas of the Head and Neck: A Clinicopathologic and Immunohistochemical Study

Raybaud-Diogène H, Fortin A, Morency R, et al (Université Laval, Québec; Hôtel Dieu de Québec; Hôpital de l'Enfant Jésus, Québec)

J Clin Oncol 15:1030–1038, 1997 12–14

Introduction.—There is currently no way to predict the response to radiotherapy for a patient with squamous cell carcinoma of the head and neck (HN-SCC). There is evidence that alterations of p53 tumor-suppressor gene expression may play a role in the development of HN-SCC, and abnormal p53 overexpression has been linked to radioresistance. Immunohistochemistry was used to evaluate *p53* and other possible markers of tumor radioresistance in HN-SCC.

Methods.—The study included 101 patients undergoing radical radiotherapy for HC-SCC. They were 87 men and 14 women; 64% had oropharyngeal tumors and 31% had oral cavity tumors. Most patients received external beam radiotherapy alone, although 37% received a brachytherapy boost. Biopsy specimens were evaluated by immunohistochemistry for expression of p3, ki-67, *c-erb* B-2, heat-shock protein-27 (HSP-27), and glutathione S transferase (GSTπ). The various markers were correlated with local control and survival.

Results.—Nuclear p53-positive staining was noted in half of the tumors studied. Expression of p53 was significantly correlated with local recurrence. Patients with p53-positive tumors had a 3-year local treatment failure rate of 56% vs. 27.5% for those with p53-negative tumors. In patients with T3–T4 tumors, these figures were 81% and 27.5%, respectively. The response to radiotherapy was also better for patients with a high proliferation rate, indicated by a ki-67 of greater than 20%. Patients whose tumors showed a low proliferation rate had a local treatment failure rate of 54%, compared with 21.5% for patients with higher proliferation rates. On multivariate analysis, the only independent prognostic factors for local recurrence were p53, ki-67, and T stage. A subsequent Cox regression model showed that the 3-year local control rate was 86% for patients with no unfavorable factors, compared with 72.5% for patients with 1 factor and 17.5% for those with 2 factors.

Conclusion.—The response of HN-SCC to radiation therapy can be predicted by p53 overexpression and low cell proliferation on immunostaining of biopsy specimens. Patients with abnormal p53 protein expression and low proliferation may be best treated by surgery rather than radiation therapy. Using these markers to predict tumor response to radiation will allow early selection of the most appropriate treatment approach.

► If one has followed the recent advances in molecular biology of head and neck cancer over the past several years, the appearance of papers such as this one is inevitable and represents perhaps the next step in analysis. What we need clinically (among many things) is a prognostic variable to select those patients who will respond to neoadjuvant therapy—either radiotherapy, chemotherapy, or both. That necessity is enhanced by the current interest in "organ preservation" by the use of combined chemoradiotherapy as the primary modality for advanced tumors, rather than surgical extirpation.

The authors have utilized an oncogene, p53, popular among head and neck researchers, as well as a cellular proliferation index, ki-67, to correlate recurrence in patients who were treated primarily with radiotherapy. The specifics of the paper are something of a clinician's nightmare, but the results hold promise.

E.A. Luce, M.D.

Assessment of Malnutrition Parameters in Head and Neck Cancer and Their Relation to Postoperative Complications

van Bokhorst–de van der Schueren MAE, van Leeuwen PAM, Sauerwein HP, et al (Free Univ, Amsterdam)

Head Neck 19:419–425, 1997 12–15

Background.—Cancer patients often suffer from cachexia. Patients with head and neck cancer have an even higher risk of malnutrition. It has been suggested that this malnutrition lowers treatment tolerance and leads to complications. This prospective study was performed to determine the efficacy of 6 nutritional parameters in predicting postoperative complications among patients with head and neck cancer.

Methods.—From 1993 to 1994, a nutritional assessment was performed for all 64 patients admitted to the department of Otolaryngology/Head and Neck Surgery of the Free University Hospital who had T2 to T4 head and neck carcinomas. The nutritional parameters assessed included: the percent weight loss during the past 6 months (PWL); the percent ideal body weight (PIW); the nutritional index (NI) calculated based on albumin, PIW, and total lymphocyte count; serum albumin (Alb); total lymphocyte count (TLC); and body fat (BF) and lean body mass (LBM). No nutritional support was offered in the preoperative period. All patients underwent major head or neck surgery with prophylactic antibiotics.

Results.—Of the 64 patients in this study group, major complications occurred in 20, including infection, anastomotic leakage, cardiac failure, pulmonary failure, septicemia, and death. Logistic regression analysis indicated that greater than a 10% weight loss over the previous 6 months was the best predictor of postoperative complications. For patients with a 10% to 15% weight loss during this period the probability of major postoperative complications was 50%, while for those with a greater than 15% weight loss the probability was almost 80%. Previous radiotherapy was also predictive of complications, although this did not reach significance. No other variables reached significance in this analysis.

Conclusions.—Among a group of prospectively studied patients with head and neck cancer, the only nutritional parameter that predicted postoperative complications was a minumum of 10% weight loss during the previous 6 months. A study is underway to determine whether preoperative nutritional support can be used to counteract the adverse effects associated with malnutrition.

► The paper is excellent and well written, particularly the discussion of the limitations of various methods of assessment of nutritional status and the relationship between nutritional status and postoperative complications. Please note that a 15% weight loss within 6 months was extremely highly predictive of postoperative complications, namely, that the majority of patients developed complications. Even 10%, the guideline selected by the authors, was predictive of one-half the patients who would sustain postoperative complications. None of the other parameters that the authors utilized were particularly reliable or consistent, although, as the authors discussed, difficulty with use of the nutritional index (NI) was the dependence of that equation partially on albumin concentrations, which were normal in over 80% of this group of patients. The variants then, in nutritional index, was with total lymphocyte count (TLC), also not particularly reliable as a predictive variable.

One can only speculate what more subtle nutritional parameters, such as the use of pre-albumin concentration, transferritin, as more sophisticated measurements of nutritional status would have demonstrated. The difficulty would probably be the too-sensitive nature of those indices.

The authors state that radiotherapy was not a predictive variable with the use of their logistic regression statistical analysis, yet this reviewer would have been much more comfortable if the authors would have broken out radiotherapy as a separate group of patients and given us information about how those patients fared vs nutritional status. This was a relatively small number of patients, and this study could be repeated by some of the higher volume institutions with larger numbers, yet the message is clear. If the patient gives a history of 10% or more weight loss over the 6 months, considerable attention must be directed toward restoration of that nutritional status before institution of radical treatment measures. The next question is, "Would such nutritional intervention make a difference?"

E.A. Luce, M.D.

Sestamibi Scanning Is Inadequate for Directing Unilateral Neck Exploration for the First-time Parathyroidectomy
Shen W, Sabanci U, Morita ET, et al (Univ of California, San Francisco)
Arch Surg 132:969–976, 1997 12–16

Background.—Some surgeons advocate the use of noninvasive localization studies before first-time parathyroidectomy. The value of sestamibi scanning in patients undergoing initial parathyroidectomy for primary hyperparathyroidism was investigated to determine whether such scanning is sufficiently accurate to permit unilateral neck exploration in these patients.

Methods.—Forty patients with primary hyperparathyroidism were included in the retrospective review. Twenty-eight patients had single adenomas; 9, multiple adenomas; and 3, hyperplasia. All underwent sestamibi scanning before first-time parathyroidectomy. Bilateral neck exploration was done in all patients, with identification of 4 parathyroid glands. The results of preoperative sestamibi scanning were compared with surgical and histologic findings.

Findings.—Scanning was correct in 71% of patients with single adenomas, 44% of those with multiple adenomas, and in none with hyperplasia. Had unilateral neck explorations been done based on localization by sestamibi scanning, parathyroidectomy would have failed in 10% of the patients overall.

Conclusions.—Although sestamibi scanning is helpful, it is not adequate for guiding unilateral neck exploration for first-time parathyroidectomy. Surgeons performing unilateral neck exploration based on the results of such scanning will have a high failure rate and incur more expense than those doing bilateral neck exploration for first-time parathyroidectomy.

► Some readers may not accept all the premises of the authors, but the paper articulates an argument that is both decision analysis based and cost based. Their patient population reflects referrals to experienced surgeons, and as such has a higher percentage of multiple adenomas than one would expect from a population of hyperparathyroid patients. That percentage just enables the authors to make their point more substantially, namely, that bilateral exploration of the neck is preferred rather than sestamibi scanning to limit dissection to 1 side of the neck only. Of interest to the readers will be the discussion of this article by several individuals at a regional surgical society meeting.

E.A. Luce, M.D.

Treatment

A Phase III Randomized Trial Comparing Concurrent Chemotherapy and Radiotherapy With Radiotherapy Alone in Resectable Stage III and IV Squamous Cell Head and Neck Cancer: Preliminary Results

Adelstein DJ, Saxton JP, Lavertu P, et al (Cleveland Clinic Found, Ohio)
Head Neck 19:567–575, 1997 12–17

Introduction.—The role of chemotherapy in patients with squamous cell head and neck cancer is not known. In a randomized trial, initial radiotherapy alone and radiotherapy with concurrent chemotherapy were compared in terms of toxicities, survival rates, and the relative possibility of organ preservation.

Methods.—One hundred patients with resectable stage III and IV squamous cell head and neck cancer were randomized to arm A with radiation alone (68–72 Gy at 1.8–2.0 Gy per day) or arm B with chemoradiation

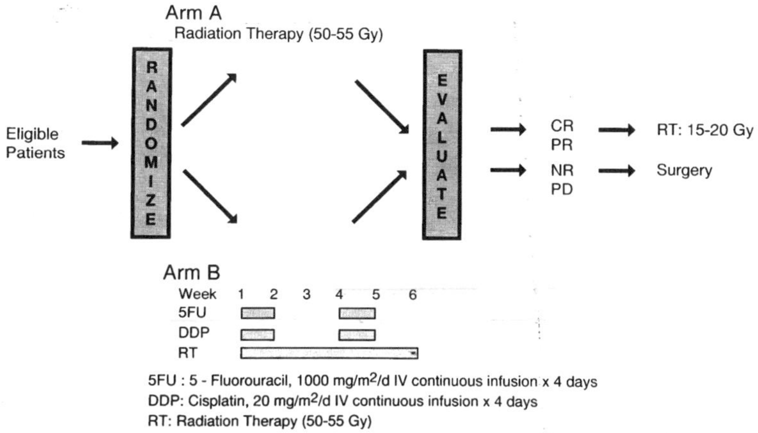

FIGURE 1.—Treatment schema. *Abbreviations: CR* complete response; *PR*, partial response; *NR*, no response; *PD*, present disease. (Courtesy of Adelstein DJ, Saxton JP, Lavertu P, et al: A phase III randomized trial comparing concurrent chemotherapy and radiotherapy with radiotherapy alone in resectable stage III and IV squamous cell head and neck cancer: Preliminary results. *Head Neck* 19:567–575, copyright 1997 John Wiley & Sons, Inc. Reprinted by permission of John Wiley & Sons, Inc.)

(identical radiotherapy with concurrent 5-fluorouracil, 1,000 mg/m²/day, and cisplastin, 20 mg/m²/day) (Fig 1). Patients were reevaluated after receiving about 50–55 Gy. Radiotherapy was completed if a response was evident. In patients with no response, radiotherapy was terminated and surgery was recommended. Salvage surgery was performed after all treatments for residual primary or nodal disease or any subsequent local-regional recurrence.

Results.—Patients receiving arm B treatment experienced the effects of toxicity more; had a higher incidence of grade III and IV neutropenia, thrombocytopenia, cutaneous reactions, and mucositis; required feeding tubes more often; and had greater weight loss. Patients receiving arm B treatment were significantly more likely to have second primary malignancies (9 had second cancers that included 4 aerodigestive tract tumors). Fifty percent of patients receiving arm A treatment and 76% of patients receiving arm B treatment had a complete response after completion of nonoperative therapy. The 36-month relapse-free survival rate was 52% for patients in arm A and 67% for patients in arm B. There were no between-group differences in overall survival rates. Overall survival rates with successful primary site preservation were 35% for patients in arm A and 57% for patients in arm B. This difference was significant in subsets of patients with laryngeal and hypopharyngeal primary malignancies but not in patients with oropharyngeal primary malignancies.

Conclusion.—Concurrent chemotherapy combined with definitive radiotherapy is significantly more toxic than radiotherapy alone in treating patients with resectable stage III and IV squamous cell head and neck cancer. Concurrent therapy can produce an improvement in relapse-free survival rates, a reduction in distant metastases, and an improvement in overall survival rates with primary site preservation.

▶ The paper addresses the issue of the use of concurrent chemotherapy plus radiotherapy to determine whether the addition of the chemotherapy has any advantage over radiotherapy alone. The study did so in terms of relapses or recurrent tumors and in the ability to preserve organs, principally the larynx and hypopharynx. Relapse rates were significantly less in the patients who received concurrent radiotherapy and chemotherapy, and the incidence of distant metastasis was less. The opportunity to preserve the larynx and/or hypopharynx was much better in this group of patients as well. The small group of patients with oral cavity or oropharyngeal lesions had no improvement in organ preservation (i.e., they required a surgical resection) with the concurrent use of chemotherapy and radiotherapy.

Several points need to be emphasized. First, the overall survival rate was not improved, and the price paid was considerable. More than one third of the patients who received both chemotherapy and radiotherapy required hospitalization vs. only 2 of 50 in the radiotherapy group. Second, the incidence of second primary malignancies was startling. Nine of the 25 patients in the combined therapy group had second primary malignancies, principally of the upper aerodigestive tract. That factor certainly would have a very profound effect on the overall survival rate. Lastly, as the authors admit, the study does not address the issue of a surgical therapy arm. This is a very small and heterogeneous group of patients, and we certainly need more data.

E.A. Luce, M.D.

Morbidity of Combined Therapy for the Treatment of Supraglottic Carcinoma: Supraglottic Laryngectomy and Radiotherapy

Steiniger JR, Parnes SM, Gardner GM (Albany Med College, New York)

Ann Otol Rhinol Laryngol 106:151–158, 1997 12–18

Background.—Both supraglottic laryngectomy (SGL) and external beam radiotherapy (XRT) are common treatment modalities for patients with supraglottic carcinoma. Both procedures, however, are often associated with significant complications as a result of abnormal laryngeal and pharyngeal function. Many surgeons have noted that morbidity is greater in patients receiving SGL if XRT is performed as well; however, documentation of this interaction has been poor. The effect of subsequent XRT on morbidity after SGL was evaluated retrospectively.

Methods.—Twenty nine patients who had been treated with SGL for supraglottic carcinoma were followed up for a mean of 64 months. External beam radiotherapy had been performed postoperatively in 17 of the 29 patients. The morbidity associated with SGL alone and SGL with subsequent XRT was evaluated, and a morbidity index score, an average

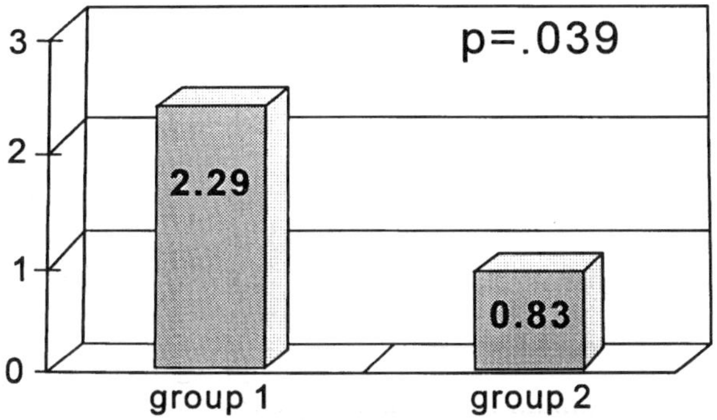

FIGURE 5.—Morbidity index, i.e., overall postoperative morbidity measured as mean of total number of morbid events per patient for each group. Statistical significance was measured by Mann-Whitney rank sum test, $P = 0.039$. *Group 1,* supraglottic laryngectomy with postoperative radiotherapy; *group 2,* supraglottic laryngectomy alone. (Courtesy of Steiniger JR, Parnes SM, Gardner GM: Morbidity of combined therapy for the treatment of supraglottic carcinoma: Supraglottic laryngectomy and radiotherapy. *Ann Otol Rhinol Laryngol* 106:151–158, 1997.)

of the total number of morbid events experienced by each patient, was created for both treatment groups.

Results.—Mortality during the 2- and 5-year period after treatment did not vary between the 2 groups. The most common cause of treatment failure was regional metastasis in the neck or the appearance of second primary tumors. The incidence of acute airway obstruction was significantly greater in patients treated with SGL and XRT (29%) than in those treated with SGL alone (0%), as was the incidence of permanent gastrostomy dependence (35% vs. 0%). Although nonsignificant, the time until independent swallowing was substantially greater in the SGL with XRT group (34.8 weeks) than in the SGL group (7.8 weeks), as was the incidence of aspiration pneumonia (35% vs. 9%) and tracheostomy dependence (24% vs. 0%). The morbidity index score for the SGL with XRT group was 2.29 events per patient, compared with 0.83 events per patient for the SGL group (Fig 5).

Conclusions.—The morbidity associated with SGL is significantly increased by subsequent radiotherapy. Although XRT is a beneficial adjunct to SGL in some patients with supraglottic carcinoma, its sequelae require that it be reserved for a strictly defined patient subset.

► The authors make a persuasive case for a tremendous increase in morbidity (perhaps an unacceptable increase) when postoperative radiation therapy is added to conservative laryngeal surgery, supraglottic laryngectomy. The authors admit to a bias in that the more severe patients received postoperative radiation therapy, yet their surgical therapy was the same for both groups, so presumably the only variable was the addition of the postoperative radiation therapy.

This operation was ***frequently*** performed by these authors, namely, 17% of all laryngeal cancer, perhaps a higher proportion than other series that use a more discrete and narrow set of criteria for performance of supraglottic laryngectomy. The findings present an interesting dilemma: what should be the management of N0 neck—radiation therapy or a complete neck dissection? If we subtract out the radical neck dissection and use radiotherapy only, would those patients now have a "morbidity index" equal to or less than the patients in this series that had surgery alone without addition of radiation therapy?

The last point to be made about this paper is that the authors really didn't break any new ground in their indications for the use of postoperative radiation therapy, yet they advocate a protocol for the N1 neck of supraglottic laryngectomy plus bilateral radical neck dissection. The problem with this protocol is that in all likelihood, the patient with the N neck will also require the addition of postoperative radiation therapy with all the attendant problems of gastrostomy and tracheostomy dependence pointed out in this article.

E.A. Luce, M.D.

Surgical Salvage After Radiotherapy for Advanced Laryngopharyngeal Carcinoma

Davidson J, Keane T, Brown D, et al (Univ of Toronto; Princess Margaret Hosp, Toronto)

Arch Otolaryngol Head Neck Surg 123:420–424, 1997 12–19

Objective.—Patients with advanced laryngopharyngeal carcinoma are generally treated with primary radiotherapy to preserve the function of the laryngopharyngeal complex. Surgery is used only if needed for salvage. The results of patients undergoing surgery after failure of radiotherapy for advanced laryngopharyngeal carcinoma were assessed.

Methods.—Three hundred thirty-six patients with T3 or T4 or N+ laryngopharyngeal carcinoma were entered into a randomized clinical trial. One group received standard fractional radiotherapy, 51 Gy in 20 fractions, whereas the other group received hyperfractionation radiotherapy, 58 Gy twice daily in 40 fractions. Salvage surgery was performed as required for recurrent disease. The patients were prospectively studied for complications, tumor recurrences, and survival.

Results.—Of 191 patients in whom primary radiotherapy failed, 163 had local or regional tumor recurrence. Salvage surgery was performed in 108 of these patients. The remaining 55 patients did not have surgery because of unresectable disease, patient refusal, medical contraindications, or death from other causes. Sixty-one patients underwent total laryngectomy and 1 had partial laryngectomy. The surgical complication rate was 27%, with considerable variation by site. The complication rate was 6% for patients having neck dissection only, 15% for those having surgery at the primary site only, and 40% for those having surgery at both sites. Actuarial survival for patients undergoing surgical salvage was 37% at 3 years and 18% at 5 years. Of 25 patients with positive resection margins, none were alive at 3 years.

Summary.—Analysis of surgical salvage after failure of primary radiotherapy for advanced laryngopharyngeal carcinoma showed that, as in previous reports, the surgical complication rate is higher, especially in patients undergoing more complex procedures. Positive resection margins were observed in one fourth of patients undergoing surgery for recurrence at the primary tumor site.

► The complication rate by these authors was actually a little lower than in other series, **except** for combined resection of primary and neck dissection, for which it was in the order of about 40%. Yet the radiotherapy dose was perhaps lower (5,200 cGy) with the obvious lessened impact on complications. Either coincident with or as a result of this lower dosage, the initial control rate was lower than in other series (42%) as well and 25% of the patients had positive resection margins.

E.A. Luce, M.D.

SECONDARY PROBLEMS

The Extent of Neck Disease After Regional Failure During Observation of the N_0 Neck

Andersen PE, Cambronero E, Shaha AR, et al (Oregon Health Sciences Univ, Portland; San Juan de Dios Hosp, San Jose Costa Rica; Mem Sloan-Kettering Cancer Ctr, NY)

Am J Surg 172:689–691, 1996 12–20

Introduction.—Apparent metastasis to the cervical lymph nodes at diagnosis of squamous carcinoma of the head and neck makes treatment of the neck mandatory. In cases without discernable metastases, the choice must be made between observation and elective treatment of the cervical lymphatics. A retrospective chart review was conducted to test the hypothesis that close follow-up after treatment of the primary tumor will detect regional failure at an early stage.

Methods.—Included in the study group were 47 patients with squamous carcinoma of the head and neck. The median age of the group was 65 years; 72% were men and 77% had a primary tumor located in the oral cavity. Staging in each case was N0 and M0. All underwent neck dissection for regional failure after surgery, which had been followed by observation of the head and neck. The median time between surgical treatment and failure in the neck was 13 months.

Results.—None of the patients had surgical treatment of the cervical lymphatics or preoperative or postoperative radiation therapy. Margins of excision of the primary tumor were negative in all cases. Neck failure was treated by comprehensive neck dissection in all patients and 30 had external beam radiation therapy. The clinical N stage of dissected necks was N1 in 37 patients at the time of neck dissection, N2A in 6, N2B in 1, and N3 in 3. Upstaging was common after pathologic examination, particularly among those initially staged as N1; 18 of those patients were found to have N2B disease. Twenty-three of the 47 patients had extracapsular

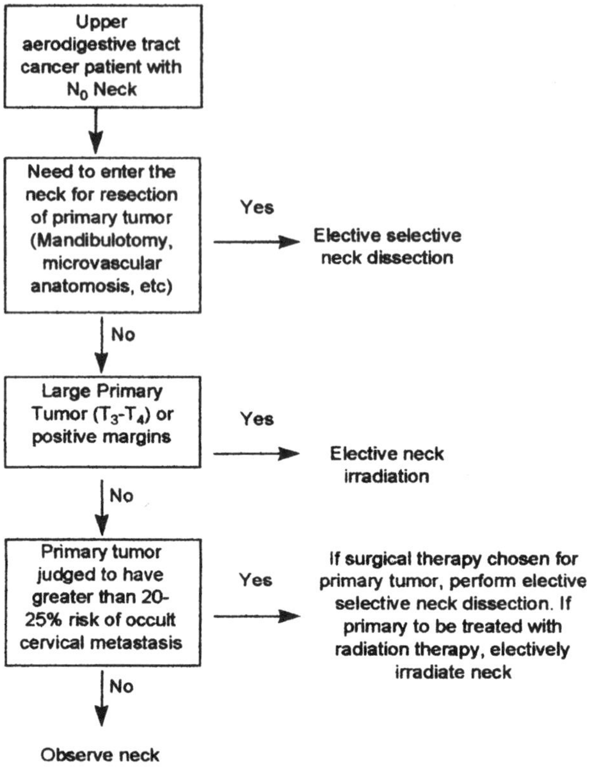

FIGURE 2.—Suggested algorithm for elective neck treatment decision making. (Reprinted by permission of the publishers, from Andersen PE, Cambronero E, Shaha AR, et al: The extent of neck disease after regional failure during observation of the N_0 neck. *Am J Surg* 172:689–691, 1996. Copyright 1996 by Excerpta Medica Inc.)

extension. Overall, 77% of patients had adverse pathologic findings at the time of neck dissection.

Discussion.—Because there is no noninvasive, accurate method for evaluating the cervical lymphatics in patients with squamous carcinoma of the head and neck, oncologists must rely on clinical judgment in deciding upon elective neck dissection. Close follow-up does not ensure that cervical metastasis will be detected at a low stage, however, and selective dissection can reduce the morbidity associated with radical dissection. Until further data are obtained, elective dissection is recommended when the risk of occult metastasis is judged to be greater than 20% to 25% (Figure 2).

▶ The authors have effectively dispelled a myth that was actually not tenable nor believed by the majority of head and neck surgeons. The myth was that observation of the negative neck on a regular and close periodic follow-up basis would enable detection of regional recurrence at an early stage.

What we need, as recommended by the authors as well, is a randomized trial to prove the efficacy of selective neck dissection for the N0 neck in patients at significant risk (greater than 25% to 30% incidence) of occult metastases and the use of radiotherapy in those patients who have adverse pathologic findings on examination of the specimen.

E.A. Luce, M.D.

Endovascular Management of Hemorrhage in Patients With Head and Neck Cancer

Morrissey DD, Andersen PE, Nesbit GM, et al (Dotter Inst for Interventional Radiology, Oregon Health Sciences Univ, Portland)

Arch Otolaryngol Head Neck Surg 123:15–19, 97 12–21

Purpose.—In patients with head and neck cancer, bleeding can be a difficult problem to control. The traditional approach is open surgical exploration with ligation of the bleeding vessel. This can be difficult and often leads to a prolonged recovery in the hospital. For some patients, endovascular embolization may be a good alternative to open surgical ligation. The use of selective endovascular embolization in the management of hemorrhage in patients with head and neck squamous cell carcinoma was evaluated.

Patients.—The experience included 12 patients undergoing angiography and selective embolization for 13 separate episodes of hemorrhage. Eleven patients had previous surgery, and 7 had preoperative irradiation. One patient had previous external beam radiation therapy, and 3 had postoperative radiation therapy. Bleeding was related to recurrent tumor in 5 patients, postoperative hemorrhage in 1, radiation necrosis in 3, and active pharyngocutaneous fistulas in 4. The external carotid artery and branches were involved in 8 patients and the common carotid artery in 4.

Treatment and Outcomes.—The bleeding vessels were embolized with a combination of inflatable balloons, platinum coils, and microparticles. A 30-minute test occlusion was performed before permanent occlusion in patients with bleeding from the common carotid artery. All bleeding vessels were successfully occluded, and there were no episodes of recurrent bleeding. The patients' average hospital stay after embolization was 8 days.

Conclusions.—Hemorrhage is a dangerous and difficult complication in patients with head and neck cancer. This experience suggests that angiography with embolization is a safe and effective alternative to surgical control of hemorrhage. Some additional complications are possible with embolization, including thrombus propagation, inadvertent detachment of embolization materials, and complications of intentional carotid occlusion.

▶ This situation is probably one of the most difficult in head and neck oncology, namely, a previously irradiated patient with recurrent cancer and/or a pharyngeocutaneous fistula in the presence of an operative field. The inevitable fibrosis distortion and friability of the tissues, and, most important, the artery, make surgical intervention in the presence of acute hemorrhage a surgeon's nightmare. We are not given information by this series on which patients were selected for surgery and which patients had selective endovascular angiography and embolization. Two thirds of the patients, though, were bleeding from the external carotid artery, perhaps a little more amenable to embolization. In addition, of the 4 patients who had the common carotid artery occluded, 2 had transient hemiplegia and 1 patient had permanent hemiplegia. To me, the principal advantage would be in the presence of a very difficult surgical field, once the patient's pressure was stabilized, then endovascular occlusion could be accomplished while maintaining pressure on the bleeding point. Frequently during the "flail" in the operating room to obtain proximal control of the vessels, significant blood loss occurs and the patient may be, despite the surgeon's best intentions, hypotensive at the time of ligation. As the authors point out, this single factor, hypotension, is responsible for a dramatic increase in the incidence of permanent neurologic complications and mortality.

E.A. Luce, M.D.

Reconstruction

Current Role of the Radial Forearm Free Flap in Mandibular Reconstruction

Zenn MR, Hidalgo DA, Cordeiro PG, et al (Mem Sloan-Kettering Cancer Ctr, New York)

Plast Reconstr Surg 99:1012–1017, 1997 12–22

Background.—Mandibular reconstruction was once associated with significant morbidity and mortality but is now a safe, common procedure. The best donor site for good functional and aesthetic results is still debated. A review of more than 150 mandibular reconstructions in almost 10 years has shown that other sites were used in more than 20% of cases. The most appropriate indications for use of the radial forearm free flap in mandibular reconstruction were defined.

Methods.—A study focused on 17 of 155 patients who had mandibular reconstruction at a cancer center. The radial forearm donor site was used in these 17 patients. The mean patient age was 55 years. Epidermoid carcinoma was the most common underlying disease. The mean follow-up was 13.5 months. The radial forearm free flap was used as an osteocutaneous flap, as intraoral lining with a reconstruction plate or for external skin coverage with a simultaneous free fibula reconstruction, or to salvage a previous fibula free flap reconstruction.

Results.—One patient died. There were no anastomotic failures. Postoperative fracture at the donor site occurred in 2 patients, and 1 patient required surgical treatment. Exposure, infection, and other hardware-related problems were seen in 3 patients. All donor sites healed without secondary procedures. The cosmetic result at the donor site was good in a few patients and fair to poor in most patients.

Discussion.—Today, the radial forearm free flap is considered a secondary option for mandibular reconstruction because of poor-quality bone stock, inadequate soft-tissue bulk, poor donor site appearance, and the possibility of radius fracture. The forearm donor site is suited to mandibular reconstruction for large posterior intraoral defects with limited adjacent mandibular involvement, for reliable coverage of reconstruction plates, and for very large defects when no single flap can provide the ideal configuration and amount of bone and soft tissue.

▶ This article came from "headquarters" for the use of the fibula free flap for mandibular reconstruction. In about 10% of the cases, they did use the radial forearm flap; in only half of those (5%) was bone actually incorporated. In addition, they had problems with the bone donor sites. My conclusion from this article is that if there are any indications for a radial forearm *osteo*cutaneous flap for mandible reconstruction, they are *extremely* few.

E.A. Luce, M.D.

Fibular Free Flap Reconstruction of the "True" Lateral Mandibular Defect

Anthony JP, Foster RD, Kaplan MJ, et al (Univ of California, San Francisco)

Ann Plast Surg 38:137–146, 1997 12–23

Purpose.—For most defects of the anterior mandible, microsurgical vascularized free tissue transfer is the reconstructive technique of choice. However, there are questions regarding the reconstruction of lateral segmental mandibular defects, including whether these defects should be reconstructed at all. Although unreconstructed lateral mandibular defects cause less problems than anterior defects, they can still interfere with function. To avoid problems with donor site morbidity, some surgeons have recommended using a reconstruction plate covered by a soft tissue flap, instead of vascularized bone flaps. An experience with the fibular free flap for reconstruction of the lateral mandibular defects was described.

Methods.—Seventeen patients with mandibular defects confined to the lateral segment underwent fibular free flap mandibular reconstruction. Thirteen patients had advanced cancer (Fig 1A, B), and all but 1 of these had received some type of radiation to the tumor bed. All patients were followed for more than 3 months. Assessments included speech quality, oral continence, chewing ability, donor site morbidity, and dental rehabilitation outcomes.

Results.—The mean defect size was 6 cm, and it took an average of 4 additional hours to perform the microsurgical and bone-plating procedures. One month postoperatively, 1 patient had a fractured fixation plate. At 1 year, another patient had malocclusion requiring rerotation of the condyle on the affected side. Five patients had recurrent tumor and died.

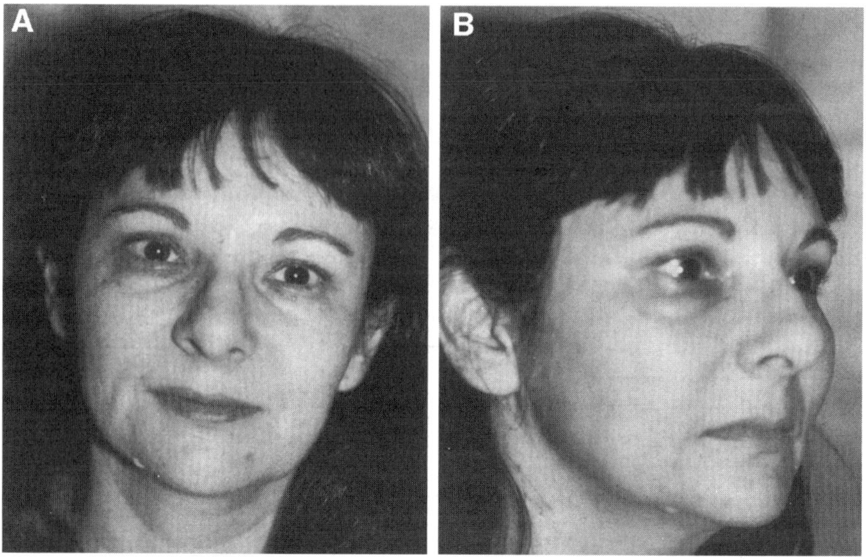

FIGURE 1.—Anterior (A) and oblique (B) views of a 45-year-old woman with squamous cell carcinoma involving the right lateral mandible. (Reprinted from *Annals of Plastic Surgery*, courtesy of Anthony JP, Foster RD, Kaplin MJ, et al: Fibular free flap reconstruction of the "true" lateral mandibular defect. *Ann Plast Surg* 38:137–146, 1997, by permission of Little, Brown and Company, Inc.)

Overall, the results were judged as good or excellent in 88% of patients. All patients but 1 could eat at least a soft diet, and 65% could chew solid foods on the operated side. Dental rehabilitation was performed in 71% of patients; about half of these patients received osseointegrated implants, often placed at the time of tumor removal.

Conclusion.—With the fibular free flap, reconstruction can achieve the same excellent cosmetic and functional results as achieved for the central portion of the mandible. The fibular free flap is easily harvested and can be shaped to fit any defect. The authors no longer use soft-tissue flaps and plate reconstructions for mandibular defects.

► This paper has been written with lucidity and clarity, and the discussion section alone is an excellent review of the rationale behind each phase in the evolution of mandibular reconstruction. The authors' point is, simply stated, that if microvascular reconstruction with the fibula is the preferred method for anterior mandibular reconstruction, then a similar thought process and conclusion can be applied to lateral mandibular defects. Of interest was that one fourth of their patients had *immediate* osseointegrated implants placed in the fibular graft at the time of reconstruction. Nevertheless, because of the small patient series, we need more accrued experience to be assured that we can select such patients for this approach.

So, what patients, if any, should receive a radial forearm osseocutaneous flap? Read on.

E.A. Luce, M.D.

Resection and Immediate Microvascular Reconstruction in the Management of Osteoradionecrosis of the Mandible

Shaha AR, Cordeiro PG, Hidalgo DA, et al (Mem Sloan-Kettering Cancer Ctr, New York)

Head Neck 19:406–411, 1997 12–24

Background.—Patients with advanced cancers of the head and neck are often treated with high dosages of radiation. This treatment can lead to the development of osteoradionecrosis (ORN) of the mandible. Advanced osteoradionecrosis of the mandible can be difficult to treat. This report describes the treatment of 6 patients who had advanced osteoradionecrosis of the mandible. They were treated with surgical resection of the affected portion of the mandible with immediate mandibular reconstruction and microvascular free-tissue transfer.

Methods.—All 6 patients had head or neck cancer and were exposed to postoperative radiotherapy, ranging in dosage from 6,000 to 7,900 cGy. From 5 months to 17 years later, these patients developed ORN. Initial treatment was conservative and included local debridement, oral irrigation, and antibiotics. In 3 cases hyperbaric oxygen was employed. Despite this treatment, the necrosis was not responsive and progressed to mucosal ulceration and bone exposure. These patients were then treated with mandibular resection, followed by an osteotomized, contoured fibular graft. The cutaneous surface was used to resurface the soft tissue defect.

Results.—The surgery was well tolerated, with no significant postoperative complications. Hospitalization duration was for a median of 15 days. Two patients had minor wound sepsis that required removal of some hardware. Cosmetic and functional results were satisfactory. All patients are now capable of eating at least a soft diet.

Conclusions.—The management of advanced osteoradionecrosis remains controversial. For these patients, radical resection of the involved portion of the mandible, followed by free microvascular reconstruction, appears to be a good option. Once the wound has healed, osseointegrated implants should be considered to improve the functional results. This was achieved for 1 patient in this series.

▶ This paper was selected because of the aggressive approach taken by the authors to advanced osteoradionecrosis (ORN). Less advanced forms of ORN (absence of a fistula, limited areas of intraoral exposure, absence of a pathologic fracture) respond to a rigorous and compulsive conservative treatment program consisting of intense oral hygiene, minimal debridement, and *perhaps,* long-term antibiotics. This reviewer views the use of hyperbaric oxygen therapy extremely skeptically, but it has its advocates.

These 6 patients, though, were at a dead end and were successfully managed with contemporary head and neck reconstruction techniques, namely the resection of involved tissues and replacement with vascularized bone and soft tissue lining and/or coverage. Total rehabilitation, though, means osteointegrated dental implants, and at the time of the writing of the paper, only 1 of the 6 patients had been implanted—a truly nit-picking criticism.

E.A. Luce, M.D.

Repair of a Complete Glottic-Subglottic Stenosis With a Fibular Osseocutaneous Free Flap

Esclamado RM, Carroll WR (The Cleveland Clinic Found, Ohio; Univ of Alabama, Birmingham)

Arch Otolaryngol Head Neck Surg 123:877–879, 1997 12–25

Background.—Reconstruction of extensive laryngotracheal stenosis remains difficult. The ideal grafting material would be well vascularized, resistant to infection, resorption and scarring, strong enough to support the airway, but flexible enough to allow contouring and airtight repair. This case report describes the use of a fibula osseocutaneous revascularized flap for reconstruction of a complex laryngotracheal stenosis.

Case Report.—Woman, 24, requested repair of severe laryngotracheal stenosis. She had been in an accident 7 years earlier and undergone 3 failed attempts at stenosis repair. Direct laryngoscopy revealed shortened and thickened vocal folds with a contracted anteroposterior glottic dimension, a posterior glottic scar with fixation of the left cricoarytenoid joint and a mobile arytenoid cartilage. The glottic stenosis was contiguous with a complete subglottic and upper tracheal stenosis associated with anterior thyroid cartilage and anterior cricoid arch loss. As standard techniques had failed, a fibular free-flap reconstruction was agreed on. The pre-epiglottic and subglottic scars were excised. The fibularosseocutaneous flap was harvested. The graft was approximately 5 cm in length and was positioned to reconstruct the anterior thyroid cartilage, as well as the anterior 180 degrees of the cricoid and upper trachea. Microvascular anastomosis was performed, and the patient healed uneventfully. When the stent was removed at 6 weeks, the patient was able to speak and breathe with her tracheostomy tube plugged. She did well for 9 months, but gradually dyspnea and difficulty speaking recurred. Direct laryngoscopy revealed restenosis of the subglottis caused by bony regrowth. Revision surgery was performed 1 year after initial reconstructive surgery. Postoperatively, the patient did well again and was able to breathe and speak. She was decannulated and continued to do well 16 months after revision.

Conclusions.—This report describes a case of the successful use of a fibular osseocutaneous free-flap to reconstruct a severe laryngotracheal stenosis. This technique may be useful in cases of severe stenosis or when traditional techniques have failed.

► The reader must balance the spectacular nature of the result in this case report with the realization that the more structurally and functionally intricate organ, the larynx, remained intact. The two vocal cords and at least one arytenoid were in place. The authors actually had to reconstruct the anterior cricoid, trachea, and a portion of the thyroid cartilage. Despite that little bit of whining on my part about the difficulty and complexity of the reconstructive problem, the result was superb.

The necessity to perform a revision procedure because of bone overgrowth and subsequent reobstruction raises the point whether lining the bone graft at the primary setting, perhaps with vascularized skin as well, would avoid this problem. Also, the debulking aspect of the procedure by removal of the perineal muscles would put the vascular supply at risk.

The most provocative aspect, as the authors discussed, is the use of vascularized tissue such as perichondrium or periosteum or periosteum and perichondrium combined for the next level, namely, the reconstruction of the structural complexity of the larynx.

E.A. Luce, M.D.

Miscellaneous

Merkel Cell Carcinoma: An Aggressive Malignancy

Pergolizzi J Jr, Sardi A, Pelczar M, et al (St Agnes HealthCare, Baltimore, Md)
Am Surg 63:450–454, 1997 12–26

Background.—The rare, aggressive skin tumor known as Merkel cell carcinoma is appropriately classified as a cutaneous neuroendocrine carcinoma. Initial reports suggested that local therapy was adequate, but experience has shown that treatment must be more aggressive. The management of Merkel cell carcinoma in 5 patients was evaluated.

Patients.—The experience included 5 patients with histologically and immunohistochemically confirmed Merkel cell carcinomas. The patients' mean age was 75 years, with the primary lesion located in the head and neck in 3 patients and the extremities in 2. The primary tumors were treated by wide excision, with clear margins. Within a mean of 10 months, 4 of the tumors recurred. Local recurrence developed in 2 patients who did not receive radiotherapy to the primary tumor site. Of 3 patients receiving adjuvant therapy to the regional lymph nodes, 2 had regional recurrences. At 23 months' follow-up, 1 patient treated with wide excision, prophylactic lymph node dissection, and adjuvant chemotherapy was alive and disease free. Three of the remaining 4 patients died with disease.

Discussion.—Merkel cell carcinoma is an aggressive tumor that must be treated aggressively. The initial treatment is wide local excision, with a margin of 2.5–3.0 cm. Adjuvant radiotherapy, to a dose of 5,000–6,000 cGy, can help to prevent local and regional recurrence. The immunohistochemical diagnosis of Merkel cell carcinoma is confirmed by positive markers for cytokeratins. Unfavorable prognostic factors include male sex, young age, lesions larger than 2 cm, lesions located in the head and neck, metastasis at diagnosis, and histologic evidence of lymphatic and vascular invasion.

► This tumor is underrated and underestimated by many clinicians. As documented in this small group of patients, wide excision and postoperative radiotherapy is probably the recommended treatment. If the initial primary presentation is small, a local excision might be the first diagnosis. Clearly, one must return to the scene of the crime and perform a radical re-resection of the site with at least 2-cm margins, which will create a substantial-sized defect for reconstruction.

E.A. Luce, M.D.

Neurotropic Cutaneous Tumors of the Head and Neck

Osguthorpe JD, Abel CG, Lang P, et al (Med Univ of South Carolina, Charleston)

Arch Otolaryngol Head Neck Surg 123:871–876, 1997 12–27

Background.—Perineural propagation of cutaneous tumors has been reported in 0.18% to 1% of basal cell carcinomas and 1% to 14% of cutaneous squamous cell carcinomas. Neurotropic behavior in a cutaneous tumor is associated with perivascular invasion, metastases, and poor prognosis. To determine the outcome of patients with neurotropic cutaneous tumors of the head and neck, a retrospective review was undertaken.

Study Design.—A chart review was performed for 7,852 patients referred between 1984 and 1995 for micrographically controlled excisions of skin cancer. In this series there were 37 patients or 0.47% with neurotropic tumors. Of these 34 patients available for follow-up, 9 had basal cell carcinomas and 25 had squamous cell carcinomas. The median size of the visible or palpable cutaneous tumor was 2 × 1 cm at presentation.

Findings.—Of the 9 patients with neurotropic propagation confined to the subcutaneous tissue, none developed further disease after surgery. Of the 16 with deep extracranial perineural propagation, 10 developed no further disease during follow-up and 1 died of other disease without evidence of tumor recurrence. Two of the remaining patients died. Of the 9 patients with neurotropic tumors extending through the foramen, only 3 underwent craniofacial resection. Of these, 1 is without evidence of disease recurrence, 1 died of other disease without evidence of tumor recurrence, and 1 developed recurrence. The 6 other patients have all had disease recurrence, and some have died.

Conclusions.—A retrospective review was undertaken to examine the outcome of patients with neurotropic cutaneous tumors of the head and neck. For those with extracranial tumors, micrographic tissue mapping, surgery, and irradiation were successful in 76% of cases. For those with neurotropic tumors that penetrated the skull base, prognosis was poor, regardless of therapy.

► This variant of skin cancer is distinctly unusual (the authors report a ½% incidence but probably understate the frequency since this paper is a retrospective review of a very *large* number of patients) but certainly an aggressive variant. I couldn't be certain of the survival rate, but the figures seem in the neighborhood of 50%, depending on which patients were either included or excluded. Although not *explicitly* stated—although the authors had sufficient evidence to do so—it was implied that positive margins are not managed successfully with radiotherapy alone. The failure of radiotherapy to control positive margins in skin cancer as satisfactorily as re-excision is a personal bias of this observer and others as well. The best cure is re-excision. Then the question must be asked whether to add postoperative radiotherapy in this particular aggressive variant. The authors state their preference in the article, and the recommendations seem consummately sensible.

What did not seem particularly sensible—at least based on the evidence available from the paper—was the recommendation for at least 1-year delay before reconstruction. I understand the rationale, but we need some hard evidence that a delay improves survival if a recurrence develops and equally as important, that the 1-year window is adequate, if delay is selected.

E.A. Luce, M.D.

Adenoid Cystic Carcinoma of the Salivary Glands: A Review of 10 Years

Sur RK, Donde B, Levin V, et al (Univ of Witwatersrand, Johannesburg, South Africa)

Laryngoscope 107:1276–1280, 1997 12–28

Background.—The overall prognosis of adenoid cystic carcinoma of the salivary gland is unfavorable. However, the 5-year survival rate may not reflect this. The actual cure rate is not well defined, because long-term follow-up is not well documented. A 10-year experience with this tumor was presented.

Methods.—Fifty patients with adenoid cystic carcinoma treated at the University of Witwatersrand, Johannesburg, South Africa, in the past 10 years were reviewed. There were an equal number of women and men, with ages ranging from 21 to 88 years. Seventeen patients had neural invasion, and 5 had metastatic disease. Thirty-four patients underwent surgery and 16 had radiotherapy as the initial management.

Findings.—At 10 years, overall survival was 29%; disease-free survival, 26%; and local control, 30%. Most recurrences happened in the first 3 years. Nine patients had metastasis after treatment, with a mean survival of 15 months after metastasis developed. Disease-free survival, overall survival, and local control were unaffected by age, site, type of salivary gland, tumor stage, node positivity, or neural invasion. Extent of surgical resection significantly affected disease-free survival and local control but not overall survival because of the tumors' slow growth. Patients with microscopic residual disease postoperatively treated with radiotherapy had better outcomes than patients who had biopsy and radiotherapy, although this difference was nonsignificant.

Conclusions.—Surgeons must make every attempt to remove all microscopic tumor in patients with adenoid cystic carcinoma of the salivary glands. Adding postoperative radiotherapy with high-energy photons apparently does not improve locoregional control or survival. However, a review of the literature indicates that neutron treatment has a place in the treatment of advanced adenoid cystic carcinoma that is inoperable or recurrent.

▶ This report confirms other studies of adenoid cystic carcinoma—namely, that complete resection is preferable, postoperative radiation therapy **may** be of benefit, and a progressive decrease in survival occurs during a 5- to 10- to 20-year period. When reading this article, remember that the authors are from radiation oncology, and many of the patients had well-advanced disease.

E.A. Luce, M.D.

Perioperative Strategies in the Management of Carotid Body Tumors

Leonetti JP, Donzelli JJ, Littooy FN, et al (Loyola Univ of Chicago)
Otolaryngol Head Neck Surg 117:111–115, 1997 12–29

Introduction.—Carotid body tumors are paragangliomas arising from chemoreceptors at the carotid bifurcation. Because these tumors grow slowly, they usually become rather large before they are diagnosed. The clinical signs are subtle, with only a nondiscrete fullness located deep to the sternocleidomastoid muscle. A series of 16 surgically treated carotid body tumors were reviewed to gain insight into the perioperative management of these challenging lesions.

Patients.—The review excluded 3 elderly patients with no other symptoms, for whom no treatment was recommended. The remaining 16 patients came to medical attention with a palpable, lateral neck mass. Ipsilateral vagal nerve paralysis was present in 4 patients, 2 of whom also had ipsilateral hyoglossal nerve paralysis; these problems were all associated with previous surgical "neck exploration." Another 2 patients had undergone previous surgery for attempted tumor removal. In the remaining patients, the diagnosis was made by fine-needle aspiration biopsy or by MRI with MR angiography.

> *Technique.*—When at least 1 cm of uninvolved carotid artery was seen below the styloid base, a lateral transcervical surgical approach was used. For patients with more superior internal carotid artery involvement, a preauricular infratemporal, transparotid approach was used. The styloid musculature was stripped away and the styloid process removed to gain superior control of the artery. The direction of dissection was posterior for the vagus

TABLE 1.—Perioperative Strategies in the Management of Carotid Body Tumors

Preoperative
Patient history
Family history
Physical examination
Catecholamine screening
CT, MRI, MRA
Cervicocerebral angiography
Intraoperative
Wide lateral neck exposure
Cranial nerve protection
Carotid artery dissection under magnification
Bipolar coagulation of tumor vasculature
Postoperative
Speech and swallow therapy
Vocal fold infection
Vocal fold medialization
Nasogastric or gastric feeding tube

(Courtesy of Leonetti JP, Donzelli JJ, Littooy FN, et al: Perioperative strategies in the management of carotid body tumors. *Otolaryngol Head Neck Surg* 117:111–115, 1997.)

nerve and superior for the hypoglossal nerve. This was followed by tumor mobilization in an inferior-to-superior direction, with the use of judicious bipolar coagulation under cool irrigation and loupe or microscope magnification. If needed to repair an area of carotid artery resection or injury, saphenous vein or synthetic graft material was used.

Outcomes.—There were no cases of stroke or major postoperative bleeding. Eight patients had a total of 11 new-onset lower cranial nerve palsies, with 6 cases of vagus nerve injury, 3 of hypoglossal neuropathy, and 2 of glossopharyngeal nerve deficit. Prolonged nasogastric feeding and speech and swallowing therapy were needed for 7 patients with postoperative loss of function of at least 2 of cranial nerves IX, X, and XII.

Discussion.—(Table 1) outlines the perioperative management of carotid body tumors. If the diagnosis of carotid body tumor is not clinically suspected, unnecessary neck exploration may be performed. The diagnosis is better made by MRI and MR angiography than by biopsy. At surgery, the emphasis is on protection of the carotid artery and lower cranial nerves. These patients are vulnerable to combined neural deficits resulting in dysfunctional speech, swallowing, and airway protection.

▶ The authors present a coherent preoperative strategy in the management of carotid body tumors (see Table 1). What was particularly alarming was the number of cranial nerve injuries that occurred as a result of "neck exploration" elsewhere, apparently without adequate preoperative workup. The sequela of these nerve injuries in some patients was prolonged difficulty in swallowing and aspiration, not a trivial complication. Any patient with a lateral neck mass in association with the carotid deserves at least a CT/MRI workup and then excision in experienced hands.

E.A. Luce, M.D.

A Clinical and Histologic Comparison of Percutaneous Dilational Versus Conventional Surgical Tracheostomy

Stoeckli SJ, Breitbach T, Schmid S (Univ Hosp of Zurich, Switzerland)
Laryngoscope 107:1643–1646, 1997 12–30

Introduction.—Conventional tracheostomy permits better tracheobronchial lavage and is more comfortable for the patient than translaryngeal intubation, but adverse events are more frequent with the former technique. The outcome and complications of percutaneous dilational tracheostomy (PDT) and conventional surgical tracheostomy were compared.

Methods.—The 83 patients included in the study required tracheostomy for prolonged mechanical ventilation in the ICU or after surgery for a large tumor in the upper respirodigestive tract. Those in the PDT group had the procedure performed with transnasal translaryngeal endoscopic guidance.

Results.—Forty-seven patients underwent PDT (group 1) and 36 had the standard surgical procedure (group 2). The groups were similar in sex, age, underlying disease, and duration of previous translaryngeal intubation. Group 1 patients were followed up for a median of 355 days and group 2 for a median of 388 days. Three patients in group 1 (6.4%) and 13 in group 2 (36.1%) had postoperative complications, a difference that was highly statistically significant. Postoperative bleeding occurred in 5 patients who had undergone conventional tracheostomy; 1 died and 2 required surgical intervention. Only 1 patient in the PDT group had minimal bleeding from the stoma site. There were 8 cases of wound infection in group 2, but none in group 1. No patient in either group had clinical signs of laryngotracheal stenosis at follow-up. A third of the PDT cases were found to have cartilage fractures with displacement of pieces of cartilage. The resulting inflammatory reaction and scarring suggest that PDT may be associated with a higher risk for late stenosis.

Conclusions.—Percutaneous dilational tracheostomy is a safe and simple procedure that results in significantly lower morbidity than the standard surgical tracheostomy. Despite more injury to the tracheal wall, PDT did not cause laryngotracheal stenosis.

► This is a study that makes sense. Percutaneous dilational tracheostomy has fewer complications than "open" tracheostomy. A key element in the avoidance of complications specific to PDT, such as off-lumen punctures or punctures through the posterior wall of the trachea, is the use of translaryngeal endoscopic guidance of the puncture and guide wire.

The authors raise the specter of fragments of cartilage, as sequestra, as a nidus for future chronic inflammation and possible stenosis. Neither in the bibliography nor cited by the authors was an experimental study of this element, a project waiting for an enterprising young resident. Please note that this study, although prospective, was not randomized in any manner, a serious criticism that must be considered when weighing the results.

E.A. Luce, M.D.

Plastic Surgery

Quality Assurance in Plastic Surgery: Reduction Mammaplasty
Berg A, Palmer B (Karolinska Hosp, Stockholm)
Scand J Plast Reconstr Hand Surg 31:327–331, 1997 12–31

Introduction.—A group of 78 patients who underwent reduction mammaplasty in 1994 were studied to develop a specific, continuous quality assessment program for this procedure. Elements evaluated were the surgical result in general, the different techniques used, and the surgeons involved. Also considered were the patients' subjective judgments.

Methods.—The mean age of the patients was 36 years. Thirty-three were operated using the Lejour's short scar technique, with or without liposuction. In the remaining 45 patients, Strömbeck's technique of a superomedial pedicle was used. A "Reduction mammaplasty quality assurance sheet" was developed to collect data before and after operation. Items on the sheet included breast volume, weight of resected tissue, complications, healing, postoperative improvement, position of the nipple-areola complex, and patient satisfaction. Data were recorded at 4–6 weeks postoperatively and at 1-year follow-up.

Results.—The mean hospital stay was 1.4 days in both groups. Most patients returned to work after a mean of 17 days. Although the rate of early complications was low overall, it was significantly higher in the Lejour group (21.1%) than in the Strömbeck group (4.4%). Symmetry was judged "very good" or "good" in 92% of patients. The ideal nipple-submammary fold distance (6–7 cm) was achieved in only 8 cases. The distance was too long in both the Strömbeck (mean 9.2 cm) and Lejour (mean 11.4 cm) groups. Half of the patients reported decreased sensitivity in the nipple-areola complex. Only 3 of 78 patients continued to have significant pain after mammaplasty. Overall satisfaction was high (90%) and did not differ between groups.

Discussion.—The "Reduction mammaplasty quality assurance sheet" proved to be easy to handle and sufficiently complete. Use of this document provides a starting point for a uniform national continuous quality assurance program for reduction mammaplasty.

▶ The authors should be lauded for their effort to utilize outcomes studies, and incorporate the results into a continuous quality improvement for practicing surgeons. The performance of outcomes studies by clinicians is a growing initiative and an important one to maintain our role in the decision-making process about clinical care.

The problem with this particular effort is the more traditional approach of the authors' focus on hospital stay, complications, and the ***surgeon's*** assessment of the result. What is needed in this study and most if not all outcomes studies, is a quality-of-life index. The authors did do some element of study with a patient rating of the result, but the study of quality of life has become a science in itself with the use of validated instruments. True "quality assurance" assesses patient satisfaction and patient function in ***addition*** to the clinician's opinion.

E.A. Luce, M.D.

13 Vascular Surgery

Introduction

The management of patients with asymptomatic, significant carotid stenosis remains problematic. Although the Asymptomatic Carotid Atherosclerosis Study (ACAS) trial showed a statistically significant benefit for carotid endarterectomy in asymptomatic patients with a greater than 60% stenosis, the stroke risk reduction was only 1% per year. The identification of carotid plaque rupture as a potential marker for the progression of a mature asymptomatic plaque to a symptomatic lesion by Carr et al. (Abstract 13–1) may in the future allow more accurate selection of asymptomatic patients at risk for stroke. Although the morphologic criteria identified by Carr et al. cannot be detected in vivo at present, as imaging techniques improve it may be possible to detect these plaque changes, thereby better identifying asymptomatic patients who will benefit from carotid endarterectomy. Until then, the recommendations of Cronenwett et al. (Abstract 13–2), that carotid endarterectomy may not be efficacious in asymptomatic patients greater than 80 years of age or if the procedure-associated stroke exceeds 3% to 5%, must be borne in mind. Furthermore, in my opinion carotid angioplasty and stenting currently have only a limited role in the treatment of either asymptomatic or symptomatic carotid stenosis, outside of randomized trials. The results of carotid angioplasty and stenting, even from the institution where this approach to the management of carotid disease was initially developed (Abstracts 13–3 and 13–4), appear to be no better, and potentially worse, than the results of carotid endarterectomy.

The endovascular management of aortic and visceral arterial disease also continues to be explored. Although the initial results of treatment of abdominal aortic aneurysms by using aortic stent grafts have been quite acceptable, the question of whether stent graft repair excludes the aneurysm long term remains unanswered. In my recent review of the published studies of endovascular aortic aneurysm repair, it appeared that the risk of development of an endoleak (which puts the patient again at risk for aneurysm rupture) during follow-up could be as much as 20%. The paper by Illig et al. (Abstract 13–5), examining the fate of the proximal aortic cuff after standard surgical repair of abdominal aortic aneurysm, adds further to this concern. They demonstrated that if the proximal aortic cuff was greater than 28 mm Hg at the time of aneurysm repair, continued cuff enlargement to over 30 mm in diameter (where an endoleak would likely develop) was highly likely. To me, much work, including more studies reporting long-term follow-up, remains to be done before endovascular aneurysm repair can become a standard technique for the management of this problem. The importance of long-term follow-up in assessing the value of endovascular treatment of atherosclerotic renal artery disease was also demonstrated in the study of Tullis et al. (Abstract 13–7). They report a high rate of restenosis after renal artery angioplasty with or without stent placement, which was directly related to the degree of residual stenosis immediately after treatment. Furthermore, they demonstrated that, although stenting improved initial results, the use of stents was associated with a higher risk of long-term restenosis compared with angioplasty alone, even if a good initial result was achieved with stenting.

Treatment of symptomatic arterial occlusive disease, particularly infrainguinal disease, continues to be associated with less than ideal results. Abbott et al. (Abstract 13–8) demonstrated no difference in the patency rate of Dacron vs. polytetrafluoroethylene grafts used for femoral to above-knee popliteal artery bypasses, but they showed that based on long-term graft patency rates, such procedures should be reserved for older, non-smoking patients with good arterial anatomy. Furthermore, they found that graft patency was significantly better when 8 mm grafts were used compared to 6 mm grafts. Stonebridge et al. (Abstract 13–9) demonstrated improved graft patency in femoral to below-knee popliteal or infrapopliteal prosthetic bypasses when a distal vein cuff was used. However, the results of prosthetic bypass to infrapopliteal arteries using a distal vein cuff were significantly worse than results of vein bypass to such arteries. Whyman et al. (Abstract 13–10) found no benefit for balloon angioplasty in patients with mild or moderate intermittent claudication compared with patients treated with exercise therapy alone and Abou-Zamzam et al. (Abstract 13–11) demonstrated infrainguinal bypass for limb salvage to be of little value (from the patients' point of view) in patients who were not ambulatory and were not living independently. It is hoped that the results of each of these well-done studies—three of which were prospective randomized trials—will be carefully considered and applied to everyday management of patients with infrainguinal occlusive disease.

The management of failed or failing dialysis access bridge grafts remains a significant problem. It has been suggested that endovascular treatment of failing or failed access grafts using balloon angioplasty will prolong graft patency. However, the well-done prospective randomized trials by Lumsden et al. (Abstract 13–16) and Marston et al. (Abstract 13–17) demonstrated balloon angioplasty of stenoses at the graft vein anastomosis before or after graft failure to be of little value. Considering results of balloon angioplasty in the treatment of stenosis in lower extremity venous bypass grafts, these findings are not surprising. In contrast, endoscopic management of incompetent perforating veins in patients with leg ulceration has been shown to be effective (Abstracts 13–20 to 13–22). However, the importance of incompetent perforating veins in the pathophysiology of venous stasis remains controversial.

Finally, Bender et al. (Abstract 13–23) showed that routine pulmonary artery catheterization does not reduce morbidity and mortality associated with elective vascular surgery procedures. Massie et al. (Abstract 13–24) demonstrated that patients undergoing coronary angiography and coronary revascularization, as indicated by positive dipyridamole thallium study findings before vascular surgical procedures, did no better than patients who simply proceeded with vascular reconstructive procedures without further cardiac evaluation and treatment. In addition, Huber et al. (Abstract 13–25) demonstrated routine use of an intraoperative autologous transfusion device in patients undergoing elective aortic reconstruction to be very expensive and to seldom prevent postoperative autologous blood transfusion. Thus, many of the practices used in the management of patients undergoing vascular surgical procedures that intuitively seem appropriate are found to be of little value when subjected to scientific scrutiny.

James M. Seeger, M.D.

Carotid Disease

Atherosclerotic Plaque Rupture in Symptomatic Carotid Artery Stenosis

Carr S, Farb A, Pearce WH, et al (Northwestern Univ, Chicago; Armed Forces Inst of Pathology, Washington, DC)

J Vasc Surg 23:755–766, 1996 13–1

Introduction.—Plaque rupture is often the precipitating event in acute coronary syndromes and similar events may be important in the development of neurologic symptoms associated with significant carotid stenosis. Forty-four patients who underwent carotid endarterectomy were studied prospectively for plaque morphologic features characteristic of symptomatic vs. asymptomatic disease.

Methods.—Study participants were 33 men and 11 women; 19 were symptomatic and 25 had high-grade (greater than 70%) asymptomatic stenosis. Patients' medical records were reviewed and 2 groups had similar risk factors, except that the symptomatic group had significantly more men. Mean stenosis was 77% for asymptomatic and 74% for symptomatic patients. Carotid endarterectomy specimens were analyzed with pentachrome staining and light microscopy for 10 morphologic characteristics. Selected for analysis were the sections with plaque ulceration or thrombus and/or sections from the most stenotic segment of the plaques.

Results.—Plaque rupture, fibrous cap thinning, infiltration of the fibrous cap with foam cells, and intraplaque fibrin were significantly more common in symptomatic compared to asymptomatic plaques. If the first 3 features were all present within a plaque, there was a 77% chance that the plaque would be from a symptomatic patient. Plaque rupture was present in 74% of plaques from symptomatic patients compared to 32% of plaques from asymptomatic patients, while fibrous cap thinning was seen in 95% of plaques from symptomatic patients vs. 48% of plaques from asymptomatic patients. Infiltration of foam cells into the fibrous cap (84% vs. 44%) and intraplaque fibrin (100% vs. 68%) were also significantly more common in symptomatic vs. asymptomatic plaques. In contrast, no differences were seen in the incidence of plaque hemorrhage, necrotic cores, luminal thrombus, smooth muscle cell infiltration, eccentric shape, or plaque type between the two groups.

Conclusion.—As in acute coronary symptoms, plaque rupture potentially plays a role in the pathogenesis of neurologic symptoms in patients with carotid artery disease. Foam-cell infiltration of the fibrous cap may contribute to rupture of the atherosclerotic plaque and may be associated with the progression of a mature asymptomatic plaque to a symptomatic lesion.

► Rupture of the fibrous cap of carotid atherosclerotic plaques is likely an important cause of neurologic symptoms related to carotid atherosclerosis. However, in vivo identification of plaques at risk for or having fibrous cap rupture is impossible at present. Regardless, the importance of detection of plaques at risk for rupture of the fibrous cap is obvious. Detection of such plaques should identify asymptomatic patients at higher risk for stroke than those selected for carotid endarterectomy using current criteria (60% to 80% or greater stenosis) in whom surgery reduces the stroke risk by only approximately 1% per year.

J.M. Seeger, M.D.

Cost-effectiveness of Carotid Endarterectomy in Asymptomatic Patients

Cronenwett JL, Birkmeyer JD, Nackman GB, et al (Dartmouth-Hitchcock Med Ctr, Lebanon, NH)

J Vasc Surg 25:298–311, 1997 13–2

Introduction.—The Asymptomatic Carotid Atherosclerosis Study (ACAS) and the North American Symptomatic Carotid Endarterectomy Trial (NASCET) have provided sufficient evidence that carotid endarterectomy (CEA) is beneficial in symptomatic and asymptomatic patients with 60% to 70% internal carotid artery (ICA) stenosis. However, it remains uncertain whether the expense of performing 19 CEAs to prevent 1 stroke in patients who are asymptomatic is justified. The cost-effectiveness of CEA in treating asymptomatic patients with 60% or greater ICA was evaluated.

Methods.—A cost-effectiveness analysis was performed using a Markov decision model to reflect the possible clinical outcomes of hypothetical asymptomatic patients with 60% or greater ICA stenosis who were initially selected for either medical management or surgical treatment. The model used the outcomes reported in ACAS and also assumed that patients who had transient ischemic attacks or minor strokes while being managed medically crossed over to surgical treatment. The NASCET data were used to model the outcome of patients who became symptomatic. The average costs of surgery and major stroke were $8,500 and $34,000 plus $18,000 per year, respectively. The incremental cost-effectiveness ratio of surgical treatment was calculated as the incremental cost per quality-adjusted life year (QALY) saved by surgical vs. medical management.

Results.—Surgical treatment improved quality-adjusted life expectancy from 7.87 to 8.12 QALYs. The incremental lifetime cost was $2,041, which produced an incremental cost-effectiveness ratio of $8,000 per QALY saved by surgical vs. medical treatment. The cost of care during medical treatment for major stroke greatly offset the initial expense of CEA in patients treated surgically. Eventual CEA was performed in 26% of patients medically managed. The relative cost of surgical treatment rose substantially with increasing age, increasing perioperative stroke rate, and decreasing stroke rate during medical management.

Conclusion.—Carotid endarterectomy was cost-effective, compared to other commonly accepted health care practices in asymptomatic patients from the ACAS with 60% or greater carotid stenosis. Surgery is not cost-effective in very elderly patients or those with very high or very low stroke risk.

► Although cost-effectiveness is not the only measure of benefit from a particular type of treatment, computer modeling of cost-effectiveness allows investigation for the influence of various factors on outcome. This decision analysis model points out that because stroke risk reduction after CEA in asymptomatic patients occurs slowly, age and the incidence of postoperative stroke affect long-term benefit significantly. Because of this, the authors show that CEA may not be cost-effective in asymptomatic patients older than 80 years of age or if the procedure-associated stroke risk exceeds 3% to 5%. In my state, the older than 85 years group has seen the greatest percentage increase in CEA since the publication of the ACAS, so I hope that these findings will be carefully considered by all of us.

J.M. Seeger, M.D.

Elective Stenting of the Extracranial Carotid Arteries

Yadav JS, Roubin GS, Iyer S, et al (Univ of Alabama, Birmingham)

Circulation 95:376–381, 1997 13–3

Introduction.—Surgical endarterectomy is considered superior to medical management of severe carotid stenosis, but it has serious risks and limitations that must be considered. Percutaneous carotid balloon angioplasty has the potential to be safer, less traumatic, more cost-effective, and usable in patients with significant carotid stenosis at high surgical risk. The outcome of percutaneous carotid angioplasty and elective stenting of the extracranial carotid arteries was prospectively evaluated in a consecutive series of 107 patients (126 vessels) with carotid stenosis 60% or more.

Methods.—After thorough clinical and imaging evaluations, patients underwent balloon angioplasty and elective stenting. Quantitative carotid angiography was performed before stenting, after stenting, and at a 6-month follow-up examination. Morbidity, mortality, and the need for repeat intervention by angioplasty or endarterectomy were recorded.

Results.—The mean stenosis was decreased from 78% to 2%. During initial hospitalization and the first 30 days after angioplasty and stenting, 7 patients had minor strokes, 2 had major strokes, and 1 died. The combined incidence of all strokes and death was 7.9%. The incidence of ipsilateral major strokes and death was 1.6%. During follow-up, no strokes occured. At a 6-month follow-up, the mean angiographic stenosis in 81 patients was 18%. Four of 81 patients (4.9%) experienced asymptomatic restenosis of ≥ 50%. Repeat interventions were performed in 5 patients who were asymptomatic; 2 of them had angioplasty for restenosis, 2 had angioplasty for stent deformation, and 1 had endarterectomy for restenosis.

Conclusion.—Patients with extracranial carotid disease can be successfully treated using percutaneous carotid angioplasty and stenting with low rates of restenosis and repeat interventions.

A Comparison of Angioplasty With Stenting Versus Endarterectomy for the Treatment of Carotid Artery Stenosis

Jordan WD Jr, Schroeder PT, Fisher WS, et al (Univ of Alabama, Birmingham)
Ann Vasc Surg 11:2–8, 1997 13–4

Background.—Carotid endarterectomy (CEA) is the standard treatment for high-grade stenosis of the extracranial carotid arteries. Percutaneous transluminal angioplasty has also been used to treat significant carotid artery stenoses. The safety and efficacy of percutaneous carotid angioplasty with stenting (PTAS) as a treatment for high-grade carotid stenosis was examined in a prospective trial at the University of Alabama, Birmingham. This study compares the patients who underwent PTAS with a retrospectively examined patient group that underwent CEA for similar disease during the same 14-month study period.

Study Design.—A review was performed of all patients who underwent treatment for carotid stenosis between August 1994 and October 1995 at the University of Alabama at Birmingham Hospital and the Birmingham VA Hospital. There were 107 patients who underwent PTAS and 166 patients who underwent CEA in the study group. The clinical end points were defined as transient or permanent neurologic deficits at 24 hours, 30 days or 6 months after the procedure. Data were collected prospectively in patients undergoing PTAS and retrospectively in patients undergoing CEA.

Results.—Death or clinical neurologic deficits that occurred or persisted beyond 24 hours occurred in 3.6% of patients who underwent CEA and

9.3% of patients who underwent PTAS. Significant nonneurologic complications occurred in 1.2% of patients who underwent CEA and in 5.6% of patients who underwent PTAS. Six-month follow-up information was obtained for 193 patients. Among these patients, there were 7 minor strokes, 1 major stroke, and 4 deaths in the PTAS group and 1 minor stroke, 1 major stroke, and 6 deaths in the CEA group.

Conclusions.—Although early results of the treatment of carotid artery stenosis with PTAS have been promising, comparison with a retrospective group of patients undergoing CEA indicates that CEA is the safer procedure. Furthermore, long-term follow-up will be necessary to determine whether PTAS may be a useful alternative treatment for carotid artery stenosis in selective high-risk patients with significant carotid stenosis.

▶ These 2 papers (Abstracts 13–3 and 13–4) are from the institution in which angioplasty and stenting in the treatment of significant carotid stenosis have been initially studied. Results from these studies demonstrate carotid endarterectomy and carotid angioplasty and stenting to be associated with equivalent major stroke incidence and death, whereas carotid PTA is associated with a significantly higher incidence of minor strokes. These results must be considered to be very preliminary because the studies were not randomized comparisons, the study of the patients undergoing surgery was retrospective, and limited follow-up information was available. However, the results of the carotid angioplasty and stenting to date are worse than the results of CEA, and the risk of long-term restenosis after carotid angioplasty and stenting (which likely will be higher than the risk of restenosis after CEA) remains to be determined. In my opinion, carotid angioplasty and stenting should remain experimental (and therefore not reimbursable) until further information, potentially including the results of large, randomized trials with long-term follow-up, are available.

J.M. Seeger, M.D.

Aortoiliac Disease

Fate of the Proximal Aortic Cuff: Implications for Endovascular Aneurysm Repair

Illig KA, Green RM, Ouriel K, et al (Univ of Rochester, NY)
J Vasc Surg 26:492–501, 1997 13–5

Background.—There has been great interest in the last few years in the repair of abdominal aortic aneurysms using endovascular techniques. All such devices currently rely on mechanical hooks or frictional engagement for secure endovascular graft positioning and to protect the aneurysmal cavity from arterial pressure. Continued secure endograft fixation depends on continued integrity of the proximal and distal cuffs and late dilation could result in graft disengagement, reestablishment of arterial pressure within the aneurysmal sac, or graft dislodgement. Because information regarding the behavior of the native artery at fixation points after intraluminal repair will not be obtained for many years, the long-term size changes of the proximal aortic cuff and iliac vessels after conventional abdominal aortic aneurysm repair were examined.

Methods.—Original and repeat CT scans of 33 patients who had repair of an infrarenal abdominal aortic aneurysm were reviewed. Repeat CT scans were performed at a mean of 88.6 months after repair.

Results.—At 5 years, the overall survival rate for these 33 patients was 73%. Computed tomography scans showed a mean preoperative infrarenal aortic cuff diameter of 24.5 mm. At an average of 89 months after repair, the mean infrarenal aortic cuff diameter had increased by 4.3 mm to 28.8 mm, and the infrarenal cuff was 30 mm or greater in 11 patients. As early as 6 years after repair, 3 of 7 patients examined during this time period had cuffs that were dilated to 30 mm or greater. Late dilation to 30 mm or greater occurred in 16% of patients who had preoperative infrarenal aortic cuffs of 27 mm or less and in 88% of patients who had preoperative cuffs of 28 mm or larger. The mean late iliac artery size was 16.9 mm, and 30% were 20 mm or greater.

Discussion.—One third of patients who survive repair of an abdominal aortic aneurysm have significant dilation of the proximal infrarenal aortic cuff over time. Proximal dilation is rare in patients with a smaller initial diameter of the aortic cuff while it is extremely common in patients with larger cuffs. Although, cuff dilation rarely causes problems after conventional suture fixation, long-term results after endoluminal repair are unknown. The results of this study indicate that endovascular aortic prostheses that can continue to self-expand many years after implantation will be required. Furthermore, these results suggest that endovascular aneurysm repair may not be the best solution for patients with a long life expectancy or preoperative proximal aortic cuffs greater than 27 mm.

► As trials of endovascular repair of infrarenal abdominal aortic aneurysms progress toward completion and potential market approval, the fundamental question of the durability of such repairs remains unanswered. This paper suggests that continued enlargement of the juxtarenal aorta is a part of the natural history of aneurysmal disease and that in a significant percentage of patients, this enlargement will be clinically significant. Aneurysm necks less than 28 mm in diameter appear less likely to enlarge over time, and restriction of endoluminal abdominal aortic aneurysm repair to patients with such anatomy seems prudent. However, this will likely limit the number of patients eligible for endoluminal abdominal aortic aneurysm repair. Obviously, much more work remains to be done before this exciting new technique can become the standard of care for patients with infrarenal abdominal aortic aneurysm.

J.M. Seeger, M.D.

Gender Differences in Abdominal Aortic Aneurysm Prevalence, Treatment, and Outcome

Katz DJ, Stanley JC, Zelenock GB (Univ of Michigan, Ann Arbor)

J Vasc Surg 25:561–568, 1997 13–6

Background.—The role of gender in the diagnosis, management, and outcome of diseases requiring peripheral vascular surgery remains poorly defined. Recent evidence suggests that women have a greater risk of mortality after repair of aortic aneurysms. Gender differences in the management of and outcome of surgery for abdominal aortic aneurysms (AAA) were investigated.

Methods.—The Michigan Inpatient Data Base was searched for records of patients admitted between 1980 and 1990 with intact or ruptured AAAs. Mode of treatment and surgical mortality rates were determined for each of the 47,739 patients identified.

Results.—Age at admission and surgery for AAA was significantly greater for women than for men. Mean patient age at admission was 73.0 and 77.4 years for women with intact and ruptured AAAs, respectively, compared with 69.4 and 71.9 years, respectively, for men. After adjustment for age, hospitalization for intact AAAs occurred at an annual rate of 108.1 men per 100,000 aged 50 years or older, whereas women were hospitalized at a rate of only 22.5 per 100,000. Hospitalization for ruptured AAAs was also more common in men than women (22.6 vs. 4.5 per 100,000). Men were 1.8 times as likely to receive surgical treatment for intact AAAs than were women, and were 1.4 times as likely as women to be treated surgically for ruptured AAAs. The risk of mortality was 1.4 times as high for women as men after surgical repair of an intact AAA, and was 1.45 times as high for women as men after repair of a ruptured AAA.

Conclusions.—The existence of differences in cardiovascular disease treatment based upon gender are clearly supported by this study. Surgical repair of both intact and ruptured AAAs is performed less commonly in women than in men, and the risk of mortality associated with surgical repair is substantially greater in women. It is not clear whether these contrasts result from biological differences or simply to gender-based differences in disease management. However, the existence and magnitude of the effects present a compelling justification for a major prospective study.

► Based on this study, it appears that women with AAAs are less likely to undergo repair and more likely to die after repair of either intact or ruptured AAAs. The reason for these differences isn't clear, but the differences appear to be very significant. Clearly, results of treatment of women with AAA need to be examined carefully by each of us.

J.M. Seeger, M.D.

Results of Percutaneous Transluminal Angioplasty for Atherosclerotic Renal Artery Stenosis: A Follow-up Study With Duplex Ultrasonography

Tullis MJ, Zierler RE, Glickerman DJ, et al (Univ of Washington, Seattle; Seattle Veterans Affairs Med Ctr)

J Vasc Surg 25:46–54, 1997 13–7

Objective.—There is little information about the short- and long-term anatomical outcomes after percutaneous transluminal renal angioplasty (PTRA). The anatomical results of PTRA were evaluated with serial duplex ultrasonographic studies.

Methods.—A total of 52 PTRA procedures were performed on 41 patients (15 women), average age 65 years, with greater than 60% diameter reduction of the renal arteries (stents were placed in 12 arteries). Patients were followed-up by renal artery ultrasonographic duplex scanning for an average of 34 months for purposes of classifying the extent of disease. (Patients underwent 5 in 10 duplex examinations.)

Results.—Immediately after PTRA, 23 arteries were classified as normal, 19 as having less than 60% stenosis, and 10 as having 60% or greater stenosis. During follow-up, restenosis developed in 29 patients. The cumulative incidence of restenosis from normal to 60% or greater was 13% at 1 year and 19% at 2 years. The cumulative incidence of restenosis from less than 60% to 60% or greater was 44% at 1 year and 55% at 2 years. The difference between restenosis rates for arteries initially classified as normal vs. less than 60% stenosis was significant. Although 83% of stented arteries and 33% of arteries not stented were normal immediately after PTRA, 1 year later, 44% of stented arteries and 18% of arteries not stented had restenosed.

Conclusion.—Duplex ultrasonographic follow-up of PTRA demonstrates that the initial anatomical result is predictive of restenosis. Furthermore, although stenting gives superior improvement initially, arteries so treated show a high early restenosis rate.

► Using serial renal artery duplex examinations, the University of Washington group has shown that the incidence of restenosis after PTRA is high, that restenosis is related to the degree to residual stenosis after angioplasty, and that renal artery stenting improves initial results but does not limit long-term restenosis. In addition, little relationship was seen between clinical outcome and the initial or continuous success of PTRA, which means that previous studies documenting continued improvement after PTRA based only on clinical grounds are of little value. The role of PTRA in the management of patients with renal artery disease remains unclear, and comparative studies (PTRA vs. surgery vs. medical therapy) with long-term anatomical follow-up will be necessary before the appropriate use of PTRA in patients with renal vascular hypertension can be determined.

J.M. Seeger, M.D.

Infrainguinal Disease

Prosthetic Above-Knee Femoropopliteal Bypass Grafting: Results of a Multicenter Randomized Prospective Trial

Abbott WM, for the Above-Knee Femoropopliteal Study Group
(Massachusetts Gen Hosp, Boston)

J Vasc Surg 25:19–28, 1997 13–8

Background.—The use of prosthetic grafts above the knee in the treatment of infrainguinal occlusive disease has become popular because of the seemingly acceptable outcomes with polytetrafluoroethylene grafts (PTFE). Knitted Dacron polyester grafts have also been used, with equivalent and sometimes superior results in some series. Dacron and PTFE were compared in a randomized, prospective, multicenter study in the United States and Canada.

Methods.—Two hundred forty-four patients underwent placement of a knitted Dacron polyester graft impregnated with collagen or a thin-wall expanded reinforced PTFE graft to the above-knee popliteal artery, usually from the common femoral artery. Follow-up included a physical examination and noninvasive hemodynamic study, sometimes with duplex scanning, for as long as 5 years.

Findings.—The procedural mortality rate was 0, and the morbidity rate was 6.5%. The patient survival rate was 77% at 3 years. At this time, the 2 grafts did not differ significantly in primary or secondary patency rates. The primary patency rate for Dacron was 62%, and for PTFE it was 57%. There were no unexpected adverse outcomes on limb status. Patency rates in both graft groups were inferior in patients receiving small (5-6 mm) grafts, in patients younger than 65 years, and in patients who smoked.

Conclusion.—The use of synthetic bypass grafts above the knee should be limited to older nonsmokers with favorable anatomy. The choice of graft material in such patients will depend on handling characteristics and cost. Above-knee prostheses should be used only selectively in younger smokers. The graft size should be carefully considered in patients undergoing this procedure.

► Although no difference was seen in the patency rates of above-knee femoral popliteal bypasses done using either PTFE or Dacron polyester grafts, several important observations were made in this prospective study. Patency was significantly better with 8-mm compared with 6-mm grafts and significantly worse in patients less than 65 years of age who continue to smoke. Surprisingly, failure of these prosthetic grafts did not increase the risk of limb loss, which is different from results from other studies. Regardless, as these authors state, above-knee femoral popliteal bypass procedures using prosthetic grafts should be reserved for older, nonsmoking patients with good arterial anatomy because use in other patients will lead to inferior long-term results.

J.M. Seeger, M.D.

Randomized Trial Comparing Infrainguinal Polytetrafluoroethylene Bypass Grafting With and Without Vein Interposition Cuff at the Distal Anastomosis

Stonebridge PA, for the Joint Vascular Research Group (Univ of Edinburgh, Scotland; Infirmary of Edinburgh, Scotland)
J Vasc Surg 26:543–550, 1997 13–9

Background.—The vein cuff developed by Miller is now favored for use with infrainguinal polytetrafluoroethylene (PTFE) bypass grafts. A randomized study was conducted to determine whether a vein cuff improves short-term and medium-term patency and limb salvage rates in patients undergoing femoral-above-knee popliteal and femoral-below-knee popliteal artery PTFE bypass procedures.

Methods.—The multicenter trial allocated patients to 1 of 2 groups: the first had an interposition vein cuff constructed at the distal anastomosis as described by Miller, and the second had a direct PTFE-to-artery distal anastomosis done. The cuff is created by taking a segment of available vein slightly longer than double the length of the distal arteriotomy. The vein is opened longitudinally, producing a panel that is sewn around the arteriotomy to produce the cuff (Fig 1). The PTFE graft is then sutured end-to-cuff. Outcome criteria were primary graft patency and limb salvage rates. Patency was assessed by the presence of distal pulses, a persistent significant rise in Doppler pressure, or a patent graft on duplex scan.

Results.—A total of 261 bypass operations were randomized, 133 to vein cuff and 128 to no vein cuff. Twelve-month patency rates were 80% for cuffed and 84% for uncuffed above-knee popliteal artery PTFE bypass grafts. Two-year patency rates in the above-knee procedures were 72% and 70%, respectively, for cuffed and uncuffed groups. Bypass grafts to below-knee popliteal arteries had 12-month patency rates of 80% for the cuffed group and 65% for the uncuffed group; 2-year patency rates were 52% and 29%, respectively (Fig 4) ($P < .003$). At the end of the follow-up period (median 617 days), there were 19 major limb amputations and 45 deaths. Differences in limb salvage rates between cuffed and uncuffed groups did not reach statistical significance.

Conclusion.—Use of a distal anastomosis interposition vein cuff did not improve the patency rate of femoral-above-knee popliteal PTFE bypass grafts but there was a statistically significant increase in patency rate when a cuff was used in femoral-below-knee popliteal PTFE bypass graft procedures.

► Controversy continues as to whether use of a vein cuff at the distal anastomosis of a prosthetic femoral popliteal or femoral tibial bypass improves graft patency. This randomized trial and one other from Europe[1] suggest that use of a vein cuff does improve results of prosthetic bypass to the below-knee arteries. However, the follow-up in these studies is limited, and even at 2 years, results of prosthetic bypasses done with a vein cuff to

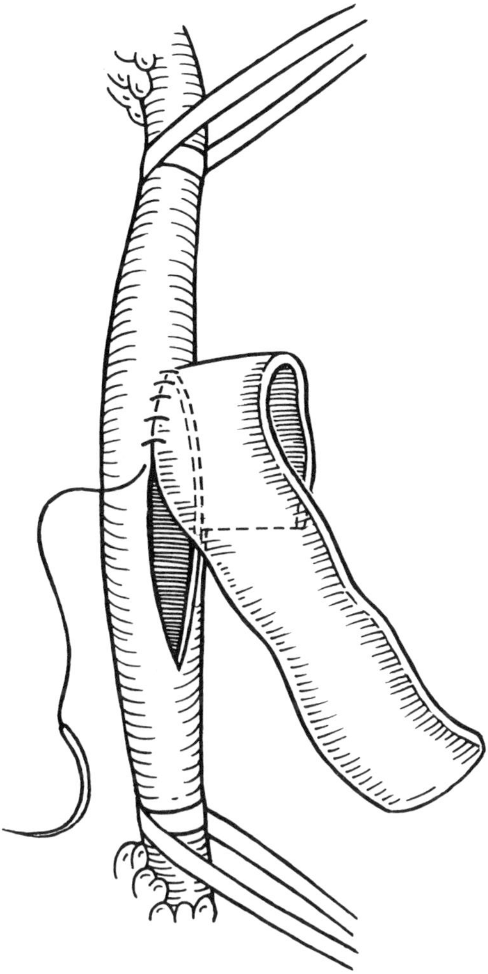

FIGURE 1.—Vein panel is sewn longitudinally around arteriotomy. (Courtesy of Stonebridge PA, for the Joint Vascular Research Group: Randomized trial comparing infrainguinal polytetrafluoroethylene bypass grafting with and without vein interposition cuff at the distal anastomosis. *J Vasc Surg* 26:543–550, 1997.)

below-knee popliteal and intrapopliteal arteries still appear significantly worse than results of vein bypass to these arteries.

J.M. Seeger, M.D.

Reference

1. Raptis S, Miller JH: Influence of a vein cuff on polytetrafluoroethylene grafts for primary femoropopliteal bypass. *Br J Surg* 82:487–491, 1995.

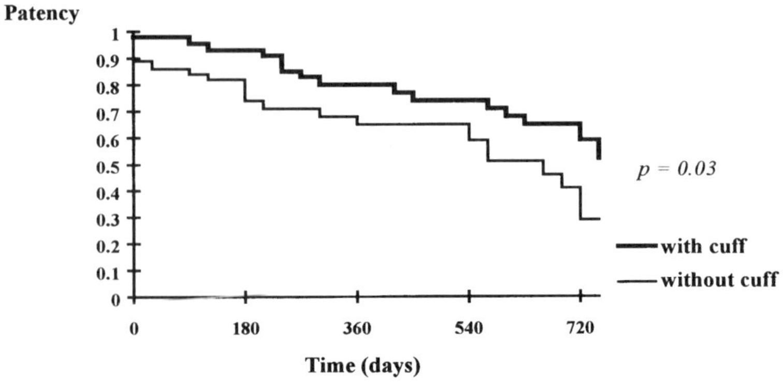

Grafts at risk

Time (months)	0	180	360	540	720
Cuff	48	38	30	25	10
No cuff	47	32	23	17	5

FIGURE 4.—Graft patency data for femoral-below-knee popliteal artery bypass grafts with and without a distal anastomosis vein cuff. (Courtesy of Stonebridge PA, for the Joint Vascular Research Group: Randomized trial comparing infrainguinal polytetrafluoroethylene bypass grafting with and without vein interposition cuff at the distal anastomosis. *J Vasc Surg* 26:543–550, 1997.)

Is Intermittent Claudication Improved by Percutaneous Transluminal Angioplasty? A Randomized Controlled Trial

Whyman MR, Fowkes FGR, Kerracher EMG, et al (Univ of Edinburgh, Scotland; Royal Infirmary of Edinburgh, Scotland)
J Vasc Surg 26:551–557, 1997 13–10

Introduction.—The use of and indications for percutaneous transluminal angioplasty (PTA) for the treatment of peripheral arterial disease are expanding. However, there have been very few controlled studies to support its benefits. A randomized, controlled trial of PTA vs. conventional medical therapy for patients with mild to moderate intermittent claudication was conducted.

Methods.—Of 600 patients with claudication screened, 62 (47 with short femoral artery stenoses or occlusions and 15 with iliac stenoses) were randomly assigned to PTA plus medical therapy, or to only medical therapy, consisting of low-dose aspirin and advice regarding smoking and exercise. After 2 years, the groups were compared for differences in outcome, including patient-reported maximum walking distance, treadmill walking distance to onset of claudication, treadmill maximum walking distance, ankle-brachial pressure index, quality of life, and duplex US assessment of occlusive disease.

Results.—Two-year outcomes were similar in terms of patient-reported maximum walking distance, treadmill distance to onset of claudication, treadmill maximum walking distance, and ankle-brachial pressure index. Number of occluded arteries and degree of stenosis of patent arteries were less in the PTA group. There was no significant difference in quality of life.

Conclusions.—Two years after treatment, patients with mild to moderate intermittent claudication treated with PTA have less extensive arterial occlusive disease than those treated by medical therapy alone. However, the PTA-treated patients have no significant advantage in terms of walking or quality of life.

▶ Although the authors of this article suggest that larger trials might demonstrate subsets of patients with claudication that would benefit from PTA, the overall conclusion from this and other randomized studies is clear: PTA does not improve claudication symptoms compared to medical therapy alone. This finding should have significant implications. Hopefully, results of this study, or larger trials if necessary, will finally lead to appropriate and likely limited use of PTA in patients whose only symptoms are claudication.

J.M. Seeger, M.D.

Functional Outcome After Infrainguinal Bypass for Limb Salvage

Abou-Zamzam AM Jr, Lee RW, Moneta GL, et al (Oregon Health Sciences Univ, Portland)

J Vasc Surg 25:287–297, 1997 | 13–11

Background.—The outcome of patients after lower extremity bypass surgery has been evaluated by parameters such as graft patency, limb salvage, and survival. However, these traditional parameters do not address the patient's functional status.

Methods.—The preoperative and 6-month postoperative living situation and ambulatory status were evaluated in 513 patients who had infrainguinal bypass for limb salvage. The effect of risk factors was evaluated by multivariate analysis.

Results.—Before having indications for surgery, 92% of patients lived independently and 91% were ambulatory. The operative mortality rate was 2.7%. Six months postoperatively, 86% of patients were alive, and the assisted primary graft patency rate was 92%. At 6 months, 99% of surviving patients who lived independently before surgery had returned to independent living, and 97% of patients who were ambulatory before surgery were ambulatory. Of 25 survivors who were not living independently before surgery, only 1 achieved independent living at 6 months. Of 29 nonambulatory patients, 6 become ambulatory postoperatively. Multivariate analysis showed that preoperative living situation and ambulatory status are important in predicting 6-month outcome. Predictors of poor ambulatory status at 6 months were amputation and loss of primary patency. At 5 years, the overall survival rate was 48.1%.

Discussion.—These results indicate that in patients who have infrainguinal bypass for limb salvage, preoperative independence and ambulation are important predictors of postoperative independence and ambulation. Infrainguinal bypass procedures for limb salvage are associated with low operative mortality, and the vast majority of independent and ambulatory patients are able to return to independent living and ambulation. In patients who have infrainguinal bypass for limb salvage, poor overall long-term outcome more often results from intercurrent illness than from infrainguinal bypass.

▶ A primary requirement for a successful lower extremity bypass has always been a patient who is likely to benefit from the procedure. This study demonstrates that patients who are ambulatory benefit significantly from infrainguinal bypass for limb salvage. In contrast, those who were not ambulatory or living independently were seldom improved and had a high mortality at 6 months. Obviously, the benefit of infrainguinal bypass in these patients was limited and arterial reconstruction in such patients should at most be used very selectively.

J.M. Seeger, M.D.

Thrombolysis of Occluded Infrainguinal Vein Grafts: Predictors of Outcome

Nackman GB, Walsh DB, Fillinger MF, et al (Dartmouth Hitchcock Med Ctr, Lebanon, NH)

J Vasc Surg 25:1023–1032, 1997 13–12

Objective.—Some reports recommend thrombolysis as treatment for thrombosed infrainguinal vein grafts, suggesting that this may permit immediate interventions to correct the cause of graft failure, or it may facilitate more focused surgical intervention. However, the late results of thrombolysis do not appear as good as those of graft replacement. A series of patients undergoing thrombolysis of occluded infrainguinal vein grafts was reviewed to determine factors affecting graft patency and limb salvage rates.

Methods.—The study included 44 patients undergoing percutaneous, catheter-directed urokinase thrombolysis of occluded infrainguinal vein bypass grafts over a 1-year period. Differences in survival and patency were assessed by life-table analysis. Patient-specific factors affecting outcomes were identified by univariate and multivariate analysis.

Results.—Thrombolysis carried a mortality rate of 2% and a nonfatal complication rate of 16%. In one fourth of the grafts, thrombolysis failed to restore graft patency. Thrombolysis was successful in the remaining 33 grafts, but 88% of those later required adjunctive surgery or percutaneous transluminal angioplasty. Primary patency rate after successful thrombolysis was 25% at 1 year and 19% at 2 years. On multivariate analysis, factors associated with a higher graft patency rate were not having diabetes and having a vein graft in place for longer than 1 year. The two-year limb salvage rate was 63% for patients with successful thrombolysis vs. 31% for those in whom thrombolysis failed. Two-year survival after thrombolysis was 89%.

Conclusions.—In patients with occluded infrainguinal vein grafts, thrombolysis has a low chance of providing durable graft patency, even with adjunctive measures. Limb salvage rate is significantly improved for patients with successful thrombolysis, however. Thrombolysis may be helpful in nondiabetic patients with mature vein grafts and no alternatives for additional autogenous revascularization.

► Despite its appeal and widespread use, the success of thrombolysis in treatment of occluded infrainguinal vein bypass grafts has been limited. This study shows that in patients without diabetes whose grafts are older than 12 months, results are potentially acceptable. In contrast, in patients without these "good" characteristics attempted thrombolysis was of little value. Additionally, even in the group with the "good" characteristics, long-term results were worse than those previously reported when a new bypass using autogenous vein conduit was done to treat an infrainguinal vein bypass occlusion. Thus, use of thrombolysis in selected patients with occluded infrainguinal vein bypass grafts may be of some value, particularly when repeat reconstruction is limited by lack of autogenous conduit. However, the "try it and see" approach is more likely to do harm than good.

J.M. Seeger, M.D.

Impact of Arterial Surgery and Balloon Angioplasty on Amputation: A Population-based Study of 1155 Procedures Between 1973 and 1992

Hallett JW Jr, Byrne J, Gayari MM, et al (Mayo Found, Rochester, Minn)

J Vasc Surg 25:29–38, 1997 13–13

Background.—Leg revascularization procedures are frequently performed with the goal of avoiding the necessity of amputation when advanced ischemia occurs. Improved limb salvage rates as a result of vascular procedures have been reported by a large number of referral practices; however referral bias, loss of patients to follow-up, and selection bias may inflate the estimate of success when based on patient records within individual practices. To avoid these biases, a population-based survey of the incidence of balloon angioplasty and arterial surgery in the legs, and of leg amputation as a consequence of arterial occlusive disease was performed.

Methods.—Databases of regional hospitals were searched for medical information regarding residents of Olmsted County, Minnesota. Patients were identified who had undergone balloon angioplasty, surgical procedures, or amputations as a consequence of arterial occlusive disease of the legs between 1973 and 1993. Clinical and demographic information were collected for each patient.

Results.—Between 1973 and 1993, 1,155 procedures were performed for occlusive arterial disease in the leg on 449 residents (57% male) of Olmsted County. Of the procedures, 733 were arterial surgery, 363 were amputations, and 59 were percutaneous balloon angioplasties. Intervention was indicated by limb-threatening ischemia in 47% of patients, and non–limb-threatening ischemia in 53%. Indications for balloon angioplasty and surgical intervention did not differ. The procedures were elective in 87.1% of cases and emergent in 12.9%. Amputations were digital in 21% of cases, and major in the remaining 79%. Surgical and angioplastic procedures were performed more commonly in men than women (141.9 and 57.4 per 100,000 person-years, respectively). The incidence rate for surgical and angioplastic procedures rose from 1975 to 1985, peaking at 109.5 per 100,000 person-years, and subsequently fell to 93.1 per 100,000 person-years in 1992. The incidence rate for balloon angioplasty increased markedly, from 1979 to 1992, from 1.4 to 17.0 per 100,000 person-years, respectively, with no evidence of a plateau. Concurrently, the incidence of major amputation decreased from 36.7 per 100,000 person-years in 1973, to 19.0 per 100,000 person-years in 1992. Minor amputation incidence did not change during the same period.

Conclusions.—The frequency of vascular surgery and balloon angioplasty for treatment of occlusive arterial disease of the leg has increased between 1973 and 1993, and has likely been an important causal factor in the reduced frequency of major amputations during the last decade. The length of this study and its population-based nature lend confidence to these conclusions.

▶ This population-based study demonstrates a decline in rate of amputation as the rate of arterial revascularization (particularly infrageniculate revascularization) has increased; this confirms my bias that arterial revascularization improves limb salvage. However, the majority of patients in this study underwent amputation without a prior revascularization procedure. Amputations in a large population of patients such as this are done for multiple different problems, and multiple factors influence the decision to attempt limb salvage even in patients with limb-threatening ischemia. Regardless, this study suggests that aggressive, appropriate use of infrageniculate bypass appears to be effective in reducing the overall risk of amputation.

J.M. Seeger, M.D.

Natural History of Infrainguinal Vein Graft Stenosis Relative to Bypass Grafting Technique

Gupta AK, Bandyk DF, Cheanvechai D, et al (Univ of South Florida, Tampa)

J Vasc Surg 25:211–225, 1997 13–14

Introduction.—A better understanding of the natural history of infrainguinal vein graft stenosis might allow grafts to be categorized in the early postoperative period according to degree of risk for vein graft stenosis. Grafts at higher risk could thus be identified and followed with intensive surveillance.

Methods.—The incidence of vein graft stenosis relative to bypass grafting technique was examined in 338 infrainguinal vein bypasses. The patient population included 242 men and 80 women with a mean age of 67 years. Four grafting techniques were used: in situ greater saphenous vein bypass (131), reversed greater saphenous vein bypass (120), nonreversed translocated greater saphenous or cephalic vein bypass (48), and reversed spliced alternative vein bypass (39). Most (83%) revascularization procedures were required because of critical limb ischemia. Intraoperative duplex scanning was performed to classify defects according to degree of stenosis and optimize bypass construction. Duplex graft surveillance was repeated before hospital discharge, 6 weeks later, and at 3- to 6-month intervals thereafter. Rates of graft patency and revision/failure were compared with grafting technique, need for operative revision, and intraoperative duplex scan results.

Results.—Three-year primary/secondary graft patency rates were significantly higher for in situ bypass grafts (85%/97%) than for reversed (57%/83%), nonreversed translocated (62%/78%), or alternative (51%/76%) vein bypass grafts. During a mean follow-up of 19 months, the incidence of graft revision was lower for in situ (10%) and nonreversed (16%) saphenous vein bypass grafts than for reversed saphenous (23%) and alternative (28%) grafts. The most common abnormality identified both at operation and postoperative surveillance was stenosis at the valve site or localized in a vein segment. Despite normal intraoperative graft duplex scans, reversed vein grafts had a revision/failure rate that was 2.5 times greater than that of in situ/nonreversed translocated vein conduits. Intraoperative duplex scanning led to the revision of 56 (16%) bypass grafts. The grafts that were modified at operation because of duplex scanning results were 2 times more likely to require postoperative revision than grafts with normal intraoperative scans.

Conclusions.—All 4 grafting techniques used for infrainguinal lower-limb revascularization were successful in achieving long-term patency. Although strictures developed with all 4 graft types, the need for revision varied with bypass grafting technique. Reversed vein bypasses and grafts modified at operation require more surveillance for the development of stenosis.

► As expected, the risk of subsequent vein graft stenosis appears to be directly related to the quality of vein used for the infrainguinal bypass. Early and intermediate bypass graft failure is lowest when in situ bypass is done with a good vein (normal hemodynamics by intraoperative duplex) and increases when intraoperative revision or use of spliced or alternative venous conduit is required. Additionally, valve lysis may decrease the risk of long-term graft failure even in reversed saphenous veins, likely a controversial observation. Regardless, these results suggest that it may be possible to tailor duplex vein graft surveillance protocols to individual patients, thereby reducing costs of surveillance without sacrificing optimal graft patency.

J.M. Seeger, M.D.

Long-term Outcome After Early Infrainguinal Graft Failure

Robinson KD, Sato DT, Gregory RT, et al (Eastern Virginia Med School, Norfolk)

J Vasc Surg 26:425–438, 1997 13–15

Background.—In an effort to avoid lower extremity amputation, increasing numbers of patients with recurrent limb ischemia are offered further attempts at revascularization after failure of previous ipsilateral bypass grafts. In some cases, however, aggressive management is unsuccessful, and the patient ultimately loses the limb after undergoing additional operative risk. The long-term outcome and prognostic factors after early (less than 30 days) infrainguinal graft failure were studied retrospectively.

Methods.—During the period of review (January 1985 through October 1995), 112 new infrainguinal bypass grafts in 102 patients occluded within 30 days of operation. Indications for surgery were ischemic rest pain (44%), tissue loss (31%), severe lifestyle-limiting claudication, and acute ischemia with rest pain (6%). In 43% of cases, the index procedure was a repeat leg bypass. Patient records were reviewed for limb salvage data, patency, and prognostic risk factors.

Results.—Most of the 112 early graft failures occurred within the first 24 hours after surgery. No further attempts at revascularization were undertaken in 9 lower extremities, 7 of which were amputated within the next month. In the 103 takeback procedures, limb salvage rates were better for patients who underwent surgery for claudication than for those with rest pain or tissue loss. For all takebacks, secondary patency rates were 70% at 1 month but only 37% at 1 year. Patients with claudication were excluded from limb salvage analysis, which left 84 threatened limbs. Life table analysis of the latter group yielded limb salvage rates of 74% at 1 month, 54% at 1 year, 40% at 3 years, and 31% at 5 years. Rates of limb salvage and graft patency were significantly lower for patients given anticoagulant therapy after the index procedure and for those who had undergone previous ipsilateral leg revascularization. Patients with a single-vessel runoff had a significantly lower limb salvage rate than those with multiple-vessel runoff. The secondary patency rate was better after thrombectomy and revision or complete graft replacement than after thrombectomy alone. Neither limb salvage nor graft patency rates were influenced by age; sex; previous inflow surgery; diabetes; hypertension; smoking; the presence of cardiac, renal, or pulmonary disease; or undergoing femoropopliteal vs. femorotibial–femoropedal bypass grafting.

Conclusion.—Although long-term rates of limb salvage and graft patency are poor for patients who have undergone takeback revascularization procedures after early graft failure, a single takeback procedure appears warranted in such cases. Multiple takebacks, however, are not generally advisable.

▶ Although the outcome after takeback procedures for early graft thrombosis is poor, it is clearly better than not attempting to salvage the graft. I would agree with the authors that a single take back procedure is justified after early graft failure because identification and correction of a technical defect (including poor decisions regarding the adequacy of the conduit or the distal anastomotic site) can lead to long-term graft patency and limb salvage in some patients. On the other hand, every effort should be made to ensure the initial technical adequacy of the bypass so that the need for takeback procedures is limited.

J.M. Seeger, M.D.

Dialysis Access

Prophylactic Balloon Angioplasty Fails to Prolong the Patency of Expanded Polytetrafluoroethylene Arteriovenous Grafts: Results of a Prospective Randomized Study

Lumsden AB, MacDonald MJ, Kikeri D, et al (Emory Univ, Atlanta, Ga)

J Vasc Surg 26:382–392, 1997 13–16

Background.—The number of individuals in the United States who depend on hemodialysis is growing at about 10% per year. The maintenance of hemodialysis access grafts is an immense social and clinical problem. Because current grafts and graft salvage techniques are inadequate, there has been much interest in minimally invasive, prophylactic catheter techniques for treating stenoses in functioning arteriovenous grafts. Prophylactic balloon angioplasty has been suggested as a means of prolonging assisted primary graft patency.

Methods.—In a prospective, randomized trial, the results in 32 patients who had percutaneous transluminal angioplasty for graft stenoses greater than 50% were compared with results in 32 control patients who had no intervention. Stenoses greater than 50% in functioning, expanded polytetrafluoroethylene grafts were detected by color flow duplex scanning. After confirmatory angiographic examination, patients with angiographic stenoses greater than 50% were randomly assigned to balloon angioplasty or observation. Duplex scanning was performed every 2 months. Outcome measures were graft thrombosis, graft dysfunction that prevented dialysis, and 6 or more percutaneous transluminal angioplasty procedures in 18 months.

Results.—The patient groups were well matched demographically, but patients in the treatment group had more previous interventions and concurrent central stenoses. The 6-month patency rates were 69% in the treatment group and 70% in the observation group. The 12-month patency rates were 51% in the treatment group and 47% in the observation group. There were no significant differences between groups. There was an 80% confidence limit for detection of a difference greater than 20%.

Discussion.—It is possible that the greater number of patients in the treatment group who had had previous intervention adversely affected the outcome. However, these findings indicate that a generic approach of percutaneous transluminal angioplasty for all polytetrafluoroethylene grafts with stenoses greater than 50% does not prolong patency. Therefore, such an approach is not supported.

► Management of failed or failing dialysis access bridge grafts remains a significant problem. It has been suggested that prophylactic balloon angioplasty (PTA) will prolong the patency of prosthetic dialysis access grafts. It has also been suggested that results of endovascular management of failed access grafts are equivalent to results of surgical repair. This nicely done prospective randomized trial shows both of these suggestions to be incorrect. Little value was seen for prophylactic PTA in the treatment of stenoses at the venous anastamosis, and surgical management of failed access grafts was found to result in improved access graft patency compared to endovascular management. Considering results of balloon angioplasty in the treatment of stenosis in lower-extremity venous bypass grafts, these findings are not surprising.

J.M. Seeger, M.D.

Prospective Randomized Comparison of Surgical Versus Endovascular Management of Thrombosed Dialysis Access Grafts

Marston WA, Criado E, Jaques PF, et al (Univ of North Carolina, Chapel Hill)
J Vasc Surg 26:373–381, 1997 13–17

Introduction.—The increasing number of patients receiving long-term dialysis has made preservation of thrombosed hemodialysis shunts a more frequently encountered problem. Salvage of the thrombosed shunt can be accomplished by surgical or endovascular means. The efficacy of these 2 methods was compared in a prospective randomized trial.

Methods.—The 91 patients included in the trial had 115 episodes of polytetrafluoroethylene shunt thrombosis. All shunts were evaluated within 1 week of thrombosis and treated within 48 hours of diagnosis.

Endovascular salvage was performed in 59 episodes of shunt thrombosis and surgical salvage in 56. The 2 randomized groups were similar in age, sex, and clinical characteristics. Restoration of graft function in the endovascular group was attempted with mechanical (82%) or thrombolytic (18%) graft thrombectomy followed by percutaneous angioplasty. Surgical salvage was attempted with thrombectomy plus graft revision in 78% of shunts and with thrombectomy alone in 22%. Patients were followed up for at least 6 months to compare shunt patency and length of graft function achieved with the 2 methods.

Results.—The initial success rate in restoring graft function was 82% in grafts treated surgically and 71% in those treated with endovascular techniques. In the months after salvage, surgery achieved a significantly better primary graft patency than endovascular therapy. At 12 months, 25% of grafts managed surgically remained patent, but only 9% of grafts undergoing endovascular treatment remained patent. Patients with venous anastomotic stenosis, had a significantly better patency rate than those with other causes of graft thrombosis. While patients with long-segment venous outflow stenosis or occlusion has significantly worse patency rates.

Conclusions.—The primary patency rate after thrombosed access graft salvage is significantly better with surgical treatment than with endovascular treatment. However, patency is low at 6 and 12 months after the salvage procedures, regardless of the type of treatment.

► Management of failed or failing dialysis access bridge grafts remains a significant problem. It has been suggested that prophylactic balloon angioplasty (PTA) will prolong the patency of prosthetic dialysis access grafts, and that results of endovascular management of failed access grafts are equivalent to results of surgical repair. These 2, nicely done, prospective randomized trials show both of these suggestions to be incorrect. Little value was seen for prophylactic PTA in the treatment of stenoses at the venous anastamosis prior to graft failure, and surgical management of failed access grafts was found to result in improved secondary access graft patency compared with endovascular management. Considering results of balloon angioplasty in the treatment of stenosis in lower extremity venous bypass grafts, these findings are not surprising.

J.M. Seeger, M.D.

Distal Revascularization–Interval Ligation for Limb Salvage and Maintenance of Dialysis Access in Ischemic Steal Syndrome

Berman SS, Gentile AT, Glickman MH, et al (Univ of Arizona, Tucson; Virginia Vascular Associates, Norfolk)

J Vasc Surg 26:393–404, 1997 13–18

Background.—About 150,000 patients in the United States are currently treated by renal replacement and hemodialysis. Maintenance of vascular access grafts and fistulas and resulting complications in this population are very costly. Ischemic steal syndrome related to a functioning dialysis access graft or fistula is traditionally treated by banding or ligation, although these methods result in inconsistent limb salvage, loss of a functional access, or both. The authors describe their experience with the distal revascularization–interval ligation (DRIL) procedure as an alternate method of limb revascularization that eliminates steal while maintaining continuous dialysis access.

Methods.—The medical records of 21 patients who underwent the DRIL procedure for severe limb ischemia related to a functioning arteriovenous access site were reviewed. Patients underwent color flow duplex scanning, digital photoplethysmography, and arteriography. Arterial ligation distal to the arteriovenous fistula origin eliminated the steal physiologic mechanism, and arterial bypass grafting from above to below the arteriovenous fistula revascularized the extremity.

Results.—Of the 21 patients, 11 had chronic ischemia with rest pain, paresthesia, or ulcerations related to 9 native fistulas and 2 prosthetic bridge grafts. Acute ischemia was seen in 10 patients related to 3 native fistulas and 7 prosthetic bridge grafts. The DRIL procedure was used in all 21 patients. Three patients were treated for ischemia at the time of arteriovenous fistula construction. Of the 21 bypass procedures, 19 were performed with autogenous vein; there were 9 brachial-brachial procedures, 3 brachial-radial, 2 radial-radial, 2 brachial-ulnar, 1 popliteal-popliteal, 1 femoral-popliteal, and 1 femoral-peroneal. Polytetrafluoroethylene grafts were used in 1 external iliac-popliteal and 1 axillary-brachial bypass graft. At 18 months, life-table analysis showed a patency rate/limb salvage rate of 100% and an access site patency rate of 94% for the DRIL procedures.

Discussion.—The results in these patients show that the DRIL procedure can restore antegrade flow to an ischemic limb, eliminate the potential pathway for the steal physiologic mechanism, and maintain continuous dialysis access. Although the DRIL procedure is given little attention in most vascular textbooks that discuss complications of arteriovenous access, it is recommended to all access surgeons as the first choice for treating steal syndrome related to a functioning arteriovenous access. None of the alternate methods for managing steal have achieved the consistent results of the DRIL technique in salvaging a viable extremity and functional arteriovenous access site.

▶ This technique for managing this difficult problem is one that we have used successfully.

J.M. Seeger, M.D.

Preoperative Vancomycin Prophylaxis Decreases Incidence of Postoperative Hemodialysis Vascular Access Infections

Zibari GB, Gadallah MF, Landreneau M, et al (Louisana State Univ, Shreveport; Univ of Florida, Jacksonville)

Am J Kidney Dis 30:343–348, 1997 13–19

Introduction.—Infection of newly placed or revised vascular access bridge grafts is hard to treat, and is one of the common causes of vascular access failure. Vancomycin prophylaxis is recommended by many investigators to reduce the incidence of polytetrafluoroethylene (PTFE) graft infection, but there are no known trials assessing the effectiveness of this practice. Preoperative vancomycin prophylaxis was evaluated in a prospective, randomized trial to determine whether it reduces the incidence of postoperative graft infection.

Methods.—Two hundred six patients who underwent 408 permanent vascular access procedures were randomly assigned during a 5-year period to either group 1 (206 procedures), a single IV dose of 750 mg of vancomycin about 6–12 hours before graft placement, or group 2 (202 procedures), no vancomycin. Patients were evaluated for access infection within 30 days of access placement and before access use for chronic dialysis.

Results.—Operative procedures included 219 primary procedures (55 native fistulas and 164 PTFE grafts) and 189 secondary procedures (161 thromboses and 28 revisions). Nine patients underwent a lower extremity Gore-Tex graft as a primary vascular procedure. Two group 1 patients (1%) and 12 group 2 patients (6%) had access infections ($p = 0.006$). All 14 infections happened in upper extremity PTFE grafts.

Conclusion.—With the increasing use of prosthetic rather than natural grafts for vascular access for hemodialysis, the rate of access infections and the subsequent loss of access sites are rising. The use of preoperative single-dose IV vancomycin prophylaxis is a simple, cost-effective approach to decreasing the rate of postoperative access infections. Vancomycin prophylaxis may not be justified in native fistulas because of their low infection rate.

► Postoperative hemodialysis access graft infection remains a significant problem. This well-done study demonstrates that a single dose of vancomycin will significantly reduce the incidence of postoperative infection. Although use of vancomycin in this manner may increase the risk vancomycin-resistant enteroccus of infection, this risk appears small and use of prophylactic vancomycin during access graft placement appears justified.

J.M. Seeger, M.D.

Venous Disease

Endoscopic Versus Open Subfascial Division of Incompetent Perforating Veins in the Treatment of Venous Leg Ulceration: A Randomized Trial

Pierik EGJM, van Urk H, Hop WCJ, et al (Hosp de Weezenlanden, Zwolle, The Netherlands; Univ Hosp Rotterdam-Dijkzigt, The Netherlands; Erasmus Univ Rotterdam, The Netherlands; et al)
J Vasc Surg 26:1049–1054, 1997 13–20

Introduction.—Venous ulceration is a common cause of serious disability. Most venous ulcers respond to conservative treatment, but recurrent ulceration is typical. Subfascial division of incompetent perforating veins can provide good long-term results, but the surgery involves long incisions through compromised cutaneous and subcutaneous layers. Postoperative wound complications are common. Endoscopic approaches have been developed that allow subfascial endoscopic interruption of incompetent perforating veins. No comparative trials have been performed between open and endoscopic subfascial explorations for perforator ligation. This comparison was accomplished in a prospective, randomized trial evaluating ulcer healing and postoperative wound complications in a cohort of patients with chronic lower leg venous ulceration.

Methods.—Of 39 patients with venous ulceration on the medial side of the lower leg, 20 were randomly assigned to endoscopic perforator ligation by use of a mediastinoscope and 19 to open perforator ligation by the modified Linton approach.

Results.—The incidence of wound infections was 53% after open perforator ligation and 0% after the endoscopic approach. Mean length of hospital stay was significantly longer for open than endoscopic procedures (7 and 4 days, respectively). At postoperative month 4, ulcers were healed in 17 patients each in the open and endoscopic groups. At a mean follow-up of 21 months, no patients in either group had recurrent ulcerations.

Conclusion.—Endoscopic and open subfascial division of incompetent perforating veins are similarly effective in the treatment of venous ulceration of the lower leg. Significantly fewer wound complications were observed in the endoscopic than in the open procedure group. Endoscopic perforator ligation is the recommended method.

Efficacy of Subfascial Endoscopy in Eradicating Perforating Veins of the Lower Leg and Its Relation With Venous Ulcer Healing

Pierik EGJM, van Urk H, Wittens CHA (Univ Hosp Rotterdam-Dijkzigt, The Netherlands)

J Vasc Surg 26:255–259, 1997 13–21

Background.—Early reports of subfascial endoscopic ligation of perforating veins in patients with venous ulceration indicate good clinical outcome in terms of newly formed varicosities, ulcer healing, and wound complications. In some cases, however, ulcers failed to heal or ulceration recurred after endoscopic treatment of incompetent perforating veins. The efficacy of subfascial endoscopy in eradicating perforating veins and the relationship between persistent incompetent perforating veins and problems with ulcer healing was prospectively determined.

Methods.—Study participants were all consecutive patients with lower leg venous ulceration who underwent subfascial endoscopic treatment of perforating veins during a 14-month period. All had class 6 chronic venous insufficiency; none had an arterial component to their ulceration. The patients underwent duplex US scans of the lower leg before and 6 weeks after operation. Findings during subfascial endoscopic perforator ligation, performed with a mediastinoscope and clipping instrument, were compared with the number and localization of the perforating veins on the mediodorsal side of the lower leg identified by venous duplex examination.

Results.—Patients were 11 men and 9 women with a mean age of 64 years. Preoperative duplex scanning identified 46 incompetent perforating veins (mean 2.3 per patient) on the mediodorsal side of the lower leg. Six competent perforating veins were found in 5 patients. A total of 54 perforating veins were identified and clipped during subfascial endoscopy. The site of 43 incompetent and all 6 competent perforating veins were confirmed during operation; 5 additional perforating veins found in 4 patients had not been visualized at preoperative duplex US. Postoperative duplex US scans identified 6 incompetent perforating veins in 4 patients, and the ulcers in 3 of these patients did not heal. All ulcers healed in the remaining 17 patients.

Conclusions.—Endoscopic subfascial division of perforating veins was confirmed to be an effective and safe procedure in the treatment of patients with venous ulceration of the lower leg. All existing perforating veins were identified and divided in 17 of 20 patients in this series. The failure of ulcers to heal after operation appears to be related to the persistence of incompetent perforating veins.

► These 2 papers (Abstracts 13–20 and 13–21)—reviewing the same group of patients—demonstrate the efficacy of endoscopic subfascial ligation of perforating veins in patients with venous ulceration. However, patients in these studies were also treated with external compression, which is equally efficacious in achieving ulcer healing. Furthermore, follow-up was for only 12 months. Now that a technique for perforator ligation associated with minimal morbidity is available, it is time to compare external compression, with and without perforation ligation, to finally determine whether perforator interruption is important in the treatment of venous ulceration.

J.M. Seeger, M.D.

Early Outcome After Isolated Calf Vein Thrombosis

Meissner MH, Caps MT, Bergelin RO, et al (Univ of Washington, Seattle)
J Vasc Surg 26:749–756, 1997 13–22

Introduction.—Patients with isolated calf vein thrombosis (CVT) are thought to have a substantially lower risk of pulmonary embolism than those with proximal deep vein thrombosis (DVT), but the optimal management of CVT remains controversial. A series of patients with acute DVT was followed up to define the natural history of CVT, with emphasis on symptoms, propagation, recanalization, and the development of valvular incompetence.

Methods.—From December 1986 to July 1996, 499 patients with acute DVT were referred as candidates for the study. In 58 patients (12%), thrombosis was confined to the calf veins of at least 1 extremity. Study participants numbered 268 patients, including 29 with an isolated CVT who underwent clinical and duplex US examinations of the lower extremities at 1 and 7 days, 1, 3, 6, 9, and 12 months, and yearly thereafter.

Results.—Median follow-up was 163 days for patients with isolated CVT and 240 days for those with proximal DVT. Thirty-five (70%) of the 50 extremities with CVT available for analysis were symptomatic (pain in 30 and edema in 21) before treatment. The prevalence of symptoms decreased to 33% at 2 weeks, but 23% continued to be symptomatic at 1 year. Although only 9% of uninvolved extremities contralateral to a CVT remained symptomatic at 1 year, the prevalence of symptoms in extremities with proximal DVT was 54%. Recanalization in CVT limbs reduced the mean thrombus load by 50% at 1 month and to zero at 1 year. Valvular incompetence progressively increased, however, and 24% of extremities with CVT had reflux at 1 year. Propagation to a more proximal level in the same extremity occurred in 4 limbs (13%) with isolated CVT. Pulmonary embolism was diagnosed initially in 11% and during follow-up in 3% of patients.

Conclusions.—The long-term prognosis after isolated CVT does not appear to be entirely benign. Approximately 25% of limbs will remain symptomatic after 1 year, and PE does develop in some patients. Anticoagulation therapy may minimize the development of postthrombotic syndrome.

► Conventional knowledge suggests that isolated CVT is not clinically significant because it is uncommonly associated with pulmonary emboli and postphlebitic syndrome. This carefully done natural history demonstrates otherwise. Furthermore, although the role of anticoagulation in reducing the sequelae of isolated CVT was not specifically addressed, these results certainly suggest that anticoagulation therapy is appropriate, particularly now that outpatient treatment with low–molecular weight heparin is possible.

J.M. Seeger, M.D.

Miscellaneous

Routine Pulmonary Artery Catheterization Does Not Reduce Morbidity and Mortality of Elective Vascular Surgery: Results of a Prospective, Randomized Trial

Bender JS, Smith-Meek MA, Jones CE (Johns Hopkins Univ, Baltimore, Md)

Ann Surg 226:229–237, 1997 13–23

Background.—Although the pulmonary artery catheter is used commonly in patients who are critically ill or undergoing major elective surgery, there are few prospective, randomized studies of the value of the pulmonary artery catheter under such conditions. The effect of preoperative placement of a pulmonary artery catheter with optimization of hemodynamic results on outcome after elective vascular surgery was determined.

Methods.—In a tightly controlled, prospective, randomized trial, 104 consecutive patients were randomly assigned to 1 of 2 groups. Group I had placement of a pulmonary artery catheter on the morning of operation and group II had placement of the catheter only if clinically indicated. In group I, patients were resuscitated to pre-established end points and kept at these points before, during, and after operation. Patients in group II were given standard care.

Results.—One patient in each group died. In group I, 13 patients had intraoperative or postoperative complications. In group II, 7 patients had intraoperative or postoperative complications. More fluid was given to patients in group I than in group II. Overall length of stay in the ICU was similar in both groups. A postoperative pulmonary artery catheter was needed only in 1 patient in group II.

Discussion.—These results indicate that routine use of a pulmonary artery catheter in patients undergoing elective vascular surgery increases the volume of fluid used but does not significantly improve morbidity or mortality or reduce length of stay or cost. Routine use of the pulmonary artery catheter should be limited to specific clinical situations.

▶ Several recent large studies have documented relatively low cardiac complication rates after aortic surgery and shown that routine extensive preoperative cardiac evaluation is unnecessary to achieve these results. This paper demonstrates that routine use of pulmonary artery catheters does not improve morbidity or mortality after elective vascular surgery. Standardized surgical and anesthetic care and the liberal use of β-blockers and prophylactic nitroglycerine may have influenced these results. However, it continues to be shown that good results can be achieved with appropriate care rather than "do everything" care.

J.M. Seeger, M.D.

Is Coronary Angiography Necessary for Vascular Surgery Patients Who Have Positive Results of Dipyridamole Thallium Scans?

Massie MT, Rohrer MJ, Leppo JA, et al (Univ of Massachusetts, Worcester)
J Vasc Surg 25:975–983, 1997 13–24

Background.—The decision to perform further invasive cardiac evaluation and to consider coronary revascularization procedures before peripheral vascular surgery is often based on positive results of a dipyridamole thallium scan. It is generally believed that treatment of anatomically significant coronary artery disease lowers the risk associated with later vascular operation. However, the benefits of aggressive diagnostic and therapeutic cardiac procedures in such patients have not been determined.

Methods.—Dipyridamole thallium scanning was performed in 934 patients scheduled for peripheral vascular surgery to help evaluate operative risk. In 297 patients, ischemic responses were noted. Ischemic responses were defined as 2 or more segments of redistribution. The medical records of 70 of the 297 patients who had coronary angiography were reviewed. Data were compared with data from 70 control subjects who did not have further cardiac evaluation but who were otherwise matched for age, gender, peripheral vascular operation, and number of segments of redistribution on dipyridamole thallium scans.

Results.—Of the 297 patients, 70 had cardiac catheterization and 25 had coronary revascularization procedures. An adverse outcome occurred in 46% of patients who had coronary angiography and 44% of control subjects. Fewer cardiac events with later vascular operations were seen in patients who had coronary angiography and who were considered for myocardial revascularization than in control subjects. Potential benefits from invasive cardiac evaluation were offset by 3 deaths and 2 myocardial infarctions that complicated the cardiac evaluation and treatment. No significant differences were seen between patients who had angiography and control subjects in perioperative nonfatal myocardial infarction, fatal myocardial infarction, late nonfatal myocardial infarction, or late cardiac death. Long-term follow-up showed that myocardial infarctions occurred later in patients who had coronary angiography than in control subjects, but this difference was not associated with improved overall survival.

Discussion.—Extensive cardiac evaluation and treatment did not improve perioperative or long-term survival in patients undergoing vascular surgical procedures. For most patients considered for vascular surgery with positive dipyridamole thallium scan results, coronary angiography does not provide additional useful information.

▶ The data demonstrating the *limited* value of extensive preoperative cardiac evaluation in patients undergoing peripheral vascular surgery procedures continues to accumulate. This study demonstrates that when the morbidity and mortality of the subsequent coronary artery bypass procedure is included, patients with a positive thallium study undergoing coronary angiography and coronary revascularization as indicated before to a vascular surgical procedure were no less likely to suffer a perioperative myocardial infarction or cardiac death than those with positive thallium studies who simply proceeded to the vascular reconstruction. In addition, only 1 patient of 70 undergoing coronary angiography had a lesion amenable to treatment using coronary angiography (another commonly used argument for such preoperative cardiac evaluation). Routine, extensive cardiac evaluation before vascular surgical procedures clearly cannot be justified and such evaluations should be limited to patients whose symptoms justify coronary revascularization apart from their need for peripheral vascular reconstructions.

J.M. Seeger, M.D.

Intraoperative Autologous Transfusion During Elective Infrarenal Aortic Reconstruction

Huber TS, Carlton LC, Irwin PB, et al (Univ of Florida, Gainesville; Gainesville VA Med Ctr, Fla)

J Surg Res 67:14–20, 1997 13–25

Background.—It is believed that intraoperative autologous transfusion (IOAT) devices may decrease the need for allogenic transfusion during major surgical procedures. The value of IOAT during cardiovascular surgeries, however, is controversial. Previous nonrandomized studies have found that IOAT is a clinically beneficial and cost-effective technique for maintaining blood volume; however, others have reported that the IOAT is not cost-effective during aortobifemoral bypass. Further, the decreased incidence of transfusion-related infectious disease transmission in recent years has lessened the need for avoidance of allogenic transfusion. The efficacy of IOAT, using the Haemonetics Cell Saver (CS) as a routine procedure during infrarenal aortic reconstruction was evaluated, and predictors of cost-efficient and/or clinically significant salvage volumes were determined.

Methods.—Medical records of patients undergoing elective infrarenal aortic reconstruction, with the use of CS, at a single hospital from 1991 to 1995 were reviewed. Blood loss, transfusion products used, CS return, cost of CS return, and predictors of cost efficient (1,250 mL or greater) and/or clinically significant (500 mL or greater) CS return were determined.

Results.—Mean blood loss during the procedure was 1,737 mL, of which a mean of 702 mL (43%) was salvaged by CS. The volume of blood salvaged by CS was considered clinically significant or cost efficient in 64.6% and 16% of cases, respectively. Blood loss and recovery were both greater in patients with aneurysms than in those with occlusive disease. In patients with aneurysms, increased aneurysm size and male gender were predictive of clinically significant blood salvage by CS. In patients with occlusive disease, low platelet count, extended operative time, and revascularization of a renal artery as an additional procedure predicted clinically significant blood return. Predictors of cost-efficient blood return by CS were present only for aneurysm repair and included performance of an additional vascular procedure, and the requirement for clamping of the suprarenal aorta. Allogenic packed red blood cells were administered to 73.8% of patients despite the use of CS, with a mean of 3.0 units required. The mean cost of blood salvage by CS added to the cost of the required additional allogenic packed red blood cells was $699.00 and $680.22 for patients with occlusive and aneurysmal disease, respectively, compared with the $346.16 and $427.42, respectively, which would have been the cost if allogenic transfusion had been the sole source of blood.

Conclusions.—Although the volume of blood salvaged by CS during elective reconstruction of the aorta is clinically significant in most cases, it is not cost efficient. The use of CS may be indicated in complex aortic reconstructions; however, routine CS use in elective reconstructions of the aorta should be discontinued.

▶ This study done at my institution has taught me 2 things. First, although blood loss during elective infrarenal aortic reconstruction is variable and somewhat unpredictable, on average the amount of blood that is salvaged by routine use of an IOAT device during such procedures is low. Second, the use of IOAT devices is expensive, particularly when compared with the cost of allogenic transfusion, even when the costs associated with long-term complications of allogenic blood transfusion are included. Based on these observations, we no longer routinely use IOAT. Rather, when concerned about the potential of blood loss during elective infrarenal aortic reconstruction, we connect the IOAT canister (cost ~$35.00) to the regular wall suction and use the entire IOAT system only if enough blood is salvaged to make return clinically valuable.

J.M. Seeger, M.D.

Nicotine and Cotinine Stimulate Secretion of Basic Fibroblast Growth Factor and Affect Expression of Matrix Metalloproteinases in Cultured Human Smooth Muscle Cells

Carty CS, Soloway PD, Kayastha S, et al (State Univ of New York, Buffalo; Roswell Park Mem Inst, Buffalo, NY)

J Vasc Surg 24:927–935, 1996 13–26

Introduction.—Both clinical and experimental studies suggest that cigarette smoking promotes the development of intimal hyperplasia, atherosclerosis, and aneurysms. Because nicotine and its metabolite, cotinine, were recently found to promote proliferation of human smooth muscle cells (SMCs) in vitro, researchers hypothesized that these chemicals may increase production of cytokines and affect the expression of matrix metalloproteinases (MMPs) in SMCs in vitro.

Methods.—The experiments used SMCs that were harvested from human arteries and grown in culture. After SMCs were grown to subconfluency, cultures were incubated in M199, which contains 0.1% fetal bovine serum, with or without nicotine or cotinine at various concentrations. Supernatants and cell lysates were then assayed by enzyme-linked immunosorbent assay for basic fibroblast growth factor (bFGF), tumor necrosis factor alpha (TNF-α), platelet-derived growth factor AB (PDGF-AB), and transforming growth factor beta (TGF-β). Expression of MMP was determined in subconfluent cultures incubated with albumin, with or without nicotine or cotinine, at 10^{-8}mol/L and 10^{-7}mol/L for 6, 12, 18, 24, and 36 hours. Northern blot analyses were conducted with human cDNA probes for collagenase-1, stromelysin-1, gelatinase A, gelatinase B, and triose phosphate isomerase. Phosphor-imaging techniques were used for quantitation of blots.

Results.—The production and secretion of bFGF was promoted in a dose-dependent manner by both nicotine and cotinine. The 2 chemicals did not significantly affect PDGF, TNF-α, and TNF-β secretions. Collagenase was up-regulated by both nicotine (4.5-fold at 18 hours and 5.8-fold at 24 hours) and cotinine (from 5.0-fold to 29-fold at 18 hours). Stromelysin-1 was up-regulated by the 2 agents at 12 and 18 hours (from 1.5-fold to 7.0-fold). Both nicotine and cotinine also up-regulated gelatinase A (from 2.0-fold to 6.5-fold), and a peak usually occurred at 12 hours.

Discussion.—Cigarette smoke, which contains a complex mixture of several thousand chemicals, may lead to injury of the vessel wall. Because nicotine and cotinine are potent regulators of bFGF and MMP synthesis in human vascular SMCs, cigarette smoking may play an important role in aneurysmal formation and in the development of restenosis after vascular reconstruction. It is possible that the nicotine products designed to aid in smoking cessation may result in comparable nicotine and cotinine serum concentrations, thus adversely affecting the cardiovascular system.

▶ This study demonstrates that nicotine and cotinine (a metabolite of nicotine) stimulate SMCs in vitro to release growth factors and MMPs that are involved in the development of intimal hyperplasia. Should further work confirm similar effects of nicotine and its breakdown products in vivo, the role of cigarette smoke in progressive atherosclerosis and revascularization failure would be clearer. Additionally, the safety of nicotine patches used for smoking prevention would be seriously questioned.

J.M. Seeger, M.D.

14 Noncardiac Thoracic Surgery

Introduction

The field of general thoracic surgery continues to undergo a renaissance. New developments in the field of minimally invasive thoracic surgery and lung volume reduction surgery (LVRS) continue to fuel major new understandings of pulmonary physiology and pathology. General thoracic surgery continues to advance on a variety of fronts, as oncologic therapies begin to include multidisciplinary approaches, bringing surgery into a variety of settings where it once had been a stranger.

A review of this year's literature shows significant signs of the vibrancy of the field of thoracic surgery, as I hope the reader will see in the abstracts and commentaries that follow. This overview is divided into four sections. The first covers LVRS and the challenges that accompany this potentially revolutionary procedure. The second section presents an update of the role of thoracic surgery in the treatment of non–small-cell lung cancer (NSCLC), which is a major focus of this review. The third section examines results of clinical studies in mesothelioma. Lastly, in the fourth section, some interesting large clinical series and therapeutic reports are included to keep the reader abreast of the latest developments in a variety of areas of oncologic thoracic surgery.

A highlight of the section is the reintroduction of LVRS as a treatment for emphysema that followed the initial studies done by Dr. Otto Brannigan. With the renewed interest in volume reduction surgery over the last 4 years, several centers have been proposing a variety of different approaches, from the standpoints of the surgical technique used and the patients to be selected for this procedure. The results from centers around the country have varied greatly in terms of morbidity, and therapeutic benefits, leading to a number of questions on the part of third-party payers. In particular, the Health Care Financing Authority (HCFA), with its large Medicare population, has asked: Can LVRS, as a new therapeutic tool for emphysema, be given the stamp of approval as a safe and efficacious procedure applicable to a large number of patients? In 1996, the HCFA in a historic collaboration with the National Institutes of Health (specifically, the National Lung and Blood Institute), developed a call for applications from centers of excellence in the field of volume reduction surgery to pilot an important trial to compare volume reduction surgery to the results of medical care and pulmonary rehabilitation alone.

Eighteen centers were selected in 1996 and 1997, and they have been meeting on a regular basis to develop this phase III randomized trial. For the first time, a surgical procedure, as well as new pharmacologic agents, will be studied in a prospective way to determine efficacy. In particular, it will be examined in the light of its prospectively determined morbidity and mortality. It is important for thoracic surgeons to understand the importance of the commitment on the part of the HCFA to provide the clinical reimbursements that cover the clinical care required for this historic trial. The commitment could set the stage for the evaluation of other innovative surgical procedures to be funded through similar mechanisms.

When the HCFA reviewed the reports from the 18 centers, which had been selected based on their clinical excellence, the range of perioperative mortality was found to be quite broad. In addition, length of hospital stay and efficacy measurements also demonstrated a wide range. It appeared that the data from the 18 centers confirmed the need for uniform selection criteria, a uniform surgical procedure, and a prospective determination of the efficacy and safety of this potentially revolutionary technique.

The following questions came out of the initial review of the literature from the steering committee of the National Emphysema Treatment (NET) Trial: Which patients would benefit most from this procedure? (Most reports showed approximately 20% to 25% of patients who underwent the procedure received no therapeutic benefit.) What is the best surgical approach to this procedure, including new minimally invasive thoracoscopic techniques being evaluated alongside standard median sternotomy as the preferred approach? Importantly, what is the durability of this procedure? How long does the procedure contribute a therapeutic benefit to patients with emphysema? What are the long-term effects of this procedure in terms of possible comorbidities, including cardiac disease or subsequent pulmonary disorders? And, specifically, how can we best predict which patients would receive the most benefit from this approach based on the topography of their disease, and what radiographic method would be best suited to determine and select patients for operative intervention?

The NET Trial represents a historic achievement on the part of the surgical community, the National Institutes of Health, and the HCFA. We look forward to the successful completion of this trial and will evaluate the following reports in the light of the important questions that have been raised by the initial review of the NET steering committee.

We wish the reader well in undertaking a review of this year's thoracic surgery literature and hope that this endeavor will continue to keep him or her stimulated and interested in this exciting field of surgery.

David J. Sugarbaker, M.D.

Lung Volume Reduction Surgery

Perfusion Scintigraphy in the Evaluation for Lung Volume Reduction Surgery: Correlation With Clinical Outcome

Wang SC, Fischer KC, Slone RM, et al (Washington Univ, St Louis)

Radiology 205:243–248, 1997 14–1

Objective.—Lung volume reduction surgery has evolved as a palliative treatment for emphysema. Yet some of these patients have a poor outcome or die after surgery. Preoperative perfusion scans in patients who underwent lung volume reduction surgery to identify scintigraphic markers associated with outcome were retrospectively evaluated.

Methods.—Ventilation-perfusion scintigraphic findings in 103 patients (47 women), aged 41 to 76, were evaluated for emphysematous heterogeneity, extent of maximally perfused lung, and lobar predominance, by readers blinded to patient identity and clinical outcome, and compared with outcome. Patients were followed for a minimum of 6 months.

Results.—During follow-up 7 patients died, 6 of respiratory failure. At 6 months, forced expiratory volume in 1 second had improved by 47%, 6-minute walking distance by 20%, and arterial oxygen-tension while breathing room improved by 20%. Outcome measures that correlated most strongly with scintigraphic measures were forced expiratory volume, artrial oxygen tension, and 6-minute walking distance (Fig 5). Surviving

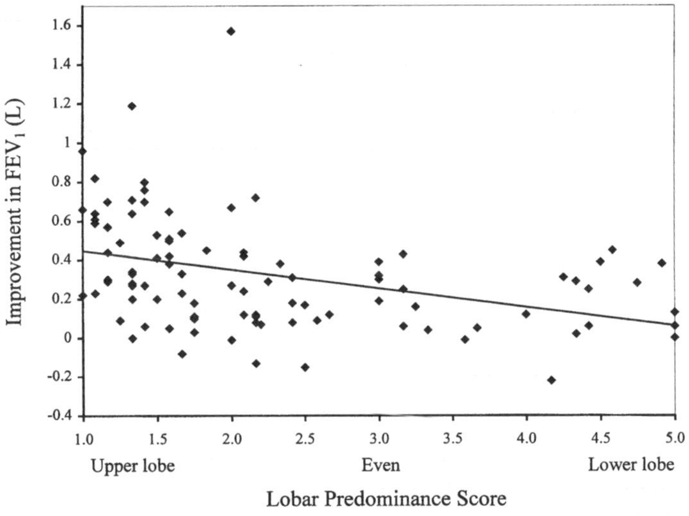

FIGURE 5.—Scatter plot of improvement in FEV_1 as a function of lobar predominance of emphysema. A low score represents predominantly upper-lobe emphysema and a high score represents predominantly lower-lobe emphysema. The best-fit line is illustrated ($r = -0.38$). *Abbreviation: FEV_1*, forced expiratory volume in 1 second. (Courtesy of Wang SC, Fischer KC, Slone RM, et al: Perfusion scintigraphy in the evaluation for lung volume reduction surgery: Correlation with clinical outcome. *Radiology* 205:243–248, 1997. Radiological Society of North America.)

patients had a significantly higher maximal perfusion than those who died (34% vs. 25%).

Conclusion.—Perfusion scintigraphy can provide additional prognostic information about outcome after lung volume reduction surgery.

▶ The authors have put forth an interesting and relatively well-known theory on the use of perfusion scintigraphy for evaluation of patients who are to undergo potential lung volume reduction surgery (LVRS). The description of the use of perfusion scintigraphy is an interesting physiologic correlate to the lack of aeration and perfusion of the upper zones of both lungs in patients suffering from emphysema. It is of interest that these patients, who have such gross abnormalities in the upper lobes that they can be easily demonstrated by scintigraphy to have altered ventilation, are the same patients who experienced improved physiologic parameters following surgery. This is an interesting analysis and confirms other clinical observations that patients with heterogeneous disease appear to be those most likely to benefit from LVRS. This well-done study simply confirms that those patients who have significant difficulties with aeration in the upper lobes due to the heterogeneous distribution of their disease are precisely the patients who received significant benefit from the relief of the compression of the adjacent, relatively more normal lung following resection of these areas.

As seen in Figure 5, the patients with predominantly upper lobe disease, as demonstrated by scintigraphy, are the ones to benefit most from LVRS. This is an important study because it confirms previous observations. However, the practical use of non-heterogeneous scintigraphy to differentiate those patients who might benefit from LVRS from those who will not limits the technology to simply a confirmatory test following a well-done chest CT scan. We will need to see improvements in the technology of scintigraphy in order to be able to demonstrate other target areas besides simply the upper lung fields, which usually are so grossly involved that plain radiographs and CT scans adequately demonstrate target zones.

D.J. Sugarbaker, M.D.

Pulmonary Emphysema: Comparison of Preoperative Quantitative CT and Physiologic Index Values With Clinical Outcome After Lung-Volume Reduction Surgery

Gierada DS, Slone RM, Bae KT, et al (Washington Univ, St Louis)
Radiology 205:235–242, 1997 14–2

Objective.—Visual interpretation of disease features of emphysema on CT scan can be influenced by a variety of factors. Quantitative CT assessment eliminates these variations. The relevant quantitative CT parameters of emphysema were defined and compared with outcomes after lung volume reduction surgery (LVRS), and the relationship between quantitative CT and preoperative physiologic values were investigated.

Methods.—Preoperative CT scans were performed in 46 patients. The quantitative CT indices determined global emphysema severity, regional emphysema severity, emphysema heterogeneity, and volume of normally attenuated lung-volume of lung with attenuation between −850 and −701 HU. Preoperative and postoperative forced expiratory volume in 1 second (FEV_1), partial pressure of arterial oxygen (PaO_2), and 6-minute walking distance were compared.

Results.—Three patients died postoperatively and were not included in the results. Postoperative FEV_1, forced vital capacity, 6-minute walking distance, and PaO_2 increased significantly (by 52%, 22%, 19%, and 15%, respectively). Patients whose attenuation-frequency histograms showed a narrow, low-attenuation peak had more improvement after surgery. Candidates for LVRS may not benefit from quantitative CT because of the extent of their disease. Correlations between quantitative CT data and pathologic findings were not maximized. The emphysema index for global and regional emphysema was defined at −900 HU, with patients with improved outcome having a mean lung attenuation greater than −900 HU, 75% or more of upper lung less than −900 HU, more than 25% of lung less than −960 HU, and a ratio of upper- to lower-lung emphysema indices of 1.5 or greater. Patients also had a better outcome if the volume of attenuated lung was more than 1 L, with full width at half maximum of the attenuation-distribution 80 HU or less. Patients with preoperative FEV_1 less than 25% of predicted and a total lung capacity of less than 150% of predicted improved their 6-minute walking distance by 2 to 3 times.

Conclusion.—Many quantitative CT scans were correlated with preoperative physiologic values but not with many outcome measures. Quantitative assessments may be useful for stratifying candidates for LVRS.

► This is another confirmatory report from the group looking at preoperative quantitative CT scanning as a useful investigative tool for determining which patients will improve after surgery. The stratification of disease into the upper lobes is demonstrated by attenuation below −900 HU in 75% or more of the upper lobe, correlating with those patients who had the best overall outcome. The use of a ratio of upper to lower lobe lung disease indexes would seem to be of value for assessing the degree of upper lobe vs. lower lobe disease. A disease ratio of 1.5 or greater in the upper lobe vs. the lower lobe would appear to be a potentially useful indicator of patients who should be selected for LVRS.

This paper is an interesting and useful study because it confirms again that one can quantify the degree of emphysema before surgical resection with the use of quantitative CT scanning and that this, indeed, will correlate to the patients' physiologic index values. It confirms the fact that the anatomy, as defined by chest CT scanning and quantified on the basis of the upper lobe-to-lower lobe emphysema index, does, indeed, correlate with the physiologic outcome after LVRS.

Again, it is imperative that we produce a more sensitive technique for determining whether there are other patients without predominant upper lobe disease who may potentially benefit from LVRS. It is also important to develop a mechanism by which lung compliance (via the anatomical structures in the lung) can be determined and used to predict those patients who would receive a longer, more durable therapeutic response from LVRS.

D.J. Sugarbaker, M.D.

Preoperative Predictors of Operative Morbidity and Mortality in COPD Patients Undergoing Bilateral Lung Volume Reduction Surgery

Szekely LA, Oelberg DA, Wright C, et al (Harvard Med School, Boston)
Chest 111:550–558, 1997 14–3

Objective.—Whereas some patients with chronic obstructive pulmonary disease (COPD) benefit from bilateral lung volume reduction surgery (LVRS), questions regarding indications and contraindication to surgery, long-term outcome, and physiologic changes after surgery remain unanswered. Findings of preoperative predictors of outcome in 47 consecutive patients with severe COPD who underwent bilateral LVRS were reported.

Methods.—Preoperative pulmonary function tests, chest radiography, cardiopulmonary exercise testing, and the 6-mile walk test (6MWT) were performed on 47 patients (22 males, average patient age 60.5 years) who also completed a questionnaire. Unacceptable postoperative outcomes included death within 6 months after discharge and a hospital stay of more than 21 days. Patients were followed for 6–12 months.

Results.—Seventeen patients were awaiting lung transplantation. All patients were former smokers. The average hospital and ICU stays were 32 and 14 days, respectively, with mechanical ventilation provided for an average of 19.1 days. Nine patients (19.1%) died. Radiologic studies revealed that 75% of patients had predominantly upper lobe emphysema, 16% had predominantly lower lobe emphysema, and 9% had both. Forced expiratory volume in 1 second, forced vital capacity, maximum inspiratory pressure, resting partial pressure of arterial carbon dioxide ($PaCO_2$), 6MWT results before and after rehabilitation, and a $PaCO_2$ at maximum oxygen consumption were correlated with hospital stay. According to multiple regression analysis, inability to walk more than 200 m in the 6MWT before or after rehabilitation and a resting $PaCO_2$ of 45 mm Hg or greater were the most significant predictors of hospital stays of more than 21 days and death. Eight patients who died had hospital stays of more than 21 days. Five of 11 hypercapnic ($PaCO_2$ of 45 mm Hg or greater) died.

Conclusion.—Inability to walk more than 200 m in the 6MWT before or after rehabilitation and a resting $PaCO_2$ of 45 mm Hg or greater were the most significant predictors of poor outcome in COPD patients with COPD undergoing bilateral LVRS.

▶ This is an important study because it demonstrates the range of patient morbidity and mortality after LVRS. The authors have done an excellent job of carefully isolating the predictors of morbidity and mortality in patients undergoing median sternotomy and bilateral LVRS. Important physiologic parameters identified include the inability to walk more than 200 meters on a 6MWT, suggesting severe physiologic impairment, and a $PaCO_2$ of 45 mm Hg or greater, again suggesting severe physiologic impairment. These 2 factors were noted to predict poor outcome in this particular study.

The authors are to be commended for examining the surgical approach to emphysema in this severely limited group of patients with severe respiratory compromise. The overall mortality rate of 19% suggests that, indeed, such patients should be reconsidered for LVRS on the basis of the 2 parameters indicated above. It is possible to conclude from this study that in general patients with an inability to walk more than 200 meters on a 6MWT walk or with a $PaCO_2$ 45 mm Hg or greater should not be considered for LVRS, at least not by the technique described (median sternotomy), which, I think, is still practiced by a large number of surgeons who are currently studying this procedure.

D.J. Sugarbaker, M.D.

Patients With Emphysema: Quantitative CT Analysis Before and After Lung Volume Reduction Surgery: Work in Progress

Bae KT, Slone RM, Gierada DS, et al (Washington Univ, St Louis)

Radiology 203:705–714, 1997 14–4

Objective.—Whether morphologic changes in the lungs after lung volume reduction surgery (LVRS) reflect changes in lung function is not completely understood. The severity and distribution of emphysema were quantitatively assessed using inspiratory and expiratory CT images before and after LVRS and compared with clinical findings and patient outcome.

Methods.—Preoperative and/or postoperative CT scans at full inspiration and expiration were performed in 10 patients with chronic obstructive pulmonary disease (COPD), aged 41 to 77 years, who underwent LVRS in 1994. By means of a semiautomated segmentation method, all lung sections were analyzed. Lung volumes were calculated and a frequency distribution of attenuation values was constructed. Attenuation and lung volumes before and after surgery were compared. Pulmonary function tests and arterial blood gas analysis were performed before and after pulmonary rehabilitation and postoperatively at 1, 3, 6, and 12 months.

Results.—Lung volume calculated by the semiautomated segmentation method was in close agreement with calculation by the manual method, the mean and standard deviation of the proportional difference being 2.4% and 4.5%, respectively. Average inspiratory and expiratory volumes were reduced by 25% and 41%, respectively. The emphysema inspiration index decreased to 38% postoperatively from a preoperative value of 60%. Likewise the emphysema expiratory index decreased to 27% postoperatively from a preoperative value of 60%. Comparison of the preoperative and postoperative histograms revealed a reduction in cross-sectional area and volume and a reduction in the percentage of lung severely involved. Preoperative and postoperative inspiratory and expiratory indices were significantly correlated with percentage predicted forced expiratory volume in 1 second (FEV_1), and postoperative inspiratory and expiratory indices were significantly correlated with FEV_1/forced vital capacity. Diffusing capacity was highly correlated with preoperative inspiratory and postoperative expiratory indices. The preoperative inspiratory index was weakly correlated with residual volume/total lung capacity.

Conclusion.—Lung volume calculated by the semiautomated segmentation method was in close agreement with volume calculated by the manual method. Lung volume reduction surgery resulted in increased airflow and improved inspiratory and expiratory emphysema indices. These findings imply the existence of a multifactorial mechanism for the improved lung function after surgery.

▶ Patients in this study underwent a quantitative CT scan analysis before and after volume reduction surgery. This study suggests that quantitative CT scans are capable of determining the amount of existing diseased lung both before and after surgery. The index was used to determine the amount of volume decrease at both inspiration and expiration and suggests that CT scans are capable of documenting this trend in parenchymal reduction with the overall reduction in emphysema vs. normal lung.

At both inspiration and expiration there is a decrease in the amount of emphysema after surgery as characterized by the emphysema index before and after the resection of diseased tissues. This emphysema index could provide a useful tool for comparing patients after a variety of surgical procedures. There remains a good deal of controversy as to whether open techniques or closed techniques are preferable in terms of their ability to reduce the emphysema index and shunt both ventilation and perfusion to a more physiologically normal parenchyma. Some refinement in the use of radiologic techniques may lead to better patient selection and also to better evaluation of patients after a variety of surgical procedures, including resection, laser ablation, and plication.

D.J. Sugarbaker, M.D.

Radiologic Emphysema Morphology Is Associated With Outcome After Surgical Lung Volume Reduction

Weder W, Thurnheer R, Stammberger U, et al (Univ Hosp, Zurich, Switzerland)

Ann Thorac Surg 64:313–320, 1997 14–5

Objective.—Lung volume reduction surgery (LVRS) benefits carefully selected patients with emphysema. Whether emphysema morphology might predict functional outcome after surgery is not known. A retrospective study was designed to define a simple, CT-based radiologic emphysema classification that can be reproducibly applied by clinicians and to evaluate whether this pragmatic classification identifies certain morpho-

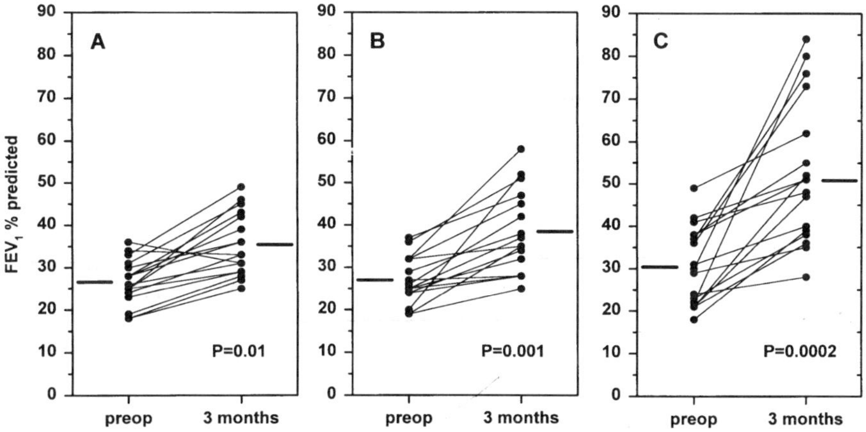

FIGURE 2.—Effect of thoracoscopic lung volume reduction on forced expiratory volume in 1 second (FEV_1) in homogeneous **A**, intermediately heterogeneous **B**, or markedly heterogeneous **C**, emphysema types. Each panel depicts individual (*dots connected with lines*) and mean (*horizontal lines*) values before (preop) and after the operation. The *P* values correspond to comparisons of postoperative with preoperative values. (Reprinted with permission from the Society of Thoracic Surgeons from Weder W, Thurnheer R, Stammberger U, et al: Radiologic emphysema morphology is associated with outcome after surgical lung volume reduction. *Ann Thorac Surg* 64:313–320, 1997).

logic types of emphysema that predict a more favorable clinical outcome after LVRS.

Methods.—Preoperative and 3-month postsurgery functional tests, and radiologic evaluations—including preoperative chest CT scans—were performed in 50 patients (16 women) with severe emphysema who underwent LVRS. Results were reviewed by 6 blinded physicians. Patients with bullae of 7 cm or greater were excluded from the study. Three main morphologic types, based on chest CT scans, were classified as markedly heterogeneous (17 patients), intermediately heterogeneous (16 patients), and homogeneous (17 patients). Additional features evaluated for heterogeneous cases included predominantly upper lobe type, predominantly lower lobe type, and bullae.

Results.—Pulmonary function, walking distance, and dyspnea improved significantly after surgery. Patients with markedly heterogeneous emphysema had the greatest improvement in forced vital capacity and forced expiratory volume in 1 second (Fig 2). Forced expiratory volume in 1 second improved by 81% in the markedly heterogeneous emphysema group, by 44% in the intermediately heterogeneous emphysema group, and by 34% in the homogeneous emphysema group.

Conclusion.—This emphysema classification system can identify patients who will benefit from LVRS and can predict functional outcome after surgery.

► This rather straightforward study from Switzerland seeks to determine the anatomical distribution of emphysema in patients undergoing surgical LVRS. It provides an interesting classification. The subjective classification from homogeneous to markedly heterogeneous disease is a useful one because of its simplicity. It can provide a means for the practitioner to immediately assess a patient's candidacy for LVRS. The morphologic type of emphysema assessed by this simplified, oriented classification did predict surgical outcome in this group of 50 patients studied retrospectively. A prospective analysis would be required for us to validate this morphologic classification.

Needless to say, however, it has continually been observed that patients with heterogeneous disease—particularly with predominantly upper lobe disease—are those who have a significant amount of parenchymal compression and therefore seem to benefit most from LVRS. This points out the fact that the patients benefiting most from LVRS are those who are functionally most similar to patients with giant bullous disease, who, for years, have enjoyed a significant improvement after bullectomy. The compression of adjacent normal lung by the large grapelike clusters of emphysema blebs suggests that the blebs are mimicking giant bullous disease. The follow-up at 3 months suggests that thoracoscopic LVRS is most beneficial in patients with marked heterogeneous disease. However, are a large number of patients, even within this subgroup, who benefit only modestly from this procedure. Most of the benefit accrued to a small number of patients who received a significant improvement. Understanding the reason certain patients, even within this subgroup, benefit and why others do not remains the focus of further study. The reader is directed to the fact that this paper gives follow-up only at 3 months; the long-term durability of this procedure remains in significant doubt.

D.J. Sugarbaker, M.D.

Changes in Lung Volume and Volume of Emphysema After Unilateral Lung Reduction Surgery: Analysis With CT Lung Densitometry

Holbert JM, Brown ML, Sciurba FC, et al (Univ of Pittsburgh, Pa)

Radiology 201:793–797, 1996 — 14–6

Background.—The physiologic mechanisms underlying the improvements achieved by lung reduction surgery are not completely understood. Changes in the volume of lungs and in the volume of emphysema after unilateral lung reduction surgery (ULRS) were investigated by CT lung densitometry.

Methods.—Computed tomography was performed in 28 patients before and 3 months after ULRS. The scans were analyzed to define the volume of the lungs and of emphysema.

Findings.—Lung volume decreased 22% after ULRS. The intact opposite lung volume increased by 4%. Emphysema in the surgically reduced lung was decreased by 14%. In the opposite lung, emphysema was unchanged. Mean CT numbers increased 26 Hounsfield Units in the surgically reduced lungs but were unaffected in the opposite lungs.

Conclusion.—The effect of ULRS on lungs can be assessed by CT lung densitometry and a 3-dimensional graphics work station. This procedure decreases emphysema and lung volume in the surgically reduced lung without significant worsening of contralateral emphysema at 3 months.

▶ This is a very interesting study because it is the first to examine the effects of volume reduction surgery in a unilateral setting. The pulmonary dynamics and chest wall volume shifts seen with a free mediastinum are, as yet, unquantified. This study is of significance because it suggests that the physiologic response to ULRS may not mimic the response seen in bilateral reduction. This is because of the increase in the lung volume of the unoperated side, after a unilateral reduction, as documented in this study. This finding may suggest that a second contralateral volume reduction may be associated with a significant physiologic improvement, which reflects the additive effect of the shift of the mediastinum back toward the contralateral side once it is volume reduced.

The problem with most of these studies is that we are studying patients with severely diseased lungs, and, therefore the amount of normal parenchyma available for recruitment after volume reduction still remains minimal. Nevertheless, this study is important because it carefully investigates the effect of volume reduction surgery by the unilateral approach. This may enhance our understanding of when to perform a unilateral vs. a bilateral reduction. This will be particularly important when we begin to get more long-term follow-up and better understand the durability of the response to surgery. It may very well be that a staged volume reduction surgery will provide significantly longer palliative improvement in this severely compromised group of patients.

D.J. Sugarbaker, M.D.

Lung Volume Reduction Surgery for Emphysema

Russi EW, Stammberger U, Weder W (Univ Hosp, Zurich, Switzerland)

Eur Respir J 10:208–218, 1997 14–7

Background.—Lung volume reduction surgery (LVRS) is a novel palliative procedure performed in a subgroup of patients with advanced emphysema. Researchers worldwide are currently determining selection criteria, searching for the best surgical treatment, and documenting the physiologic changes and long-term effects of LVRS.

Lung Volume Reduction Surgery for Emphysema.—Lung volume reduction surgery may be done to relieve dyspnea in selected patients with severe pulmonary emphysema, thus improving their pulmonary function, ability to perform daily activities, and quality of life. The resection of destroyed areas of the lung may decrease hyperinflation, resulting in amelioration of diaphragm and chest wall mechanics; increased elastic recoil pressure, augmenting expiratory flow rates; and potentially improving gas exchange. Through meticulous patient selection, refinement of operative

TABLE 3.—Functional Results After Lung Volume Reduction Surgery

Author	Pts No.	Approach	Procedure	ΔFEV_1 %
Cooper *et al.* [17] 1995	20	MS	Bilateral stapled resection	82
Demertizis and co-workers [35] 1996	20	MS	Bilateral stapled resection	32
Eugene *et al.* [36] 1995	28	VATSu	KTP laser and/or Nd-YAG laser, discretely bullous areas and hyperinflated areas were stapled	34
Keenan *et al.* [30] 1996	67	VATSu	Nd-YAG laser (10), stapled resection (23), stapled resection with modest laser ablation (34)	27
Little *et al.* [37] 1995	81	VATSu	Nd-YAG	15
McKenna *et al.* [28] 1996	72	VATSu	Nd-YAG (33) or stapled resection (39)	33 stapler group, 13 laser group
Miller and co-workers [27] 1996	53	46 MS, 7 Tu	Stapled resection	93
Naunheim and co-workers [31] 1996	50	VATSu, 5 patients operated on contralateral side	Staled resection	35
Wakabayashi [32] 1995	483	VATSu, in 57 cases subsequently operation of the opposite side	Nd-YAG laser, type 4 bullae were excised and sutured or stapled	62 in group with preoperative FEV_1 <14% pred (n=33) 28 in group with preoperative FEV_1 ≥15% pred (n=191)
Yusen and co-workers [34] 1996	84	MS	Bilateral stapled resection	58

Abbreviations: Pts, patients; *ΔFEV_1*, change in forced expiratory volume in 1 second from preoperative to postoperative; *MS*, median sternotomy; *VATSu*, unilateral video-assisted thoracoscopic surgery; *Tu*, unilatral thoracotomy; *KTP laser*, potassium titanyl-phosphate laser: *Nd-YAG laser*, neodymium-yttrium aluminum garnet laser; *% pred*, percentage of predicted value.

(Courtesy of Russi EW, Stammberger U, Weder W: Lung volume reduction surgery for emphysema. *Eur Respir J* 10:208–218, 1997.)

techniques, and improved anesthesiologic and postoperative management, perioperative mortality has been reduced to less than 5%. Bilateral resection produces the best functional results. Such resection can be done by either median sternotomy or video-assisted thoracoscopy. The mean increase in forced expiratory volume in 1 second obtained by bilateral resection in patients already receiving optimal medical therapy ranges from 32% to 93% (Table 3). The decrease in hyperinflation, determined by a reduction in total lung capacity, ranges from 15% to 20%. In most patients, the benefits of LVRS are maintained for at least 1 year.

▶ This report is of interest because it provides a careful review of the literature and a comparison of the various surgical techniques available for the performance of LVRS. It is interesting that in the author's review, there was no significant difference in outcome between median sternotomy and bilateral thoracoscopic stapled resection. The percentage increase in forced expiratory volume in 1 second (FEV_1) appears to vary significantly within both techniques. It remains to be seen whether the thoracoscopic approach—intuitively less morbid—will indeed provide a significant advantage over median sternotomy. Certainly, however, one can conclude from some of the graphics presented that, indeed, both of these approaches—as well as the use of the Nd-YAG laser—do appear to have a physiologic effect. It will be important to further study this, particularly regarding lasers, as this particular technique has begun to lose a significant number of advocates in the thoracic surgery community.

Also of note in this particular study is the fact that the most important effect of LVRS appears to relate to the amelioration of shortness of breath. In this study, dyspnea decreased from a mean of 3.4 to 1.8, as assessed by the Medical Research Counsel dyspnea score. This fact indicates, again, that this approach primarily alleviates the symptoms of COPD and severe respiratory discomfort and that the actual physiologic improvements may be more difficult to assess, particularly in the long term. The lack of sustained, long-term follow-up, as noted in this review, also makes the durability of the response in this group of patients difficult to assess.

D.J. Sugarbaker, M.D.

Effect of Surgical Lung Volume Reduction on Breathing Patterns in Severe Pulmonary Emphysema

Bloch KE, Li Y, Zhang J, et al (Univ Hosp of Zurich, Switzerland)

Am J Respir Crit Care Med 156:553–560, 1997 14–8

Objective.—Lung volume reduction surgery (LVRS) can benefit patients with emphysema. How these benefits affect breathing patterns is unknown. Respiratory inductive plethysmography (RIP) was used for the nonobtrusive study of natural breathing patterns in patients with severe, diffuse pulmonary emphysema before and several months after LVRS to identify preoperative breathing pattern characteristics associated with greatest improvement in lung function after surgery.

Methods.—Unilateral or bilateral video-assisted thoracoscopic resection was performed on 19 patients (6 women), aged 42 to 75 years, with advanced emphysema. Respiratory inductive plethysmography performed before and 1.5 to 7 months after LVRS measured changes in rib cage and abdominal volumes. Measurements were made for 20 to 60 minutes during natural at-rest breathing. Lung function and dyspnea were evaluated.

Results.—Whereas average time, volume, and flow components remained essentially unchanged after LVRS, abdominal volume displacement contributions to V_T were significantly increased and the amounts of paradoxical abdominal and rib cage movement during inspiration were

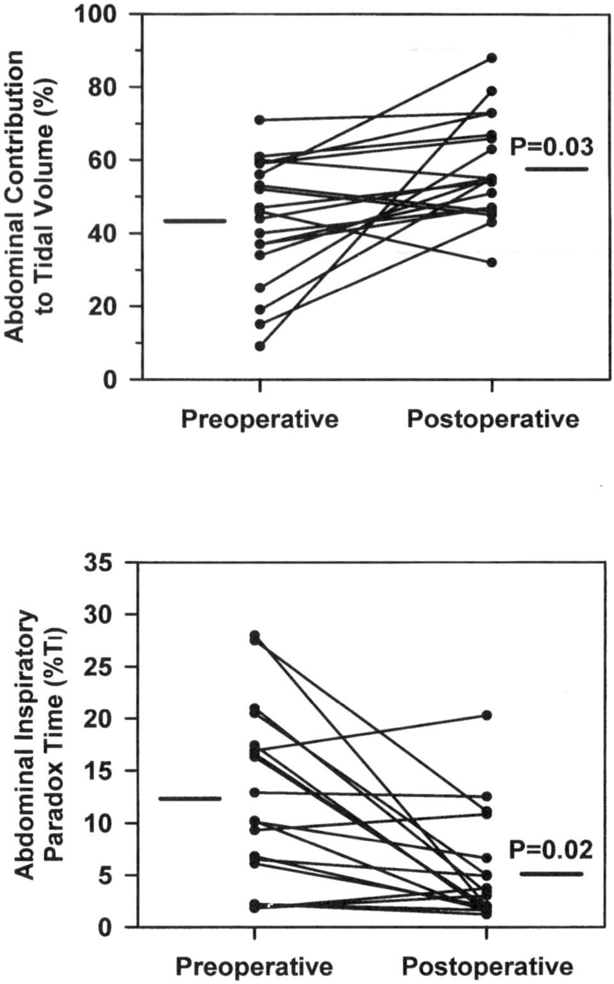

FIGURE 3.—Effect of surgical lung volume reduction on contribution of abdominal volume changes to tidal volume (**top panel**) and on the fraction of inspiratory time with paradoxical abdominal motion (**bottom panel**). Individual values of 19 patients and group means (*horizontal lines*) are displayed. (Courtesy of Bloch KE, Li Y, Zhang J, et al: Effect of surgical lung volume reduction on breathing patterns in severe pulmonary emphysema. *Am J Respir Crit Care Med* 156:553–560, 1997). Official Journal of the American Thoracic Society. Copyright 1997, American Lung Association.)

reduced, indicating improved synchronization of rib cage–abdominal motion (Fig 3). Abdominal volume changes increased tidal volume from an average preoperative value of 43% to 58% postoperatively. The amount of inspiratory time taken up by paradoxical abdominal motion declined from a preoperative value of 12.3% to a postoperative value of 5.1%. Phase shift between rib cage and abdominal motion, hyperinflation, airway obstruction, and subjective dyspnea scores improved significantly after surgery.

Conclusion.—These findings suggest that LVRS reduces the strain on respiratory muscles and improves hyperinflation, airway obstruction, and elastic recoil. A better understanding of these mechanisms should improve patient selection criteria.

► This report is of interest because it demonstrates that there are alterations in the physiologic pattern of breathing in patients who have had successful LVRS. This is important because we can show that the body's physiologic breathing patterns are altered in a positive way, proceeding toward normalcy. The increase in the percentage of the abdominal contribution to breathing is particularly important, as is the decrease in the percentage of abdominal paradoxical movements—a finding that is seen in patients with severe hyperinflation and flattening of the diaphragm. The effects of the abdominal contribution to total volume are increased after successful surgery, as is the time for abdominal inspiratory paradox.

I think that the most important contribution this paper has made to this field is to demonstrate that, indeed, there are physiologic responses and that one can alter the pattern of respiratory function after volume reduction surgery. This suggests that a restoration of normal physiology might be the result of a more perfect operation if, indeed, more micro-ablation of emphysematous disease were possible.

D.J. Sugarbaker, M.D.

Lung-volume Reduction Improves Dyspnea, Dynamic Hyperinflation, and Respiratory Muscle Function

Martinez FJ, Montes de Oca M, Whyte RI, et al (Univ of Michigan, Ann Arbor; Tufts Univ, Boston)

Am J Respir Crit Care Med 155:1984–1990, 1997 14–9

Background.—Pulmonary function and elastic recoil improve in patients with emphysema after lung-volume reduction surgery (LVRS), even though forced vital capacity and forced expiratory volume in 1 second (FEV_1) remain unchanged in some patients.

Methods.—Pulmonary function, exercise capacity, dynamic lung volume, preoperative dyspnea, and respiratory muscle (RM) function were prospectively evaluated before and at least 3 months after LVRS in 17 patients (6 women), with an average age of 61 years, with severe emphysema and hyperinflation.

Results.—After LVRS there were significant changes in FEV_1 from 26.7% to 39.0% of predicted, in total lung capacity from 134.7% to 118.3% of predicted, and in respiratory volume from 239.6% to 180.3% of predicted. The average 6-minute walking distance increased significantly from 620 feet before surgery to 1,259 feet after surgery. Both resting and isowork end-expiratory lung volumes and end-inspiratory lung volumes decreased significantly. Dyspnea, as measured on a visual analogue scale, decreased in 10 of 12 patients from an average of 79.6 before surgery to 49.3 after surgery. After surgery, maximal voluntary ventilation improved significantly. Whereas resting RM function remained essentially unchanged, isowork RM function improved significantly. Except for 1 patient, changes in the Borg-scale score at equivalent workloads were significantly correlated with changes in end-expiratory lung volume, both before and after surgery, and with changes in end-expiratory pleural pressure.

Conclusion.—Functional status, static pulmonary function, and elastic recoil improve significantly after bilateral LVRS as a result of improved diaphragm function and respiratory pressure generation.

▶ This report, together with the one previously examined, suggests that LVRS will improve dyspnea and dynamic hyperinflation and that, interestingly enough, RM function will be improved. This is, again, an important verification of the fact that the effects of LVRS go beyond a mere reduction in dyspnea, resulting in a significant improvement in the physiologic activity in breathing.

This is an extremely well-done study. I think the conclusions are sound and provide the basis for further tailoring of the surgical technique to maximize these new parameters observed in patients both before and after surgery. The improvement in respiratory muscle strength, in particular, suggests that a significant amount of physiologic recovery is possible in this group of patients and that the changes from long-term chronic respiratory insufficiency are not irreversible.

D.J. Sugarbaker, M.D.

Lung Volume Reduction Surgery Improves Maximal O_2 Consumption, Maximal Minute Ventilation, O_2 Pulse, and Dead Space-to-Tidal Volume Ratio During Leg Cycle Ergometry

Benditt JO, Lewis S, Wood DE, et al (Univ of Washington, Seattle)

Am J Respir Crit Care Med 156:561–566, 1997 14–10

Objective.—Whereas lung volume reduction surgery (LVRS) improves exercise capacity in patients with emphysema, the specific physiologic effects of LVRS that result in improved exercise performance are not known. A progressive exercise test was used to evaluate a consecutive series of patients with emphysema before and 3 months after LVRS.

Methods.—Spirometry and arterial blood gas determinations were performed in 21 patients (6 female) at rest and at peak cardiopulmonary exercise before and after bilateral LVRS. Patients scored their at rest and peak exercise dyspnea levels on a visual analogue scale.

Results.—After surgery, maximal work improved significantly by a median of 17.5 watts (46%), expired volume per unit time improved by 6.6 L/min (27%), heart rate at isowatt exercise decreased significantly by 3.5 beats/min, and dead-space gas volume to tidal gas volume at peak exercise decreased significantly by 0.07 (13%) because of a significant increase in tidal volume. Dyspnea visual analogue scale measurements at rest declined from a median of 29 to 9 and at peak exercise declined from a median of 82 to 47. Respiratory acidemia developed at peak exercise in 16 patients before surgery and in 13 after surgery.

Conclusion.—Exercise performance improves in emphysema patients after LVRS as a result of improved maximal ventilation.

► This study is of interest because it carefully examined the respiratory function of a group of patients undergoing LVRS by measuring oxygen consumption, maximum minute ventilation, oxygen pulse oximetry, and dead space–to–tidal volume ratio during leg cycle ergometry. Of particular importance is the fact that despite successful LVRS, limited ventilatory capacity remained the primary problem limiting exercise in these patients. The tendency for a majority of subjects to have acute respiratory acidemia at peak exercise was not significantly reduced after surgery. This suggests that patients receive a modest-to-minor benefit from LVRS surgery on a physiologic basis and that after surgery, even though the sensation of dyspnea has been substantially improved, patients may still have a physiologic impairment.

Also of interest is the study of the power output in watts before and after surgery, which suggests an improvement, and the maximal oxygen consumption, which suggests a modest improvement. The real challenge will be to use these tools of physiologic measurement to define and design treatments that ablate more emphysematous lung in a finer way than gross surgical resection, thus enhancing the remaining, more normal pulmonary segments.

D.J. Sugarbaker, M.D.

Functional and Oximetric Assessment of Patients After Lung Reduction Surgery

Bousamra M II, Haasler GB, Lipchik RJ, et al (Med College of Wisconsin, Milwaukee)

J Thorac Cardiovasc Surg 113:675–682, 1997 14–11

Objective.—The mechanism by which lung volume reduction surgery (LVRS) decreases an emphysema patient's dependence on supplemental oxygen is not definitively known. Before and after LVRS, patients underwent a detailed oximetric assessment to determine the effect of the procedure on the need for supplemental oxygen.

Methods.—Preoperative and postoperative arterial blood gas values, lung volumes, dyspnea scores, 6-minute walk test, exercise oximetry scores, and diffusion capacity of carbon dioxide were recorded and spirometry was performed in 37 patients with heterogeneous emphysematous disease.

Results.—At 3 months postoperatively, forced vital capacity and forced expiratory volume in 1 second had improved by 37% and 59%, respectively, and at 6 months, by 33% and 48%, respectively. In 16 patients, maximal inspiratory and expiratory pressure increased significantly. Performance on the 6-minute walk test improved from 913 feet before surgery to 1,108 and 1,202 feet at 3 and 6 months, respectively. At 3 and 6 months, respectively, after surgery, percent resting had declined significantly to 11% and 4%, and Borg scores had declined significantly to 12 and 11. Self-rated dyspnea improved from 0.83 before surgery to 2.4 at latest follow-up, with mild improvement in 15 patients, moderate improvement in 11, major improvement in 7, and mild worsening in 1. Before surgery, 83% of patients met American Thoracic Society criteria for supplemental oxygen, and after surgery 70% met the criteria. Ten patients with exercise desaturation were able to discontinue supplemental oxygen after surgery.

Conclusion.—Whereas LVRS significantly improves symptoms in patients with emphysema, the need for supplemental oxygen remains for most as a result of hypoxemia during exercise, despite a subjective improvement in dyspnea scores.

▶ This important report points out that in these well-studied patients, a large number who had significant improvement after LVRS still required oxygen as defined by the American Thoracic Society criteria for supplemental oxygen. Important is the fact that 10 of these patients with exertional desaturation while breathing room air discontinued supplemental oxygen because of the reduction in dyspnea. This suggests, first, that in certain patients there will be a disconnect between the significant subjective improvements and those functional improvements related to LVRS, and second, that exercise-induced hypoxia was not reversed in a large number of these patients. Therefore, the discontinuation of supplemental oxygen because of the reduction in the subjective sense of dyspnea may not be warranted. The authors caution against the discontinuation of oximetric evaluations in these patients. It is clear that hypoxic patients undergo myocardial deterioration, and we might, therefore be hastening their demise by relieving them of their adherent warning system for hypoxia—namely dyspnea—through the physiologic alteration, still poorly understood, that results from LVRS.

D.J. Sugarbaker, M.D.

Bilateral Lung Volume Reduction Surgery for Advanced Emphysema: A Comparison of Median Sternotomy and Thoracoscopic Approaches

Kotloff RM, Tino G, Bavaria JE, et al (Univ of Pennsylvania, Philadelphia)

Chest 110:1399–1406, 1996 14–12

Background.—At the authors' center, lung volume reduction surgery in patients with advanced emphysema has been performed by median sternotomy (MS) and by video-assisted thoracoscopic surgery (VATS), according to individual surgeons' preferences. The short-term outcomes of the procedures done by MS and VATS were compared.

TABLE 2.—Mortality Before Hospital Discharge by Procedure Type and Age

Procedure	Mortality: No. Died/Total (%) <65 yr	≥65 yr
MS	2/37 (5.4)	9/43 (20.9)*
VATS	0/29 (0)	1/11 (9.1)

*P < 0.05 compared with median sternotomy group more than 65 years of age.
Abbreviations: MS, median sternotomy; *VATS,* video-assisted thoracoscopic surgery.
(Courtesy of Kotloff RM, Tino G, Bavaria JE, et al: Bilateral lung volume reduction surgery for advanced emphysema: A comparison of median sternotomy and thoracoscopic approaches. *Chest* 110:1399–1406, 1996.)

Methods.—Eighty patients underwent surgery by MS and 40 by VATS. In all patients, preoperative assessment included pulmonary function testing, arterial blood gas determination, and a 6-minute walk test. Pulmonary function testing and the walk test were repeated 3 to 6 months after surgery.

Findings.—At the end of surgery, all patients were extubated, but 17.5% of those in the MS group and 2.5% in the VATS group later needed reintubation. The mortality rates at 30 days were 4.2% and 2.5% in the MS and VATS groups, respectively. Although this difference was nonsignificant, the total in-hospital mortality rate was 13.8% for the MS group and remained unchanged in the VATS group. Deaths occurred mainly among elderly patients (Table 2). The 2 groups did not differ significantly in the duration of air leaks or length of hospital stay. The functional outcomes associated with the 2 methods were similar.

Conclusion.—Bilateral lung volume reduction surgery by MS and VATS results in comparable improvement in pulmonary function and exercise tolerance. VATS is associated with a significantly reduced incidence of respiratory failure and a trend toward lower in-hospital mortality. Thus, this may be the preferred technique, especially in high-risk patients.

► This is a very important study because it is one of the first studies to provide a head-to-head comparison of median sternotomy vs. VATS within the same hospital. Of note is the fact that although the physiologic responses to the 2 approaches were very similar with improvements approximating those in the literature, the mortality rate—particularly in the over-65 age group—was significantly improved in patients undergoing a VATS. The surgeons involved are well trained in both techniques, and this suggests that there may be some inherent advantage to thoracoscopic resection. As seen in Table 2, the take home message of this particular study is that a well-performed VATS may be beneficial to those patients over the age of 65 because it appears to result in about half the mortality rate of those undergoing MS. This is significant and, I think, provides the basis for further investigation into technique refinement, particularly in the video-assisted approach.

D.J. Sugarbaker, M.D.

Thoracoscopic Lung Volume Reduction Surgery Reduces Dyspnea and Improves Exercise Capacity in Patients With Emphysema

Keller CA, Ruppel G, Hibbett A, et al (St Louis Univ)

Am J Respir Crit Care Med 156:60–67, 1997 14–13

Objective.—Whereas lung volume reduction surgery (LVRS) improves exercise performance in patients with emphysema, the reason for, and duration of, the improvement is not precisely known. Measures of inspiratory and expiratory flows and changes in exercise capacity were compared after preoperative pulmonary rehabilitation and within 6 months after unilateral LVRS.

Methods.—Pulmonary function, exercise (6 mile walk and bicycle ergometer), and dyspnea scores were recorded for 25 patients aged 44 to 73 years.

Results.—Exercise time improved significantly from 4.43 to 5.71 minutes, maximum workload increased from 37.1 to 52.4 W, maximum oxygen consumption increased from 9.71 to 11.84 mL/kg/min, minute ventilation during maximum exercise increased from 24.4 to 28.5 L/min, tidal volume increased from 951 to 1,145 mL, average minute ventilation increased from 0.89 to 1.06 L/s, average minute ventilation increased from 0.77 to 0.90 L/sec, dyspnea index improved from 82% to 72%, and 6-minute walk test improved from 934 to 1,071 feet. Inspiratory to total cycle time remained unchanged. These improvements were the result of increased inspiratory flows after the surgically decreased residual volume. Baseline Focal and Transition Focal scores were 3.36 and 6.12, respectively. Changes in maximum voluntary ventilation were correlated with improvements in dyspnea scores.

Conclusion.—Subjective improvements in dyspnea scores were related to changes in maximum voluntary ventilation but not to improvement in exercise performance. Additional studies need to be performed to determine what parameters are responsible for improvements in exercise capacity after LVRS.

▶ This report by Keller et al. is of interest because it demonstrates the lack of correlation between shortness of breath and exercise variables following LVRS. The study found that the carefully examined physiologic response to LVRS did not uniformly correlate with the patient's subjective impression of improvement of dyspnea. Specifically, the changes in the maximum volume ventilation, resting PaO_2 and FEV_1 reduction appeared to correlate best with the patient's subjective improvement in dyspnea.

Importantly, however, exercise variables did not correlate significantly with subjective markers indicating improvement in dyspnea (with only 1 exception). Again, this points out the importance of discerning the subjective response to LVRS reduction surgery vs. the physiologic response, which would most likely be predictive of improved long-term survival. We are always cautious of procedures that simply improve one's sense of well being when, indeed, there is no sustained physiologic improvement. I think this study suggests that all patients undergoing LVRS need to have both physiologic and exercise evaluations before and after surgery, as well as routine pulmonary function tests and subjective dyspnea scores.

D.J. Sugarbaker, M.D.

Functional Comparison of Unilateral Versus Bilateral Lung Volume Reduction Surgery

Argenziano M, Thomashow B, Jellen PA, et al (Columbia-Presbyterian Med Ctr, New York)

Ann Thorac Surg 64:321–327, 1997 14–14

Introduction.—As a tenable option in the treatment of end-stage emphysema, lung volume reduction surgery (LVRS) has recently reemerged. It can provide significant improvements in respiratory function and dyspnea with low perioperative morbidity and mortality. Although bilateral LVRS is considered the procedure of choice, many patients with end-stage emphysema are not considered ideal candidates for this procedure and, thus, may benefit more from a unilateral procedure. Results of unilateral LVRS were reviewed.

Methods.—In 92 patients selected on the basis of severe hyperinflation with air trapping, diaphragmatic dysfunction, and disease heterogeneity, LVRS was performed during a 20-month period. There were 28 patients who had the unilateral procedure because of asymmetric disease, concomitant tumor resection, or previous thoracic operation.

Results.—In exercise capacity and dyspnea, unilateral LVRS resulted in improvement comparable with the bilateral procedure and had similar

TABLE 6.—Comparison of Functional Results in Unilateral Vs. Bilateral Lung Volume Reduction With at Least 3 Months of Follow-up

Category	FEV_1 (mL)	FVC (mL)	6MW (ft)	DI
Bilateral (n = 45)				
Preoperative	557 ± 215 (22 ± 8)	1,737 ± 673 (49 ± 17)	584 ± 325	4.1 ± 0.8
Postoperative*	851 ± 415 (34 ± 14)	2,219 ± 800 (64 ± 17)	908 ± 381	1.7 ± 1.4
Difference†	70% ± 79%‡	48% ± 63%	289 ± 320	−2.3 ± 1.4
Unilateral (n = 21)				
Preoperative	493 ± 131 (22 ± 8)	1,508 ± 460 (49 ± 17)	530 ± 395	4.1 ± 0.8
Postoperative*	644 ± 250 (34 ± 14)	1,888 ± 585 (64 ± 17)	839 ± 341	1.5 ± 1.2
Difference†	28% ± 28%	29% ± 338%	315 ± 270	−2.6 ± 1.4

Note: All data given as mean ± standard deviation. Numbers in parentheses are percent predicted.

*Postoperative results represent data collected between 3 and 6 months after operation.

†Expressed as percent change for forced expiratory volume in 1 second (*FEV_1*) and forced vital capacity (*FVC*), and as absolute change for 6-minute walk distance (*6MW*) and modified Medical Research Council dyspnea scale (*DI*).

‡$P < 0.02$ compared with unilateral lung volume reduction. (Reprinted with permission from the Society of Thoracic Surgeons courtesy of Argenziano M, Thomashow B, Jellen PA, et al: Functional comparison of unilateral versus bilateral lung volume reduction surgery. *Ann Thorac Surg* 64:321–327, 1997.)

perioperative mortality rates and actuarial survival at 24 months. Improvements in spirometric indices of pulmonary function, however, were less than in patients having the bilateral procedure (Table 6).

Conclusion.—Unilateral lung volume reduction surgery provides functional and subjective benefits in selected patients that are comparable in magnitude with those associated with a bilateral operation. In patients with asymmetric disease distribution, a previous thoracic operation, or contraindications to sternotomy, unilateral LVRS is an option in the therapy of end-stage emphysema and may have a role as a bridge to transplantation in selected patients.

► This is an important study because it examines the appropriate use of unilateral vs. bilateral LVRS. There has been debate, particularly between the proponents of VATS and those who favor median sternotomy, on the usefulness of unilateral staged thoracoscopic resection. There may be patients who, because of intraoperative instability or severe respiratory compromise, would be best served by unilateral resection—and the accompanying postoperative recovery and improvement in respiratory function—before the performance of a second LVRS procedure. When a second unilateral procedure immediately follows the first, during the second procedure, high-pressure positive ventilation is placed against the previous staple lines and one might intuitively predict that more air leaks and potentially longer hospitalization could result. A second advantage of the unilateral staged approach is that patients experiencing intraoperative instability could, by avoiding the trauma of an additional procedure, gain a potential reduction in hospital stay and a reduction in overall morbidity and mortality.

Perioperative mortality, in this study, was greater in patients undergoing bilateral procedures than in those having unilateral procedures. In addition, overall improvement with the bilateral procedure included 289 ft in the 6-minute walk test compared with 315 ft with the unilateral procedure (Table 6). This suggests there is a potential improvement in physiologic parameters after unilateral LVRS that is not necessarily reflected in the limited (28%) improvement in FEV_1 after a unilateral procedure compared with a bilateral procedure (70% improvement). The reader is directed to the previous study that suggests there may be a disconnect between the physiologic functional variables after volume reduction surgery and those static measurements composed of standard pulmonary function testing, such as the FEV_1.

Coupled with the improvement in perioperative mortality rate—which was only 3.6% for the unilateral patient group vs. 7.4% in the bilateral group—the suggestion could be made that a unilateral approach makes sense for a select group of patients. Combined with the potential for the durability of the response to be limited with a bilateral approach, these 2 factors could provide a basis for approaching most patients with a staged thoracoscopic resection. Assessment after a unilateral approach might lead to enough physiologic or functional improvement that one could reasonably delay the second of the staged procedures until the physiologic and subjective responses to the first began to wane.

D.J. Sugarbaker, M.D.

Lung Function 12 Months Following Emphysema Resection

Gelb AF, Brenner M, McKenna RJ Jr, et al (Univ of California, Los Angeles; Univ of California, Irvine; Univ of Toronto)
Chest 110:1407–1415, 1996 14–15

Objective.—Lung function, including elastic recoil, was evaluated at 6 and 12 months after bilateral lung volume reduction surgery (LVRS) in patients with emphysema.

Methods.—Lung function tests and lung elastic recoil pressures were recorded for 10 male patients, (average age, 67 years) 2 weeks before and 6 and 12 months after surgery.

Results.—Compared with preoperative measures, total lung capacity at 12 months was reduced significantly from 9.5 to 8.5 L, forced expiratory volume in 1 second at 12 months was reduced from 0.71 to 0.95 L, functional residual capacity was decreased from 7.5 to 6.2 L, residual volume was decreased from 6.8 to 5.5 L, residual volume/total lung capacity had declined from 71% to 65%, diffusing capacity had increased from 5 to 10, diffusing capacity/alveolar lung volume had increased from 0.9 to 2.2, P_{STAT} FRC rose from 1.3 to 3.0, and static lung elastic recoil pressure total lung capacity increased from 11 to 15. Compared with values at 6 months, lung volumes had increased significantly and expiratory airflow and lung elastic recoil pressures had decreased significantly. Conductance of the S airway segment increased from 0.20 preoperatively to 0.28 L/sec/cm at 12 months and critical transmural pressure in the collapsible segment improved over the same period from 3.2 to 2.5 cm H_2O.

Conclusion.—Improvement in lung elastic recoil at 12 months after LVRS resulted in significant increases in expiratory airflow because of increased airway conductance, increased conductance of the S airway segment, and lowered critical transmural pressure in the collapsible segment. Improvements seen in lung function and elastic recoil are higher at 6 months than at 12 months.

▶ This study provides a very important first glimpse at long-term follow-up in patients undergoing emphysema resection. Of vital interest is the report that physiologic response peaked at 6 months and, thereafter, began to deteriorate. At 1 year, there was a significant deterioration in the improvement in lung function and elastic recoil improvement when compared with measurments at 6 months. The study indicates that the effects of LVRS are going to be limited in the long term. It provides, I think, a rational basis for the ongoing National Emphysema Treatment Trial, which seeks a prospective validation of the technique in terms of its immediate efficacy for both subjective and physiologic improvements, as well as its long-term durability.

D.J. Sugarbaker, M.D.

Incidence of Lung Nodules Found in Patients Undergoing Lung Volume Reduction

Hazelrigg SR, Boley TM, Weber D, et al (Southern Illinois Univ, Springfield; St Louis Univ)

Ann Thorac Surg 64:303–306, 1997 14–16

Introduction.—The most frequent cause of death in men and women is lung cancer. Difficult clinical decisions are created with patients who have severe obstructive lung disease, an extensive smoking history, and a new lung nodule. Patients having lung volume reduction surgery are a population at high risk for cancer. In a group of patients being evaluated for lung volume reduction surgery, diagnosis and management of incidental lung nodules were investigated.

Methods.—A lung volume reduction operation was performed over a 2-year period in 281 patients with severe obstructive lung disease with hyperinflation. Before surgery, all patients had chest roentgenograms, chest CT, echocardiography, pulmonary function testing with arterial blood gases, ventilation perfusion scans, and exercise testing. Video-assisted techniques were used for the unilateral procedures and median sternotomy or thoracoscopy were used for the bilateral procedures. Recordings were taken of all lung nodules identified on radiologic examination or identified in resected specimens. An analysis was conducted on the incidence of lung nodules and their management.

Results.—At least 1 lung nodule was identified in 39.5% of the 281 patients. Typical benign calcification patterns were seen in 52 nodules. Of the remaining nodules, 78 were resected and 20 were followed up. Cancer was seen in 17 resected nodules, 13 of which were primary lung cancers. Twenty-eight of the resected nodules were not identified by the preoperative radiologic evaluation.

Conclusion.—In patients having lung volume reduction operations, nodules are frequently seen. There was an overall incidence of cancer of 6.4% of patients, and several were identified only at the pathologic examination. For those with primary lung cancer, survival at short-term follow-up has been excellent. There should be aggressive diagnosis and managment of nodules found in this group of patients. To help stratify the risk of a nodule being malignant, nodule enhancement studies in the CT scan have been recently used, but results are short term.

► This carefully done, multi-institutional trial points out the important, previously described fact that patients with long-standing emphysema appear to be at greater risk for the development of bronchogenic carcinoma than patients with other effects of long-term cigarette smoking. The fact that 39% of these patients seen for volume reduction surgery had at least 1 lung nodule identified at workup suggests that these patients need to be carefully screened for possible malignancies. It is of interest that the overall cancer rate in this group was 6.4%, with 13 of 281 patients (4.6%) having a primary malignancy of the lung identified.

This suggests that patients undergoing volume reduction surgery need a careful assessment and that any lung nodule—no matter how large or small—needs to be fully evaluated. Based on the data presented here, those patients with calcified nodules can be evaluated in a routine fashion. Should a benign calcific distribution be identified, one could expect a very low likelihood of malignancy. However, noncalcified nodules in this group of patients, regardless of size, appeared to require full evaluation. In probably the majority of cases, this evaluation should include a surgical resection, often performed in combination with volume reduction surgery. The debate as to whether a limited parenchymal resection or a more extensive lobectomy is the best treatment for primary bronchogenic carcinoma would appear to be moot in this group of patients whose severely compromised pulmonary function could not afford the more aggressive resection.

D.J. Sugarbaker, M.D.

Advances in Staging of Non–Small-Cell Lung Cancer

Non–Small Cell Lung Cancer: Nodal Staging With FDG PET versus CT With Correlative Lymph Node Mapping and Sampling

Steinert HC, Hauser M, Allemann F, et al (Univ Hosp, Zürich, Switzerland)
Radiology 202:441–446, 1997 14–17

Background.—Choosing appropriate treatment for cancer depends on accurate tumor staging. Surgical resection is preferred for early stages of bronchogenic carcinoma. Mediastinoscopy can accurately assess mediastinal nodes, although CT and MRI have major limitations in depicting mediastinal lymph node metastases. Positron emission tomography (PET) with 2-[fluorine-18] fluoro-2-deoxy-D-glucose (FDG) can potentially differentiate lymph nodes with metastases from those without. Most studies comparing the accuracy of PET and CT in the staging of mediastinal metastases of lung cancer have included a small sample size or a limited number mediastinal lymph nodes or have encountered limited surgical correlations. This prospective study compared the accuracy of state-of-the-art partial-body FDG PET with state-of-the-art contrast material–enhanced CT in nodal staging of mediastinal metastases.

Methods.—Contrast material–enhanced CT and FDG PET were performed in 47 patients with non–small-cell lung cancer; 23 patients had spiral CT and 24 patients had conventional CT. Images were interpreted before surgical staging. A lesion was considered malignant if it had a nodular appearance and intense FDG uptake similar to that of the brain. Nodal stations were localized according to the American Thoracic Society mapping system. Extensive lymph node sampling of 599 nodes from 191 nodal stations was performed.

Results.—Nodal metastases were confirmed at histopathologic analysis in 29% of patients after mediastinoscopy or thoracotomy. The sensitivity was 89% for PET and 57% for CT for the staging of N2 or N3 disease in mediastinal nodes. The specificity was 99% for PET and 94% for CT. The positive predictive value was 96% for PET and 76% for CT. The negative predictive value was 97% for PET and 87% for CT. Accuracy was 96% for PET and 85% for CT. Positron emission tomography was able to assign the correct N stage in 96% of cases; CT was correct in 79% of cases. Differences between spiral and conventional CT were not significant.

Discussion.—In these patients, FDG PET was superior to CT in nodal staging of non–small-cell lung cancer. For exact localization of lymph node metastases, emission- and transmission-corrected PET scans are needed. These data support using the brain as a reference standard for the thorax. It is likely that lesions with FDG activity similar to the FDG activity in the brain are malignant. If these results are confirmed in other studies with larger populations, FDG PET may be considered superior to CT in nodal staging of patients with non–small-cell lung cancer.

▶ This paper is one of the first to compare CT scanning with FDG PET scanning in the early detection of nodal metastases for non–small-cell lung cancer. The important component of this paper pertains to the correlation of both PET scanning and CT scanning with subsequent nodal mapping from surgical resection and biopsy. Of significance, PET scanning is highly specific and sensitive in its predictive value for determining the presence of metastatic disease. Positron emission tomography scanning could be very important in the treatment of patients with locally advanced non–small-cell lung cancer. Specifically, stage IIIA patients who undergo induction therapy could be re-examined with PET scanning to determine the effect of induction therapy on downstaging mediastinal disease.

As seen in a Southwest Oncology Group study and the Cancer and Leukemia Group B 8935 trial, the presence of persistent N1 disease after induction therapy is a poor prognostic indicator. The possibility of saving patients with this disease stage unnecessary thoracotomy is an appealing one. Current national trials are looking at the role of surgery vs. nonsurgery in stage IIIA disease, and this may, indeed, withhold potential curative surgery for patients who have had N2 disease eradicated by induction therapy. Therefore, the use of PET scanning for subsequent restaging in the mediastinum may hold more promise because it would appropriately identify downstaged patients for resection while indicating high-dose radiotherapy or other nonresectional treatment strategies for patients with persistent N2 disease.

D.J. Sugarbaker, M.D.

The Prognostic Significance of Tumor Cell Detection in Intraoperative Pleural Lavage and Lung Tissue Cultures for Patients With Lung Cancer
Buhr J, Berghäuser KH, Gonner S, et al (Justus Liebig Univ, Giessen, Germany)
J Thorac Cardiovasc Surg 113:683–690, 1997 14–18

Background.—Previous studies of pleural lavage in patients undergoing surgery for lung cancer have found malignant cells in the lavage fluid of 9% to 33% of patients. However, these studies have not considered the prognostic significance of intraoperative pleural lavage. A prospective study of intraoperative pleural lavage in lung cancer was reported.

Methods.—Three hundred forty-two patients underwent intraoperative pleural lavage during surgery for primary lung cancer. Lavage was performed with 300 mL of physiologic saline solution before and after tumor resection and lymph node dissection. Lung tissue cultures of the tumor-free lung parenchyma were performed to study how tumor cells enter the pleural cavity before resection.

Results.—Lavage performed in 99 patients with nonmalignant lung disease (controls) yielded no positive results. The rate of positive results in the initial intraoperative lavage in 132 patients was 39%. Of the 132 patients with positive results on the first lavage, 99 also had positive results on the second lavage. Just 9 patients had positive results only on the second lavage (Fig 3). Intraoperative peritoneal pleural lavage was more likely to be positive in patients with more advanced disease. Distant metastases were more common in patients who had a positive initial lavage. The 4-year survival rate was 24% for patients in whom the initial

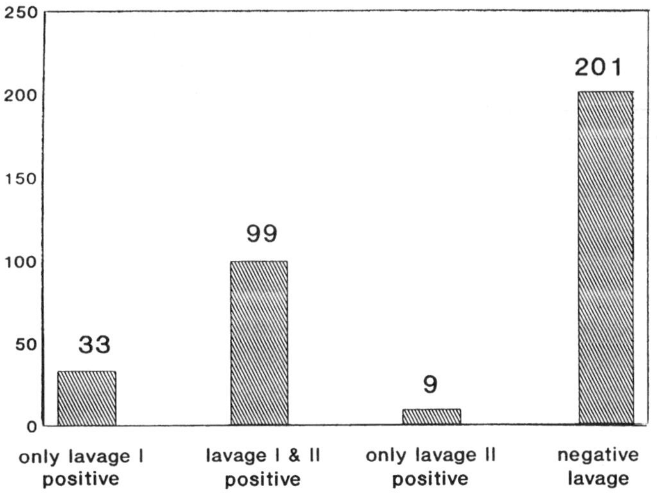

FIGURE 3.—Cytologic results in intraoperative pleural lavage (342 patients). (Courtesy of Buhr J, Berghäuser KH, Gonner S, et al: The prognostic significance of tumor cell detection in intraoperative pleural lavage and lung tissue cultures for patients with lung cancer. *J Thorac Cardiovasc Surg* 113:683–690, 1997.)

lavage was positive and 52% of those in whom the lavage was negative. The survival difference was significant for patients with stage I and stage IIIA disease, but not for stage II disease. Seventy percent of patients studied had tumor cells detected in cultured lung parenchyma. The tumor cells were always found in lymphatic vessels.

Conclusion.—Many patients with lung cancer undergoing intraoperative pleural lavage have tumor cells in the lavage fluid. The positive results do not result from surgical manipulation of the lung. The spread most likely occurs via the lymphatic vessels, through preformed stomas connecting the subpleural lymphatics with the pleural space. Positive results on intraoperative pleural lavage are an additional prognostic factor for patients with lung cancer.

Pleural Lavage Cytology Immediately After Thoracotomy and Before Closure of the Thoracic Cavity for Lung Cancer Without Pleural Effusion and Dissemination: Clinicopathologic and Prognostic Analysis

Higashiyama M, Doi O, Kodama K, et al (Osaka Med Ctr for Cancer and Cardiovascular Diseases, Japan)

Ann Surg Oncol 4:409–415, 1997 14–19

Background.—Cytologic examination of pleural lung fluid is often performed, and its results are useful in staging and managing disease. But are the cytologic results of fluid analyses themselves prognostic of the clinicopathologic course? Positive and negative results of pleural lavage cytology were compared in patients with lung cancer.

Methods.—Lung resection for primary lung cancer was used in 325 patients who also underwent cytologic examination of their pleural lavage fluid. After thoracotomy but before surgery, if no lesions were visible, 200 mL of physiologic saline solution was introduced into the pleural cavity. After the lung resection and a routine flushing with 2,000 mL of saline, another 200 mL of saline was used to wash the pleural cavity. After both 200-mL washes, the fluids were collected for cytologic analyses in glass bottles containing heparin. On the basis of positive (including borderline positive) and negative staining results, patients were placed in 1 of 4 groups: group A (control; 262 patients) had negative results both after thoracotomy and before closure, group B (19 patients) had positive results after thoracotomy but negative results before closure, group C (22 patients) had negative results after thoracotomy but positive results before closure, and group D (22 patients) had positive results both after thoracotomy and before closure. After a median follow-up of 43 months (range, 1–90 months), information on disease recurrence was available in 306 patients.

Findings.—Compared with group A, groups C and D had significantly advanced disease; group C had more aggressive nodal involvement, and group D had more aggressive nodal involvement, tumor stage, and pleural involvement. Recurrence rates were 35%, 42%, 61%, and 68% in groups

A, B, C, and D, respectively, and recurrence rates correlated significantly with the lavage results. Survival rates at 5 years were 71%, 69%, 45%, and 33%, respectively, with survival in groups C and D significantly worse compared with group A. Even though univariate analysis showed that lavage results correlated significantly with survival, multivariate analysis did not reveal lavage fluid positivity or negativity to be an independent prognostic factor of survival.

Conclusion.—Cytologic analysis of pleural lavage fluid does help with staging of disease and the prediction of recurrence, but results are not, by themselves, predictive of recurrence. Other factors are obviously involved.

► These 2 papers (Abstracts 14–18 and 14–19) are important because they investigate at the prognostic significance of tumor cell detection in the fluid lavaged interoperatively in the chest, both before and after surgical resection in patients with non–small-cell lung cancer. Specifically, the paper by Buhr et. al. shows that in a large number of patients, detection of tumor cells in pleural lavage before resection proves that tumor cells have spread into the pleural cavity. When detected, these cells were a negative prognostic predictor that was independent of subsequent stage. This was, indeed, an independent predictor. In the paper by Higashiyama et. al., the detection of disease through pleural lavage at the time of thoracotomy was, again, highly predictive of poor outcome. However, it was not independent of stage, suggesting that no prognostic value was added to conventional the TNM staging system after resection.

An interesting strategy would be to perform pleural lavage before operative therapy and, if the lavage was positive, to consider some form of induction therapy before surgical resection in an effort to sterilize intrapleural contents and to downstage the tumor from a microscopic stage IIIB (positive pleural effusion) to a resectable stage. We await the outcome of larger, multi-institutional trials currently underway to definitely conclude the value of pleural lavage cytology during and after thoracotomy in the treatment of patients with non–small-cell lung cancer.

D.J. Sugarbaker, M.D.

Mediastinal Lymph Node Metastasis in Patients With Clinical Stage I Peripheral Non–Small-Cell Lung Cancer

Takizawa T, Terashima M, Koike Y, et al (Niigata Cancer Ctr Hosp, Japan)
J Thorac Cardiovasc Surg 113:248–252, 1997 14–20

Objective.—Whether radical systemic lymphadenectomy in the mediastinum for lung cancer patients is merited is controversial. The surgeon's intraoperative observation of lymph nodes and the locations of diseased lymph nodes in patients with clinical stage I peripheral non–small-cell lung cancer (NSCLC) were investigated.

Methods.—Between 1984 and 1994 systematic mediastinal lymphadenectomy was performed in 575 patients (253 female), aged 29 to 83 years, who underwent lobectomy for clinical stage I NSCLC.

Results.—There were 79 (14%) patients with positive N2 nodes with metastases not detected in 54 (68%) of them at surgery. In 26 patients with N2 disease, no nodal metastases were found in the hilar or lobar region, a 33% skip rate. Mediastinal lymph node metastases were found in all N2 patients with cancer of the right upper lobe, in all N2 patients but 1 with cancer of the right middle lobe, in all N2 patients but 1 with cancer of the right lower lobe, in all N2 patients with cancer of the left upper lobe, and in all N2 patients but 1 with cancer of the left lower lobe.

Conclusion.—Systematic staging of mediastinal lymph nodes should be performed in all patients with clinical stage I NSCLC.

► For many years it has been difficult to map reliably the lymphatic drainage of the lung. Lower lobe tumors, particularly, have a propensity for crossover metastasis. This study very nicely documents the incidence of skip metastases from tumors of the lung to mediastinal lymph nodes, an occurrence that makes full assessment of all mediastinal nodes mandatory in patients with clinical stage I disease before resection.

The most interesting data from this article demonstrated that mediastinal lymph nodes were positive in 79 patients with clinical stage I disease making up a total of 14% of the cohort. Interestingly, involved lymph nodes appeared normal intraoperatively in 68% of these patients. Thirty-three percent of patients with positive N2 mediastinal nodes had negative lobar N1 nodes.

This very well done and documented study indicates the need for assessment of the mediastinum in patients with clinical stage I disease. Specifically, the use of mediastinoscopy would appear to be indicated in patients with clinical stage I disease given the overall poor survival of this group when resected with surgery alone. Indeed, the use of mediastinoscopy to determine those patients with microscopic N2 disease could identify an ideal cohort for the use of induction therapy in the hope of eradicating N2 disease before surgical resection, because of the lack of bulk disease in these patients.

D.J. Sugarbaker, M.D.

Wedge Resection Versus Lobectomy for Stage I (T1 N0 M0) Non–Small-Cell Lung Cancer

Landreneau RJ, Sugarbaker DJ, Mack MJ, et al (Allegheny Univ for the Health Sciences, Pittsburgh, Pa; Harvard Univ, Boston; Med City Hosp, Dallas; et al)

J Thorac Cardiovasc Surg 113:691–700, 1997 14–21

Background.—The value of nonanatomical wedge resection in the treatment of stage I non–small-cell lung cancer vs. the current gold standard—anatomical lobectomy—has not been established definitively. Also, the

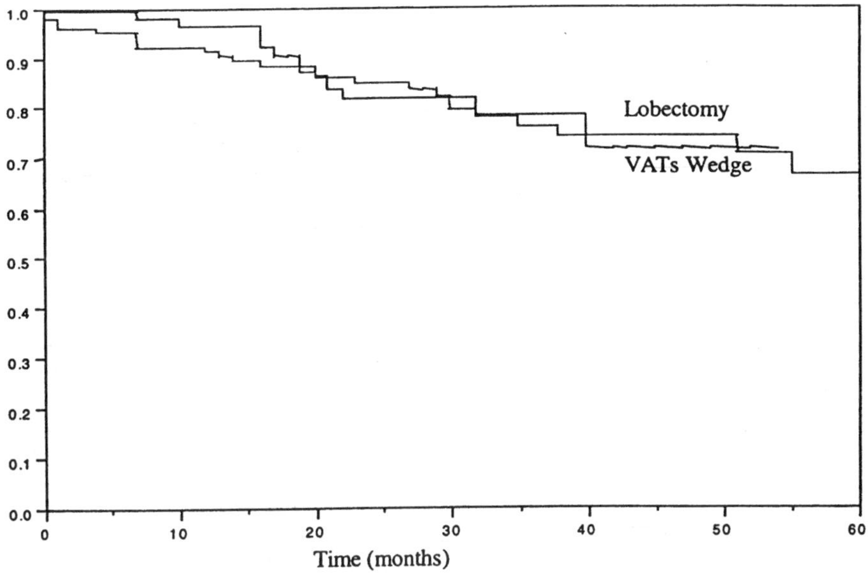

FIGURE 3.—Five-year actual survival differences between patients having video-assisted thoracic surgical (*VATS*) wedge resection and those having lobectomy are shown. (Courtesy of Landreneau RJ, Sugarbaker DJ, Mack MJ, et al: Wedge resection versus lobectomy for stage I (T1 N0 M0) non–small-cell lung cancer. *J Thorac Cardiovasc Surg* 113:691–700, 1997.)

efficacy of the video-assisted thoracic surgical approach to wedge resection of peripheral lung cancers has not been studied directly.

Methods.—The outcomes of 219 consecutive patients with pathologic stage I (T1 N0 M0) non–small-cell lung cancer were analyzed. Resection was performed in 42 patients, video-assisted wedge resection in 60, and lobectomy in 117.

Findings.—The operative mortality rate was 3% in patients undergoing lobectomy and 0% in those having wedge resection. The 5-year survival rate was 58% for patients undergoing open wedge resection, 65% for those having video-assisted wedge resection, and 70% for those undergoing lobectomy. Survival rates among patients having video-assisted thoracic surgical wedge resection and those having lobectomy were similar (Fig 3). In log rank testing, significant differences were noted among survival curves during the 5-year study, a result of a significantly greater non–cancer-related death rate by 5 years among patients undergoing wedge resection.

Conclusion.—In patients with cardiopulmonary physiologic impairment, wedge resection by open thoracotomy or the video-assisted thoracic surgical approach appears to be a viable "compromise" treatment for stage I T1 N0 M0 non–small-cell lung cancer. Because the risk for local recurrence with these methods is increased, anatomical lobectomy continues to be the surgical treatment of choice for such cancer in patients with adequate physiologic reserve.

▶ This paper attempts to address the continuing debate on whether wedge resection or lobectomy is the better treatment for lung cancer. The debate needs to be settled, and I think this paper goes a long way toward doing so. Of note is the 3% operative mortality rate among patients supposedly considered good risks for undergoing lobectomy. This stands in counterdistinction to the 0% mortality rate in those getting a wedge or video-assisted resection. In exchange for this increase in perioperative mortality, there was a 5% improvement in survival at 5 years in this group of patients. (However, the survival benefit of the lobectomy group is less dramatic when contrasted with the video-assisted group, probably because of the small T1 lesions better suited to video-assisted resection. Interestingly, the increased death from noncancer causes in the wedge resection and video-assisted resection groups testifies to the need to strive for lowered operative mortality in these groups.

The final conclusion really is that a wedge resection or video-assisted thoracoscopic resection is appropriate for patients who have impaired cardiopulmonary reserve or have other significant medical co-morbidities that make the risk of lobectomy higher. One can conclude from this paper that lobectomy carries a higher operative mortality rate, even in good-risk patients and that it is also accompanied by a better long-term survival. Therefore, in patients who are considered at high risk for thoracic procedures, a video-assisted resection or wedge resection by conventional open techniques would appear to represent a viable alternative to standard lobectomy.

D.J. Sugarbaker, M.D.

Feasibility of Mathematical Models to Predict Success in Video-assisted Thoracic Surgery Lung Nodule Excision

Demmy TL, Wagner-Mann CC, James MA, et al (Univ of Missouri, Columbia)
Am J Surg 17:20–23, 1997 14–22

Objective.—Whether video-assisted thoracic surgery (VATS) or open thoracotomy should be the procedure of choice for difficult-to-remove pulmonary nodules was assessed. A mathematical model was established for predicting operative success using preoperative computerized tomography (CT) measurements.

Methods.—Preoperative CT was performed in 50 patients who underwent VATS lung nodule excision or biopsy. Three mathematical equations were used to predict operative success. Nodules were classified as visible if they could be seen with the telescope alone and further classified as resectable by VATS or not. Resectability was assessed on the basis of size and depth. Procedures were classified as simple if the nodules were visible and resectable. All other procedures were classified as complex. The validity of the 3 equations was assessed based on operative experience.

Results.—Three patients were unable to undergo VATS. Age, sex, COPD, chest dimension, and nodal pathology were unrelated to localization, resectability, or simplicity in the remaining 47 patients (72% male), mean age 57.1 years. The mathematical expression S/(D + 1) where S = nodule size (cm) and D = distance (cm) to the nearest visceral pleura yielded significantly larger values for nodules that were visible. Nodules were visible in 35 (74%) patients and palpable and/or needle localizable in 4 (9%). Eight were not located because they were significantly deeper. The expression 1/(S + D + 1) yielded a significantly higher value for nodules that were resectable. Of the 39 VATS-located nodules, 21 (54%) were resectable. Those that were not resectable were located deeper and were significantly larger than resectable nodules. Simple cases had significantly higher scores than complex cases in the simplicity expression [1/S(D + 1)]. Procedures were classified as simple for 19 (40%) nodules and complex in 28 (60%) nodules. According to the results of logistic regression analysis, the mathematical expressions used were independent predictors of resectability and simplicity.

Conclusion.—Mathematical models using CT measurements can be used to predict the feasibility of success of VATS for removing pulmonary nodules.

▶ This article is included in this year's YEAR BOOK out of interest. The authors have used a very novel method for determining resectability of subpleural nodules. While it is not expected that most practicing surgeons calculate the ability to see a nodule based on its depth within the parenchyma expressed as a visibility quotient, I think it is of interest that there is a relationship between the depth of a nodule from the surface of the pleura and the probability of successful removal.

D.J. Sugarbaker, M.D.

Video-assisted Thoracic Surgery: Has Technology Found Its Place?

Mack MJ, Scruggs GR, Kelly KM, et al (Columbia Hosp, Dallas; Montreal Gen Hosp; Allegheny Gen Hosp, Pittsburgh, Pa)

Ann Thorac Surg 64:211–215, 1997 14–23

Objective.—Because video-assisted thoracic surgery decreases pain and shortens hospital stay, concern about its cost and overuse have raised questions. A group of thoracic surgeons whose practice is devoted mainly to noncardiac thoracic surgery was surveyed to assess the impact of VATS on the practice of thoracic surgery.

Methods.—A questionnaire was sent to the 229 members of the General Thoracic Surgery Club in November 1995 soliciting demographic information and opinions about frequency of use of VATS, its role in their practices, limitations of the procedure, and appropriateness of its use in various procedures. A second mailing was made to nonresponders.

Results.—Of the 200 questionnaires returned 189 (94.5%) were completed. Although most responders (66.3%) were employed in an academic or government environment, 33.7% were working in private practice. More than half (51.5%) had practiced thoracic surgery 15 years or more and more than 90% had practiced at least 5 years. Although VATS was used in 20% or less of procedures by most surgeons (60.2%), and 38.1% of surgeons believed the technique was significantly overused, 62.6% believed the role of VATS had stabilized, 51.9% believed the use of VATS was about right, and approximately 33% felt that the use of VATS would increase. VATS was the technique of choice by more than 50% of respondents for management of pleural disease, lung biopsy, recurrent pneumothorax, sympathectomy, early empyema, clotted hemothoraces, secondary pneumothorax, limited lung cancer treatment, and benign esophageal disease, and was also preferred for diagnosis of indeterminate pulmonary nodules and of anterior and posterior mediastinal masses. Most respondents would not use VATS for thymectomy, lobectomy, or lung volume reduction surgery.

Conclusion.—There is significant interest in VATS as a minimally invasive technique for specific thoracic procedures.

▶ This is an interesting review of the practice patterns and opinions of a group of practicing noncardiac thoracic surgeons. It is particularly interesting regarding the role of VATS; it appears that this approach is now standard for the majority of practicing thoracic surgeons in the management of pleural disease, lung biopsy, recurrent pneumothorax and sympathectomy. VATS is also thought to be acceptable for the approach and diagnosis of indeterminate pulmonary nodules and also for anterior and posterior mediastinal masses where biopsy and diagnosis are an important component of management. In addition, the use of VATS in the early management of empyema, hemothoraces and secondary pneumothoraces has also been accepted by the majority of thoracic surgeons. As well, the use of thoracoscopic techniques for benign esophageal disease, particularly myotomy is increasing in popularity.

There is still some reluctance on the part of the thoracic surgery community to perform video-assisted lobectomies, thymectomies, or lung volume reduction procedures. Most of these techniques are limited by the rather archaic instrumentation we are using currently in our thoracoscopic and video-assisted procedures. When techniques are worked out and instrumentation developed that can enable a surgeon to perform equivalent anatomic procedures with a high degree of safety, then it is expected that video-assisted lobectomy will become more commonplace.

D.J. Sugarbaker, M.D.

The Impact of Surgical Adjuvant Thoracic Radiation Therapy for Patients With Nonsmall Cell Lung Carcinoma With Ipsilateral Mediastinal Lymph Node Involvement

Sawyer TE, Bonner JA, Gould PM, et al (Mayo Clinic and Mayo Found, Rochester, Minn)

Cancer 80:1399–1408, 1997 14–24

Background.—Recurrence rates and survival in non–small-cell lung carcinoma are generally worse for patients with ipsilateral mediastinal (N2) lymph node involvement than for those with less nodal involvement (N0 or N1). Perhaps this poorer outcome is the result of retained subclinical local disease; if so, then adjuvant thoracic radiotherapy (TRT) to treat sites of retained disease may help improve outcomes in such patients. These authors put this hypothesis to the test.

Methods.—Complete surgical resection for lung carcinoma was performed in 224 patients (143 men and 81 women) with squamous cell, adenosquamous, or large cell carcinoma or adenocarcinoma. All patients had at least 1 involved N2 lymph node station. No patient had metastatic disease before the thoracotomy, nor had any patient received prior radiation or chemotherapy. Adjuvant TRT was used in 88 patients (39%) at a median dose of 50.4 Gy.

Findings.—At a median follow-up of 3.5 years, 158 of 224 patients (71%) had died, for an overall survival rate of 29%. Local recurrence rates at 4 years were significantly better in the group treated by surgery and TRT (17%) than in the group treated by surgery alone (60%) (Fig 1). Local recurrences were the first site of failure in 50% of the patients who received surgery alone; local disease recurrence occurred in only 16% of patients who also received TRT (a statistically significant difference) Overall survival at 4 years was also significantly better in the group treated with

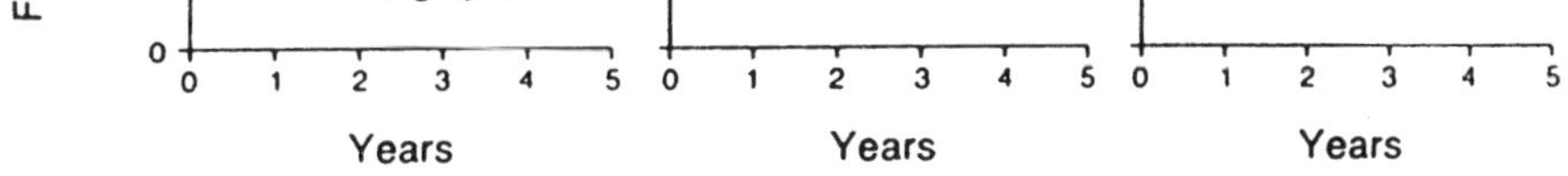

FIGURE 1.—The addition of postoperative thoracic radiotherapy (*TRT*) was associated with a significantly higher rate of freedom from local recurrence compared with surgery alone for (left) the entire group of patients (*P* less than 0.0001), (center), patients with 1 involved N2 lymph node (*P* = 0.02), and (right) patients with more than 1 involved N2 lymph node (*P* less than 0.0001). (Courtesy of Sawyer TE, Bonner JA, Gould PM, et al. The impact of surgical adjuvant thoracic radiation therapy for patients with nonsmall cell lung carcinoma with ipsilateral mediastinal lymph node involvement. Cancer 80:1399–1408, ©1997, American Cancer Society. Reprinted by permission of Wiley-Liss, Inc., a subsidiary of John Wiley & Sons, Inc.)

surgery and TRT (43%) than in the group treated by surgery alone (22%). Multivariate analysis indicated that TRT, the absence of superior mediastinal lymph node involvement, and less N1 lymph node involvement were significant independent predictors of outcome in these patients.

Conclusion.—Resection plus adjuvant TRT improved not only local recurrence rates, but also overall survival compared with patients undergoing resection alone in these patients with N2 lymph node involvement. The recurrences that did develop with TRT were more often at a site distant from the primary site, further supporting the role of TRT in improving local disease control. Further research is needed to define the role of TRT in prolonging disease-free control and survival in patients with non–small-cell lung cancer with N2 lymph node involvement.

► This is an important paper because it gives us some important insights into the possible role of adjuvant radiation therapy, even though the study is retrospective and the 2 cohorts of patients (1 receiving radiotherapy and 1 not receiving radiotherapy in the adjuvant setting) were not prospectively randomized. The standard understanding of thoracic surgeons and medical oncologists has been that adjuvant radiotherapy will increase the local control rate but will not translate into increased patient survival. This thinking comes from the results of the Lung Cancer Study Group's prospective, randomized trial completed in the late 1980s.

In the study abstracted here, the markedly reduced local recurrence rate—from 60% in the nonradiotherapy arm to 17% in the radiotherapy arm—was of note. In this study, the reduction did translate into a statistically significant survival advantage. Postoperative radiotherapy was associated with significantly higher freedom from local recurrence. It was quite marked in this cohort of patients and undoubtedly represents the major reason there was a survival advantage with adjuvant radiotherapy.

It appears that the role of adjuvant radiotherapy needs to be addressed again in a prospective randomized way. Unlike the technology of the 1970s and 1980s, radiotherapy has recently become less morbid and potentially more effective given the new CT-guided tight field delivery systems. I think we should look forward to a new prospective trial for examining chemoradiotherapy combinations in the adjuvant setting.

D.J. Sugarbaker, M.D.

Cost of Combined Modality Interventions for Stage III Non–small-cell Lung Cancer

Evans WK, Will BP, Berthelot J-M, et al (Univ of Ottawa, Ont, Canada; Ottawa Regional Cancer Centre, Ont, Canada; Statistics Canada, Ottawa, Ont, Canada)

J Clin Oncol 15:3038–3048, 1997 14–25

Introduction.—Treatment interventions are under fiscal scrutiny, especially in areas in which therapeutic efficacy is modest. A small, but definite, survival advantage has been demonstrated with the use of chemotherapy in stage IV lung cancer. Reported was the economic impact of new treatment interventions being used with increasing frequency in the management of stage III non–small-cell lung cancer (NSCLC), using a costing model of lung cancer developed by Statistics Canada of Ottawa.

Methods.—The lung-costing model is part of a larger project of the POpulation HEalth Model (POHEM) that has been used to estimate the total cost of managing all stages of lung cancer in the Canadian health care system. Recent findings have shown that combined modality therapy gives a survival advantage for patients with stage III NSCLC. The lung-costing model was used to evaluate the cost effectiveness in Canadian dollars of chemotherapy interventions with and without radiotherapy in patients with stage IIIA disease and chemoradiotherapy for patients with stage IIIB disease. Figures were based on 1993 Canadian health care costs with the government as payer in a universal health care system. Survival data were collected.

Results.—The standard cost of radiation treatment for patients with stage IIIA and stage IIIB NSCLC was assessed at $34,595 and $31,928 per person, respectively. The cost of treating patients with stage IIIA NSCLC with preoperative and postoperative therapy would increase by $15,886 (intervention 1) and the addition of postoperative radiotherapy would increase the cost by $22,963 (intervention 2). Chemoradiotherapy for stage IIIB disease (intervention 3) would increase the cost by about $8,912 per patient. The cost effectiveness based on life-year gained for interventions 1, 2, and 3 was $9,348, $14,985, and $3,348, respectively. Outpatient chemotherapy could significantly improve cost effectiveness.

Conclusion.—Neoadjuvant therapy for stage IIIA NSCLC and combined modality therapy for stage IIIB NSCLC are cost effective interventions that compare well with commonly accepted medical interventions, such as mammography for women over 50 years of age, hemodialysis, or zidovudine for AIDS. Economic barriers should not impede adoption of this treatment approach for patients with NSCLC.

► I have included this paper because it makes a very important point. Even when comparing chemoradiotherapy with radiotherapy alone in stage IIIA disease, the cost of treatment for patients enjoying an increased survival is justified. There is nothing more powerful from an economic standpoint, than returning a patient to work and allowing that patient to become a premium-paying member of an insurance plan and a tax-paying member of society. All too often, our society indicts the high cost of medical care based on some isolated economic analysis. This paper simply shows that when you look at the cost of sickness, it is relatively small compared with the benefits of wellness.

D.J. Sugarbaker, M.D.

Mesothelioma Update

Surgically Debulked Malignant Pleural Mesothelioma: Results and Prognostic Factors

Pass HI, Kranda K, Temeck BK, et al (NIH, Bethesda, Md)
Ann Surg Oncol 4:215–222, 1997 14–26

Objective.—As a result of a revision of the staging system for malignant pleural mesothelioma (MPM), renewed interest has developed in re-examining the role of surgery in managing this disease. Current morbidity and mortality rates are reported for a pleurectomy-decortication and extrapleural pneumonectomy debulking effort, recurrence patterns, survival after surgery, and preoperative and postoperative risk factors for debulking.

Methods.—Preoperative tumor volume was calculated in 60 (63.2%) of 95 patients (17 female), aged 30 to 77 years, using 3-dimensional computerized reconstructions of CT images. Pleurectomy (*n* = 39) or extrapleural pneumonectomy (EPP) (*n* = 39) was performed. Tumors were not resectable in 17 (17.9%) patients. Survival time and time to progression were recorded. Factors significantly associated with survival were identified using the Cox proportional hazards model.

Results.—Platelet counts were 404,000 for patients undergoing EPP, 344,000 for patients having pleurectomy, and 434,000 for patients with unresectable cancers. Tumor volumes averaged 491, 114, and 304 mL, respectively. Complications occurred in 34 patients, the most common being supraventricular tachycardia in 14 EPP patients and 2 in pleurectomy patients. There were 2 surgery-related deaths. Median followup was 33.7 months. Median survival was 11.2 months. Median survival for pleurectomy patients was significantly longer (14.5 months) than for EPP patients (9.4 months) and for unresectable patients (5.0 months). The median survival for debulked patients was 7.2 months. Local, distant, and local plus distant recurrence rates for EPP patients were 38%, 25%, and 5%, respectively. For pleurectomy patients, the same recurrence rates were 69%, 8%, and 3%, respectively. Univariate analysis identified tumor volume and platelet counts as predictive of survival in all 3 groups and predictive of progression-free survival in the operative groups. According to multivariate analysis, tumor volume greater than 100 mL, biphasic histology, male sex, and elevated platelet count were predictive of decreased survival.

Conclusion.—The mortality rate after debulking operations in this study was low. Patients with high platelet counts and biphasic histology should be considered for experimental therapies that involve only minimal surgery (tissue biopsy) and permit accurate assessments of results.

► This is an interesting article in that it demonstrates a fact I think most surgeons who deal with mesothelioma have thought was true clinically for some time; that is, the amount of tumor present appears to correlate with overall survival. Dr. Pass has demonstrated the safety of extrapleural pneumonectomy when performed in a controlled setting. He has also demonstrated the recalcitrant, relentless clinical course of this disease. The overall median survival in this group, 11.2 months, was only slightly increased to 14.5 months for patients undergoing pleurectomy and decreased to 9.4 months for patients undergoing extrapleural pneumonectomy. This article also points out the need for effective adjuvant therapies if we are, indeed, going to increase survival in this dreaded disease.

Also of interest was the fact that elevated platelet counts, biphasic histology, and male sex were all associated with decreased survival in this group. This echoes similar reports by our group and others that epithelial subtype patients with negative lymph nodes appear to be the primary beneficiaries of an aggressive multimodal approach to malignant pleural mesothelioma.

D.J. Sugarbaker, M.D.

Patterns of Failure After Trimodality Therapy for Malignant Pleural Mesothelioma

Baldini EH, Recht A, Strauss GM, et al (Dana-Farber Cancer Inst, Boston; Harvard Med School, Boston)

Ann Thorac Surg 63:334–338, 1997 14–27

Introduction.—As the incidence of diffuse, malignant pleural mesothelioma increases, there is still no standard approach to treatment. Recommended treatments have included supportive care only, single-modality approaches, and aggressive combination therapies. The results and patterns of failure of an aggressive, trimodality treatment approach to malignant pleural mesothelioma were evaluated.

Methods.—The study included 49 patients with malignant pleural mesothelioma treated during a 6-year period. All patients underwent extrapleural pneumonectomy; 2 died in the perioperative period, and 1 died 5 weeks later. Of the 46 survivors, 35 underwent adjuvant chemotherapy, in most cases consisting of cyclophosphamide, doxorubicin, and cisplatin. Chemotherapy was followed by hemithorax radiation therapy (RT). Chemotherapy, but not RT, was given to 10 patients, and 1 patient received no adjuvant therapy. Patterns of failure in the 46 assessable patients were analyzed.

Results.—The recurrence rate was 54%, with a median time to first failure of 19 months. Thirty-five percent of patients had a local site of first recurrence and 26% had an abdominal site. The contralateral thorax was the site of first recurrence in 17% of patients, and other distant sites were involved first in 8%. Twenty-one patients with recurrence died, with a median time from relapse to death of only 3 months. In the series overall, median survival was 22 months and 34% reached 3-year survival.

Conclusion.—In patients receiving aggressive treatment (cytoreductive extrapleural pneumonectomy, adjuvant chemotherapy, and consolidative

RT) for malignant pleural mesothelioma, the ipsilateral hemithorax is the most common site of failure. There are few isolated distant failures. Future treatments for this uncommon tumor should focus on improving local control, such as by radiation modifiers, concurrent administration of RT and chemotherapy, intrapleural chemotherapy, and earlier delivery of RT.

▶ This important contribution to the literature demonstrates from clinical study that malignant pleural mesothelioma has a unique tumor biology. Unlike most solid tumors in which hematogenous metastases represent the primary site of failure after surgical resection, in malignant pleural mesothelioma it is relentless local recurrence that is the primary cause of death for most patients undergoing aggressive therapy. This is important because as we begin to develop new treatment strategies for the control of this disease, it appears that aggressive local therapies—whether they be photodynamic therapy, local regional chemotherapy, or other means of controlling local recurrence—hold the most promise in the treatment of this disease in the near term.

However, one could consider that once local control has been achieved in this malignancy, we might see an altered natural history, with the entry of patients seen with hematogeneous metastases. Nevertheless, this study suggests that malignant pleural mesothelioma does have a relatively low metastatic potential, with local regional recurrence representing a primary site of recurrence.

D.J. Sugarbaker, M.D.

Long Survival After Pneumonectomy for Pleural Malignant Mesothelioma With Metastasis to Infradiaphragmatic Lymph Node

Nomori H, Horio H, Kobayashi R, et al (Saiseikai Central Hosp, Tokyo)
Scand J Thorac Cardiovasc Surg 31:237–239, 1996 14–28

Objective.—Although malignant mesothelioma is virtually incurable, a case is presented of a woman with a 63-month survival after extrapleural pneumonectomy with infradiaphragmatic lymph node metastases. Factors influencing survival are discussed.

Case.—Woman, 47, with no exposure to asbestos, was diagnosed with malignant epithelial mesothelioma in July 1990. In November, extrapleural pneumonectomy with resection of the diaphragm and pericardium (replaced with Dacron velour) was performed. Two enlarged lymph nodes between the diaphragm and kidney, and surrounding the abdominal aorta were found and resected. The tumor, pathologic Butchart stage III, had not spread to mediastinal sites or chest wall. The patient received cisplatin and adriamycin chemotherapy and has had no recurrence.

Conclusion.—Low tumor invasiveness, noninvolvement of the mediastinum, chest wall, peritoneum, and pericardium, and complete resection of the metastasis-bearing infradiaphragmatic lymph nodes contributed to this patient's long-term survival.

► This article makes the same point based on a case report that Baldini et al. made in the previous article namely, that aggressive local management of malignant pleural mesothelioma may result in extended survival. With survival of patients receiving treatment or supportive care alone hovering in the 9- to 12-month range, it is interesting to see a report of a patient treated with extrapleural pneumonectomy and radical extended lymph node dissection who is alive and well 63 months postresection. I think the major point of this paper is that extended survival is possible in patients with pleural mesothelioma. This is an important realization if we are to develop treatment strategies that extend our ability to control local regional disease.

D.J. Sugarbaker, M.D.

Thoracic Oncology Update

Recurrence of Thymoma: Analysis of Clinicopathologic Features, Treatment, and Outcome

Ruffini E, Mancuso M, Oliaro A, et al (Univ of Torino, Italy)

J Thorac Cardiovasc Surg 113:55–63, 1997 14–29

Objective.—Although surgical resection of thymoma improves survival, recurrence several years later is not infrequent. Frequency of recurrence, disease-free survival, treatment modalities, and outcome in relation to clinicopathologic characteristics of the tumor, associated myasthenia gravis (MG), and patients without recurrence are reported.

Methods.—Between 1974 and 1993, 310 patients underwent surgery for thymoma. The tumor was totally resected in 266 patients. Thirty patients (14 women), aged 20 to 71 years at surgery, had a recurrence.

Results.—For the 30 patients with recurrent disease, rates were 5% with encapsulated stage I tumors, 10% with stage II, 30% with stage III, 33% with stage IVa, and 20% with invasive tumors. Recurrence rates, disease-free survival, and overall survival were not affected by the presence of MG. Disease-free survival was significantly longer for encapsulated thymomas than for invasive thymomas (132 vs. 71 months) and was significantly longer for patients not receiving adjuvant therapy than for those receiving adjuvant therapy (110 vs. 57 months). Eleven patients had a local recurrence, and 17 patients had a distant recurrence. Extent of recurrence was not determined in 2 patients. Reoperation was performed in 16 of 17 patients with recurrence, and total resection was performed in 10. Eleven patients received radiotherapy alone. Overall 5- and 10-year survivals were 48% and 24%, respectively. Factors predictive of increased survival after recurrence were extent of recurrence, total resection of recurrent tumor, and absence of adjuvant therapy after initial resection.

Conclusion.—Resection of recurrent thymoma increases survival. Distant recurrence and inability to resect all of the recurrent tumor carry a poor prognosis.

► This study is important because it does demonstrate that there is a salvage therapy for patients with recurrent malignant thymoma who recur locally. The interesting part of this study was that only 30 recurrent thymomas were noted out of a total of 266 completely resected thymomas. Of note was the fact that an inability to resect and evidence of distant metastatic disease were associated with a very poor survival. This disease, particularly thymic epithelial carcinoma, is well known for its propensity for drop metastases. In my experience, occasional en bloc resections, including mediastinal exenteration and concomitant extrapleural pneumonectomy, have been successful in controlling disease. Obviously, the importance of this study is that it underscores the fact that extensive surgical procedures will be required in cases of recurrent thymoma, but they can be expected to yield a certain salvage rate, particularly when coupled with adjuvant radiotherapy.

D.J. Sugarbaker, M.D.

Bronchial Carcinoid—Twenty Years' Experience Defines a Selective Surgical Approach

Chughtai TS, Morin JE, Sheiner NM, et al (McGill Univ, Montreal)

Surgery 122:801–808, 1997 14–30

Objective.—A review of the clinical behavior of bronchial carcinoids and clarification of a surgical approach are presented.

Methods.—Records from 1975 to 1996 of 84 patients (28 male), aged 19 to 80 years, with resected bronchial carcinoids were retrospectively reviewed for clinicopathologic variables, surgical treatment, and outcome. Mean follow-up was of 6.8 years.

Results.—For most asymptomatic patients an abnormal chest x-ray was the first indication of disease. Common symptoms in patients were recurring or persisting pneumonia despite antibiotic treatment, cough, and hemoptysis. One patient had carcinoid syndrome. CT predicted tumor extent and location in most patients. CT predicted lymph node status with a sensitivity of 67%, a specificity of 97%, a positive predictive value of 80%, and a negative predictive value of 94%. Bronchoscopy was diagnostically successful in 70% of patients, cytology in 2%, and transthoracic needle biopsy in 23%. Patients with central tumors were significantly younger by 10 years than patients with peripheral lesions. Resection was aggressive in 82% of patients and conservative in 18%. One patient died perioperatively. Twelve (15%) patients had atypical carcinoids, 10 (12%) had lymph node metastases, and 6 (7%) had tumorlets. Whereas overall survival at 5 and 10 years was 93% and 83%, survival at 5 and 10 years for patients with atypical disease was significantly lower (44% and 44%).

Survival rates for patients with typical disease were 97% and 95%. The presence of tumorlets and metastatic disease also decreased survival.

Conclusion.—Survival is decreased in bronchial carcinoids with atypical histology, lymph node metastases, and presence of tumorlets. Bronchoscopy with biopsy, CT scan, intraoperative assessment, and frozen section analysis can be used to assess histopathologic features. Conservative surgery should be considered in patients without negative features.

► Bronchial carcinoid is an interesting tumor that occasionally enters the practice of most general thoracic surgeons. The majority of patients presenting with bronchial carcinoid will have a benign tumor, and poor prognosis is only associated with atypical histology, the presence of tumorlets, or lymph node involvement as demonstrated in this study. Typically, the diagnosis is made on bronchial inspection of the tumor because biopsy is often accompanied by significant hemorrhage. Following surgical resection, an assessment of the presence or absence of lymph node metastases will establish whether one is dealing with a typical or atypical carcinoid.

This particular article is of interest because most of the patients in this study underwent a bronchoscopic biopsy, which is recommended by the authors. In my own experience, I have found bronchial biopsy rarely necessary to make an accurate diagnosis of bronchial carcinoid, and I have found CT scan to be of only limited value in determining the presence or absence of lymph node metastases. An important note in this study was the overall survival rates of 93% and 82% at 5 and 10 years, respectively.

D.J. Sugarbaker, M.D.

Adenoid Cystic Carcinoma of the Airway: Thirty-Two–year Experience

Maziak DE, Todd TRJ, Keshavjee SH, et al (Univ of Toronto)

J Thorac Cardiovasc Surg 112:1522–1532, 1996 14–31

Background.—Because of the rarity of adenoid cystic carcinoma of the trachea, few centers have been able to report treatment outcomes in significant numbers of patients. The management and follow-up of 38 patients with a diagnosis of primary adenoid cystic carcinoma treated at 1 center between 1963 and 1995 were reported.

Methods.—The patients had a mean age of 44.8 years (range, 15 to 80 years) and a male-female ratio of 1:1.1. Thirty-two patients underwent resection and reconstruction; 26 of these received adjuvant radiotherapy. Six patients with unresectable tumors received radiotherapy only as the primary treatment.

Outcomes.—All patients were found to have local invasion beyond the wall of the trachea on pathologic examination. Forty-four percent of the patients had metachronous hematogenous metastases, and 33% had pulmonary metastases. Half of the resections performed were complete and potentially curative. Two patients died within 30 days of surgery. The remaining 14 had a mean survival of 9.8 years. Of the 16 patients undergoing incomplete resection, 1 died operatively, and 15 had a survival of 7.5 years. The mean survival in the 6 patients treated with primary radiation was 6.2 years. Those with pulmonary metastases had a mean survival of 37 months from the diagnosis of metastases.

Conclusion.—Although late local recurrence after resection is characteristic of adenoid cystic carcinoma of the upper airway, excellent long-term palliation can be achieved after both complete and incomplete resection. Radiotherapy alone can result in long periods of control. Adjuvant radiotherapy is assumed to positively affect survival.

▶ This is a very interesting study of 38 patients treated by Dr. F.G. Pearson over his career. This individual and the entire staff at the Toronto General Hospital have contributed greatly to our understanding of adenoid cystic carcinoma of the airway. The most significant feature elucidated in this report is the fact that patients with completely or incompletely resected disease can be expected to live a long time, hence, neglect of airway disease may lead to premature death from obstruction. Also of note is the fact that this is a very indolent disease, even when metastatic disease is present. Thus, radical surgical resection appears to be indicated, given the long-term patient survival associated with metastases when they are present.

Also of interest is the use of adjuvant radiotherapy. In a majority of cases, radiotherapy was used in the adjuvant setting, as it is well known that radiotherapy before tracheal resection may impair the subsequent healing of the trachea. We are indebted to Dr. Pearson and colleagues for this excellent review and for their contribution to our understanding of adenoid cystic carcinoma and its appropriate therapy.

D.J. Sugarbaker, M.D.

Long-term Results of Lung Metastasectomy: Prognostic Analyses Based on 5206 Cases

Pastorino U, for the International Registry of Lung Metastases (Royal Brompton Hosp, London)

J Thorac Cardiovasc Surg 113:37–49, 1997 14–32

Background.—In 1991, the International Registry of Lung Metastases was established to determine the long-term outcomes of pulmonary metastasectomy. The first analysis of the data collected was reported.

Methods.—Between 1991 and 1995, 5,290 patients undergoing metastasectomy over more than 4 decades were enrolled in the database. The patients had been treated at centers in Europe, the United States, and Canada. Eighty-eight percent of the patients underwent complete surgical resection. The primary lesion was epithelial in 2,260 patients, sarcoma in 2,173, germ cell in 363, and melanoma in 328.

Findings.—After complete metastasectomy, actuarial survival was 36% at 5 years, 26% at 10 years, and 22% at 15 years (Fig 1). After incomplete resection, the 5- and 10-year survival rates were 13% and 7%, respec-

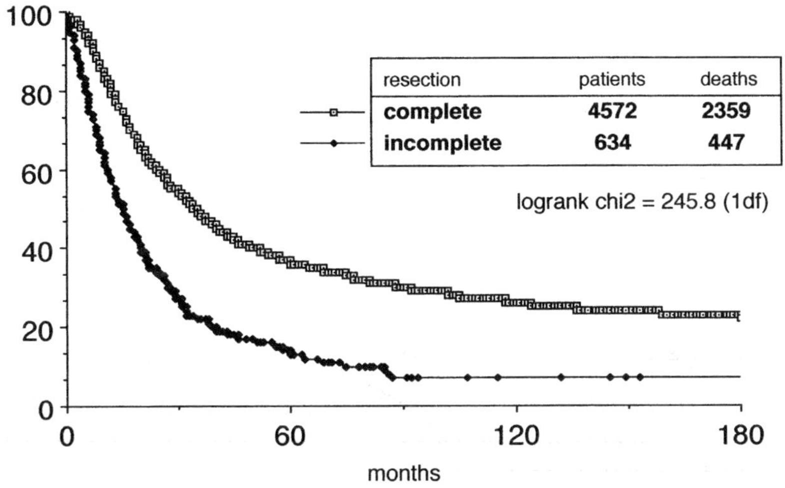

Patients at risk:

complete	809	254	78
incomplete	35	5	1

FIGURE 1.—Overall actuarial survival after lung metastasectomy: complete resection vs. incomplete resection. The number of patients at risk at 5, 10, and 15 years is reported at the **bottom**. (Courtesy of Pastorino U, for the International Registry of Lung Metastases: Long-term results of lung metastasectomy: Prognostic analyses based on 5206 cases. *J Thorac Cardiovasc Surg* 113:37–49, 1997.)

tively. Pathologic study showed that 46% of the patients had single metastases and 52% had multiple metastasis. The radiologic determination of the number of lung metastases was accurate in 61%, too low in 25%, and too high in 14%. A multivariate analysis indicated that patients with germ cell tumors, disease-free intervals of 36 months or more, and single metastases had a better prognosis.

Conclusion.—Lung metastasectomy is a safe procedure that is potentially curative. However, radiologic staging appears to be inaccurate in a large percentage of patients. Intraoperative exploration by an experienced surgeon would optimize resection.

► This paper has an interesting study design in that a variety of centers in Europe and the United States entered existing cases into a large database. This large, retrospective review is hamstrung by all the problems that attend retrospective analyses. Nevertheless, some important facts come out of this particular study, the first being that there is an absolute 5-year survival for a significant proportion of patients undergoing metastasectomy. I think the confirmation of the fact that the number of metastases, the length of disease-free interval, and the cell type (particularly germ cell tumors) indicate better prognosis is an important contribution. It is important to emphasize that the difference between complete and incomplete resection is not a technical operative difference left to the skill of the surgeon, but is primarily a marker of disease biology. Patients who undergo incomplete resection of pulmonary metastases are usually patients who have an overwhelming amount of disease in which smaller micronodules were not determined preoperatively.

D.J. Sugarbaker, M.D.

Factors Influencing Long-term Survival After Lung Metastasectomy

Robert JH, Ambrogi V, Mermillod B, et al (Geneva Univ; Royal Brompton Natl Heart and Lung Hosp, London)
Ann Thorac Surg 63:777–784, 1997 14–33

Introduction.—Reported survivals for patients undergoing resection of lung metastases are sometimes even better than those reported after surgery for primary lung cancer. However, the available data are insufficient to draw conclusions about how metastasectomy works and in whom it should and should not be done. Toward identifying those patients most likely to benefit, the authors reviewed their 14-year experience with lung metastasectomy.

Methods.—From 1980 to 1993, 276 patients underwent 1 or more lung metastasectomies. The patients were 193 men and 83 women (mean age, 38 years). In each patient, complete excision of all intrathoracic disease was considered feasible, and reliable control of primary disease had been achieved. Sixty-three patients went on to have a second-stage metastasectomy, 12 had 3 stages, and 2 had 4 stages. On univariate and multivariate analyses, disease-free interval and size and number of resected metastases were assessed for predictive value.

Results.—Forty-six percent of patients had primary sarcoma, 32% had teratoma, and 53% had carcinoma. The 2-year actuarial survival rate was 69%, with a 95% confidence interval of 62% to 74%. Survival decreased to 48% at 5 years (95% confidence interval, 40% to 55%) and 35% at 10 years (95% confidence interval 23% to 44%). On multivariate analysis, almost all useful predictive information was obtained from histologic examination. The median disease-free interval was 21 months; this parameter had no effect on survival. The number of metastases had some predictive value.

Conclusion.—Some patients undergoing lung metastasectomy achieve long-term survival. The major determinant of survival is histologic tumor type. Metastasectomy may be considered even for patients with a short disease-free interval, numerous metastatic lesions, or even recurrent tumor deposits after a first or second metastasectomy.

▶ The facts are worth reviewing that patients who are candidates for pulmonary metastasectomies are those who (1) have had their primary tumor controlled surgically, (2) have no evidence of other systemic metastases, (3) do not have a melanoma, and (4) have adequate pulmonary reserve to undergo the planned resection. This study looks at a small cohort of patients treated at Geneva University Hospital and the Royal Brompton

Hospital in London. Of interest is the fact that disease-free survival was not a significant prognostic factor in the multivariate analysis and that the primary predictors of survival related to the tumor's primary histology.

In addition, a marker of tumor biology would appear to be the number of metastases presenting at the time of surgical resection. Indeed, in this trial, the number of metastases resected did contribute, although less significantly, to long-term prognosis. It is important to realize that for the majority of patients, the pattern of metastatic spread is a marker of the aggressiveness of the tumor and that surgical resection, although removing visible disease, has no impact on the underlying biology of the tumor, particularly when the tumor has manifested itself systemically, as in patients undergoing pulmonary metastasectomy.

The actual surgical technique of pulmonary metastasectomy also remains the focus of significant study. A national trial within the Cancer and Leukemia Group B currently seeks to randomize patients between treatment with median sternotomy vs. unilateral/bilateral video-assisted resections to determine the difference in not only long-term therapeutic efficacy, but in cost, length of stay, and other parameters of surgical morbidity and mortality.

D.J. Sugarbaker, M.D.

Pulmonary Resection as an Adjunct in the Treatment of Multiple Drug-Resistant Tuberculosis

Van Leuven M, De Groot M, Shean KP, et al (Univ of Cape Town, South Africa; MDR-TB Clinic, Cape Town, South Africa)

Ann Thorac Surg 63:1368–1373, 1997 14–34

Background.—Pulmonary disease resulting from multiple drug–resistant *Mycobacterium tuberculosis* is particularly difficult to treat, with recurrence rates as high as 50%. Combinations of drug therapy and surgery can improve the outcome in some patients with localized disease. An experience using this combination in patients at a Cape Town, Africa hospital was evaluated.

Methods.—Over almost 6 years, of 241 patients with lung disease resulting from *M. tuberculosis* infection, 62 had infection that was resistant to at least isoniazid and rifampicin; these 62 formed the study group. Chest radiographs and, in some cases, CT were used to identify the extent of resection. Stapling was used to secure all pneumonectomy stumps, and no muscle flap or thoracoplasty was used on bronchial stumps. To avoid contaminating the pleural space, an extrapleural approach was used to remove damaged lung areas. Antituberculous drug therapy was started before the surgery and continued until the patient was disease-free. Postoperative follow-up included regular sputum cultures and chest radiographs.

Findings.—Patients ranged in age from 16 to 72 years (average age, 34 years), with about equal numbers of men and women (53% and 47%, respectively). One death occurred as a result of massive pulmonary em-

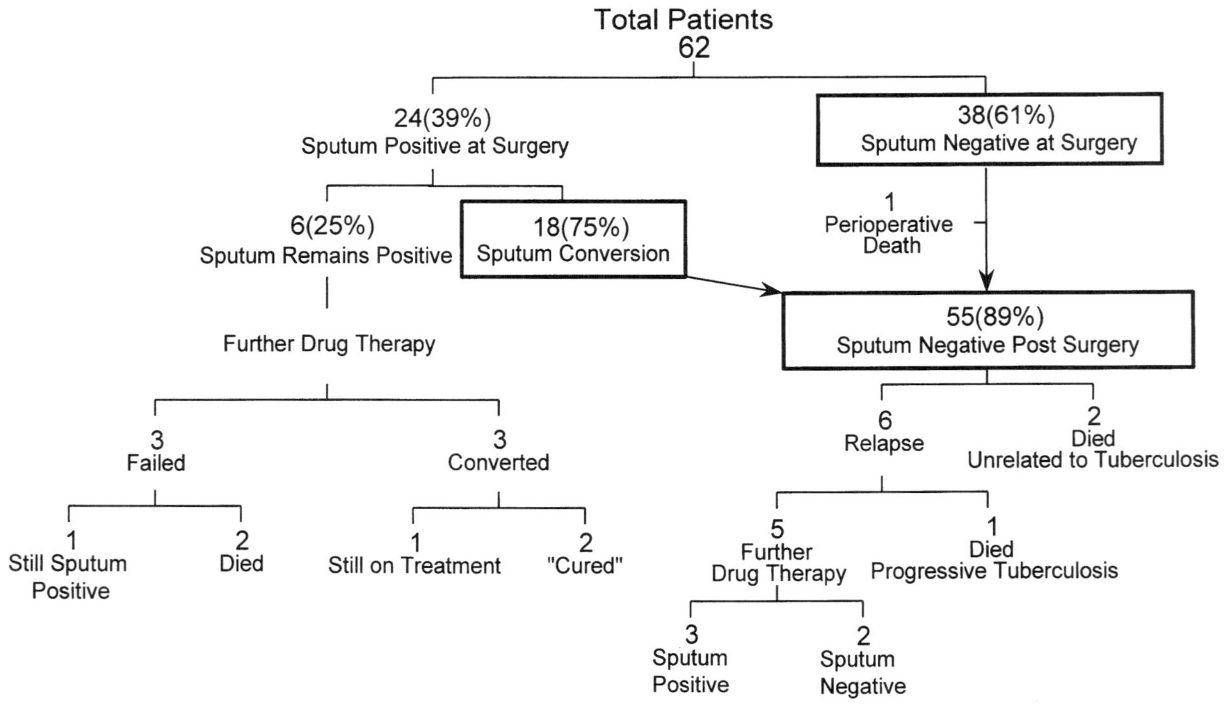

FIGURE 1.—Results of surgery for 62 patients undergoing pulmonary resection for drug-resistant strains of *Mycobacterium tuberculosis*. (Reprinted with permission from the Society of Thoracic Surgeons courtesy of Van Leuven M, De Groot M, Shean KP, et al: Pulmonary resection as an adjunct in the treatment of multiple drug-resistant tuberculosis. *Ann Thorac Surg* 63:1368–1373, 1997.)

bolism (mortality rate, 1.6%), and 14 patients experienced complications (morbidity rate, 23%). Overall, 18 of 24 patients (75%) who had positive sputum cultures before the operation converted immediately to negative cultures after surgery. In these 24 patients, the more extensive the resection, the greater the conversion rate. Eighty percent of patients with negative sputum results at or after the operation were disease-free 3 years later, but 11% had a relapse (Fig 1).

Conclusion.—Drug therapy combined with surgical resection was effective in treating 75% of patients, with only an 11% relapse rate. Preoperative and postoperative antituberculous drug therapy is crucial. Also, a greater resection carries with it a greater chance of successful conversion.

▶ The subject of this study, performed at the University of Capetown, South Africa, is becoming more relevant to the general thoracic surgeon's practice in the United States in the late 20th century. The significant increase in the number of cases of multiple drug-resistant tuberculosis in the United States continues to escalate. The surgeon is now more frequently called in to backstop the failure of multiple drugs. It is important to realize that the surgical approach is most warranted in patients who have an anatomical defect in a particular lobe that can be pointed to as the source of the continuing sputum positivity. The most important factor contributing to patients being returned to a disease-free state here was sputum conversion, either before or after surgery. Despite aggressive surgical management, a large fraction of these patients will continue to be sputum positive.

D.J. Sugarbaker, M.D.

Subject Index

A

B

C

F

G

H

I

J

K

L

M

N

O

Q

R

S

T

W

X

Z

Author Index

A

B

C

S

T